# IAP-AHA Textbook of
## ADOLESCENT MEDICINE

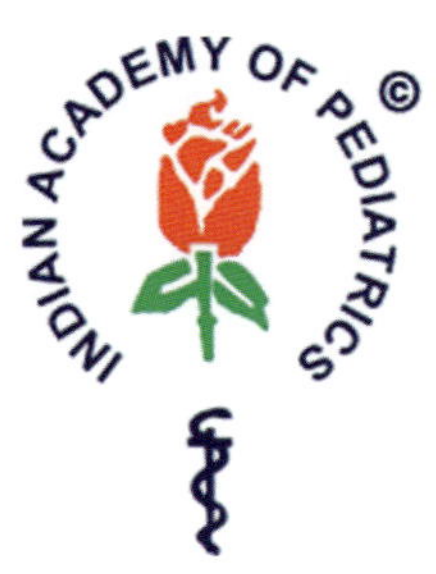

**Indian Academy of Pediatrics**

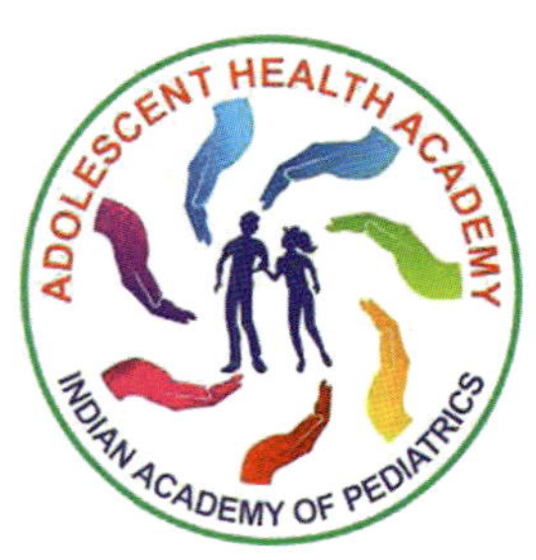

# IAP-AHA Textbook of
# ADOLESCENT MEDICINE

**Academic Editors**

**Geeta Patil**
**Atul Kanikar**
**Newton Luiz**
**Sukanta Chatterjee**

**Executive Editors**

**R N Sharma**
**Samir Shah**
**Poonam Bhatia**

**IAP**

**G V Basavaraja**
**Upendra Kinjawadekar**
**Yogesh N Parikh**
**Vineet Saxena**

**Forewords**

MKC Nair · Swati Y Bhave · C P Bansal · Piyush Gupta
G V Basavaraja · Upendra Kinjawadekar
Yogesh N Parikh · Vineet Saxena

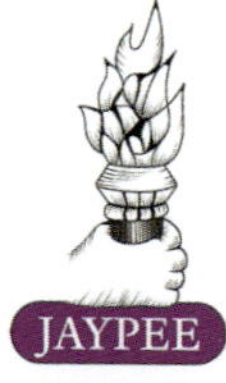

JAYPEE

**JAYPEE BROTHERS MEDICAL PUBLISHERS**
*The Health Sciences Publisher*
**New Delhi | London**

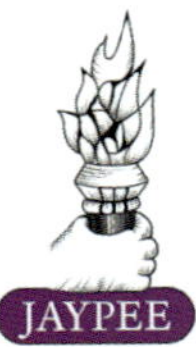 **Jaypee Brothers Medical Publishers (P) Ltd.**

**Headquarters**
Jaypee Brothers Medical Publishers (P) Ltd
EMCA House, 23/23-B
Ansari Road, Daryaganj
New Delhi 110 002, India
Landline: +91-11-23272143, +91-11-23272703
+91-11-23282021, +91-11-23245672
Email: jaypee@jaypeebrothers.com

**Corporate Office**
Jaypee Brothers Medical Publishers (P) Ltd
4838/24, Ansari Road, Daryaganj
New Delhi 110 002, India
Phone: +91-11-43574357
Fax: +91-11-43574314
Email: jaypee@jaypeebrothers.com

**Overseas Office**
JP Medical Ltd.
83, Victoria Street, London
SW1H 0HW (UK)
Phone: +44 20 3170 8910
Fax: +44 (0)20 3008 6180
Email: info@jpmedpub.com

Website: www.jaypeebrothers.com
Website: www.jaypeedigital.com

© 2024, Indian Academy of Pediatrics



*IAP-AHA Textbook of Adolescent Medicine*

*First Edition:* **2024**

ISBN: 978-93-5696-995-7

*Printed at: Samrat Offset Pvt. Ltd.*

# Academic Editors

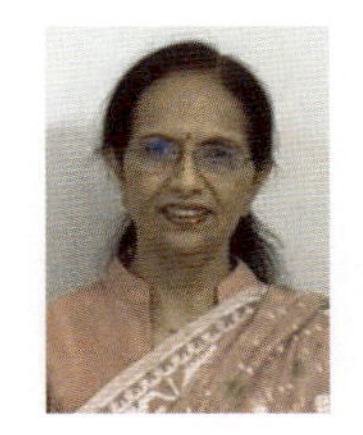

**Geeta Patil**

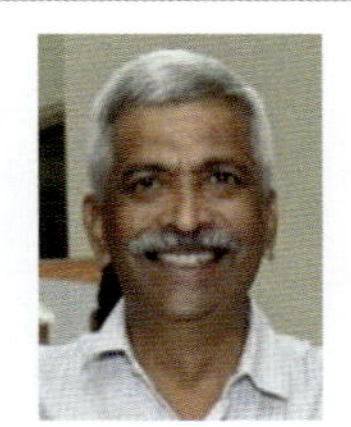

**Atul Kanikar**

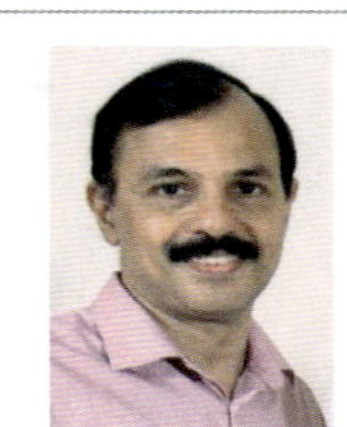

**Newton Luiz**

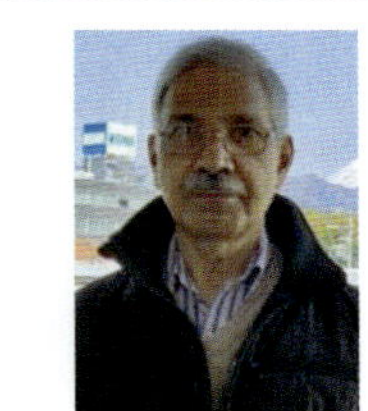

**Sukanta Chatterjee**

# Executive Editors

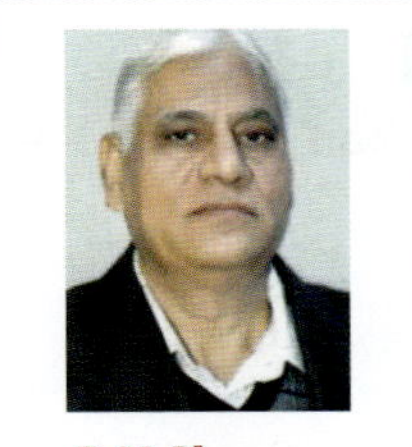

**R N Sharma**

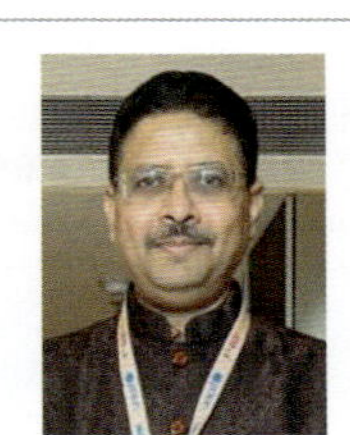

**Samir Shah**

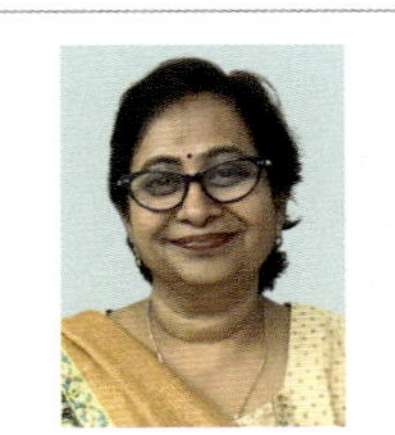

**Poonam Bhatia**

# Editorial Board

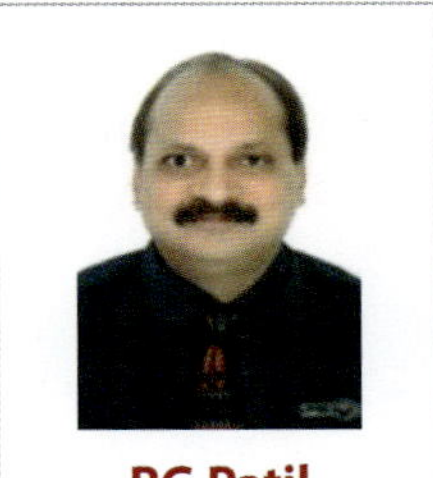

**RG Patil**

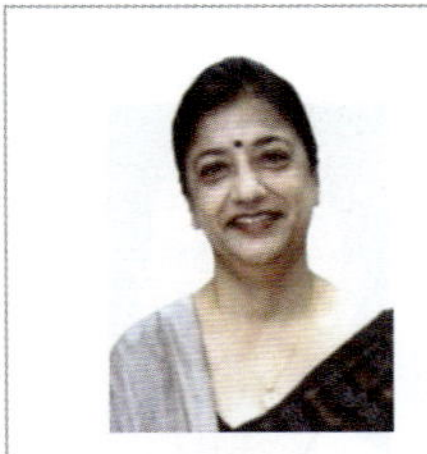

**Piyali Bhattacharya**

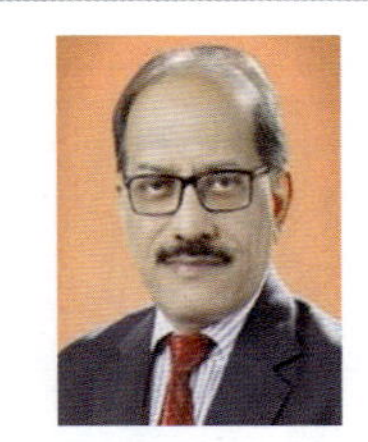

**Harish Pemde**

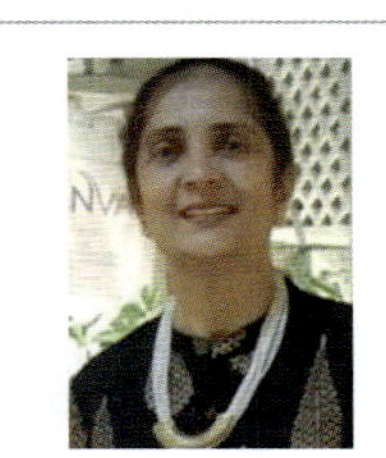

**Sushma Desai**

# Section Editors

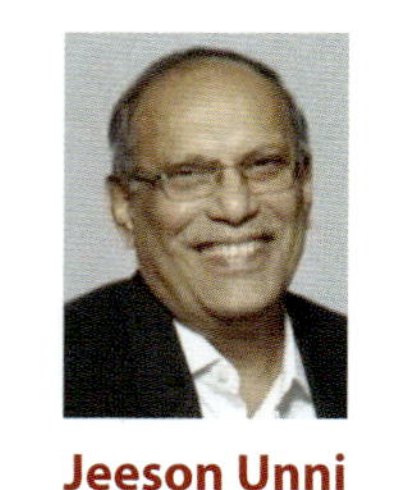

**Jeeson Unni**

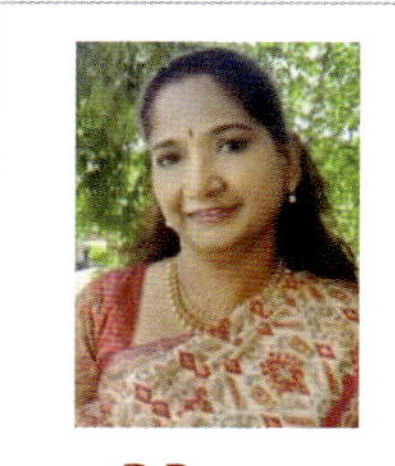

**R Prema**

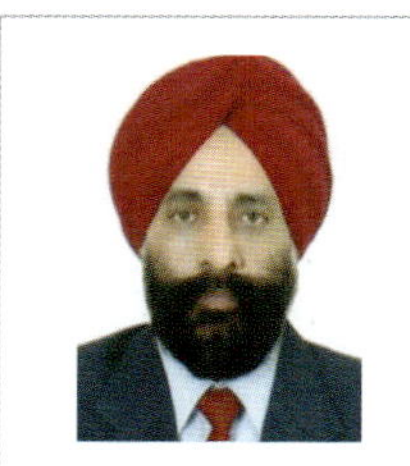

**Harmesh Bains**

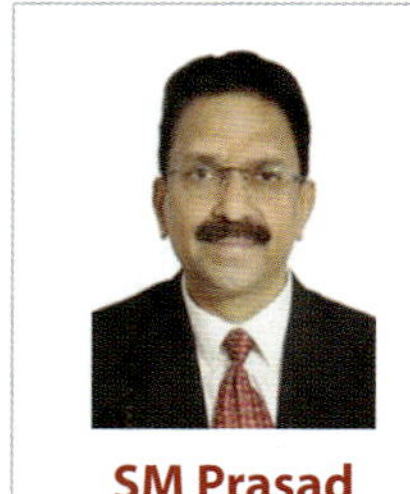

**SM Prasad**

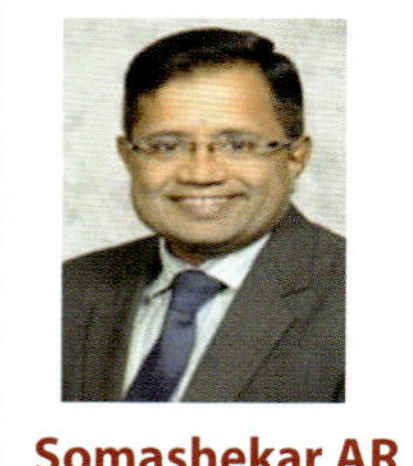

**Somashekar AR**

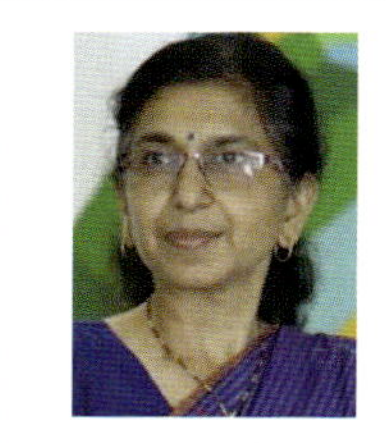

**Swati Ghate**

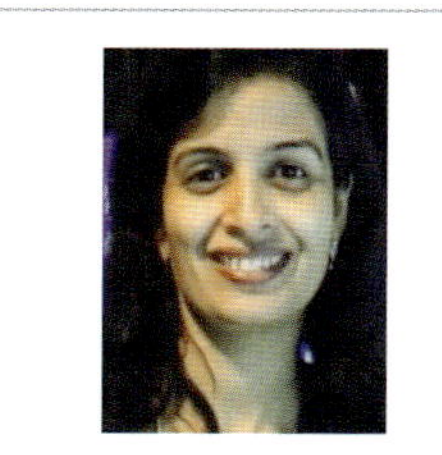

**Deepa Janardhanan**

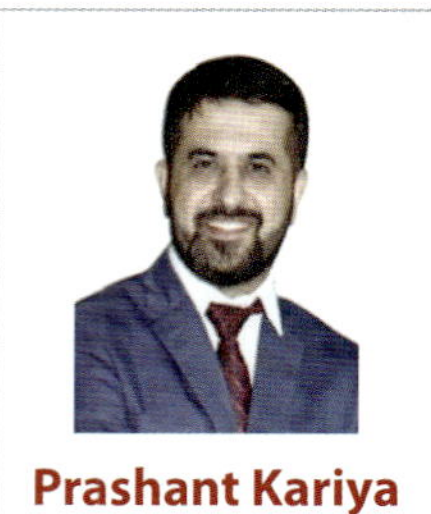

**Prashant Kariya**

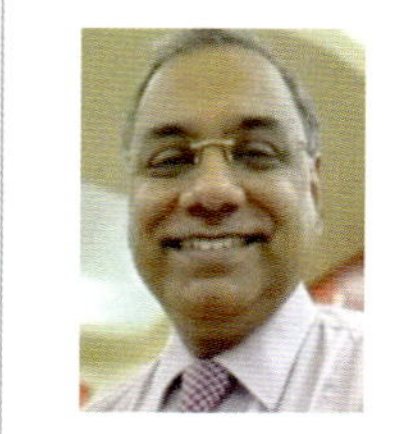

**Shamik Ghosh**

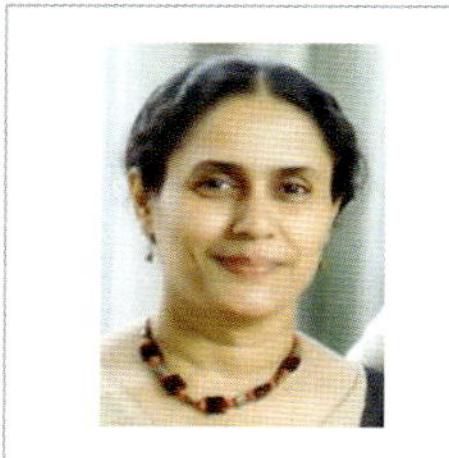

**Vaishali Deshmukh**

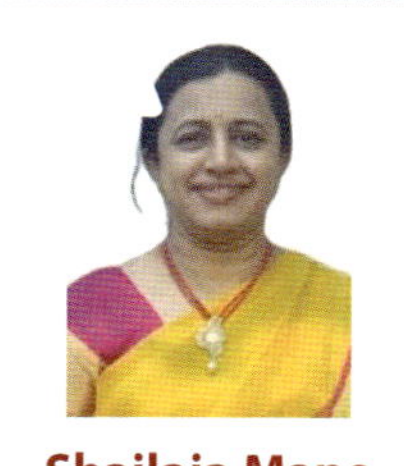

**Shailaja Mane**

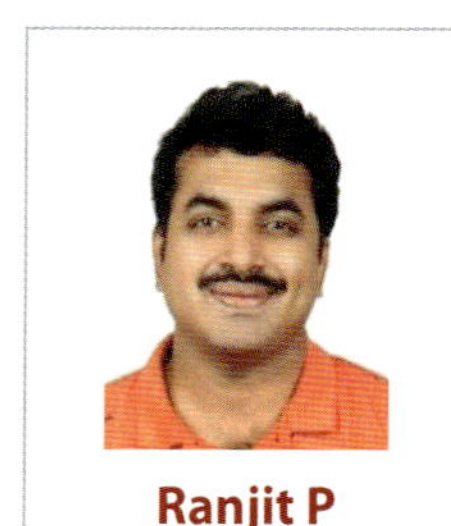

**Ranjit P**

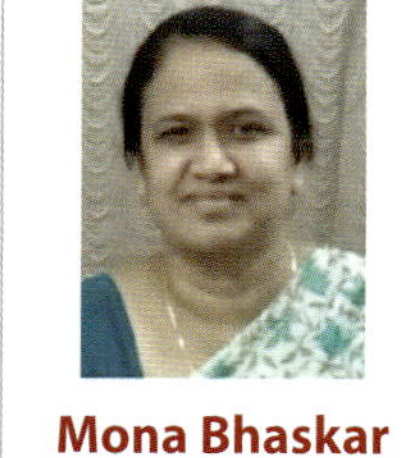

**Mona Bhaskar**

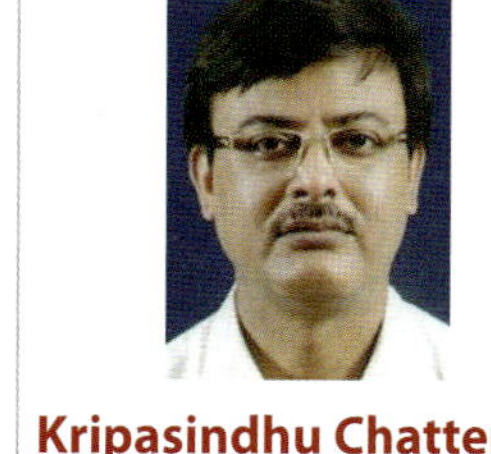

**Kripasindhu Chatterjee**

# Contributors


**Abheet Gupta**
BS (Psychology)
Counselor
Hospital Diversion Program
Northeastern Family Institute
Vermont, USA

**Afreen Khan**
MD (Pediatrics)
Associate Professor
Department of Pediatrics
Hamdard Institute of Medical Sciences
and Research Institute (HIMSR) and
associated HAHC Hospital
Noida, Uttar Pradesh, India

**Aishwarya Kulkarni**
BDS MDS (Prosthodontics and Implantology)
Senior Lecturer
Department of Prosthodontics
SMBT—Institute of Dental Science and
Research
Nashik, Maharashtra, India

**Ajit Singh Chawla**
MD FIAP
Consultant Pediatrician and Adolescent
Practitioner
Chawla Hospital
Ludhiana, Punjab, India

**Amruthvarshini Inamadar**
MBBS MD (Pediatrics) Fellowship in Rheumatology
(EULAR) Fellowship in Clinical Immunology
Senior Resident
Department of Pediatrics
MS Ramaiah Medical College
Bengaluru, Karnataka, India

**Anuradha Bansal**
MD (Pediatrics)
Specialist (Pediatrics)
ESIC Hospital
New Delhi, India

**Anuradha HS**
MBBS DNB (Pediatrics) PG Diploma in
Adolescent Pediatrics
Director and Pediatrician
Tots 2 Teens Healthcare, Bengaluru
Senior Consultant
Gunasheela Infertility and Maternity Hospital
Bengaluru, Karnataka, India

**Anuradha Singh**
MBBS MD (Paediatrics) PG Certification in
Adolescent Pediatrics
Consultant Pediatrician
ESIC Hospital, Okhla
New Delhi, India

**Anurag Bajpai**
MD FRACP SCE
Pediatric Endocrinologist
Regency Center for Diabetes,
Endocrinology and Research
Kanpur, Uttar Pradesh, India

**Aram Chenthil**
DCH PGDAP
Director/Senior Consultant
Ulagamathi Hospital, Neyveli
Gandhi Nagar, Tamil Nadu, India

**Arun B Nair**
MBBS MD
Professor
Department of Psychiatry
Government Medical College
Thiruvananthapuram, Kerala, India
Hon Consultant Psychiatrist
Sree Chitra Tirunal Institute for Medical
Sciences and Technology
Thiruvananthapuram, Kerala, India

**Ashim Kumar Ghosh**
MBBS DCH PGDAP
Practicing Pediatrician and Adolescent
Pediatrician
Private Clinic
Asansol, West Bengal, India

**Ashok Banga**
MBBS MD (Pediatrics)
Consultant Pediatrician
Department of Pediatrics
Astha and Chirayu Hospital
Gwalior, Madhya Pradesh, India

**Atul Kanikar**
MBBS DCH
Consulting Adolescent Health Care
Pediatrician
Dr Kanikar Clinics
Nashik, Maharashtra, India

**Ayushi Soni**
MD (Psychiatry) (SAMC & PGI, Indore)
Senior Resident
Department of Psychiatry
Sri Aurobindo Medical College and
PG Institute
Indore, Madhya Pradesh, India

**Bharath Reddy**
MBBS MD DNB Fellowship in Pediatric
Pulmonology and Sleep DMLE DCRL
Consultant, Pediatric Pulmonologist and
Sleep Specialist
Shishuka Children's Hospital
Bengaluru, Karnataka, India

**Bimlesh Kumar**
MD
Assistant Professor
Department of Pediatrics
Government Medical College
Badaun, Uttar Pradesh, India

**Bindusha S**
MD DCH DNB
Professor
Department of Pediatrics
Government Medical College
Thrissur, Kerala, India

**Chandrika Rao**
MD PGDAP PGD-Medical law and Ethics
Professor
Department of Pediatrics
Ramaiah Medical College
Bengaluru, Karnataka, India

**Chinmay Kinjawadekar**
MD DNB (Psychiatry) Fellowship in Child
Psychiatry
Consultant
Department of Psychiatry
KJ Somaiya Hospital
Sion, Maharashtra, India

**Chitra Dinakar**
MBBS DCH DNB (Paed) PGDAP (Adol Paed)
Professor and Head
Department of Pediatrics
St Martha's Hospital
Bengaluru, Karnataka, India

**Chitra Sankar**
MBBS DCH MRCP PGD DN FIAP
Consultant Developmental Pediatrician
Manipal Hospitals
Bengaluru, Karnataka, India

**C P Bansal**
MD SIAP PGDAP
Consultant Pediatrician
Director, Shabd Pratap Ashram
Gwalior, Madhya Pradesh, India

**DB Kadam**
MD (General Medicine)
Professor
Department of Medicine
SKN Medical College, Narhe, Pune
Emeritus Professor
BJ Government Medical College
Pune, Maharashtra, India

**Deepa Janardhanan**
DNB MNAMS PGDAP
Specialist Pediatrician
ESIC Hospital
Ernakulam, Kerala, India

**Deepa Passi**
MBBS MD (Pediatrics) FIMSA
Senior Consultant
Department of Pediatrics
Apollo Hospitals
Noida, Uttar Pradesh, India

**Dhanya Soodhana**
MD (Pediatrics) Fellowship in Pediatric and
Adolescent Endocrinology
Pediatric and Adolescent Endocrinologist
Department of Pediatrics
Aster MIMS (Malabar Institute of Medical
Sciences)
Kozhikode, Kerala, India

**Diksha Shirodkar**
MBBS MD (Pediatrics) MRCPCH (UK)
Assistant Professor
Department of Pediatric Endocrinologist
Yenepoya Medical College and Hospital
Mangaluru, Karnataka, India

**Elizabeth KE**
MD DCH PhD FIAP FRCPCH
Professor and Head
Department of Pediatrics
Sree Mookambika Institute of Medical
Sciences
Kanyakumari, Tamil Nadu, India

**Gayatri Bezboruah**
MD
Professor and Head
Department of Pediatrics
Gauhati Medical College and Hospital
Guwahati, Assam, India

**Geeta Patil**
MD FIAP
Senior Consultant Pediatrician
Adolescent Health Care Specialist and
Counselor
Chaitanya Hospital, Bengaluru
Visiting Consultant
Manipal Hospital
Bengaluru, Karnataka, India

**Gibby Koshy**
FRCPCH FRCP (London) PhD MBBS MPH
MTropPaed FHEA MRCPS Glasgow
Consultant Pediatrician
Parkview Family Health Care
Kollam, Kerala, India

**Gurmeet Kaur**
MD DCH MBBS
Professor and Head
Department of Pediatrics
Christian Medical College and Hospital
Ludhiana, Punjab, India

**G V Basavaraja**
MBBS MD DNB FIAP
Professor of Pediatrics and Head
Department of Pediatric
Intensive Care Unit
Indira Gandhi Institute of Child Health
Bengaluru, Karnataka, India
National President, IAP-2024
National Honorary Secretary
General, IAP-2020–21

**Harikishan Kumar Y**
MD DVL
Professor and Unit Head
Department of Dermatology
Rajarajeswari Medical College and Hospital
Bengaluru, Karnataka, India

**Harinder Singh**
MBBS MD PGDAP
Consultant Adolescent Pediatrician
Bhagat Clinics
Ludhiana, Punjab, India

**Harish Pemde**
MD (Pediatrics) FIAP
Director, Professor of Pediatrics
In-Charge, Centre for Adolescent Health
Lady Hardinge Medical College and
Kalawati Saran Medical College
New Delhi, India

**Harmesh Singh Bains**
MD PGDHHM MAMS FIMSA FIAP FNNF Heinz
Fellow RCPCH
Professor and Head
Department of Pediatrics
Punjab Institute of Medical Sciences
Jalandhar, Punjab, India

**Himabindu Singh**
MD (Ped) PGDAP FIAP
Dean
Shadan Institute of Medical Sciences (SIMS)
Government of Telangana
Hyderabad, Telangana, India

**Hiral Kotadia**
MD (Psychiatry) (IHBAS, Delhi) Post Doctoral
Fellowship in Child & Adolescent Psychiatry
(JIPMER, Puducherry)
Associate Professor
Department of Psychiatry
Sri Aurobindo Medical College and PG
Institute
Indore, Madhya Pradesh, India

**Intezar Mehdi**
MBBS DNB MRCPCH FRCPCH (UK)
Director and Head
Consultant Pediatrics Hematologist,
Oncologist and Bone Marrow Transplant
Department of Pediatric Oncology,
Hematology and BMT
Bengaluru, Karnataka, India

**Jayant Pandharikar**
MBBS MD (Ped) PGDAP
Consultant Pediatrician and
Adolescent Physician
Director
Sushrut Children and Maternity Hospital
Amravati, Maharashtra, India

**JC Garg**
MBBS DCH
Consultant Pediatrician
Garg Nursing Home
Gwalior, Madhya Pradesh, India
Past Chairman, AHA IAP

**Jeeson C Unni**
MD FIAP
Senior Consultant
Department of Pediatrics
Aster Medicity
Kochi, Kerala, India

**Jugesh Chhatwal**
MBBS MD DCH
Professor
Department of Pediatrics
School of Medical Sciences and Research,
Sharda University
Greater Noida, Uttar Pradesh, India

**JS Nikhil Ram**
MBBS MD (Dermatology)
Consultant
Department of Dermatology
Rajarajeswari Medical College and Hospital
Bengaluru, Karnataka, India

**Kajal Taneja**
MD (Psychiatry) Post-Doctoral Fellow (PDF) in
Child & Adolescent Psychiatry
Senior Resident
Child Psychiatry Unit
Department of Psychiatry
Christian Medical College
Vellore, Tamil Nadu, India

**Kalpana Datta**
MBBS MD (Pediatrics)
Professor and Head
Department of Pediatrics
Government Medical College
Kolkata, West Bengal, India

**Kalyani Patra**
MBBS DCH PGDAP
Consultant Adolescent Expert
MGM New Bombay Hospital and
Adolescent Wellness Centre
Navi Mumbai, Maharashtra, India

**Kamlesh Parekh**
MD DCH
Chief Pediatrician
Amruta Hospital
Surat, Gujarat, India

**Kripasindhu Chatterjee**
MD DCH FIAP
Professor and Head
Department of Pediatrics
Santiniketan Medical College
Bolpur, Birbhum, West Bengal, India

**Krutika Arunachalam**
FICOG FCPS DFP DGO MBBS
Consultant
Department of Obstetrics and Gynecology
Dr Khopkar Hospital
Navi Mumbai, Maharashtra, India

**Lakshmi Shanthi**
MBBS DCH PGDAP
Consultant Pediatrician and Adolescent
Health Specialist
Health and Wellness Centre
Coimbatore, Tamil Nadu, India

**M Vijayarani**
MBBS DCH PG-DAP
Pediatrician and Adolescent Consultant
SNEHAM—Guidance Center for Children
and Adolescents
Ranipet, Tamil Nadu, India

**Madhura Karguppikar**
MD PDCC (Paediatric and Adolescent
Endocrinology)
Consultant Pediatric Endocrinologist
Department of Pediatrics
SKN Medical College
Pune, Maharashtra, India

**Madhushree Deshpande**
MBBS DCH FCGP
Consultant Pediatrician and Adolescent
Advisor
Deshpande Hospital
Bilaspur, Chhattisgarh, India

**Manini Moudgal**
MBBS FAAP
Consultant Pediatrician
Kid's Care Clinic
Mysuru, Karnataka, India

**Manmeet Sodhi**
MD (Paed)
Professor and Head
Department of Pediatrics
Government Medical College
Amritsar, Punjab, India

**Merlin Thanka Jemi**
MSc MPhil (Clinical Psychology)
Lecturer in Clinical Psychology Grade I
Child Psychiatry Unit
Department of Psychiatry
Christian Medical College
Vellore, Tamil Nadu, India

**MKC Nair**
DSc
Emeritus Professor-Research
Former Vice-Chancellor
Kerala University of Health Sciences
Director
NIMS Spectrum-CDRC
Thiruvananthapuram, Kerala, India

**Mona M Basker**
DCH MD (Pediatrics) PGD-AP PGD-AP (PG
Diploma in Adolescent Pediatrics, Kerala)
Clinical Fellowship in Adolescent Medicine
The Hospital for Sick Children (Toronto)
Professor
Adolescent Medicine
Department of Pediatrics
Christian Medical College
Vellore, Tamil Nadu, India

**Mothi SN**
MBBS DCH MD
Consultant and Pediatrician
Founder Trusty
Ashakirna Hospital
Bengaluru, Karnataka, India

**Narmada Ashok**
DNB MRCPCH FIAP PGDDN DAA MBA
(Hosp Admin)
Consultant Pediatrician and Director
Nalam Medical Centre and Hospital
Vellore, Tamil Nadu, India

**NC Prajapati**
MD
Principal
Government Medical College
Badaun, Uttar Pradesh, India

**Neema Sitapara**
MD (Pediatrics) PG Dip Adol Pediatrics PG Dip
Clinical Hypnosis PG Dip Value Education and
Spirituality
Consultant Pediatrician
Adolescent Counselor
Director
Maa Sharda Child Care Hospital
Rajkot, Gujarat, India

**Neeti Soni**
MBBS DCH PGDAND
Consultant and Director
Soni Hospital
Aurangabad, Maharashtra, India

**Neetu Taneja**
BSc MSc Nursing
Senior Nursing Officer and Counsellor
Centre for Adolescent Health
Kalawati Saran Children's Hospital
Lady Hardinge Medical College
New Delhi, India

**Newton Luiz**
MD DCH DNB FIAP
Head
Department of Pediatrics
Dhanya Mission Hospital
Thrissur, Kerala, India

**Nirmala Joshi**
BSc MBBS MD (Pediatrics)
Consultant Pediatrician
Department of Pediatrics
Chiranjiv Clinic and Associate Hospitals
Lucknow, Uttar Pradesh, India

**Nishchal Bhatt**
MD (Pediatrics) PGD
Consultant Pediatrician and Teenagers
Health Expert
Dr Nishchal V Bhatt Children Hospital
Ahmedabad, Gujarat, India

**Nishikant Kotwal**
MBBS BCH CAHC
Director
Department of Pediatrics
Colours Childrens Hospital and
Manorama Children Hospital
Nagpur, Maharashtra, India

**Paula Goel**
MD DCH PGDAP PGP Diabetology
(John Hopkins School of Medicine) Diplomate
IBLM (US Board Certified in Lifestyle Medicine)
PGP Psychiatry
Founder and Director
Fayth Clinic
Mumbai, Maharashtra, India

**Payal Mittal**
DNB (Pediatrics) MNAMS
Associate Professor
Department of Pediatrics
FH Medical College and Hospital
Agra, Uttar Pradesh, India

**Piyali Bhattacharya**
DCH MD (Ped) FIAP FRCP (London)
Consultant Pediatrician
Sanjay Gandhi Postgraduate Institute of
Medical Sciences
Lucknow, Uttar Pradesh, India

**Poonam Bhatia**
DCH PGDAP PGPN
Director
Tot's 2 Teens Child Guidance Clinic
Dewas, Madhya Pradesh, India

**Prashant Kariya**
MD (Peds) PGDHHM
Associate Professor
Department of Pediatrics
Kiran Medical College
Surat, Gujarat, India

**Prashanth Inna**
MS DNB Fellowship in Paediatric Orthopedics
(UK and Korea)
Consultant in Pediatric Orthopedics
Manipal Hospitals
Bengaluru, Karnataka, India

**Prashanth MR**
MBBS DCH DNB PG-DAP
Associate Professor
Department of Pediatrics
Mysore Medical College
Mysuru, Karnataka, India

**Preeti Galagali**
MD PGDAP FIAP
Consultant Adolescent Health Specialist
and Pediatrician
Director
Bengaluru Adolescent Care and
Counselling Centre
Bengaluru, Karnataka, India

**Prerna Kukreti**
MBBS MD (Psychiatry)
Professor
Department of Psychiatry
Lady Hardinge Medical College
New Delhi, India

**Pukhraj Bafna**
MD DCH FIAP PhD
Head
Department of Medicine
Adolescent Health Consultant
United Hospital
Rajnandgaon, Chhattisgarh, India

**R Prema**
MBBS MD (Psychiatry)
Professor
Department of Pediatrics
Rajarajeswari Medical College and
Hospital
Bengaluru, Karnataka, India

**Rachna George**
MD (Psychiatry) MRCPsych Post-Doctoral
Fellow (PDF) in Child & Adolescent Psychiatry
Senior Resident
Child Psychiatry Unit
Department of Psychiatry
Christian Medical College
Vellore, Tamil Nadu, India

**Rahul Pengoria**
MBBS MD (Ped) MAMS
Associate Professor
Department of Pediatrics
Government Medical College
Firozabad, Uttar Pradesh, India

**Ramakant Dajiba Patil**
MD (Pediatrics)
Consultant Pediatrician
Antara Hospital
Nashik, Maharashtra, India

**Ramesh B Dampuri**
MBBS DCH PGD-AP PGD-AP FPPC
Consultant Pediatrician and
Adolescent Physician
I/C RMO, Medical Records Department
Niloufer Hospital, Hyderabad
Dampuri Child and Adolescent Clinic
Secunderabad, Telangana, India

**Ranjith P**
DNB MNAMS PGDAP
Consultant
Department of Pediatrics and
Adolescent Health
Kozhikode, Kerala, India

**Rashmi Gupta**
MD FIAP PGDAP FICMCH
Director
Department of Pediatrics
Vatsalya Hospital and Mishthi Foundation
Gwalior, Madhya Pradesh, India

**Ravi Bhatia**
MBBS DNB (Pediatrics) PGD-AP PGDAP MNAMS
Professor and Head
Department of Pediatrics
Pacific Medical College and Hospital
Udaipur, Rajasthan, India

**Ravishankara Marpalli**
MBBS DCH DNB (Paed)
Senior Consultant and Head
Department of Pediatrics
SS Sparsh Hospital
Bengaluru, Karnataka, India

**Rekha Harish**
MD FIAP
Former Professor and Head
Department of Pediatrics
Government Medical College Jammu and
Hamdard Institute of Medical Sciences
and Research (HIMSR)
New Delhi, India

**Reshmi YS**
MD (Pediatrics)
Assistant Professor
Adolescent Medicine
Department of Pediatrics
Christian Medical College
Vellore, Tamil Nadu, India

**RG Patil**
DCH PGDAP
Pediatrician
Adolescent Expert and Counsellor
Nagpur, Maharashtra, India

**Ritu Gupta**
MBBS DCH (MAMC, Delhi)
Consultant Pediatrician, Adolescent
Health Expert
Certified Parent and Teen Coach from Jay
Shetty Coaching School, USA
Friends Eye and Childcare Centre
Noida, Uttar Pradesh, India

**R N Sharma**
MBBS DCH
Consultant Pediatrician and
Adolescent Health Expert
R N Sharma Clinic
Agra, Uttar Pradesh, India

**Ruth Etzel**
MD PhD
Professor
Milken Institute School of Public Health
George Washington University
Washington, DC, USA

**S Sitaraman**
MD (Pediatrics) Fellow Pediatric Neurology (UK)
Director
Babylon's Newton Institute of Child and
Adolescent Development
Jaipur, Rajasthan, India

**Saloni Seth**
MBBS MD DNB (Psychiatry)
Senior Resident
Department of Psychiatry
Lady Hardinge Medical College and
Associated Hospitals
New Delhi, India

**Samir Shah**
MB DCH FIAP
Consultant Pediatricians and
Adolescent Practitioner
Samir Hospital and Holistic
Adolescent Care Center
Vadodara, Gujarat, India

**Sandeep Kavade**
DNB (Peds) PGD Developmental Neurology, CC
Adolescent Medicine
Director
Vatsalya Mother Child Care
and Manomay Child Development Centre
Pune, Maharashtra, India

**Sanghamitra Ray**
MD (Pediatrics)
Assistant Professor
Department of Pediatrics
Vardhman Mahavir Medical College and
Safdarjung Hospital
New Delhi, India

**Sangita Lodha**
MBBS DCH
Senior Pediatrician
Director and CEO
Arihant Multi Specialty Hospital
Nashik, Maharashtra, India

**Santosh S Bhide**
MBBS MS DNB
Senior Consultant
Ophthalmologists Ruby Hall Clinics, Pune
Founder and Director
Bhide Clinic
Pune, Maharashtra, India

**Saurabh Uppal**
MD (Ped) MRCPCH (UK) Fellowship in Pediatric
Endocrinology ESPE Fellowship in Pediatric
Endocrinology (Alder Hey Children's Hospital,
Liverpool, UK)
Consultant Pediatric Endocrinologist
Endo-Kidz Centre for Growth, Diabetes
and Hormones for Children
Jalandhar, Punjab, India

**SG Kasi**
MD DCH
Consultant Pediatrician
Kasi Clinic
Bengaluru, Karnataka, India

**Shaila S Bhattacharyya**
MD DCH DM MRCP
Professor
Department of Pediatrics and
Pediatric Endocrinology
Shivajoyti Clinic
Bengaluru, Karnataka, India
Founder President Pediatrics Association
of Karnataka PEAK 2022–2023
Past President ISPAE 2021–22

**Shailaja Mane**
MD (Pediatrics) PHD PGDAP IBCLC
Professor and Head
Department of Pediatrics
Dr DY Patil Medical College, Hospital and
Research Centre
Pune, Maharashtra, India

**Shamik Ghosh**
MBBS DCH (AFMC, Pune) DNB (Paediatrics)
MRCP (Edinburgh) MRCPCH (London) Certificate
Course in Basics of Adolescent Addiction
Management (NIMHANS)
Senior Consultant Paediatrician with a
Special Interest in Adolescent Health
Department of Paediatrics
Bhagirathi Neotia Woman and
Child Care Hospital
Newtown, Kolkata, West Bengal, India

**Shilpi Siddhanta Talukdar**
MBBS DNB (Ped) DCH (UK) MRCPCH (UK)
Department of Pediatrics
Eastern Railway Hospital
Liluah, West Bengal, India
Divisional Medical Officer (Pediatrics)

**Shivananda S**
MD (Pediatrics)
Retired Director
Indra Gandhi Institute of Child Heath
Bengaluru, Karnataka, India

**Shreeya Kulkarni**
MBBS MS (ENT) DNB (ENT)
Professor and Head
Department of ENT
Dr Vasantrao Pawar Medical College
Hospital and Research Center
Nashik, Maharashtra, India

**Shrihar Atul Kanikar**
BSMS IISER Pune
Practicing Adolescent Care Pediatrician
Nashik, Maharashtra, India

**Shubhada Khirwadkar**
MD (Pediatrics) Masters in Clinical Psychology
Chief Pediatrician, Project Director of
SEHAT (Strategic Enhancement of Health
in Adolescent in Tribal Area)
Mahatma Gandhi Hospital
Nagpur, Maharashtra, India

**Shyamkant Chaudhari**
MBBS DCH
General Pediatrician
Director
Nelson Memorial Children's Hospital
Nashik, Maharashtra, India

**SM Prasad**
MBBS DCH MD (Ped)
Professor
Department of Pediatrics
Akash Institute of Medical Sciences and
Research Centre
Bengaluru, Karnataka, India

**Sneha Jay Bhalerao**
BASLP MSc SLP
Hon Consultant
Department of Audiology and Speech
Language Pathology
Shree Guruji Rugnalaya
Nashik, Maharashtra, India

**Somashekhar AR**
DC DNB PGDAP PGDHHM Fellow in Respiratory
Disease (KKH, Singapore)
Professor and Head
Department of Pediatrics
MS Ramaiah Medical College
Bengaluru, Karnataka, India

**Sonia Bhatt**
MD (Pediatrics) PGCAP (Adolescent Pediatrics)
DAA (Diploma Allergy and Asthma)
Professor and Head
Department of Pediatrics
FH Medical College
Agra, Uttar Pradesh, India

**Sonia S Kanitkar**
DCH (Peds) Fellow Neonatology (Germany)
PGDAP FIAP
Director and Consultant
Kinder Clinic and Adolescent Care Center
Bengaluru, Karnataka, India

**Sucheta Kinjawadekar**
MD (Obs/Gyne)
Consultant
Kamalesh Mother and Child Hospital
Navi Mumbai, Maharashtra, India

**Sudhir Mishra**
MD (Pediatric) FIAP
Consultant Pediatrician/Former Head
Pediatrician
Tata Main Hospital
Jamshedpur, Jharkhand, India

**Sukanta Chatterjee**
MD FIAP
Former Professor and Head
Department of Pediatrics
Medical College
Kolkata, West Bengal, India

**Sulbha Amol Pawar**
MBBS DCH PGDAP IBCLC PGPN
Director
Department of Pediatrics
Anurag Children's Hospital
Nashik, Maharashtra, India

**Suma TL**
MBBS DCH DNB Fellowship in PHO (Kidwai)
Consultant Pediatrics
Hematology Oncology and BMT
HCG Cancer Center
HCG Hospital
Bengaluru, Karnataka, India

**Sumitha Nayak**
MD DNB FIAP Adv Certificate in Vaccinology-IVI,
S. Korea and CMC Vellore PGD-Guidance and
Counseling, PGD-Medical Law and Ethics
Consultant Pediatrician
Shishu—The Children's Clinic
Bengaluru, Karnataka, India

**Sunita Manchanda**
MBBS DCH PGDAP MA (Counselling Psychology)
Consultant Pediatrician and Adolescent
Specialist
Jain Sant Phool Chand Ji Charitable
Hospital
Gurugram, Haryana, India

**Sushma Desai**
MD DCH PGDAP
Consultant Pediatrician
Adolescent Physician and Counsellor
Mental Health First Aider-Specialized in
Suicide Prevention
Director
Gopi Children Hospital and Adolescent
Health Care Centre
Surat, Gujarat, India

**Swati Ghate**
MBBS DCH PGDAP MA (Clinical Psychology)
Joint Director
Babylon's Newton Institute of Child and
Adolescent Development
Jaipur, Rajasthan, India

**Swati Y Bhave**
MD DCH FCPS FIAP FAAP (Hon)
Professor Emeritus in Adolescent
Medicine
Senior Consultant in Adolescent
Pediatrics and Head and In-Charge of
Family Guidance Center and
Adolescent Wellness
Department of Pediatrics
Dr DY Patil Medical College
Pune, Maharashtra, India

**Swetha Madhuri**
MD (Psychiatry)
Assistant Professor
Child Psychiatry Unit
Department of Psychiatry
Christian Medical College
Vellore, Tamil Nadu, India

**Sylvia James**
BOT MSc (Psychology)
Tutor in Occupational Therapy
Child Psychiatry Unit
Department of Psychiatry
Christian Medical College
Vellore, Tamil Nadu, India

**Tanu Shree**
MBBS
PG Resident
Department of Psychiatry
Ram Manohar Lohia Hospital
New Delhi, India

**Thrupti S**
MD FRGUHS (IGICH)
Consultant Pediatrics and Adolescent
Endocrionlogist
Avant BKG Multispecialty Hospital
Mysuru, Karnataka, India

**Upendra Kinjawadekar**
MD DCH
Pediatrician
Kamlesh Mother and Child Hospital
Apollo Hospital
Nerul, Maharashtra, India

**Usha Banga**
MD (Pediatrics)
Consultant
Astha Clinic and
Prayaas Hospital
Bhopal, Madhya Pradesh, India

**Utkarsh Bansal**
MD (Pediatrics) MAMS FACEE (Peds EM)
Professor and Head
Department of Pediatrics
Hind Institute of Medical Sciences
Lucknow, Uttar Pradesh, India

**Vaishali Deshmukh**
MBBS DCH DNB (Paed) PGD-AP
In-Charge
Nine-to-nineteen Clinic
Deenanath Mangeshkar Hospital
Pune, Maharashtra, India

**Vaman Khadilkar**
MD DNB DCH FIAP MRCP
Professor Pediatric Endocrinology
Hirabai Cowasji Jehangir Medical
Research Institute (HCJMRI)
Pune, Maharashtra, India

**Vibha Yadav**
MD
Consultant, Pediatric and Adolescent
Endocrinolgy
Regency Center for Diabetes
Endocrinology and Diabetes
Kanpur, Uttar Pradesh, India

**Vijayakumar M**
MD DNB FRCP
Professor and Head
Department of Pediatrics
Government Medical College
Kozhikode, Kerala, India

**Vipin Vashistha**
MBBS MD (Pediatrician)
Director and Consultant Pediatrician
Mangla Hospital and Research Center
Bijnor, Uttar Pradesh, India

**Yatesh Pujar**
MBBS MD (Paediatrics) DNB (Paediatrics)
PGD-AP
Consultant in Pediatrics and
Adolescent Guide
Dr Pujar Hospital
Rabkavi, Bagalkot, Karnataka, India

# Foreword

Adolescent Pediatrics Chapter was formed with 12 members by myself as Founder Secretary and Dr Swati Y Bhave as Chairperson in 2000. The initial Adolescent Care Program were as follows; (i) Adolescent Module for Director of Health Services, Kerala (1997); (ii) Family Life Education Module and Teenage Screening Questionnaire, Trivandrum and First Teenage Care Clinic at Medical College Health Unit with UNICEF Support (1999); (iii) Adolescent Care Model at panchayath—teen clubs, adolescent clinic and teenage day celebrations with UNICEF Support (2001); (iv) Anganwadi based Family Life Education Program with the Support of European Commission (2001); (v) Life Education and Counseling Program at 152 schools with the support of Trivandrum district panchayath (2002); (vi) The "State Plan of Action for the Child in Kerala-2004" chapter on Adolescent Care (2004); (vii) Postgraduate Diploma in Adolescent Pediatrics and Child Adolescent Family Counseling under University of Kerala (2004); (viii) Module for International Training Program on Adolescent Health at Jaipur, Management Institute (2004); (ix) Adolescent Reproductive Sexual Health (ARSH) need assessment study done in three districts with the support of UNFPA (2005); (x) Adolescent Reproductive Sexual Health Education with the support of ICMR support (2006); (xi) Adolescent Health District Plan Project (AHDP)—combined training program with the support of European Commission and NRHM Kerala (2006); (xii) Adolescent Care Counseling Camps held in 999 panchayaths covering 150 thousand Adolescents (2012–2013); and (xiii) The major books published on adolescent care include: *Handbook of Adolescent Gynecology and ARSH, Adolescent Pediatrics, Adolescent Counselling, SRH of Young People, Adolescent Gynecology.*

*IAP-AHA Textbook of Adolescent Medicine* on adolescent health care is for practicing pediatricians, academicians, and postgraduates. Chapters included in this book, mostly authored by *Postgraduate Diploma in Adolescent Pediatrics* holders from University of Kerala, range from basic adolescent health care to advanced concepts. The content is authenticated with appropriate references by experts in the field. All the sections have been carefully prepared by pediatricians across the country and abroad, peer reviewed by equally illustrious colleagues and ably edited by stalwarts of adolescent health academy. The main focus is on practical approaches and can be implemented in clinics, schools, and community.

I am sure that this textbook will serve as an indispensable companion for students, educators, healthcare professionals, and anyone interested in adolescent growth and development with a rich foundation of knowledge and insights into this critical field.

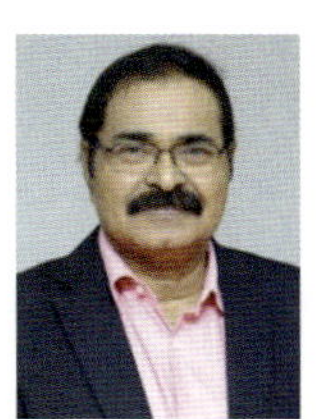

**MKC Nair**
DSc
President, CIAP–2004
Emeritus Professor-Research and Formerly Vice-Chancellor
Kerala University of Health Sciences (KUHS)
Emeritus Professor, Child Adolescent and Behavioral Pediatrics
Founder Director, CDC
Director, NIMS-SPECTRUM
Child Development Research Centre (CDRC), NIMS Medicity
Neyyattinkara, Thiruvananthapuram, India

# Foreword

I am delighted and honored to be asked to write the foreword for the *IAP-AHA Textbook of Adolescent Medicine.*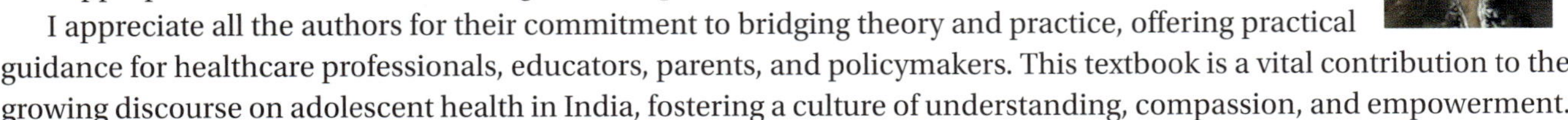

This book will be a valuable resource not only for practicing pediatricians, but also for academicians and postgraduates, as it covers all aspects from basic of adolescent health care to advanced concepts. with appropriate references from distinguished experts in the field.

I appreciate all the authors for their commitment to bridging theory and practice, offering practical guidance for healthcare professionals, educators, parents, and policymakers. This textbook is a vital contribution to the growing discourse on adolescent health in India, fostering a culture of understanding, compassion, and empowerment.

I congratulate the team—
- *Academic Editors*: Geeta Patil, Atul Kanikar, Newton Luiz, Sukanta Chatterjee
- *Executive Editors:* R N Sharma, Samir Shah, Poonam Bhatia
- *Editorial Board:* RG Patil, Piyali Bhattacharya, Hairsh Pemde, Sushma Desai, and all 14 *Section Editors* and 126 *Contributors* and the *IAP Office Bearers:* Dr G V Basavaraja, Dr Upendra Kinjawadekar, Dr Yogesh N Parikh, Dr Vineet Saxena for this herculean task.

May this textbook be embraced by all those who are dedicated to the health and well-being of the adolescent and serve as a reference of excellence.

My blessings and best wishes

**Swati Y Bhave**
MD DCH FCPS FIAP FAAP (Hon)
Professor Emeritus in Adolescent Medicine
Senior Consultant in Adolescent Pediatrics and Head and
In-Charge of Family Guidance Center and Adolescent Wellness
Department of Pediatrics
Dr DY Patil Medical College
Pune, Maharashtra, India
President, IAP 2000
Chairperson, IAP Subchapter on Adolescent Health (2003–2006)
Chairperson, IAP Taskforce on Adolescent Health (2000–2005)
IPA TAG, Adolescent Health (2007–2013)
Member, WHO HQ Geneva TSC—Child and Adolescent Health (2009–2010)
IAAH Regional Vice President, SE and Asia Middle East (2009–2017)

# Foreword

*Empowering Pediatricians to Navigate the Complexities of Adolescent Health*

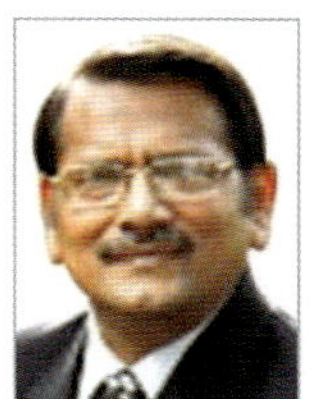

*Adolescence:* A whirlwind of change, a rollercoaster of emotions, a crossroads brimming with both potential and pitfalls. For those who dedicate their lives to nurturing children, this transformative phase presents a unique set of challenges, often met with limited training and lingering uncertainty.

That's where this ground-breaking textbook, the *IAP-AHA Textbook of Adolescent Medicine*, steps in. It marks a pivotal moment in our collective effort to empower pediatricians to confidently navigate the intricate world of adolescent health.

Born from the Adolescent Health Academy's mission to equip every pediatrician with the necessary knowledge and skills, this tome stands as a comprehensive testament to the dedication of esteemed experts across the nation. Each carefully crafted chapter, covering fundamental principles to cutting-edge concepts, is meticulously woven with practical guidance.

No longer will the unique concerns of teenagers, from physical development to mental health, from social pressures to emerging illnesses, remain shrouded in obscurity. This book dispels the shadows, offering in-depth insights and practical tools for managing everything from acne to anxieties, from nutrition to substance abuse.

The beauty of this resource lies in its practical focus. Its chapters are not mere academic treatises; they are actionable manuals designed to seamlessly integrate into everyday practice, be it in bustling clinics, bustling schools, or vibrant communities. It empowers doctors to become trusted confidantes, effective educators, and skilled caregivers, fostering a holistic approach to adolescent well-being.

For students yearning to master this specialized field, this book serves as a comprehensive guide, demystifying even the most complex topics. For practicing pediatricians seeking to fill knowledge gaps or refine their approach, it is a treasure trove of fresh insights and evidence-based practices.

Finally, it is a beacon of hope for teenagers themselves. With information readily available and accessible, they can approach this critical phase with greater awareness and understanding, armed with the knowledge to navigate challenges and embrace their immense potential.

I wholeheartedly commend the creators of this seminal work—Drs Geeta Patil, Atul Kanikar, Newton Luiz, Sukanta Chatterjee, and the entire team. The *IAP-AHA Textbook of Adolescent Medicine* is not just a book; it is a transformative tool, a bridge between knowledge and action, a catalyst for positive change. It has the power to empower not only pediatricians but also the adolescents they serve, ultimately shaping a healthier, happier future for generations to come.

Let this be the beginning of a new era in adolescent health care, characterized by confidence, competence, and compassion. Turn the pages, embrace the journey, and witness the extraordinary potential to empower both yourselves and the vibrant young lives entrusted to your care.

**C P Bansal**
MD SIAP PGDAP
Consultant Pediatrician
Director, Shabd Pratap Ashram
Gwalior, Madhya Pradesh, India
Co-chair, IPA Subgroup on Adolescent Health (2021–2023)
Former President, IAP, SAPA, AHA

# Foreword

It is a great honor for me to write foreword for the book—*IAP-AHA Textbook of Adolescent Medicine*.

Adolescence is a very important period of life, which is a period of opportunity as well as vulnerability. This is a transition period from childhood to adulthood.

The adolescent period is considered a healthy time of life. But the health problems faced during teenage are unique which require different approach.

Because of industrialization and urbanization, climate change adolescents are facing more challenges which create lot of stress in their life.

They are curious, impulsive, and rebellious. Neurodevelopmentally, they are not mature as frontal cortex is last to mature till the age of 25 years.

This book will help pediatricians tackle mental and physical health problems of adolescence more confidently, appropriately.

*IAP-AHA Textbook of Adolescent Medicine* on Adolescent Health Care is for practicing pediatricians, academicians, and postgraduates. Chapters included in this book range from basic adolescent health care to advanced concepts. The content is authenticated with appropriate references by experts in the field. All the sections have been carefully prepared by pediatricians across the country and abroad, peer-reviewed by equally illustrious colleagues and ably edited by stalwarts of Adolescent Health Academy (AHA). The main focus is on practical approaches and can be implemented in the clinics, schools and community.

This book will empower pediatricians to tackle all adolescent health problems.

I congratulate the team—

- *Academic Editors:* Geeta Patil, Atul Kanikar, Newton Luiz, Sukanta Chatterjee
- *Executive Editors:* R N Sharma, Samir Shah, Poonam Bhatia
- *Editorial Board:* RG Patil, Piyali Bhattacharya, Hairsh Pemde, Sushma Desai, and all 14 *Section Editors* an *IAP Office Bearers:* Dr G V Basavaraja, Dr Upendra Kinjawadekar, Dr Yogesh N Parikh, Dr Vineet Saxena for involving in this mission which will benefit all the pediatricians.

Congratulations and all the best to IAP-Adolescent Health Acdemy (AHA) for bringing out this book which will help to improve adolescent health care in our country.

**Piyush Gupta**
IAP President, 2021

# Foreword

Dear IAPians,

*Heartiest Congratulations!*

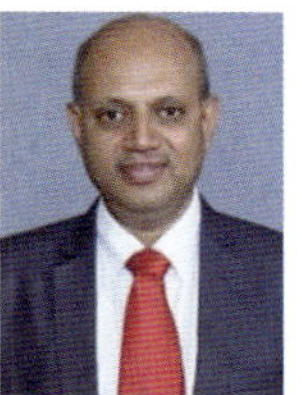

It brings immense joy and pride for the Adolescent Health Academy (AHA) of the Indian Academy of Pediatrics (IAP) to present its groundbreaking achievement—the *IAP-AHA Textbook of Adolescent Medicine*. This endeavor is the realization of a long-standing dream, driven by a commitment to addressing the unique challenges faced by adolescents, a demographic that was regrettably overlooked in the past.

Established with a modest membership, the AHA has burgeoned into a community of 3,100 pediatricians across IAP subchapters, underscoring the growing recognition of the imperative need for understanding adolescent health issues. The outdated notion of adolescence as a benign phase has been replaced by a heightened awareness of the distinct challenges that characterize this crucial period of development. There is now a palpable thirst for knowledge on how best to navigate and manage the intricacies of adolescent health, and this textbook serves as a comprehensive response to that demand.

This textbook is designed to be an indispensable resource for practicing pediatricians, academicians, and postgraduates, offering a thorough exploration of Adolescent Health Care—from fundamental principles to advanced concepts. Each chapter is meticulously crafted, drawing on the expertise of renowned professionals both within the country and abroad. The content is rigorously authenticated with appropriate references, ensuring the highest standards of accuracy and reliability.

What sets this textbook apart is its practical orientation, making the knowledge gleaned from its pages readily applicable in clinics, schools, and communities. The collaborative effort of pediatricians nationwide and abroad, coupled with thorough peer review, guarantees a wealth of insights that can be seamlessly integrated into diverse healthcare settings.

As we celebrate this milestone, I extend my heartfelt congratulations to Dr Geeta Patil, the visionary Chairperson of AHA 2024, whose dedication and passion have played a pivotal role in bringing this textbook to fruition. I commend the efforts of Dr Sukanta Chatterjee, AHA Chairperson, 2023; Dr R N Sharma, Honorary Secretary (2022–2023); and the distinguished editorial team, led by Dr Newton Luiz and Dr Atul Kanikar, for their unwavering commitment to excellence.

It is my honor to endorse this *Textbook of Adolescent Medicine*, confident that it will serve as an invaluable reference for all those committed to enhancing the health and well-being of adolescents.

Warm regards,

**G V Basavaraja**
MBBS MD DNB FIAP
Professor of Pediatrics and Head
Department of Pediatric
Intensive Care Unit
Indira Gandhi Institute of Child Health
Bengaluru, Karnataka, India
National President, IAP-2024
National Honorary Secretary
General, IAP-2020–21

# Foreword

Dear All,

One thing is certain! Adolescents must be nurtured cautiously as well as delicately to meet their ever-growing potential as we truly want them to play a pivotal role in the health of our nation. This period of transition from childhood to adulthood involves significant mental, emotional as well as physical challenges. The intentional or many a times nonintentional choices that an adolescent makes during this period can have profound ramifications on their health and well-being. The desire for a fast and adventurous life and risk taking can put an adolescent at risk for long term, even lifelong health 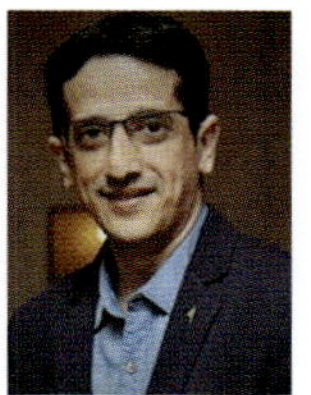 consequences. To add to it, valuing social connections is of supreme importance to them so naturally the demands of peer-group acceptance or other relationships can definitely influence healthy decision making. At the same time, it is extremely reassuring to know that if the parents, siblings, extended family, teachers as well as the medical professionals are made to understand the intricacies of this fascinating phase of life, they can surely provide that tender loving care which will help every adolescent to evolve into a productive healthy citizen.

The experts of the Adolescent Health Academy (AHA) of IAP are well aware of this and therefore keeping that as a sole aim have ventured into publishing this *IAP-AHA Textbook of Adolescent Medicine* which will be useful to all the stakeholders as stated above. It encompasses topics like road safety, environment to sports medicine, from school, parenting to nutrition and from basic prerequisites to physical and mental health, etc.

I am extremely happy to write this foreword for this book. Academic editors Drs Geeta Patil, Atul Kanikar, Newton Luiz, Sukanta Chatterjee; the executive editors Drs R N Sharma, Samir Shah, Poonam Bhatia; and the editorial board of Drs RG Patil, Piyali Bhattacharya, Harish Pemde, Sushma Desai, and all the authors have tremendous abilities to grasp and understand the problems of adolescents and their families for a major change in cultural and environmental aspects. I am certain that this book will contribute substantially to the understanding of adolescent health and thus to accelerate the health of adolescents.

Happy Reading,

**Upendra Kinjawadekar**
MD DCH
Pediatrician
Kamlesh Mother and Child Hospital
Apollo Hospital
Nerul, Maharashtra, India
IAP President, 2023

# Foreword

Health problems during adolescent period are unique, which we rarely encounter during childhood. Due to an immature prefrontal cortex in adolescence, adolescents are rebellious, argumentative, curious, impulsive, and try to seek instant gratification without thinking about consequences.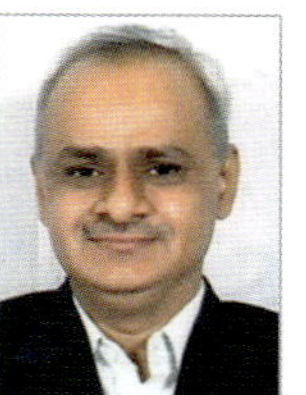

Adolescents constitute 21% of India's population. Common adolescent health problems include mental health disorders like depression, anxiety, behavioral problems, conduct disorders, substance abuse, poor school performance, and eating disorders.

Obesity, which is on the rise, will lead to early hypertension and heart problems. Puberty and sexuality issues are commonly encountered during this period.

All the caretakers—pediatricians/adolescent health specialists, parents, and teachers' community workers have to be empowered to tackle these issues.

Many problems are often rooted in high-risk behaviors and lifestyle, that are diagnosed not with laboratory tests but with detailed careful history, physical examination, through counseling.

Industrialization, globalization, nuclear families, increasing stress of day-today life, over expectation by the parents and teachers are the challenges faced by the adolescents.

This book will be reference book for pediatricians, postgraduate students nationally, internationally, and will help the pediatricians to tackle mental, physical health problems of adolescence more confidently, appropriately.

All the topics are written with Indian context, covering basic to advanced concept.

This knowledge can be used to tackle these issues in clinics, schools, and community.

I congratulate the entire team of AHA lead by Geeta Patil, Atul Kanikar, Newton Luiz, Sukanta Chatterjee as the Academic Editors. R N Sharma, Samir Shah, Poonam Bhatia are the executive editors who have coordinated and involved eminent authors in the country and outside the country.

*Editorial board members:* RG Patil, Piyali Bhattacharya, Hairsh Pemde, Sushma Desai have played vital role during all the proceedings.

*IAP office bearers:* Dr G V Basavaraja, Dr Upendra Kinjawadekar, Dr Vineet Saxena have extended helping hand when ever necessary.

Congratulations and all the best to IAP-Adolescent Health Acdemy (AHA) for bringing out this book which will help to improve adolescent health care in our country.

**Yogesh N Parikh**
IAP Hon Secretary General, IAP (2024–2025)

# Foreword

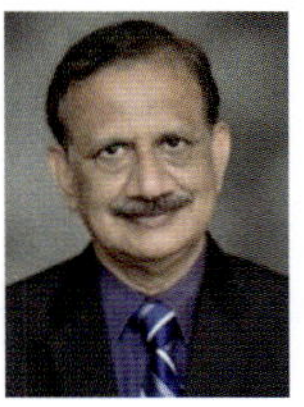

Adolescence is a critical link between childhood and adulthood, characterized by significant physical, psychological, and social transitions. These transitions carry new risks but also present opportunities to positively influence the immediate and future health of young people. This age group was ignored in the past because of the complacent belief that adolescence is a benign period.

Today we are all conscious of the unique issues of the adolescent age group and there is a thirst for information on how to handle them. India has the largest adolescent population in the world, 253 million, and every fifth person is between 10 and 19 years. India stands to benefit socially, politically, and economically if this large number of adolescents are safe, healthy, educated and equipped with information and life skills to support the country's continued development. Despite it beginning to receive more attention, there are still major gaps in both knowledge and action. IAP is proud that of its one of the best subspecialty chapter, AHA with maximum members which was nurtured by stalwarts like Dr JS Tuteja, Dr Swati Y Bhave, Dr C P Bansal, Dr SS Kamath and now being taken forward by very hardworking team of Dr Geeta Patil, AHA Chairperson, 2024; Dr Sukanta Chatterjee, AHA Chairperson, 2023; Dr R N Sharma, Hon Secretary (2022–2023) and many more who are working overtime to fill these gaps. It is a great initiative of AHA to bring out a complete book on Adolescent Health Care, which will be a great asset for practicing pediatricians, academicians, and postgraduates. This textbook covers all the key concepts right from basic to advanced. It is prepared by the masters of the subject. What is even more exciting is that besides clinics, it can be implemented in schools and at the community level. Most definitely this book will make a marked positive impact in the shaping of tender minds of India and for that the contribution of Drs Newton Luiz and Atul Kanikar, the editors of this book will always be remembered.

**Vineet Saxena**
IAP Hon. Secretary General, 2022–2023

# Preface

Adolescence is a unique stage of development and an important time for laying the foundations of good health.

It is a formative phase when they go through key mental, socioemotional, physical, sexual development and growth milestones. In the course of their development, they also face numerous physical and mental health challenges. Many physical as well as mental health problems are preventable. Many issues are often rooted in high-risk behaviors, lifestyle that are diagnosed not with laboratory tests but with detailed history of, careful physical examination, through counseling.

Adolescents constitute 21% of India's population and their health problems are magnified by industrialization and globalization. This is more pronounced in our country due to lack of access to information, counseling, and services to manage these problems.

Under the best of circumstances, providing appropriate and comprehensive health services to adolescents poses many challenges.

Over the past decade, interest in adolescent health has shown remarkable surge.

A steady decline in infectious diseases, reduced under five mortality and morbidity, improved economic status, and craving for better living has contributed to increased care seeking for adolescents.

All the stakeholders, policy makers, government, NGOs have realized that investing in health and wellbeing of this critical age group will help to have triple dividend.

All the caretakers—pediatricians/adolescent health specialists, parents, teachers have to be empowered to tackle adolescent health problems efficiently.

Indian Academy of Pediatrics (IAP) has been in forefront of training of more than 40,000 pediatricians across the country to equip them with clinical skills and recent developments.

The demand for training on Adolescent Health Care was perceived by many, and Adolescent Health Academy (Subchapter of IAP) has undertaken this project in mission mode to fulfill this demand.

The intention was to create a reference book which can give practical tips to academicians, practitioners, and postgraduate students and conceived the idea of making of *"IAP-AHA Textbook of Adolescent Medicine"*.

This textbook is organized into 14 sections that offer in depth knowledge about individual topic in Indian context. This book is a complete book on Adolescent Health Care for practicing pediatricians, academicians, and postgraduates. The chapters included in this book have tried to cover basic adolescent health care to advanced concepts.

The content is authenticated with appropriate references by experts in the field. All the sections have been carefully prepared by pediatricians across the country and abroad and peer reviewed by equally illustrious colleagues.

The main focus is on a practical approach and can be implemented in the clinics, and schools' community. This will be a perfect reference book providing all the details.

**Geeta Patil**
Chairperson, AHA 2024
Academic Editor

**Samir Shah**
Executive Editor

# Synopsis

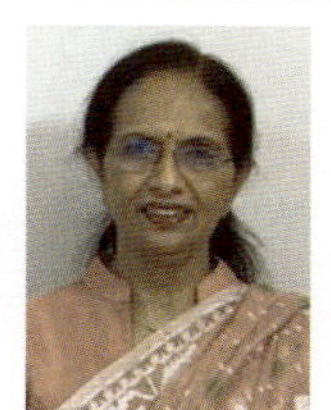

**Geeta Patil**

This book is a complete book on Adolescent Health Care for practicing pediatricians, academicians, and postgraduates. Chapters included in this book have tried to cover from basic Adolescent Health Care to advanced concepts. The content is authenticated with appropriate references by experts in the field. All the sections have been carefully prepared by pediatricians across the country and abroad and peer reviewed by equally illustrious colleagues. The main focus is on practical approach and can be implemented in the clinics, schools, and community. This will be a perfect reference book providing all the details.

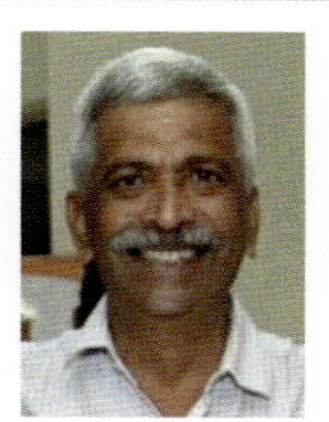

**Atul Kanikar**

With over a dozen well-segregated sections on different aspects of adolescent and youth well-being and precious contributions from experts working in the field of teen care all over the country, this book brings out everything that an undergraduate, postgraduate, and a pediatrician need to learn. A very handy book full of latest updates, useful annexure and neat presentations, this book is truly pediatrician friendly.

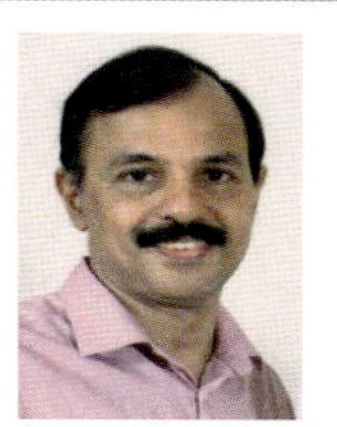

**Newton Luiz**

Pediatricians are understandably wary of managing the unique problems of teenagers, as Adolescent Medicine has always received scant attention during the postgraduate days in the past. This textbook should go a long way in filling in the knowledge gap of postgraduate students and practicing pediatricians.

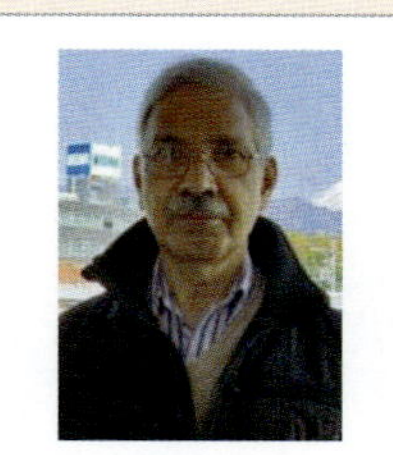

**Sukanta Chatterjee**

The *IAP-AHA Textbook of Adolescent Medicine* is the official publication of the Adolescent Health Academy (AHA) of Indian Academy of Pediatrics (IAP). The concept of this textbook was taken up as an action plan to fulfil the Theme of the Chapter for 2023, *Empower Pediatricians on Adolescent Health*. The process started on developing the recommendation from the scientific committee of AHA, then approved by the Executive Board of AHA followed by formation of a committee to take this mission forward. The Editorial Board formation and other standard process of developing a textbook was followed. I hope this publication will empower pediatricians on adolescent health practice.

# Acknowledgments

We wish to express our sincere appreciation to each contributor whose profound insights and tireless dedication have significantly enriched the content of this book.

A special note of thanks goes to our esteemed organization Indian Academy of Pediatrics and Adolescent Health Academy (IAP-AHA) whose cooperation and encouragement has been instrumental in the realization of this project.

We especially appreciate the constant support and encouragement of Shri Jitendar P Vij (Group Chairman) and Mr Ankit Vij (Managing Director) of M/s Jaypee Brothers Medical Publishers (P) Ltd, New Delhi, India, in publishing the book and also their associates, particularly Ms Chetna Malhotra (Senior Director—Professional Publishing, Marketing, and Business Development), and Mr. Naman Singh (Development Editor), who have been prompt, efficient, and most helpful.

We would like to extend a special thank you to Shubha Badami (MD) Senior Consultant Pediatrician and Adolescent Health Specialist, Rangadore Memorial Hospital, Bengaluru, Karnataka, India for graciously sharing the idea for the book cover.

# Contents

| **SECTION 3** | **MENTAL HEALTH** |
| --- | --- |

**MENTAL HEALTH**
*Section Editors:* Sushma Desai, Swati Ghate

### Part A: General Mental Health
*Sub-section Editors:* Swati Ghate, Sushma Desai



### Part B: Mental Health Disorders
*Sub-section Editors:* Swati Ghate, Sushma Desai

### Part C: Therapeutic Interventions for Mental Health Concerns
*Sub-section Editors:* Swati Ghate, Sushma Desai



**SECTION 4**   **PHYSICAL HEALTH**
*Section Editors:* Samir Shah, Poonam Bhatia, Shailaja Mane

### Part A: Endocrine Issues
*Sub-section Editors:* Harmesh Singh Bains, R Prema

## Part B: Systemic Conditions
*Sub-section Editors:* Samir Shah, Poonam Bhatia, Shailaja Mane



## Part C: Seemingly Trivial Health Issues
*Sub-section Editors:* Poonam Bhatia, Samir Shah, Shailaja Mane



## Part D: Infections
*Sub-section Editors:* Shailaja Mane, Poonam Bhatia, Samir Shah



## Part E: Adolescents with Distinctive Circumstances
*Sub-section Editors:* Samir Shah, Poonam Bhatia, Shailaja Mane

**SECTION 9** — **SOCIAL MEDIA**
*Section Editors:* Shamik Ghosh, Kripasindhu Chatterjee



**SECTION 10** — **ADOLESCENT AND THE SCHOOL**
*Section Editors:* R N Sharma, Mona M Basker

| SECTION 13 | ADOLESCENT HEALTH AND THE ENVIRONMENT |
|---|---|
| | *Section Editor:* **Somashekar AR** |



| SECTION 14 | ROAD SAFETY |
|---|---|
| | *Section Editor:* Piyali Bhattacharya |



## ANNEXURES

# Introduction

***Section Editors:*** *Jeeson C Unni, Ranjith P*

## 1.1    Adolescence

*Jeeson C Unni*

### ■ INTRODUCTION

The journey of adolescence is a phase of transformation wherein the seeds of adulthood are sown and the contours of identity begin to take shape. The children are bombarded with many negative and positive influences as they traverse the tunnel of adolescence to emerge, more often than not, as well-adjusted adults. This chapter explores the complex physical, biological, psychological and social dimensions that define this pivotal stage of human development.

Adolescence (from Latin word adolescere "to mature") is a transitional stage of physical and psychological development that transforms a child into an adult through the various stages of puberty. Adolescence is usually the teenage years but its physical, psychological or cultural expressions may begin earlier and/or end later— puberty beginning in preadolescence, especially in girls, and physical growth (mainly in males), and cognitive development continuing past teenage. Age provides only a rough marker of adolescence, and scholars have not agreed upon a precise definition. Some definitions start as early as 10 years and end as late as 26 years. The World Health Organization definition officially designates an adolescent as someone between the ages of 10 and 19 years.

To avail various schemes of our National youth Policy 2021, Government of India, youth is defined as those in the 15–35 years age group and adolescents as 13–19 years.

"Adolescence" is recognized as a phase rather than a fixed time period in an individual's life. Adolescents are the citizens of tomorrow. Behavioral patterns followed by a person during adolescence will last a lifetime. They will influence the health and well-being of the individual. Positive health of adolescents is strongly linked to their development. Their physical, psychological, and social abilities decide what they do, how they act, and whom they associate with. Technological advances have made the world a global village.

Technology has also made education and training necessary. This in turn has made the adolescents depend on their parents economically for a longer period, more than in the earlier agricultural era. At the same time, today's adolescents/youth are exposed to more information and cultural alternatives than in earlier periods. These provide the adolescent with culturally diverse choices, which cannot be easily exercised due to economic dependence. Ironically, therefore, the adolescent of today has to prepare for a global life of competition, comparison and independent functioning in a dependent environment. The "Individual" rather than the "System" is recognized as the basic unit of today's society.

Rapidly changing social, moral, ethical and religious values usher in certain "Life Styles." These affect health and behavior significantly—poor eating habits, poor oral hygiene, lack of rest, need for quick results, pleasure-seeking behavior, and stress. Certain in-built buffers of the society (both as support and control) are no longer available to the today's adolescents/youth. The stress, therefore, could result in the "Unholy Triad"—substance abuse, violence, and early sexual experimentation. Growing suicide rates and rising crime among young persons are also concerns.

Despite abilities such as reasoning and abstraction, the adolescent's behavior are often colored more by emotions rather than rationality. There is emotional heightening to contend with which more often than not, are unaware of. Frequently, they find themselves in an emotional fix of wanting to be guided by the parents, yet be free from them and be more aligned to the peers. And complex situations to contend with are plenty—puberty, dealing with sexuality and gender issues, tackling emotional upheaval, finishing basic schooling and the need to make future educational or career choices, facing responsibilities as an individual, etc.

And it is our responsibility to incorporate evidence-based methods to help the adolescent to develop the required abilities to deal with the demands and challenges of everyday life. This book will provide some of these strategies.

## ■ KEY MESSAGES

- Behavioral patterns followed by a person during adolescence could last a lifetime.
- This will influence the health and well-being of the individual.
- Positive health of adolescents is strongly linked to their development.
- Their physical, psychological and social abilities decide:
  - What they do
  - How they act
  - With whom they associate.

## ■ RECOMMENDED READING

1. Alderman E, Rieder J, Cohen M. The History of Adolescent Medicine. Pediatr Res. 2003;54:137–47. https://doi.org/10.1203/01.PDR.0000069697.17980.7C
2. Bhave's Textbook of Adolescent Medicine. Eds. A Parthasarathy, Swati Y Bhave, MKC Nair, PSN Menon, Donald E Greydanus. 2006. Jaypee Brothers Medical Publishers.
3. Patra S. Introduction to Adolescence in India: Issues, Challenges, and Possibilities. In: Patra S (Ed). Adolescence in India. Springer, 2022; Singapore. https://doi.org/10.1007/978-981-16-9881-11

<table>
<tr><td>1.2</td><td># Teenage: The Golden Epoch of Our Life Span</td></tr>
</table>

*Sukanta Chatterjee*

## ■ INTRODUCTION

Teenage literally means 13–19 years of age. The medical and social importance of this age lies in the process of transition of a child into adulthood. The World Health Organization (WHO) designates this age as adolescence. Chronologically, it includes 10–19 years of age, although the anatomical changes in adolescent starts even earlier, particularly in girls. Similarly, mental maturation to adulthood continues beyond 19 years in many adolescents. The maximum changes of transition occur between 10 and 19 years although it does not start sharply at 10 years nor it finishes abruptly at 19 years. That is why the WHO chronological age definition of adolescence between 10 and 19 years holds well.

Traditionally, illness meant physical health problems, which the individual feels and describes as symptom.

On the other hand, regarding the mental health issues, the thoughts, feelings, and behaviors which an individual develops are not considered abnormal by them; however, the family and the society feel and recognize them. This is an important fact that the healthcare providers need to recognize and act accordingly in the clinical management of adolescents. Physical health illness is less common in such adolescents in comparison to that seen in all other age groups. It is often called the "honeymoon" period of life. Mental health issues are the most common health problem in adolescents but these are not readily recognized in this period and parents bring them to medical attention at a late stage.

*Is it the Golden period of Life:* To answer this question, we have to say both YES and NO. To elaborate either the YES or the NO further, we have to describe it in three perspectives:

(1) at individual or adolescent level, (2) at family level, and (3) at social level.

## ■ YES, IT IS A GOLDEN EPOCH

### At Adolescent Perspective

Adolescents enter a new world of their own. They enjoy being exposed to the society often without direct parental supervision and develop peer relation of their choice. They love to make independent decisions. They get opportunity to explore everything available in the adult world and use them in their own way. They do not care about the adult-established social norms; rather they want to bring in new norms and feel happy to be seen as the agent of the change. The physical growth adding to the power and beauty of an adult man or woman becomes an item to showcase among peers and society. They set new style in everything—dress code, spoken language, new code texting, and choice of songs, tunes, and movies. Sexuality is another new feather in the cap. Sexuality implies reactions of the mind associated with maleness or femaleness that regulates behavior in relation to sex. It includes erotic thoughts and fantasies, emotions and desires that finally regulate behaviors and languages related to sex. They start with sexual fantasies and proceed toward experimentation without considering its consequences. Finally, each and every adolescent dreams to be someone big in the society with a lot of respect, love, affection, power, and money. Every achievement, whatever small it may be, by their own effort is always cheered by them.

The out-of-school, out-of-family, and other marginalized adolescents enjoy the liberty of being released of school and family discipline. They often start earning early as child labor to enjoy economic liberty. They get easy and early access to underworld activities, which are considered a privilege at this age.

### At Family Perspective

Parents consider their offspring to be their upcoming representatives in the society. They dream and expect their son or daughter to become more successful than themselves. Every family is making investment for the academics of their children. Adolescents get lot of opportunities not only in academics but also in sports, cultural, and many other extracurricular activities to become an all-rounder personality in the society. The number of coaching centers, be it subject-specific coaching or different state-/national-level entrance-oriented coaching, is rapidly increasing with a huge number of parents waiting outside. It reflects the golden valuation of the adolescent given by the family. The picture is nothing different at cricket coaching centers, swimming clubs, and music schools. The opportunity of adolescents in achievement of dress materials and cosmetics is also getting priority from parents only to make their children better accepted amongst peers and in the society. Parents are always aware of the possessions of different gadgets and appliances of the friends of their offspring. Nowadays, having a cell phone for an adolescent is not a dream but a reality. Coming to the growth and nutritional requirements, parents are constantly in search of new and newer food products that promote height, good figure, and fair complexion. Advertisement of DHA in food products is doing brisk business as it offers the promise of better brain development. Parents even approach medical professionals to promote brain functional capacity. They often go beyond their capacity to offer opportunities to the adolescent realizing that their child will not get a second chance to appear in school-leaving examination if leveled as a nonachiever. This is the period when an adolescent needs to be placed in a renowned institute and assured the path to a good position in the society.

The out-of-school, out-of-family, and other marginalized adolescents may have a mixed feeling of missing the family benefits and early employability.

### At Society Perspective

Adolescents are the future citizens of the country. The society creates a lot of opportunities for the future stakeholders at both government and NGO levels. The family and the society join hands to offer creative support to the adolescents within the framework of social discipline. Besides academic facilities, a lot of investments are done for the sports, recreational, and other welfare activities for the adolescents and youth. Many state governments are providing Tabs and internet connection to senior school students to facilitate their studies. Programs such as "Sabuj Sath" and "Kanyashree" in West Bengal are to name a few. Rashtriya Kishor Swasthya Karyakram (RKSK), programs of the Ministry of Women and Child Development (MWCD), and school health programs are few examples of adolescent welfare. The Protection of Children from Sexual Offences Act 2012 (POCSO) offers prevention of sexual exploitation of adolescents. The Mental Health Care Act 2017 provides mental healthcare and services to adolescents having mental health problems. It decriminalized attempted suicide. The Indian Information Technology Act 2000 (amended in 2008) increased the online transactions by a large section of adolescents and offers them cyber security. Industries are also not lagging behind; they take a "catch them young" policy to attract them and make them future customers. Companies of junk food, soft drinks, and other consumables are coming up with adolescent-focus product and advertisement.

A section of the society has a feel—good sensation in developing a support system for the out-of-home and marginalized adolescents. Arrangement of homes, joyrides during festival, and offering gifts are few examples covering a portion of them.

## ■ NOT A GOLDEN EPOCH

### Adolescent Perspective

Rigors of discipline, high expectation of parents, and early-morning to late-evening tight academic schedule steal away their play time, peer relation, and entertainment. Even the most serious students get concerned of the unpredictable outcome they see for their friends who study in the same coaching center but only few get high score or entry in a good institution. Underachievers are blamed by their parents and teachers without empowering them to be a good performer. Nobody tells him/her why he/she got low scores—5 out of 10—and how to get full scores—10 out of 10—in each and every assessment in all stages of life. They get confused of the proverb—"Failures are the pillars of success." They start losing self-confidence, the primary requirement of both making the effort and achieving the success. They need to be empowered rather than blamed or leveled as failure. There should be stage-specific empowerment training. A student getting 50% should be taught how to get 60% and then assessed to identify that he reached stage of 60% achiever; then only the lesson/training of getting 70% should be given. This implies that underachievers need more time from a skilled trainer. Unfortunately, the reverse happens—the best boy gets more attention from

the teacher. In the modern society, parents do have less time but most of them also do not retain the stage-specific skill required for the student. They give general advice like do not neglect or work hard like your friends. They fail to understand that at this formative developmental stage of adolescence, brain empowerment skill training works better than giving advice. Analyzing the advice and executing it in a positive skill direction needs maturity of the brain which is yet to complete. School-going students face another heartbroken reality while leaving school when they find that most of them do not get a chance in good institution or assured career path. Parents are unhappy like themselves; they face the real status difference being made in the society. They, at times, feel that there is no way forward and self-harm increases at this age.

The power of physical growth with an immature and impulsive mind pulls them to risk-taking behaviors leading to accidental injuries. They need to be empowered by protective device rather than being advised not to do it. Growth of sex organs with arousal of sexuality drives them to risky sexual behavior leading to immediate criminal consequences or long-term consequences such as social stigma and sexually transmitted infection (STI). Since the understanding of social norms and the consequences of their behavior are not yet developed, they should be protected rather than punished. Through news agencies, we all know this is a challenge area of the society which the judiciary is constantly struggling to resolve. The Indian society is yet to be supportive to the victims of such sexual act, who have an impulsive mind. Healthcare providers have an important role to play here by making advocacy for empowering adolescents to protect them by providing comprehensive sexuality education, access to contraceptive measures, and other sexual and reproductive health services.

For out-of-home, out-of-school, and other marginalized adolescents, this is definitely not a golden epoch. They struggle for food and shelter and lose protection of family and opportunity of education. They become a target of exploitation—sexual, child labor, and involvement in antisocial activities.

### From Family Perspective

How parents can call it a golden epoch when the defiance is maximum. An adolescent tries to put logic to his behavior which the mother takes as an argument. An adolescent takes an independent decision which the mother takes as overstepping into adult life. Every difference of choice puts parents and the adolescent in tussle; scholar or sportsman friend, same sex friend or opposite. Regarding dress code, parents plead for social permissibility or decency and the adolescent insists on his friends' choice. Every teenager dreams to be a great performer but gradually he does not find ways and means and brings down the expectation although parents keep their expectation level high, thus straining the relation constantly. A 16-year-old adolescent finds the behavior of the parents surprisingly different than what when he was 6 years of age.

## At Social Perspective

The society in general considers adolescents as future citizen but when they face adolescence in real life, they often consider this group difficult to manage. Different rules and regulations are imposed on them in institutional and noninstitutional settings. Moral policing often comes as news. Their behavior in public park and loitering places with girlfriend or boyfriend is considered a matter of nuisance. Change in dress code and style is often objected to at schools and colleges. Mental health issues including depression and anxiety are the most common health problem of this age group. The society looks at them with stigma and does not consider that mental health problems are reversible. Availability, accessibility, and affordability of treatment for this age group are still poor. Drugs and addiction are another common cause of sufferings of adolescents. The society does not have adequate treatment and prevention facilities for such addiction. The services for sexual and reproductive health needed for this group are prevented by social inhibitions and legal bindings.

## ▪ KEY MESSAGES

- The adolescent period is the most promising period of life. It's a temporary impulsive behavior phase due to yet to complete maturity of the brain.
- At this age they do many risks taking behavior, putting them in multiple health and social hazards.
- We need to nurture them, protect them from any short term or long term health consequences which could minimize their potential as this period will be timed out to adulthood with mature judgement.
- The Society need to change a lot to prevent any damage to them and the family need to be appropriately supportive to make this teenage really a golden epoch.

## ▪ RECOMMENDED READING


1. Grover S, Raju VV, Sharma A, Shah R. Depression in Children and Adolescents: A Review of Indian studies. Indian J Psychol Med. 2019;41(3):216-27.
2. https://www.indiatoday.in/law/story/adolescent-girls-should-control-their-sexual-urges-and-calcutta-high-court-2451236-2023-10-19
3. International Labour Office. (2022). World report—A future without child labour. https://www.ilo.org/wcmsp5/groups/ public/—dgreports/—dcomm/—publ/documents/publication/wcms_publ_ 9221124169_en.pdf. [Last accessed March, 2024].
4. Transport Research Wing (TRW); Ministry of Road Transport & Highways. (2021). Road accidents in India. Available from https://morth.nic.in/sites/default/files/RA_2021_Compressed.pdf. [Last accessed March, 2024]
5. Trivedi D. (2022). State of adolescent learning. Available from https://www.thehindu.com/opinion/op-ed/state-of-adolescent-learning/article65312061.ece.april.2022. [Last accessed March, 2024].
6. World Health Organization. Maternal, newborn, child and adolescent health and ageing. Available from https://platform.who.int/data/maternal-newborn-child-adolescent-ageing/static-visualizations/adolescent-country-profile. [Last accessed March, 2024].

<table>
<tr><td>**1.3**</td><td># Local, Regional, National, and International Programs for Adolescent Health</td></tr>
</table>

*Swati Y Bhave, Deepa Janardhanan, Narmada Ashok*

## ■ INTRODUCTION

Positive youth development programs engage adolescents in a constructive way by recognizing and enhancing their core strengths. They also increase networking, positive relationships and give the support the young people need in order to prevent risk-taking behaviors. There are several such programs at national and international levels that have ensured that our young people are adequately supported. Several studies have also pointed out that these programs have been effective in improving social and emotional outcomes. This chapter will elaborate on the important programs carried out throughout the world and in India for the welfare of the adolescents and young adults. Adolescents are the future of our nation, and therefore mechanisms to address and deal with adolescent issues effectively are very important for the progress of any country.

## WORLD HEALTH ORGANIZATION AND ADOLESCENCE

The World Health Organization (WHO) believes that adolescents, despite being thought of as a healthy stage, is still characterized by significant death and disability specific for this age. Adolescents in order to grow and develop in good health need information, age-appropriate sexuality education, life skills, and appropriate equitable and effective services to help them attain their maximum potential. Hence, several programs have been launched by the WHO for the benefit of the adolescents.

**Table 1** describes the various programs.

## ■ PROGRAMS BY UNICEF

The United Nations Children's Fund (UNICEF) believes that the second decade of life is a time of transformation. It believes that when the adolescents venture beyond their family to form powerful connection with peers they search for ways to stand out and belong, and hence it is the society's duty to support which is often ignored by policy makers. Hence, it is imperative that the adolescents need a good quality environment, relationship, and experience to have a good prospect **(Table 2)**.

## ■ NATIONAL PROGRAMS FOR ADOLESCENTS

With a nation pulsating with energy and vitality, India believes that the youth hold the key to realize the vision of Dream India 2047. India's huge youth population is an unparalleled demographic advantage and possess untapped wellspring of creativity, innovation, and resilience. Hence, a lot of innovative programs have been launched for the benefit of youth **(Table 3)**.

## ■ STATE-LEVEL PROGRAMS

Youth have an immense potential and all states are also keen to invest a lot in their youth. Five of the states in India have pioneering programs for the youth. The youth of India can play a pivotal role in addressing pressing social issues, such as gender inequality, poverty, and environmental degradation and these programs are targeted to support them in the same **(Table 4)**.

## MENSTRUAL HYGIENE PROGRAMS BY VARIOUS MINISTRIES

Onset of menstruation is a new phase and creates new vulnerabilities for adolescent girls. Every year millions of girls, women, and transgender are unable to manage their menstrual cycle in a dignified way. Many of their needs go unmet due to lack of basic services like toilet, sanitary pads and cultural taboos. Menstrual health and hygiene intervention programs can help overcome these obstacles. The programs adopted by various ministries are given in **(Table 5)**.

## PROGRAMS BENEFITING EARLY ADOLESCENTS

The WHO definition of adolescence includes age group of 10–19 years. **Table 6** summarizes the government of India programs which also cover this age group.

**TABLE 1:** WHO programs for adolescents.

| Name of the program | Year of launching | Objectives of the program | Age and gender of the beneficiaries | Benefits |
| --- | --- | --- | --- | --- |
| Global School Health Initiative (GSHI) | 2002 | • Reduce the number of adolescent deaths from preventable causes, such as road traffic accidents, suicide, and violence<br>• Increase the number of adolescents who are healthy and thriving, both physically and mentally<br>• Reduce the number of adolescents who are affected by sexual and reproductive health problems<br>• Reduce the number of adolescents who are affected by noncommunicable diseases, such as obesity, diabetes, and heart disease<br>• Improve the health literacy and health-seeking behaviors of adolescents<br>• Empower adolescents to participate in decision-making about their health and well-being<br>• Strengthen health systems to deliver adolescent-friendly healthcare services, including confidential and affordable access to contraception and other sexual and reproductive health services | • *Students:* Students are the primary beneficiaries of GSHI. These initiatives can help to improve students' physical and mental health, reduce absenteeism and dropout rates, improve academic performance, and reduce healthcare costs<br>• *Schools*: This initiative helps to create a healthier school environment, improve student morale, and reduce the burden on teachers and other school staff<br>• *Communities:* By reducing crime and violence, and increasing productivity<br>• *Governments*: By reducing the health care costs and creating a more productive workforce | • Improved health outcomes for students<br>• Reduced absenteeism and dropout rates by promoting healthy behavior and by providing students with the support they need to succeed<br>• Improved academic performance by promoting healthy lifestyles and by providing students with the support they need to learn effectively<br>• Reduced healthcare costs by preventing diseases and injuries<br>• Created a healthy school environment |
| Global Strategy for Women's, Children's and Adolescents' Health (2016–2030) | 2016 | • End preventable deaths of newborns, children, and adolescents<br>• End all forms of malnutrition<br>• Ensure that all women of reproductive age have access to quality reproductive, maternal, newborn, child, and adolescent health care services<br>• End preventable deaths of women from reproductive causes<br>• Eliminate gender disparities in health and achieve universal effective coverage of quality essential health services<br>• Reduce adolescent mortality by one-third by 2030 | Women, children, and adolescents | • Improved health for women, children, and adolescents<br>• Reduced poverty and inequality<br>• Increased economic productivity<br>• A more just and equitable world |

*Contd...*

Contd...

| Name of the program | Year of launching | Objectives of the program | Age and gender of the beneficiaries | Benefits |
| --- | --- | --- | --- | --- |
| Global Accelerated Action for the Health of Adolescents (AA-HA!) | 2017 | • Reduce adolescent mortality, by two-thirds from 2015 levels by 2030<br>• Improve adolescent sexual and reproductive health<br>• Prevent violence against adolescents<br>• Promote adolescent mental health<br>• Ensure adolescents thrive | Adolescents | • Improved health outcomes for adolescents<br>• Reduced health inequities<br>• Empowered adolescents<br>• Stronger health systems |
| Helping Adolescents Thrive (HAT) Initiative | 2019 as a joint initiative by WHO and UNICEF | • *Promote mental health and prevent mental health conditions:* This includes raising awareness of mental health, reducing stigma, and promoting healthy lifestyles<br>• *Help prevent self-harm and other risk behaviors:* This includes providing adolescents with the skills and knowledge they need to cope with stress and difficult emotions<br>• Improve access to affordable, quality mental health care | Adolescents | • Improved mental health for adolescents and thereby improved academic performance, reduced absenteeism and dropout rates, and improved relationships with family and friends<br>• Reduced risk of self-harm and other risk behaviors<br>• Improved access to affordable, quality health care |
| LIVE LIFE Initiative | 2021 | • Advance political will for suicide prevention<br>• Promote national strategic action for suicide prevention<br>• Deliver key effective interventions for suicide prevention | • People who are at risk of suicide will be helped by implementing effective suicide prevention interventions<br>• People who have attempted suicide by helping them to recover and live healthy and fulfilling lives<br>• Families and friends of people who have died by suicide by helping them to cope with their grief and loss<br>• *Communities:* The LIVE LIFE initiative can help to create communities that are more supportive and inclusive. This can help to reduce the stigma associated with suicide and mental illness<br>• *Governments:* The LIVE LIFE initiative can help governments to reduce the costs of suicide, such as healthcare costs and lost productivity | • Reduced suicide rates<br>• Improved mental health outcomes<br>• Reduced stigma associated with suicide and mental illness<br>• Increased access to suicide prevention and mental health care services<br>• Reduced economic costs |

Contd...

**TABLE 2:** UNICEF programs for adolescents.

| Name of the program | Year of launching | Objectives of the program | Age and gender of the beneficiaries | Benefits |
|---|---|---|---|---|
| UNICEF's Adolescent Girls Programme | 2003 | • *Health and nutrition:* UNICEF works to ensure that adolescent girls have access to quality healthcare, including sexual and reproductive health services, and that they are eating a nutritious diet<br>• *Education and skills:* UNICEF supports adolescent girls to stay in school and to develop the skills and knowledge they need to succeed in life and work<br>• *Protection:* UNICEF works to protect adolescent girls from violence, exploitation, abuse, and harmful practices<br>• *Participation:* UNICEF supports adolescent girls to participate meaningfully in decision-making at all levels | Adolescent girls | • Helping to reduce child marriage and early pregnancy<br>• Increasing access to secondary education and skills training for girls<br>• Reducing gender-based violence<br>• Promoting adolescent girls' participation in decision-making<br>• In India, UNICEF is working with partners to provide adolescent girls with life skills training, such as financial literacy and decision-making. This training helps girls to develop the skills they need to succeed in life and to protect themselves from violence and exploitation |
| UNFPA-UNICEF Global Programme to Accelerate Action to End Child Marriage | 2016 | This program aims to end child marriage by 2030 | Girls and adolescents | It supports programs that address the root causes of child marriage, such as poverty, gender inequality, and lack of education |
| UNFPA-UNICEF Global Programme to Accelerate Action to End Gender-Based Violence | 2016 | This program aims to end gender-based violence by 2030 | Girls and adolescents | It supports programs that address all forms of gender-based violence, including violence against adolescent girls and young women |
| Youth Lead | 2018 | Global program that supports young people to lead social change | Young people | Global program that supports young people to lead social change |
| StartUp! | 2019 | Program that helps young people to develop entrepreneurial skills and to start their own businesses | | The program provides young people with training, mentorship, and access to funding |
| UNICEF Youth Power | 2020 | • *Education and skills:* UNICEF supports young people to access quality education and to develop the skills and knowledge they need to succeed in life and work<br>• *Health and well-being:* UNICEF works to ensure that young people have access to quality healthcare, including sexual and reproductive health services, and that they are living in safe and healthy environments | Young people | • It is a youth-led program<br>• Provides gender equality and also social justice<br>• Helping young people to reach their full potential regardless of their background or circumstances<br>• UNICEF Youth Power is also empowering young people to take action on climate change, mental health, and other important issues facing the world today |

*Contd...*

Contd...

| Name of the program | Year of launching | Objectives of the program | Age and gender of the beneficiaries | Benefits |
|---|---|---|---|---|
| | | • *Participation:* UNICEF supports young people to participate meaningfully in decision-making at all levels, from their communities to the global stage<br>• *Protection:* UNICEF works to protect young people from violence, exploitation, abuse, and harmful practices | | |
| UNICEF U-Report | 2020 | Free, anonymous mobile messaging platform that gives young people a voice on issues that matter to them | Young people | • U-Reporters respond to polls, report issues, and support child rights. Feedback is given to the communities regarding the data and insights and also needed communications are made with the policy makers who make decisions that affect young people<br>• U-Report is an important tool for UNICEF to engage with young people and to learn about their priorities and concerns. It is also a way for young people to hold their governments and other decision-makers accountable<br>• In India, U-Reporters helped to identify the main challenges facing adolescent girls in their communities. This information was used to design and implement programs to address these challenges |
| Adolescent Girls' Initiative (AGI) | 2022–2025 | Global initiative that aims to accelerate progress toward gender equality and the empowerment of adolescent girls | Adolescent girls | AGI supports programs that help adolescent girls develop their life skills, access Sexual and reproductive health and rights (SRHR) information and services, and participate in decision-making |
| Safe Spaces | 2022 | Community-based safe spaces where young people can access information and services on sexual and reproductive health, life skills, and gender equality | Young people | It provides a safe and supportive environment for young people to socialize and participate in activities |
| Youth Councils | | Young people work with UNFPA and other partners to develop and implement programs and policies that affect their lives | Young people | Play an important role in advocating for the rights and needs of young people |

Contd...

**TABLE 3:** India—national programs for adolescents.

| Name of the program | Year of launch | Objectives | Beneficiaries | Benefits |
| --- | --- | --- | --- | --- |
| National Service Scheme (NSS) | 1969 | National program that aims to develop the social and civic responsibility of youth | Youth | The program is implemented by the Ministry of Youth Affairs and Sports in collaboration with state governments |
| Balika Samridhi Yojana | 1997 | Program that provides financial assistance to adolescent girls | Adolescent girls | • The program aims to improve the education and empowerment of adolescent girls |
| Rajiv Gandhi Scheme for Empowerment of Adolescent Girls (RGSEAG)—SABLA | 2011 | • Enable adolescent girls' self-development and empowerment<br>• Improve their nutrition and health status<br>• Promote awareness about health, hygiene, nutrition, Adolescent Reproductive and Sexual Health (ARSH) and family and child care<br>• Upgrade home-based skills, life skills, and vocational skills<br>• Mainstream out-of-school adolescent girls into formal/nonformal education<br>• Provide information/guidance about existing public services such as primary health center (PHC), community health center (CHC), post office, bank, police station | Adolescent girls in the age group of 11–18 years, with a focus on out-of-school girls | • Improved health and nutrition<br>• Reduced risk of early marriage and childbearing<br>• Increased access to education and employment opportunities<br>• Improved life skills and self-confidence<br>• Increased participation in social and community activities |
| RMNCH+A Strategy | 2013 | • Reduce maternal mortality<br>• Reduce neonatal mortality<br>• Reduce under-five mortality<br>• Improve the health and well-being of adolescents and women<br>• Promote universal access to quality health care services for all women, children, and adolescents | • Pregnant women and new mothers<br>• Newborns and children under the age of 5 years<br>• Adolescents (aged 10–19 years)<br>• Women of reproductive age (aged 15–49 years)<br>• People living in poverty<br>• People living in rural areas<br>• Indigenous peoples<br>• People with disabilities | • Nutrition of adolescents—Weekly Iron Folic acid Supplementation (WIFS)<br>• Facility-based Adolescent Reproductive and Sexual Health services (ARSH) Adolescent Friendly Health Services (AFHS) information and counseling<br>• Menstrual hygiene<br>• Preventive health checkups |
| National Programme for Youth and Adolescent Development (NPYAD) | 2014 | Program that aims to promote the development of youth and adolescents | Youth and adolescents | The program provides a range of services, including vocational training, sports and cultural activities, and life skills training |

Contd...

*Contd...*

| Name of the program | Year of launch | Objectives | Beneficiaries | Benefits |
|---|---|---|---|---|
| Rashtriya Yuva Sashaktikaran Yojana (RYSK) | 2014 | National program that aims to develop the skills and capacities of youth | Youth | The program is implemented by the Ministry of Youth Affairs and Sports in collaboration with state governments |
| Rashtriya Kishore Swasthya Karyakram (RKSK) | 2014 | • Improve the health and well-being of adolescents in India<br>• Enable adolescents to make informed and responsible decisions about their health and well-being<br>• Reduce the prevalence of malnutrition, iron-deficiency anemia, and other health problems among adolescents<br>• Improve access to quality health services for adolescents<br>• Promote adolescent participation and leadership in health<br>• Strengthen the health system to respond to the needs of adolescent | *253 million adolescents (10–19 years):* Male and female, rural and urban, married and unmarried, in and out of school | • Healthy lifestyle<br>• Violence-free living<br>• Improved nutritional status<br>• Substance misuse and prevention<br>• Reproductive and Sexual health<br>• Mental and emotional well-being |
| Swachh Bharat Abhiyan | October 2, 2014 | | This sanitation and cleanliness initiative has indirect benefits for adolescents by providing a cleaner and healthier environment | • It provides skill training to adolescents and young adults to improve their employability<br>• The Swachh Bharat Mission has three main components:<br>1. *Open defecation free (ODF):* This component aims to make India an ODF country, where no one defecates in the open<br>2. *Sanitation and hygiene:* This component aims to make India a clean country with clean water, clean toilets, and a clean environment<br>3. *Social change:* This component aims to raise awareness about the importance of cleanliness in India |
| National Youth Policy (NYP) | Adopted in 2014 and was revised in 2021 | • NYP is a policy document of the Government of India that outlines the government's vision and priorities for youth development<br>• Although not a program in itself, this policy framework guides the development and implementation of programs and initiatives for the holistic development of the youth | Youth | • These programs and initiatives are designed to address the needs of youth in different areas, such as education, employment, health, leadership development, social justice, and sustainable development<br>• The NYP-2021 is an important policy document that provides a roadmap for youth development in India. The NYP-2021 has the potential to make a significant impact on the lives of millions of young people in India |

*Contd...*

Contd...

| Name of the program | Year of launch | Objectives | Beneficiaries | Benefits |
| --- | --- | --- | --- | --- |
| National Skill Development Mission (Skill India) | 2015 | • Empower youth with market-relevant skills<br>• Create a pool of skilled workforce to support India's economic growth<br>• Reduce the skill gap between the demand and supply of skilled workers<br>• Promote lifelong learning and upskilling<br>• Encourage entrepreneurship and innovation | • School and college dropouts<br>• Unemployed youth<br>• Rural youth<br>• Urban youth<br>• Women<br>• Persons with disabilities<br>• Ex-servicemen | *Benefits for youth:*<br>• Increased employability<br>• Higher wages<br>• Better job satisfaction<br>*Benefits for society:*<br>• Reduced unemployment<br>• Increased economic productivity<br>• Reduced social problems.<br>*Benefits for the economy:*<br>• Increased economic growth<br>• Increased foreign investment<br>• Improved trade competitiveness |
| Beti Bachao, Beti Padhao | 2015 | • Improve the child sex ratio (CSR) across India<br>• Prevent female infanticide and feticide<br>• Promote the education of girls<br>• Empower women and girls<br>• Reduce gender inequality | Any resident Indian girl <10 years old | • *Financial security*: Sukanya Yojana (SSY), a tax-free account providing 8.1% interest rate per annum<br>• Create awareness on issues of girls and women<br>• Improved delivery of welfare services for women<br>• Address declining CSRin critical states and regions<br>• Better education and inclusion of women |
| Saubhagya Scheme | 2017 | The Saubhagya Scheme is a program that provides free sanitary napkins to adolescent girls | Adolescent girls | The program aims to improve menstrual hygiene awareness and practices among adolescent girls |
| Khelo India- National Program for development of sports | 2017–18 | • Promote sports and fitness at the grassroots level<br>• Identify and nurture sporting talent<br>• Create a strong sporting ecosystem in the country<br>• Develop sports infrastructure<br>• Improve the performance of Indian athletes at international competitions | Children and youth | *Benefits for athletes*:<br>• Increased access to training and competition<br>• Financial support<br>• Better coaching and support<br>• *Benefits for the sports ecosystem*: Increased participation in sports<br>• Improved infrastructure<br>• *Increased awareness of sports*:<br>• *Benefits for society*:<br>• Improved health and fitness<br>• Reduced social problems<br>• National pride |

Contd...

*Contd...*

| Name of the program | Year of launch | Objectives | Beneficiaries | Benefits |
|---|---|---|---|---|
| Samagra Shiksha Abhiyan | 2018 | • Ensure that all children have access to quality education<br>• Bridge social and gender gaps in school education<br>• Ensuring equity and inclusion at all levels of school education<br>• Ensuring safe, secure, and conducive learning environment and minimum standards in schooling provisions<br>• Promoting vocationalization of education<br>• Support states in implementation of Right of Children to Free and Compulsory Education (RTE) Act, 2009<br>• State Council of Educational Research and Training (SCERT)/State Institute of Education (SIE) and District Institute of Education and Training (DIET) | 6–14 years | • Access to education for all children<br>• Improvement in the quality of education<br>• Promoting equality<br>• Increased attendance and retention of children in early years<br>• Increased training for teachers<br>• Increased monitoring of the learning process<br>• Increased enrolment in schools<br>• Improved learning outcomes<br>• Reduced gender gap in education |
| *Government of India's programs for specially challenged youth* | | | | |
| National Trust for the Welfare of Persons with Disabilities (NTWPD) | 1999 | Nodal agency under the Ministry of Social Justice and Empowerment that works for the welfare of persons with disabilities | People with disabilities | NTWPD provides a range of services to specially challenged youth, including education, training, employment, and rehabilitation |
| Deendayal Disabled Rehabilitation Scheme (DDRS) | 2003 | DDRS is a flagship program of the Ministry of Social Justice and Empowerment that provides comprehensive rehabilitation services to persons with disabilities | Voluntary organizations | DDRS provides assistance for education, training, employment, rehabilitation of specially challenged youth |
| Pradhan Mantri Jan Dhan Yojana (PMJDY) | 2014 | Financial inclusion program that provides banking services to the poor and marginalized | People below poverty line | PMJDY provides a number of benefits to specially challenged youth, including zero balance accounts, overdraft facilities, and insurance coverage |
| Pradhan Mantri Mudra Yojana (PMMY) | 2015 | PMMY is a microfinance scheme that provides loans to small businesses and entrepreneurs | Noncorporate, nonfarm small and microentrepreneur | PMMY provides loans at low interest rates to specially challenged youth to start their own businesses |
| Skill India Mission | July 15, 2015 | Skill India Mission is a national mission that aims to train 500 million people in various skills by 2022 | Youth of the country | Skill India Mission provides a number of skills training programs to specially challenged youth, including vocational training, apprenticeship programs, and on-the-job training |

**TABLE 4:** India—various state-specific programs.

| Name of state | Name of the program | Year of launch | Objectives | Beneficiaries | Benefits |
|---|---|---|---|---|---|
| Maharashtra | Maharashtra Adolescent Health Programme (MAHP) | 2009 | MAHP is a comprehensive program that aims to improve the health and well-being of adolescents in Maharashtra | Adolescents | • The program provides various services like health screenings<br>• Immunizations<br>• Nutritional supplements<br>• Health education<br>• Counseling and support services<br>• Referral services<br>• The MAHP is implemented by the government of Maharashtra and is funded by the World Bank. The program is expected to benefit over 10 million adolescents in the state<br>• The MAHP is a significant step toward improving the health and well-being of adolescents in Maharashtra<br>• The program is expected to help adolescents stay healthy and reach their full potential |
| Karnataka | Yuva Karnataka Plus (YKP) | April 1, 2013 | YKP is a state-specific program that aims to develop the skills and capacities in Karnataka | 15–35-year-old youth | The program is implemented by the government of Karnataka in collaboration with the Ministry of Youth Affairs and Sports. It provides services like:<br>• Education and skills training<br>• Employment opportunities<br>• Entrepreneurship development<br>• Health and well-being<br>• Social and cultural development |
| Tamil Nadu | Tamil Nadu Adolescent Health Programme (TNAHP) | January 2014 | Aims to improve the health and well-being of adolescents in Tamil Nadu | 10 million adolescents | • TN-AHP is implemented through a network of adolescent health clinics, which are located in primary health centers, district hospitals, and government medical colleges. The clinics provide a range of services, including:<br>  – Health screenings<br>  – Immunizations<br>  – Nutritional counseling<br>  – Reproductive health counseling<br>  – Mental health counseling<br>  – Referral services<br>• TN-AHP also provides training to healthcare workers on adolescent health issues. The program also works with schools and communities to promote adolescent health |
| Kerala | Kerala Adolescents' and Youth Programme (KAYP) | 2016 | State-specific program that aims to improve the health and well-being of adolescents and youth in Kerala | 5 million adolescents | *The program provides the following services:*<br>• Health promotion and education<br>• Clinical services<br>• Counseling and support services<br>• Referral services |
| Odisha | Kishore Kishori Swasthya Yojana (KKSY) | July 2, 2022. | State-specific program that aims to improve the health and well-being of adolescents in Odisha | Young people and adolescents | • The program is targeted at adolescents between the ages of 10 and 19 years. The program provides a range of services, including health screenings, immunizations, nutritional supplements, and health education<br>• The program is funded by the government of Odisha and is implemented by the State Health Department |

**TABLE 5:** Menstrual hygiene programs by various ministries.

| Name of the ministry | Ministry of Women and Child Development (MoWCD) | Ministry of Education (MoE) | Ministry of Jal Shakthi (MoJS) | Ministry of Health and Family Welfare (MoHFW) | Ministry of Tribal Development | Ministry of Panchayati Raj | Ministry of Youth Affairs and Sports (MoYAS) |
|---|---|---|---|---|---|---|---|
| Name of the program | Beti Bachao Beti Padhao | Swachh Vidyalaya component under Samagra Shiksha | Swachh Bharat Mission Gramin | RKSK SHWP | Embedded within schemes | National Rural Livelihood scheme | Embedded within schemes |
| Activities under the program | Anganwadi workers (AWW) and/or super-visors and workers across states are trained to conduct session on Menstrual Hygiene Management (MHM) for out-of-school adolescent girls | State-specific projects on various interventions on menstrual health and hygiene like installation of sanitary pad vending machines and incinerators | Awareness generation on menstrual waste management | Counseling services for adolescent girls on puberty and menstrual hygiene | Training of teaches and staffs in Ashram Schools and Ekalavya schools (schools for tribal students) | Empowering and financially supporting Self Help Groups (SHGs) to set up and produce sanitary napkins | Provision of separate and functional toilets and access to sanitary pads for female sportsmen in institutions supported by MoYAS |
| | Training of out-of-school girls by Anganwadi workers (AWWs) and supervisors | Separate toilet for girls with facility for safe disposal of pads | Disposal of menstrual waste, including incineration | Educational session for adolescent boys and girls by medical team visiting schools | Awareness generation activities with students of Ashram Schools and Ekalavya schools | Marketing and demand generation of sanitary napkins production at village level by SHG-run units | Nehru Yuva Kendras and Bharat Scouts and guides are involved in MHM awareness initiatives |
| | Shelter homes, obser-vation of children in conflict with law: MHM promotional activities and supply and proper disposal mechanisms of sanitary napkins. WASH related facilities supporting MHM | Swachh Vidyalaya Program trains nodal officer on MHM in day schools and residential girls' schools like Kasturba Gandhi Balika Vidyalaya (KGBVs) | Installation of sanitary pad vending machines and incinerators in schools | Anemia control program for adolescent girls | Regular supply of sanitary napkins in Ashram Schools and Ekalavya schools | MHM awareness among women and mothers who attend meetings of SHGs and village organizations under National Rural Livelihood Mission (NRLM) | |
| | Promotion of awareness on MHM among women and mothers/caregivers of adolescent girl | Access to absorbents at the school level and teachings to make absorbents for self-use in schools and KGBVs | Separate toilets for women and girls at home for safely managing menstruation | • Community-level MHM promotional activities<br>• Distribution and supply of sanitary napkins, disposal mechanisms, training of ASHA workers | Disposal mechanisms | Finance Commission of the Gram Panchayat allocates funds for setting up solid waste disposal mechanisms in Gram Panchayats which include component of menstrual waste management | |

Contd...

*Contd...*

| Name of the ministry | Ministry of Women and Child Development (MoWCD) | Ministry of Education (MoE) | Ministry of Jal Shakthi (MoJS) | Ministry of Health and Family Welfare (MoHFW) | Ministry of Tribal Development | Ministry of Panchayati Raj | Ministry of Youth Affairs and Sports (MoYAS) |
|---|---|---|---|---|---|---|---|
| | Adolescent Resource Centre under Anemia Control Program | Sensitizing of the school management committee (SMCs) to take gender-sensitive decisions so as to help girls cope with puberty and menstruation | For out-of-school girls, MHM awareness provided through women Swachhagrahis | | WASH-related facilities supporting MHM | | |
| | Counseling of the adolescent girls on puberty and MHM, on diet, weekly iron and folic acid supplementation | School Health and Wellness Ambassador Initiative-MHM is addressed and adolescents are supported in the safe management of their menstruation | Provision of funding for IEC and training | | | | |

(RKSK: Rashtriya Kishor Swasthya Karyakram; SHWP: School Health and Wellness Program)

**TABLE 6:** National programs benefiting 10–12 years.

| Name of the Program | Year of launch | Objectives | Beneficiaries | Benefits |
|---|---|---|---|---|
| Bharat Scouts and Guides | • *Scouts:* 1909<br>• *Guides:* 1911 | • Develop the character of young people and help them to become responsible citizens<br>• Promote the physical, intellectual, and spiritual development of young people<br>• Encourage young people to be of service to their communities and to the world | Boys and girls aged 6–25 years | • Leadership development<br>• Team building<br>• Outdoor skills<br>• Community service<br>• Friendship |
| National Cadet Corps | 1948 | • Develop character, discipline, leadership, a secular outlook, the spirit of adventure, and ideals of selfless service among young citizens<br>• Create a pool of organized, trained, and motivated youth with leadership qualities in all walks of life, who will serve the nation regardless of which career they choose<br>• Provide a suitable environment to motivate young Indians to join the armed forces | Students of both genders, between the ages of 12 and 26 years | • Patriotism<br>• Leadership development<br>• Team building<br>• Outdoor skills<br>• Community service<br>• Physical fitness<br>• Discipline and self-control<br>• Academic benefits<br>• Career opportunities |
| Pradhan Mantri Poshan Shakti Nirman Scheme | • September 2021<br>• Originally launched in 1955 as Mid Day Meal Program | • For the eligible children in government and government-aided schools. Improve the nutritional status<br>• Encourage regular school attendance. The scheme is also aimed at reducing the prevalence of stunting, underweight, anemia, and low birth weight in children | All children enrolled in government and government-aided schools from preprimary to Class 8. As of March 2023, the scheme covers over 11.8 crore children across India | *Improved nutritional status:*<br>• This includes reducing the risk of stunting, underweight, anemia, and low birth weight<br>• Increased school attendance<br>• Reduced dropout rates |

### ■ KEY MESSAGES

- Knowledge of effective adolescent health programs empowers pediatricians to advocate for improved healthcare for teenagers, ensuring more adolescents receive the necessary support.

- Sharing successful strategies among regions and nations enables us to develop customized health solutions that meet the unique needs of adolescents in various communities.

- Educating teens about health programs empowers them to make informed decisions, promoting their well-being and fostering a sense of empowerment over their health.

- Studying effective teen health programs assists governments in crafting policies and allocating resources where they can have the greatest impact, ultimately benefiting the health of adolescents.

- Collaboration among countries in addressing teen health issues allows for the collective resolution of significant challenges, guaranteeing that every young person has an equal opportunity for a healthy future.

### ■ RECOMMENDED READING


1. Department of School Education and Literacy. Samagra Shiksha. [online] Available from https://dsel.education. gov.in/scheme/samagra-shiksha. [Last accessed March, 2024].
2. Nag K, Patra M. RMNCH+A: A strategic approach to reproductive, maternal, newborn, child and adolescent health in India: a new initiative in health care delivery system. J Compr Health. 2014;2(1):3-10.
3. Park K (Ed). Health Programs in India. In: Park's Textbook of Preventive and Social Medicine, 26th edition. Jabalpur: Banarsidas Bhanot Publishers; 2021. pp. 464-539.
4. Press Information Bureau. Ministry of Women and Child Development. (2023). Menstrual hygiene practices. [online] Available from https://pib.gov.in/PressRelease IframePage.aspx?PRID=1945842 [Last accessed March, 2024].
5. United Nations International Children's Emergency Fund. About U-Report. [online] Available from https://ureport.in/ about. [Last accessed March, 2024].
6. World Health Organization, United Nations International Children's Emergency Fund. WHO-UNICEF Helping Adolescents Thrive Initiative. [online] Available from https:// www.who.int/teams/mental-health-and-substance-use/ promotion-prevention/who-unicef-helping-adolescents-thrive-programme. [Last accessed March, 2024].


## 1.4 | Partnering with Adolescents and Young Adults

*Poonam Bhatia*

### ■ INTRODUCTION

With 1.8 billion adolescents and young adults (AYA), the world now caters largest AYA population in history. Rather than seeing youth as problems to be managed, adults must consider them as caring and capable individuals who have the potential for bringing positive change.

With appropriate rights of participation, AYAs are effective agents for change as they are free from pre-conceived notions and biases that often plague adults. Meaningful engagement of young people gives them the sense of ownership and they happily work for the community. Involving them in global issues such as environment change, illiteracy, poverty, healthcare, human rights, and LGBTQ enhances their abilities, shape their perspectives, attitudes, and thoughts.

### ■ DEFINITION

A Youth-Adult Partnership (YAP) embodies an equal alliance where both young individuals and adults actively engage and hold equal authority. It thrives on mutual listening, joint determination of program objectives, and collaborative decision-making. This framework empowers young people to directly tackle their challenges, engage with their realities, and cocreate lasting solutions alongside adults. Through such programs teens and youth who have ideas and energy to find innovative solutions to complex problems play key role in community building.

**What is the need?**

In 2003, the United Nations (UN) recognized the participation of AYA in their personal and community development as a fundamental right of youth [United Nations Children's Fund (UNICEF), 2003]. Empowering AYA breaks the cycle of poverty and helps in reducing incidence of gender-based violence, teen pregnancy, sexually transmitted diseases, etc. Engaging AYA in social reforms is a major protective factor against mental health disorders, many of which begin during adolescence.

On the other hand, absence of such opportunities draws them into antisocial engagements such as violence, substance abuse, engaging in unprotected sex, which negatively impacts not only their health but, the well-being of community as a whole.

Historically, young people like Raja Ram Mohan Rai, Ahilya Bai Holkar, and Swami Vivekanand have used their passion, energy, enthusiasm, to bring social change stopping Sati Pratha, prohibiting untouchability, made reformatory laws for widows etc. Internationally, global icons like Malala Yousafzai and Greta Thunberg are well recognized for their work on education and climate change, respectively.

Numerous studies provide evidences that show active involvement of AYA in decision-making and equipping them with essential opportunities and supports, such as challenges, relevance, voice, cause-based action, skill development, adult guidance, and affirmation, which lead to the achieving mastery, becoming compassionate, and improving overall health.

Policies concerning adolescents and young adults should harness their considerable potential. Research indicates that engaging youth in community discussions increases the likelihood of them assuming influential roles in the future. The way they evolve and mature will carry implications that will resonate through generations.

## COMPONENTS OF EFFECTIVE PARTNERSHIP

Effective Youth–Adult partnerships encompass several key components:

- *Equitable participation:* Both youth and adults engage on equal footing, sharing responsibilities and decision-making power.
- *Mutual respect and trust:* Creating an environment where opinions and contributions from both parties are valued and trusted.
- *Open communication:* Encouraging transparent dialogue where everyone feels comfortable expressing their thoughts and ideas.

- *Shared goals and objectives:* Collaboratively defining aims and objectives for programs or activities, ensuring alignment with the needs and perspectives of both youth and adults.
- *Capacity building:* Providing resources, training, and opportunities for skill development for both young individuals and adults involved in the partnership.
- *Sustainability and commitment:* Fostering long-term relationships and sustained commitment to the partnership's goals and outcomes.
- *Flexibility and adaptability:* Being open to evolving needs and circumstances, adjusting strategies as required for effective collaboration.
- *Supportive environment:* Creating a safe and supportive space that encourages creativity, innovation, and inclusivity for all participants.
- *Evaluation and feedback:* Regularly assessing progress, seeking feedback, and making necessary adjustments to enhance the partnership's effectiveness.
- *Empowerment and recognition:* Empowering youth and adults alike by recognizing their contributions and providing opportunities for leadership and recognition within the partnership.

True partnership is one in which each party has the opportunity to make suggestions and decisions. The contribution of each is recognized and valued. It ultimately promotes social inclusion, peace, and social harmony.

## BARRIERS IN PARTNERING

In past 30 years, there has been significant advancement in adolescent and young adult participation but challenges still persist, like lack of involvement in decision-making or bare representation or tokenism of AYA in important matters related to them.

Hierarchy in decision-making, i.e., elders or adults are put over AYA, creates uneven power dynamics. The true sharing means adults rising above their traditional roles, listening rather than telling, and working with, rather than for youth. To be effective partners, adults must have confidence and respect for young people.

The perception among youth that their voices are not heard or respected poses a significant hurdle in developing partnership. Additionally, lack of resources for training and capacity building, both for adults and adolescents, presents another obstacle in effective collaboration.

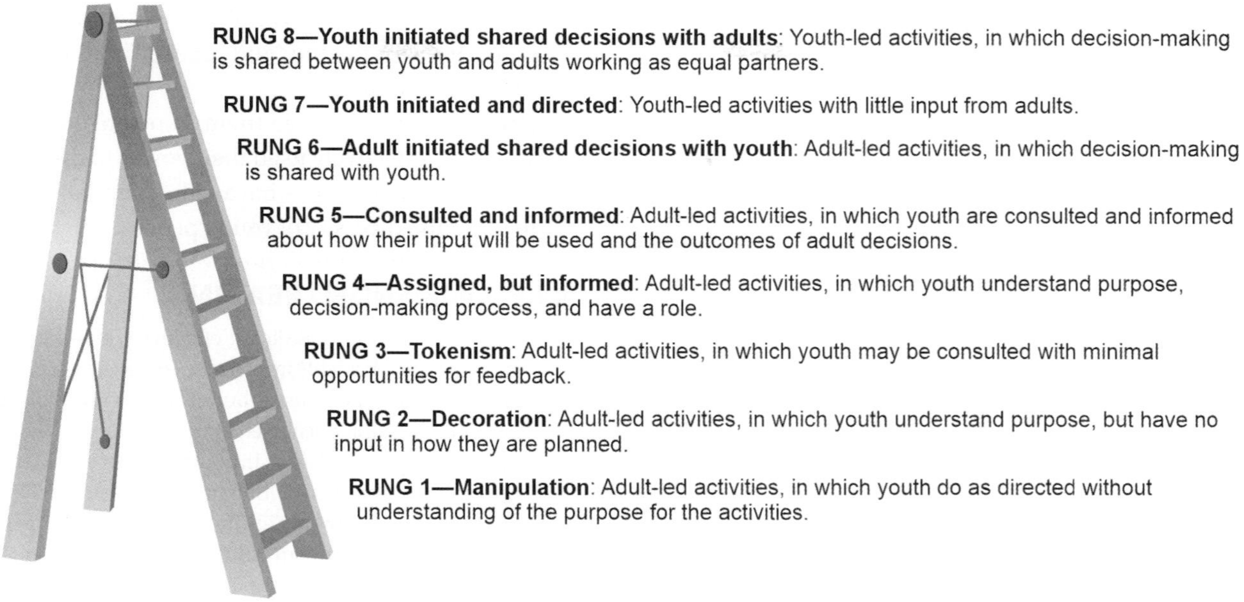

**Fig. 1:** Hart's ladder of participation.
*Source:* Adapted from Hart, R. (1992). Children's Participation from Tokenism to Citizenship. Florence: UNICEF Innocenti Research Centre, as cited in www.freechild.org/ladder.htm

## ■ WAYS TO IMPROVE AYA'S PARTICIPATION

When engaged, adolescents demonstrate internal motivation, self-efficacy, and a desire for mastery. Hence, the goal should be to promote environment that acknowledges adolescents as valuable resource. Efforts directed to provide choices and responsive environments with connections to "real life" experiences help in building confidence and engaging them. Introducing measures to explore their emerging identities, beliefs, sexualities, and opportunities will help them thrive well.

Hart's ladder of participation **(Fig. 1)** is an excellent model that can be very well adopted. In the year 1992, the International Child Development Centre of the UNICEF, first published Children's Participation: From Tokenism to Citizenship, Roger Hart's Ladder of Children's Participation applied the conceptual framework of Sherry Arnstein's Ladder of Citizen Participation to the participation of children in adult projects, programs, and activities, including forms of work, advocacy, and citizenship. In this model, youth participation can be between no participation to full participation. Hart's ladder ascends sequentially: the bottom three rungs are for youth involvement that is not true participation, while the top five rungs involve AYA genuinely.

When organizations use Hart's ladder model, they automatically get rid of nonparticipation practices and start working on ways, where they can engage youth genuinely in higher level of participation.

*Some of the ways are:*

- Empowerment starts from home, which gives them the freedom to express and choose like what to eat, what to wear negotiate on few choices such as spending time on digital media and going out with peers. Many a time, their choices might not be appropriate but learning to live with the consequences of choices will make them resilient.
- Involving them with various projects such as taking care of environment and empathizing with the weaker sections of society
- Capacity building or building skills for livelihood/ education should be the focus and should be economically viable.
- Listening and implementing on their ideas teaches self-advocacy to them.
- Community-based youth forums allow youth to discuss and find solutions of local issues.

When AYAs are actively involved (in rung 6–7 of Hart's ladder), they feel that they belong, are valued, and their contribution matters. Infact, UN (2007) also emphasizes on recognizing young people's knowledge, perspectives, and experience as valuable contributions to decision-making at all levels and calls for action by adults to support them.

## CONCLUSION

Recognizing AYAs as legitimate, crucial component of society is a win–win situation for community. To ensure their active participation and well-being, providers must establish trust, adapt communication methods, and provide age-appropriate care. Through meaningful engagement and dialogue, they can develop stronger problem-solving skills, which will ultimately prepare them to become responsible adults. Adults too get acquainted with the needs and concerns of youth, also they get fresh ideas from different perspectives thereby addressing real needs. The byproduct of this partnership is development of programs and services which will address real concerns of AYAs.

Partnering with adolescents and young adults in Healthcare is crucial to addressing their unique needs and improving health outcomes. By overcoming the challenges and employing effective collaboration strategies, healthcare professionals can play a significant role in supporting the health and well-being of adolescents and young adults as they transition into adulthood.

The bottom line for effective partnership is: Empower, Enable, and Elevate young voices.

## KEY MESSAGES

- *Active listening:* Encourage adults to actively listen non-judgmentally and not being dismissive. Such behavior fosters a sense of being heard and valued.
- *Validation:* Creating an environment where they can validate their experiences and emotions. This way AYAs feel their perspective is acknowledged and respected.
- *Encourage critical thinking:* By asking open-ended questions, brainstorming sessions, and encouraging decision-making.
- *Building trust:* Taking out time to understand one another and sharing personal stories help to build trust.

- *Constructive feedback:* Provide feedback that is constructive, specific, and focused on improvement rather than criticism.
- *Role models:* Introduce them to positive role models who have effectively used their voices to drive change.
- *Be inclusive:* Strategies have to be planned by keeping in mind the diversity of young people.

## RECOMMENDED READING


1. Advocates for Youth. Building effective youth-adult partnerships. [online] Available from https://www.advocatesforyouth.org/resources/fact-sheets/building-effective-youth-adult-partnerships/. [Last accessed March, 2024].
2. Family Planning High Impact Practices. Meaningful Adolescent and Youth Engagement. [online] Available from https://www.fphighimpactpractices.org/guides/meaningful-adolescent-and-youth-engagement/. [Last accessed March, 2024].
3. International Institute for Population Sciences (IIPS). Report: Youth in India: An NFHS-based Study 2021. [online] Available from https://www.iipsindia.ac.in/sites/default/files/Report_Youth_in_India_An_NFHS_based_Study_2021.pdf. /#. [Last accessed March, 2024].
4. Lansdown G. (2001). Promoting children's participation in democratic decision-making. UNICEF Innocenti Research Centre. [online] Available from https://www.unicef-irc.org/publications/pdf/childrens_participation.pdf. [Last accessed March, 2024].
5. National Academies of Sciences, Engineering, and Medicine. (2019). The promise of adolescence: Realizing opportunity for all youth. [online] Available from https://www.ncbi.nlm.nih.gov/books/NBK545472/#. [Last accessed March, 2024].
6. UNFPA India. Ministry of Youth Affairs and Sports, YuWaah, and UN Agencies Join Hands for Empowering Young People. [online] Available from https://india.unfpa.org/en/news/ministry-youth-affairs-and-sports-yuwaah-and-un-agencies-join-hands-empowering-young-people. [Last accessed March, 2024].
7. United Nations. Policy Guide: Youth in the Global Development Agenda. [online] Available from https://social.un.org/youthyear/docs/policy%20guide.pdf. [Last accessed March, 2024].
8. YouthDoIT. YAPs Toolkit [Internet]. [online] Available from: https://www.youthdoit.org/assets/YAPs-toolkit.pdf. [Last accessed March, 2024].

# 1.5 Peer Education Program

*Ajit Singh Chawla*

## ■ INTRODUCTION

India hosts the largest number of adolescents in the history of this planet and the number is still rising. Unfortunately, the gatekeepers (parents, teachers, doctors, and policy makers) lack the awareness about the importance of health of adolescents which is largely neglected.

The important factors responsible for this issue include the following:

- The changing family structure and social norms
- Urge for instant gratifications
- Media impact
- Disproportionate expectations
- Tremendous competitions
- Materialistic attitudes
- Diminishing resilience.

These factors have further widened the gap between parents and teenagers who are now seeking pleasure and solace outside families in the form of substance abuse, suicidal ideation, sexual experimentations, and social media addiction.

A peer is a person who has equal standing with another as in age, background, social status, and interests. Peers play a critical role in the psychosocial development of most adolescents. They, in fact, provide opportunities for personal relationships, social behaviors, and a sense of belonging. Therefore, peer education is considered as a health promotion strategy in adolescents. Peer educator program is of the teens, for the teens, and by the teens. This program will cause a behavior change in peer group with the help of peer educator.

## ■ PEER EDUCATOR

A peer educator is a member of a peer group that receives special training and information and tries to sustain positive behavior change among the group members. Peer educators should receive adequate training enabling them to understand the purpose of the program

- Be good listeners; provide encouragement, motivation; and support healthy decisions and behaviors. They should also know other sources of information and counseling so as to refer other peers to appropriate help.
- Peer educator should have leadership skills, sufficient confidence, technical competency, compassion, and communication skills and who are accepted by other peers are crucial aspects of program success.
- Respect others' feelings and opinions. Be polite.
- *Be nonjudgmental:* Do not impose your opinion of right and wrong on others. Maintain confidentiality; avoid sharing with others or making fun of any individual's opinion that was shared in the context of the session.
- Be on time. Do not use mobile phones; in case of an emergency, keep ringer on silent mode.
- Peer educators should allow that emotions, feelings, attitudes, and beliefs to be expressed and discussed openly.
- Build rapport with the group members.

### Prerequisites of Peer Educator Program

- Careful planning
- Identification and training of peer educator
- Follow-up evaluation.

### Aims of Peer Educator Program

- Creating awareness of adolescent problems
- Enhancing knowledge
- Offering choices
- Stimulating some introspection in the adolescents to take responsible decision in future life
- This 1/2 days' exhibition (youth festival) may be aimed at creating awareness, enhancing knowledge, offering choices, and stimulating some introspection in adolescents and caretakers to take responsible decisions and actions in future life. Understanding the preferences of teenagers to learn from other teenagers, we can conduct this program as a complement to "Mission School Uday," in which a group of 50 trained adolescents (peer educators) will impart scientific information to the visiting teenagers and caretakers in every city/town.

## Steps for Conducting Peer Education Program

- The peer educators with two male and two female teachers who have good communication skills and who are popular in the school/college and park will be selected by well-reputed schools in the city.
- Around 25 girls and 25 boys selected from 9th to 11th grades will undergo 3-hour intense training by their own certified Peer Educator Trainers (Pediatricians, Doctors, and trained adolescent health professionals).
- The reading material and homework will be issued to the peer educators after the training program.
- After 2–3 days, these 50 peer educators will be gathered again with their teachers to see the posters at each workstation through slide show along with a rapid revision session.
- An exit test will be conducted and instructions for the actual program will be given.
- Each batch of around 150 high school and college students along with 4 male and female teachers will visit the exhibition area covering various work stations on adolescent issues (Total 600 students and 200 PTA members) followed by a panel discussion by the experts on each days.
- The schools and college students may depict various issues through role plays and skits.
- A simultaneous posters and slogans competition (pertaining to adolescent health) will also be arranged and prize winning entries sent by various school students will be awarded.
- Adequate media coverage and involving maximum number of educational institutes will ensure the expected response. Schools can arrange this program during annual gathering.
- These peer educators will act as the foremost physical, mental and social "health buddies" during their remaining tenure with early referral to school counselor and local peer educator trainers. A cross-sectional as well as longitudinal data can be collected from various cities/towns to assess the long-term impact of this useful activity. World over "Peer educators" are considered as the front-line physical, mental and social health workers for teenagers.
- The work stations will hold attractive posters and visual aids (if possible) to depict these.
- Four adolescent care pediatricians will supervise the program and assist the peer educators who will be imparting knowledge to visiting students and answering their queries.

- The experts in the field of media, nutrition, mental health, education, sociology, law, medicine, etc., will give scientific information through various panel discussions and question–answer sessions.
- Our own experts will be the moderators.
- Parents and teachers may visit the work stations after the students have been sent for panel discussions and question answer sessions.
- Other pediatricians, parents, teachers, and media personnel can also attend the panel discussions but they will be sitting on back rows. Adequate social distancing and cleanliness will be ensured.

## Further Requirements of this Program

### Stalls

- Nutrition (with special emphasis on "JUNCS"), personal hygiene, immunization and physical fitness.
- Mental health issues
- Life skills education
- Road safety and traffic manners
- Substance abuse
- Social media education and cyber ethics
- Study skills.

### Preludes

- Skits
- Mini films/documentaries/shadow plays
- Role plays
- Power point presentations.

### Needs

- Selection of enthusiastic "Trainers of Peer educators" from various cities
- Joint effort of local branches of Indian Academy of Pediatrics (IAP) and Adolescent Health Academy (AHA) with supervision and guidance from the National team
- Final list of schools/colleges with conformations and willingness to collaborate actively
- Number of students and teachers
- Any school, which has Poster exhibition area with conference hall in the same premises
- Arrangements for transportation of visiting school/college students and teachers
- Assurance from our trainers of peer educators to supervise and sustain the activity further.

### Equipment Needed at the Venue

- Banners and posters

- Question boxes
- Microphones of various types and Green room for invitees
- Traffic controls by volunteers and school teachers
- Water-proof area for stalls with Tea/Coffee stalls and central dividing curtain for posters and slogans
- Stage arrangements for inaugural function and healthy snacks for peer educators.

## USEFULNESS OF PEER EDUCATION

It enhances the student's level of creativity in expressing ideas as well as in grabbing new concepts, as the student may not feel hesitant to clear his queries. This will also uplift his knowledge limit and thus, allow a greater level of his understanding. Feeling at ease with a peer tutor, allows a student to concentrate better on the tasks of the lesson, which may transfer into higher achievements in the future. To an extent, the student will start questioning his own doubts, and will later find a way to resolve it himself, which will enable the student to improve his critical thinking. Peer teaching involves direct interaction between the learner student and the teacher–student; this will help them to promote the active learning along with interpersonal skills, with which they can actually bid adieu to the so-called boring lectures and classes. It will ease the teacher's burden of responsibility because she is sharing her duties with her kids, which are beneficial to them. But on the other side, it will increase the teacher's role in monitoring and administering the students.

## CHALLENGES DURING ITS CONDUCTION

### Amateur/Aspirant Student

In spite of the fact that the teacher shares her tips and guidelines with the students, it will not build an expert teacher (student). There are also chances of a communication gap within the student and the teacher, which may often lead to the failure of assigned activities.

### Reluctance of Students

Toughest responsibility that lies upon the shoulders of a teacher is the reluctance of students to initiate the assigned duty. Just like the two sides of a coin, there may be students who are actually willing to teach and on the other side, there may be students who are hesitant to work out of their comfort zone. Hence, this becomes a challenge.

## Annoyed Parents

When the parents come to know about peer teaching, there may be chances for them to misinterpret the concept of peer teaching. Parents may take it in a derogate manner that their kid is being taught by some other kid of the same age and that the teacher is sitting idle. So, there may be complaints from the side of the parents until and unless they are completely given the justification behind the concept of peer teaching.

## KEY MESSAGES

- The gatekeepers (parents, teachers, doctors, and policy makers) lack the awareness about the importance of health of adolescents.
- Peer educator program is of the teens, for the teens, and by the teens. This program will result in behavior change in peer group with the help of peer educators.
- There is involvement of pediatrician, teachers, and parents along with teens.
- It includes stalls (Nutrition) (with special emphasis on "JUNCS") and personal hygiene.
- This program also includes skits, mini-films/documentaries/shadow plays, role plays, and power point presentations.

## RECOMMENDED READING


1. Abdi F, Simbar M. The peer education approach in adolescents. Narrative Review Article. Iranian J Public Health. 2013;42:1200-6.
2. Al-Iryani B, Basaleem H, Al-Sakkaf K, Kok G, van den Borne B. Process evaluation of school-based peer education for HIV prevention among Yemeni adolescents. SAHARA J. 2013;10(1):55–64.
3. Alavi Manizheh PK, Khosravi A. Puberty health: knowledge, attitude and practice of the adolescent girls in Tehran, Iran. Payesh. 2009;8(1(29):59–65.
4. Golchin NA, Hamzehgardeshi Z, Fakhri M, Hamzehgardeshi L (2012). The experience of puberty in Iranian adolescent girls: a qualitative content analysis. BMC Public Health, 12:698.
5. Main DS. Commentary: understanding the effects of peer education as a health promotion strategy. Health Educ Behav. 2002;29(4):424-6.
6. Rashtriya Kishor Swasthya Karyakram and Peer Educ, NHM, GOI.
7. Rodgers J. Guidance on delivering effective group education. Brit J Community Nurs. 2006;11:476-82.
8. Salimi H, Mirzamani M, Reisi F, Niknam M. A Survey Study on Behavioral Problems in Adolescence. Journal of Behavioral Sciences. 2007;1(2):163–70.
9. WHO Adolescent peer education in formal and non formal setting. 2005. pp. 1-37.

<table>
<tr><td>**1.6**</td><td><h1>Future of Adolescent and Youth Well-being in India</h1></td></tr>
</table>

*RG Patil*

## ■ ADOLESCENT

Adolescent is the stage where young individuals transition from childhood to adulthood. It is a critical phase of life marked by physical, psychological, and social changes. There are 1.2 billion adolescents (10–19 years) in the world, and half of the world population is under 25 years of age. India has the largest adolescent population in the world, who hold the key to the country's future. They are the resource person of the country. About 22% of the Indian population is adolescent. Adolescents are the future of the nation forming demographic and economic force.

There are three stages of adolescents—10 to 13 years—early adolescent, 14 to 16 years—middle adolescent, 17 to 21 years—late adolescent. Despite progress many Indian adolescent still lack access to quality education especially in rural areas, the quality of schools remains a significant concerns, where there are no transport facilities, poor qualities of road or no roads and most adolescent attain schools in a long way, early dropout of girls due to economic conditions or gender disparity and early marriages and household works. Now most young people are receiving formal education and lot of skills, this can be filled by job market demands, so the youth employment gap can be fulfilled.

Mental illness is a major issue. The quality of life of adolescents can be affected by depression, psychosis, and anxiety disorder, which have an impact on their development, hence exposing them to various risk-taking behavior, such as rash driving, substance abuse, violence, media addiction, teenage pregnancy, dropout from school, and delinquent behavior. Thus, early detection, anticipatory guidance, awareness, parental support, and proper treatment are the need of hour.

Major challenges are the stigma associated with mental health problem in India. Many adolescent fears seeking health from the professional due to societal taboos, breaking down the stigma and attending health professional at early stage will be helpful. Major risks of depression are suicidal thoughts and suicidal attempts, so prevention of suicide is important by awareness and education through schools, colleges, parents and teachers, and community. Developing brain during adolescence is more vulnerable to neuroplastic changes; repeated exposure to toxic influences can cause changes in brain which are likely to be more intensive and long-lasting. Half of the globally young adolescents who start smoking continue to smoke to adulthood and half of the adolescent smokers are expected to die prematurely due to smoking-related diseases. 5% of death in young people aged 15–29 years is attributable to alcohol use [national survey by Ministry of Social Justice and Empowerment (MOSJE) as per Global youth Tobacco Survey 4 (GYTS-4)]; 0.3% females and 1.9% males aged 15–29 years in India use tobacco [National Family Health Survey 5 (NHFS-5), 2019–21]. Pediatricians have an important role in identifying the risk and should collaboration with a mental health professional.

AHA-IAP Action plan—Ensure inter departmental collaboration like health, education, social welfare encourage intergenerational dialogue reduce social stigma around adolescent sexuality, scale up. Current programs like AEP, RKSK, SHWP training of teachers. Create resource and teaching materials link adolescent health services like AFHS, SRH, RKSK and monitor to know the progress. Concern related to digital safety, adolescent may be victims of perpetrators of cyber bulling, cyber stalking, trolling, doxing, hacking, phishing, creation of fake accounts sexting. Financials frauds, blackmailing knowledge regarding cyber safety and media literacy should be imparted to adolescent so that they are not involved or entangled in such situations. Most of adolescent they are addicted to digital media affecting physical and mental health awareness regarding harmful effects of digital addictions and provide appropriate guidance treatment and referral when needed.

The risk of substance misuse during adolescence can be reduced by 5%, if the first use is delayed to 25 years.

Hence, early detection is very important by screening, brief intervention, referral treatment, awareness from the family, and promoting awareness regarding substance abuse in school, colleges, and societies. Adolescents have a high risk of unhealthy eating habits and lack of physical activities, leading to obesity as well as comorbidities such as type-2 diabetes, obstructive sleep apnea, dyslipidemia, slipped capital femoral epiphysis, Blount disease, and nonalcoholic steatohepatitis (NASH). Obesity in pregnancy causes increased morbidity and mortality to mother and infant, and most of the adolescents in India are addicted to digital media thus causing health problems. It is important to empower an adolescent girl regarding education and health awareness so that she can stand on her own feet.

Environment-related illness can be nonspecific. It is important to consider environmental etiologies in differential diagnosis. Management should focus on educating parents, adolescents, and community to remove the source of exposure from their environment. Awareness regarding how to avoid environmental hazards should be incorporated in collaboration with nongovernmental organizations (NGOs), schools, colleges, and corporate bodies.

## ADOLESCENT IMMUNIZATION

Most of the parents are aware of childhood vaccination which are administered during a well baby visit in India. However, we still do not have the concept of well adolescent clinics. Adequate immunization is most important protective health services, there is a reason to immunity that is waning, catchup vaccination, for missed vaccination in childhood.

## NONGOVERNMENTAL ORGANIZATION AND PRIVATE SECTOR INVOLVEMENT

Role of NGOs like Indian Academy of Pediatrics—Adolescent Friendly Health Services (AFSI) and Adolescent Friendly School Initiative (AFHS), and Mission Kishor Uday are helpful for the adolescent health.

## NATIONAL HEALTH MISSION

It focuses on improving health care services of adolescents and ensuring the well-being of mothers and children. It indirectly impacts the health of the adolescent. A private company plays a vital role in the growth and overall development of the adolescent through corporate social responsibility programs. These companies support various educational and skill development projects. They also encourage youth entrepreneurship supporting starting business, youth-led movements, and activism.

The importance of gender equality in youth development is essential. Gender biases, early marriages, and unequal opportunities for education must be addressed. Adolescence can be benefited from the policies and programs that discourage child marriages and emphasize on promotion of female education. Overcoming caste-based discrimination and social disparity is equally important. Special attention should be given to empowering youth from marginalized communities.

## CONCLUSION

Adolescents constitute 22% population. They are the resource and demographic force. Their physical and mental health problems need awareness and proper management.

Lifestyle diseases, digital addiction, substance abuse are showing an upward trend. Early recognization awareness and management is need of hour.

Preventive measures for early marriages, safe pregnancy and delivery nutritional education to rural girls and boys. Menstrual hygiene education should be imparted. Save the girl child and her education should be included as part of the school curriculum.

## KEY MESSAGES

- The well-being of the adolescent and youth in India is crucial for the nation's progress. Adolescents are the demographic force and resource persons of the country.
- Mental health issues and lifestyle diseases are showing an upward trend. Proper awareness and anticipatory guidance are necessary.
- Suicides among adolescents is a multifactorial problem and needs a multidimensional approach.
- Girls' education and their health are important. Early marriages should be avoided.
- Risk-taking behavior and substance abuse are to be addressed through NGOs and corporate sectors and life skill education programs should be encouraged.
- Gender disparity and social stigma should be avoided.
- Family life education should be part of school curriculum.

- Focus regarding education and health should be on the urban adolescent as well as on the rural adolescent.
- Media literacy is the need of hour regarding avoiding of digital addiction, mental health issue, and lifestyle diseases.
- Job-oriented education should be encouraged for youth employment.

## ■ RECOMMENDED READING

1. Adolescent Health Division, Ministry of Health and Family Welfare, Government of India. (2014). Strategy Handbook. Rashtriya Kishor Swasthya Karyakram. [online] Available from https://nhm.gov.in/images/pdf/programmes/rksk-strategy-handbook.pdf [Last accessed May, 2024].

2. Adolescent Health Division, Ministry of Health and Family Welfare, Government of India. (2014). Strategy Handbook. Rashtriya Kishor Swasthya Karyakram. [online] Available from https://www.nhm.gov.in/images/pdf/programmes/RKSK/Medical_Officer_Training_Manual/Resource_Book_Medical_Officer.pdf. [Last accessed May, 2024].

3. Bhave SY, Menon PSN, Parthasarathy A, Greydanus DE (Eds). Bhave's Textbook of Adolescent Medicine, 2nd edition. New Delhi: Peepee Publishers and Distributors (P) Ltd; 2016.

4. Ministry of Health and Family Welfare, Government of India. National Family Health Survey (NFHS-5) 2019-21. [online] Available from https://main.mohfw.gov.in/sites/default/files/NFHS-5_Phase-II_0.pdf [Last accessed May, 2024].

# Basic Prerequisites for Practicing Pediatricians

**Section Editor:** Prashant Kariya

## 2.1 Adolescent-friendly Health Clinics and Services

Swati Ghate, Kamlesh Parekh

### ◼ INTRODUCTION

Adolescents, who constitute around 18% of our population, harbor many a physical and mental health problems that significantly affect their growth and maturation, productivity, and consequently their future. Yet, this phase of life is often considered as a golden period of rapid growth, good physical health, and well-being. The common and treatable problems like anemia, malnutrition, mental health issues, reproductive health disorders, etc., get generally overlooked only to get worsen with time. The resultant reduction in the quality and expectancy of life is detrimental not only to the adolescents and their current and future families but also to the community and the nation. Hence, investing in "adolescent-friendly health services (AFHS)" wisely and mindfully is very essential. AFHS comprise developmentally appropriate comprehensive health services for health promotion, disease prevention, and treatment of adolescents. They constitute a range of preventive, promotive, and curative services, especially designed for the adolescents and are provided as under one roof by private, governmental, and nongovernmental organizations (NGOs).

Poor health-seeking behavior and their shunning away from healthcare facilities are big obstacles in reaching to adolescents. These stem from many reasons as follows:

- Adolescents, in their journey of cognitive evolution, pass through a phase of feeling "invincible". This means that an adolescent believes that nothing can go wrong with him and he is foolproof. Since the prefrontal cortex is yet to develop, adolescents cannot think of the long-term consequences and miss out on behaving thoughtfully. Hence, they are relatively carefree about their health.
- As the immune system is relatively much mature by this age, there are negligible acute or severe infectious problems as compared to childhood. There are hardly any occasions to visit the healthcare providers. Going to a doctor appears kiddish to them.
- The everchanging bodies and minds make them confused regarding their own perceptions of their concerns. Many times, they do not realize their problem or if they do, they cannot judge its severity.
- Adolescents are secretive, and privacy is very crucial for them. They simply may not like to share their problems with anyone.
- Sometimes, they may fall short of words to exactly describe their issues. How to communicate with the doctor may be a big question for them.
- They are generally skeptical about the doctors' capacity to understand and deal with their concerns. They think of pediatricians as doctors who treat babies and physicians who look after elderlies. They may not know whom to approach.
- Easy availability of information makes them turn to the internet or else they prefer to seek advice from

their friends. Both these sources are more likely to offer unscientific or hazardous guidance.

- Many times, financial constraints stop them from visiting a doctor, as the adolescents may not wish to share their problems with their parents who bear their expenses.

Thus, it becomes imperative on the part of the healthcare system that it makes its delivery to adolescents available in an attractive and appropriate adolescent-friendly style. In addition, such services should be easily accessible, approachable, affordable, appropriate, and effective to show their results.

## COMPONENTS OF ADOLESCENT-FRIENDLY HEALTH SERVICES

Adolescent-friendly health services constitute four domains:
1. Physical infrastructure
2. Trained manpower
3. Services rendered and referral network
4. Advocacy of the services among the beneficiaries

### Physical Infrastructure

- *Location:* AFHS services could be a part of a government or private healthcare facility. In India, it is increasingly made available in all the government hospitals till the primary health care (PHC) subcenter levels through *Rashtriya Swasthya Kishor Karyakram* (RSKS) and Ayushman Bharat Schemes. At the district level, a holistic adolescent health center is run by a multidisciplinary team of experts. Adolescent health clinics are a part of most of the pediatrics departments in medical colleges. In private setups, adolescent health clinic is either an integral part of a multispecialty hospital, a child development center (CDC), or run independently by pediatricians trained in the field. Adolescent clinics are better run on a particular day/time slot especially kept aside for this population, since they do not like to go to a place surrounded by kids.

An adolescent health clinic should be placed ideally in such a center that is easy to approach and does not hold a tag of taboo topics like a mental or sexual health clinic. It should be a part of the general healthcare provider facility for typically growing children and adolescents so as to minimize the adolescents' apprehension of walking into it.

- *Ambience:* Adolescents relate themselves to adults. They hate being seen as children. Hence, the ambience should be more like that of an adult office. It should not be very colorful and should be devoid of animals/cartoons and other child-friendly caricatures and toys. The furniture should be adult sized. The waiting area could be used to display services offered. Posters and handouts on various issues of adolescent concern can be used to disseminate scientific information.

The examination/counseling room should provide adequate privacy. It is a good idea to conduct history-taking and counseling sessions in a room that is soundproof yet maintains visibility. Physical examination should always be done with a chaperone around.

- *Tools:* An adult-sized couch, adult stethoscope, stadiometer, weighing machine, blood pressure (BP) apparatus with cuffs of all sizes, orchidometer, and Snellen chart are some of the basic tools needed for a routine physical examination. Adolescent immunization charts, growth charts for height, weight and body mass index (BMI), blood pressure and waist circumference centile charts, and sexual maturity rating (SMR) charts for both sexes should be available and put to use for every adolescent that visits the clinic.

Some validated and easy-to-administer psychological questionnaires come in handy in screening and diagnosing adolescents with mental and academic concerns. Some of them are: Perceived Stress Scale, Teen Screen Questionnaire-Mental Health (TSQ-M), Patient Health Questionnaire (PHQ 2, PHQ 9), Screen for Child Anxiety Related Disorders (SCARED), Beck's Depression Inventory, CRAFT questionnaire (for substance abuse), Young Internet Addiction Scale, Screening to Behavior Intervention (S2BI), Ask Suicide-Screening Questionnaire (ASQ), Vanderbilt ADHD Scale, Tamil Nadu Learning Disability (LD) scale, Grade Level Assessment Device (GLAD) (for Learning Disability), Vineland Social Maturity Scale (VSMS), for adaptive functional maturity, etc.

### Trained Manpower

Healthcare professionals (HCPs) looking after adolescents should be well versed with their medical problems and should possess the balanced attitude and approach required for dealing with adolescents. They should get trained in basic communication and counseling skills to address common adolescent psychosocial problems. They should be aware of important laws related to adolescents. They should know how to partner with parents, peers, and teachers and develop a multidisciplinary network of adolescent-friendly experts in other related specialties like gynecology, orthopedics, etc.

Continued training of healthcare providers on unique and common physical and psychosocial health concerns of adolescents, their early detection, and management is very crucial for the success of AFHS. These concerns fall into the following six main categories which are:

1. Nutrition
2. Noncommunicable diseases
3. Mental health
4. Reproductive and sexual health problems
5. Substance abuse
6. Injuries and violence (including gender-based violence)

### *Dealing with an Adolescent*

The approach with which the healthcare providers should deal with adolescents is very different from that of children or adults. Training in this peculiar skill should mandatorily be acquired by all the concerned HCPs, so that adolescents find it easy to connect with and remain in touch with the healthcare system, which is very important for a good outcome. Not only the doctors but also the paramedic staff like nurses, receptionists, psychologists, therapists, etc., all need to be competent in handling the adolescents in an adolescent-friendly and sensitive manner. All adolescents, 10 years and above, should be talked with in privacy for some time in every visit by the treating doctor, to develop a connection with them and to emphasize their need for privacy to their parents.

Adolescents want to be treated as adults and seek direct communication. They hate baby talks. Unlike children where parents are the main communicators, adolescents appreciate if the HCP directly talks with them.

They seek privacy and confidentiality. There is always a fear of disclosure and embarrassment. Hence, the HCP should always declare the privacy policy of the clinic. The adolescent should be ensured that none of his information will be shared with anyone without his consent, the exceptions being harm to his own or anyone else's life, conflict with law, sexual abuse, and requirement of hospitalization.

### *Consent and Assent*

- As per Indian laws, a child is anyone who is under the age of 18 years.
- Anyone who is more than 12 years of age can give consent for history taking and physical examination. An adolescent should always be asked beforehand if he is willing to share his information and ready for a physical checkup. He should never be taken for granted even if the parents have consented.
- In case of individuals between 12 and 18 years of age, a parent's/legal guardian's consent is required for investigations/treatment. Any invasive procedure including taking samples or administering medicines should be undertaken only with the parent's willingness.
- Anyone >18 years of age can enter into a contract and independently decide regarding his treatment plan. Many times, adolescents are financially dependent on their parents, and thus parents become the primary decision-makers.
- For most of the treatment plans, only verbal consent is enough.
- Written consent is mandatory for undergoing a medicolegal examination, any surgical procedures, or medical termination of pregnancy (MTP).
- Consent is not needed for any kind of medical emergencies.
- Assent is the willingness of the adolescent to follow the treatment plan. It is advisable that the HCP involves the adolescent in decision-making so that he complies and gets the desired results.

## Services Rendered by Adolescent-friendly Health Services

Some of the services that are beneficial and required for adolescents are as follows:

- "Annual wellness visits" starting from 10 years of age, wherein the following activities are taken up:
  - Eliciting any concerns and clarifications
  - Screening for psychosocial stressors, high-risk behavior, mental disorders, and immunization status
  - *Physical and systemic examination:* Weight, height, BMI, BP, pubertal changes, visual acuity, and dental examination
  - Anticipatory guidance for adolescents and parents

- *Investigations:*
  - Hemoglobin
  - *In sexually active adolescents:* Annual screening for human immunodeficiency virus (HIV) and syphilis—first void urine for leukocytes in boys [screening test for sexually transmitted diseases (STD)] and swab for Gram stain/culture/KOH and wet mount for girls
  - Oral glucose tolerance test (OGTT) and lipid profile if obese and/or family history of metabolic syndrome
  - Deworming and iron and calcium supplementation
- Life skill training on various topics like normal development, nutrition, physical activities, sexual health, drug abuse, gender issues, study skills, etc.
- Addressal of routine physical health issues using conventional history taking, examination, investigations, and treatment
- Reproductive health services like distributing sanitary napkins, menstrual hygiene training, addressing gynecological and obstetric care, STD detection and management, and premarital counseling
- Mental health support for adolescents in distress in the form of evaluation and diagnosis using Diagnostic and Statistical Manual of Mental Disorders (DSM) and various psychological tools and their pharmacological and psychotherapeutic management including timely referral
- Substance-abuse screening using CRAFT and S2BI formula
- Screening, investigations, and treatment for noncommunicable diseases
- *Addressing educational concerns:* Career guidance is done using aptitude tests and interest inventories, evaluation of poor school performance through interviews, psychological testing, and educational assessment. Collaborating with educationists and vocational trainers when needed should be done.
- *Sports clinic:* Preparticipatory sport evaluation and prevention/management of sports injury in collaboration with physical therapist and orthopedic surgeon
- Forming and promoting support groups of adolescents with similar problems, for example, polycystic ovary syndrome (PCOS) support group
- Conducting group empowerment sessions for adolescents, parents, and teachers.

## Advocacy of the Services Among the Beneficiaries

Adolescent-friendly health services  should make their presence felt in the community. Schools, colleges, sports clubs, etc., are good entry points to introduce the availability of these all-inclusive services exclusively designed for adolescents. Print and electronic media should be used to spread awareness about adolescent issues in the community. Earmarked days like Adolescent Health Week, Menstrual Hygiene Day, Obesity Prevention Day, Mental Health Day, etc., should be utilized to reach to masses.

## EXPANDED ADOLESCENT-FRIENDLY HEALTH SERVICES

Hitherto, we discussed the AFHS at a pediatric care setup.

If AFHS is provided by other HCPs, it is termed an expanded AFHS. It could be either superspeciality pediatric services or delivered by other specialty branches apart from pediatrics.

## Specialty Care

Pediatric subspecialty specialists such as pediatric endocrinologists, pediatric orthopedic surgeons, pediatric dermatologists, etc., should undergo a basic training of adolescent-related common issues. They should acquaint themselves with the adolescent-sensitive approach and basics of communication.

Each indoor and outpatient department (OPD) patient should be attended by a pediatrician with adolescent health delivery training. "Adolescent Job Aid", a book, and a handy desk reference mobile application tool for primary-level health workers, is an excellent learning source developed by World Health Organization (WHO), which addresses many common issues of adolescents.

Vice versa, an existing AFHS can be expanded to include specialty care, for example, dermatology, obstetrics and gynecology (OBG), etc., on a visiting basis to run specialty clinics. Thus, multidisciplinary care can be provided to an adolescent during his single visit under one roof.

## Extended Delivery Platforms

Not only the clinics, but also various other social platforms such as schools, colleges, community establishments,

NGOs, and other associations can work in tandem with Adolescent Health Academy (AHA)/Indian Academy of Pediatrics (IAP) or pediatricians to provide a base for all the AFHS activities.

The youth-friendly media, podcasts, blogs, social media platforms, telehealth, mHealth, etc., can be judiciously utilized in expanding the reach of AFHS delivery. Adolescent pediatricians can make use of the electronic platforms or social groups and can fill the gap between the needy adolescents and their quality care.

## ■ KEY MESSAGES

- Adolescents seek a different age-specific approach and dealing by the healthcare providers.
- It is crucial that HCPs learn this unique style of delivery to maintain their connect with healthcare system.
- It can be acquired through relevant reading and from the IAP/AHA practical training modules.
- Partnering with fellow doctors, paramedics, other gatekeepers, schools, social organizations, and media is beneficial for optimum delivery of services.

## ■ RECOMMENDED READING

1. Adolescent Health Division, Ministry of Health and Family Welfare, Government of India. (2014). Strategy Handbook. Rashtriya Kishor Swasthya Karyakram. [online] Available from https://nhm.gov.in/images/pdf/programmes/rksk-strategy-handbook.pdf [Last accessed March, 2024].
2. Bhave SY, Parthasarathy A, Nair MKC, Menon PSN, Greyganus (Eds). Bhave's Textbook of Adolescent Medicine. New Delhi: Jaypee Brothers Medical Publishers (P) Ltd; 2006.
3. Galagali PM, Rao C, Dinakar C, Gupta P, Shah D, Chandrashekaraiah S, et al. Indian Academy of Pediatrics Consensus Guidelines for adolescent friendly health services. Indian Pediatr. 2022;59(6):477-84.
4. Indian Academy of Pediatrics. AYA module Adolescent Health Academy (AHA), (2020). [online] Available from https://aha.iapindia.org/wp-content/uploads/2021/04/Awesome-AYA-Manual-2020.pdf [Last accessed March, 2024].
5. National Health Systems Resource Centre. (2023). Training Manual on Adolescent Health Care Services for Community Health Officer at Ayushman Bharat–Health and Wellness Centers. [online] Available from https://nhsrcindia.org/sites/default/files/2021-10/Adolescent%20Health%20Care%20Training%20Manual%20%28CHO%29.pdf [Last accessed March, 2024].
6. World Health Organization. (2015). Global standards for quality health-care services for adolescents: Standards and Criteria. [online] Available from https://www.who.int/publications/i/item/9789241549332 [Last accessed March, 2024].
7. World Health Organization. (2018). The global strategy for women's, children's, and adolescents' health (2016-2030). [online] Available from https://www.who.int/publications/i/item/A71-19 [Last accessed March, 2024].

<table>
<tr><td>**2.2**</td><td></td></tr>
</table>

# 2.2 Transitional Care

*Nishchal Bhatt*

## ■ DEFINITION

"Transition is the purposeful, planned movement of adolescents and young adults with chronic physical and medical conditions from child-oriented to adult-oriented health care systems." (Blum et al, 1993)

"Transitional care" is the preparation of adolescents and young adults to become more involved in their own healthcare, help them learn how to make medical decisions, and eventually assist them in a planned move from pediatric healthcare providers to adult providers.

## ■ WHY IS IT NEEDED?

Adolescents aged between 10 and 19 years account for over 22% of the Indian population. An increasing number of children with long-term conditions and complex care needs are surviving into young adulthood. So, there is a growing need for specialized care to ensure seamless transfer and transition from children to adult healthcare services. Currently, there is a lack of specific, discrete provisions for transfer. This leads to feelings of being "dumped, cutoff, and abandoned". The current options for

## ▌ TIMELINE FOR INTRODUCING SIX CORE ELEMENTS INTO PEDIATRIC PRACTICE

| Core | Core element | Action | Age (years) |
|---|---|---|---|
| Core 1 | Transition policy | Discuss transition policy | 12–14 |
| Core 2 | Transition tracking and monitoring | Track progress | 14–18 |
| Core 3 | Transition readiness | Assess skills | 14–18 |
| Core 4 | Transition planning | Develop HCT plan, including a medical summary | 14–18 |
| Core 5 | Transfer and/or integration into adult care | Integration into adult practice | 18–21 |
| Core 6 | Transition completion and ongoing care with an adult physician | Confirm transfer completion and get consumer feedback | 18–21 |

(HCT: healthcare transition)

## ▌ KEY MESSAGES

- A healthcare transition occurs when an adolescent or a young adult changes from pediatric to adult care.
- Healthcare transitions in youth with chronic illnesses and physical and mental disabilities can prove challenging and sometimes be unsuccessful if not properly planned and executed by the patient (when possible), family, and clinicians.
- The majority of adolescents and parents accept transition care from pediatrics to adult services, but only a small proportion has ever received transition information from doctors.

## ▌ RECOMMENDED READING


1. Blum RW, Garell D, Hodgman CH, Jorissen TW, Okinow NA, Orr DP, et al. Transition from child-centered to adult health-care systems for adolescents with chronic conditions. A position paper of the Society for Adolescent Medicine. J Adolesc Health. 1993;14(7):570-6.
2. Children and Young People's Health Outcomes Forum. (2012). Children and young people's health outcomes strategy: Report of the children and young people's health outcomes forum. [online] Available from https://assets.publishing.service.gov.uk/media/5a7c3d87ed915d76e2ebc051/CYP-report.pdf [Last accessed March, 2024].
3. Crowley R, Wolfe I, Lock K, McKee M. Improving the transition between pediatric and adult healthcare: A Systemic review. Arch Dis Child. 2011;96(6):548-53.
4. Duke NN, Scal PB. Adult care transitioning for adolescents with special health care needs: A pivotal role for family centred care. Matern Child Health J. 2011;15(1):98-105.
5. Gleeson H, Turner G. Transition to adult services. Arch Dis Educ Pract Ed. 2012;97(3):86-92.
6. Kaehne A. Transition from children and adolescent to adult mental health services for young people with intellectual disabilities: A scoping study of service organisation problems. Adv Mental Health Intell Disab. 2011;5(1):9-16.
7. McIntosh N, Helms P, Smyth R, Logan S (Eds). Forfar and Areneil's Textbook of Pediatrics, 7th edition. Amsterdam: Elsevier; 2008. pp. 1577-8.
8. McMillan I. Bridging the gap between children and adult services. Mental Health Pract. 2011:15(2):6-7.
9. Royal College of Nursing. (2011). Learning from the past–setting out the future: Developing learning disability nursing in the United Kingdom. [online] Available from https://www.choiceforum.org/docs/rcnld.pdf [Last accessed March, 2024].
10. White PH, Cooley WC; Transitions Clinical Report Authoring Group; American Academy of Pediatrics; American Academy of Family Physicians; American College of Physicians. Supporting the health care transition from adolescence to adulthood in the medical home. Pediatrics. 2018;142(5):e20182587

# 2.3  School Health Interventions as Entry Points

*Utkarsh Bansal*

## ■ INTRODUCTION

The onset of adolescence not only brings physical changes in individuals, but also exposes them to novel vulnerabilities like nutritional deficiencies, sexual-health issues, injuries, and cybercrimes. Adolescent well-being is dependent on many interlinked factors, and access to quality health services and information is pivotal **(Fig. 1)**. The humongous efforts of healthcare workers leading to a reduction in under-5 child mortality in low- and middle-income countries (LMICs) have substantially increased the worldwide school-aged children and adolescent population. The high-income countries (HICs) have multiple services for adolescents, which are preventive interventions to promote a healthy lifestyle and are delivered through various health system-based, school-based, community-based, and digital platforms. But such services are limited in LMICs where about 90% of the global adolescent population dwells. Experience from HICs has shown that schools can be utilized for public health activities and impact the community. Imparting health education to school children has a cascading effect by improving not only the individual health but also the health of peers and family.

India is the home of 243 million adolescents, the largest population in the world. As per the National Mental Health Survey 2015–16, the prevalence of mental disorders in the age group of 13–17 years was 7.3% and nearly equal in both genders. Approximately 59% of the girls and 31% of boys in the age group of 15–19 years are anemic in India [National Family Health Survey (NFHS-5)]. Early marriages and sexual relations increase the risk of sexually transmitted diseases (STDs), unwanted pregnancies, and unsafe abortions. This compounds the fact that acquired immunodeficiency syndrome (AIDS)-related deaths have increased in adolescents despite a fall in every other age group. NFHS-4 data showed that in the age group of 15–19 years, 4.2% of girls and 4.8% of boys were obese while 42% of girls and 44% of boys were thin.

The World Health Organization (WHO) is pursuing the program "Health-Promoting Schools" and utilizing school-health methods in public health and medical services. The UNESCO's FRESH (Focusing Resources on Effective School Health) Initiative is a comprehensive model for health education **(Box 1)**. A health-promoting school (HPS) is "a school that constantly strengthens its capacity as a safe and healthy setting for living, learning, and working" **(Fig. 2)**. The schools have a crucial role in the development of children and adolescents and they can play a key role in health promotion.

## ADVANTAGES OF SCHOOL HEALTH INTERVENTION PROGRAM

- Food supplementation for improving growth
- Micronutrient supplementation to correct nutritional deficiencies
- Improved learning and cognition by improving nutrition
- Promote healthy lifestyle and habits early on in life
- Increased school enrolment and attendance
- Removing barriers to education
- Decreasing economic burden
- Prompt recognition and treatment of common diseases
- Reduce emergency room visits

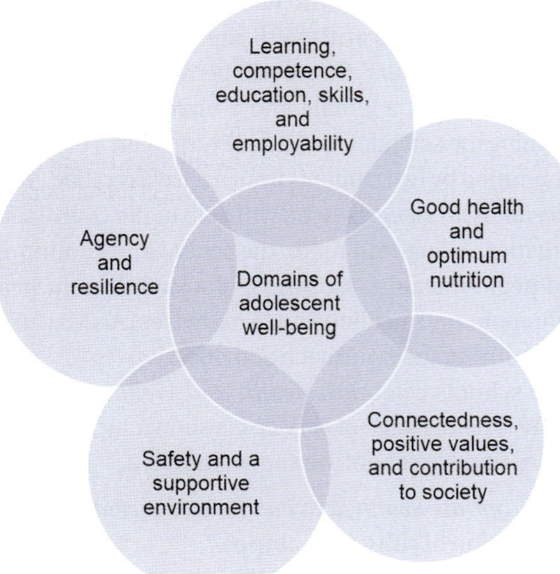


**Fig. 1:** Components of adolescent well-being.

**BOX 1:** Pillars of the Focusing Resources on Effective School Health (FRESH) 2014 framework.

- *Health-related school policies:* Nondiscriminatory, protective, inclusive, and gender sensitive to promote the physical and psychosocial health
- *Safe learning environment:* Access to safe water and provision of separate sanitation facilities; a safe, healthy, clean, and emotionally supportive environment
- *Skill-based health education:* Life-skills education that addresses health, nutrition, and hygiene issues
- *School-based health and nutrition services:* Simple, safe, and familiar health and nutrition services

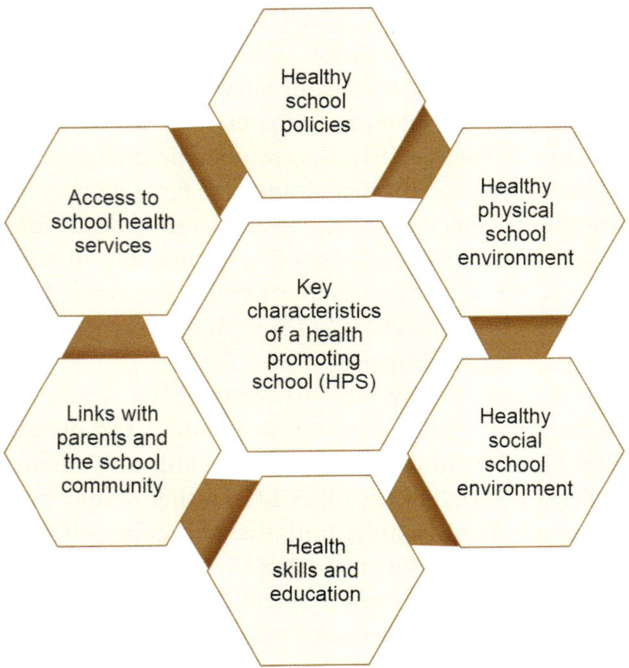


**Fig. 2:** Six key characteristics of a health promoting school.

- Improve the knowledge and practice regarding hygiene and sanitation
- Provide mental health services and positive development.

## INDIAN SCHOOL HEALTH PROGRAM

Various global and national school-based interventions have formed the basis of the development of the Indian School Health Program. The operational guidelines were released in April 2018. It aims to amalgamate health education, health promotion, and disease prevention and improve access to health services. It has a keen focus on the recent soaring morbidities like substance abuse, violence, mental health problems, and metabolic health problems.

**TABLE 1:** Package of services under the school health program.

| | |
|---|---|
| School health promotion activities | • Age-appropriate incremental learning for the promotion of healthy behavior and prevention of various diseases<br>• Delivered through school teachers/health and wellness ambassadors trained in each school in collaboration with students/health and wellness messengers |
| Health screening | The screening of children for 30 identified health conditions (4 "D"s, namely defects at birth, deficiencies, diseases, development delays including disability) for early detection, free treatment, and management through dedicated RBSK mobile health teams |
| Provision of services | • Provision of IFA (tablets of 100 mg elemental iron and 500 µg of folic acid) and albendazole tablets by teachers through WIFS and NDD* programs respectively<br>• Provision of sanitary napkins<br>• Age-appropriate vaccination<br>• Physical and mental fitness by yoga and meditation |
| Electronic health records | Electronic health records for each child |
| Imparting skills of emergency care | Training of teachers on basic first aid. |

*August 10 and February 10 every year, respectively.
(IFA: iron folic acid; NDD: national deworming days; RBSK: Rashtriya Bal Swasthya Karyakram; WIFS: weekly iron folic acid supplementation)

The school teachers who will be trained in the health promotion activities will be designated as "*health and wellness ambassadors*". There will be two teachers in each school, preferably a female and a male, and they will be performing the activities for 1 hour every week. The teachers are supported by two students from each class called "*health and wellness messengers*" who will help in the coordination of activities. Along with them, the school and community-based peer educators/*saathiyas*, block adolescent health coordinators, and auxiliary nurse midwives (ANMs) further support during their outreach activities.

The schools celebrate *Health and Wellness Day* each Tuesday. The package of services is shown in **Table 1** and activities done at school are shown in **Box 2**.

*Age-appropriate health activities for adolescents include:*
- Prevention of substance abuse
- Sexual and reproductive health
- Violence prevention

> **BOX 2:** Activities in school.
>
> - *Weekly:*
>   - Classroom transactions by health and wellness ambassadors
>   - Administration of IFA tablets
> - *Fortnightly/monthly:*
>   - Thematic school assembly
>   - Question box responses
> - *Quarterly:*
>   - Thematic adolescent health days
>   - Parent–teacher meetings
> - *Bi-annually:* Administration of albendazole tablet (National Deworming Day)
> - *Middle school:*
>   - Puberty and related changes
>   - Eye care and oral hygiene
>   - Nutrition
>   - Bullying prevention
>   - Meditation and yoga
>   - Internet safety and media literacy
>   - Prevention of substance abuse
>   - HIV/AIDS
>   - Mental health
> - *High school:*
>   - Prevention of substance abuse
>   - Sexual and reproductive health
>   - Violence prevention
>   - Unintentional injury
>   - Road safety
>   - Nutrition
>   - Meditation and yoga

(AIDS: acquired immune deficiency syndrome; HIV: human immunodeficiency virus; IFA: iron folic acid)

- Unintentional injury
- Road safety
- Nutrition
- Meditation and yoga

*School Feeding Program:* The government of India initiated the midday meal program to provide 500 kcal for 200 school days per year to students.

## SUGGESTED SCHOOL HEALTH PROMOTION ACTIVITIES

- Oral health promotion promotes the right brushing technique, access and use of appropriate fluoride-containing pastes (1,200–1,500 ppm), brushing teeth twice a day for 2 minutes, and routine oral checkups.
- Screening for disabilities including but not limited to vision, hearing, secondary to trauma, and common ailments.

- Mental health support through school-based anti-bullying programs, gender-based violence prevention, gender inclusion, resilience building, positive psychology, mindfulness, and relaxation.
- Sex education and education regarding STDs involving peers and family members to prevent sexual abuse and illnesses.
- Education regarding various addictions and their ill effects and the development of resilience to say no to drug abuse.
- Immunization activities to increase coverage of common school-age vaccines (such as human papillomavirus and diphtheria-tetanus toxoids pertussis boosters), catch-up immunization in partially or completely unvaccinated children, and special immunization drives (such as measles, rubella, and Japanese encephalitis vaccine).
- Menstrual hygiene sessions to increase knowledge, bust taboos, and enhance acceptance of the normal growth phenomenon.
- Addressing diarrhea by point-of-use water treatment and filtration and zinc supplementation.
- Control of vector-borne diseases by inculcating habits of wearing full-sleeved clothing, use of mosquito repellent creams, removing stagnant water, and promotion of mosquito nets.
- Prevention of obesity and undernutrition by education about nutritious food, increasing fruit and vegetable consumption, and promoting physical exercise; regular anthropometry to guide early interventions.
- Screening of vision to detect myopia or other visual defects, early referral, and treatment.
- Limiting screen time by educating about the problems, improving productive media usage, and involvement in other purposeful activities.
- Limiting unintentional injury, such as road traffic or cycling injuries, and drowning; promoting helmet use, road traffic rules, swimming lessons, fire and other emergency escape plans, first-aid, and resuscitation.

## CONCLUSION

Schools can be utilized in several key health interventions for children and adolescents. This can include infectious disease screening and prevention, immunization, hygiene education, healthy lifestyle promotion, micronutrient supplementation, screening of noncommunicable diseases, mental health promotion, prevention of substance abuse, violence, and internet addiction, and promotion of safety rules and first-aid measures. Age-appropriate sexual and reproductive health education along with prevention of abuse can be imparted.

## KEY MESSAGES

- Schools can play a pivotal role in health education, and promotion and screening of common diseases.
- HPSs increase the health awareness of not only the individual students but also the community as a whole.
- School health programs can target mental health problems, substance abuse, sexual-health issues, and internet addiction.
- School-based midday meal program improves nutrition and school attendance as well.
- Supplementation of vital micronutrients and minerals can prevent nutritional deficiencies and their adverse effects.
- Education about pubertal changes and reproductive health empowers adolescents to curb the taboos and myths associated with puberty.
- Schools are an ideal place for large-scale immunization drives and the completion of immunization schedules in partially or unvaccinated students.
- A healthy lifestyle adopted during adolescence is carried for life, preventing future metabolic diseases.
- School children are messengers of health and hygiene for their families and society.
- In countries where health services are limited and overcrowded, the government should focus on school-based health programs to improve the delivery of preventive services.

## RECOMMENDED READING

1. Bundy DAP, Schultz L, Sarr B, Banham L, Colenso P, Drake L. The school as a platform for addressing health in middle childhood and adolescence. In: Bundy D, de Silva N, Horton S, Jamison D, Patton G (Eds). Child and Adolescent Health and Development, 3rd edition, Volume 8. Washington, DC: The International Bank for Reconstruction and Development/The World Bank; 2018. pp. 269-86.
2. Ministry of Health & Family Welfare, Ministry of Human Resource & Development, Government of India. Operational Guidelines on School Health Programme under Ayushman Bharat. (2018). [online] Available from https://nhm.gov.in/New_Updates_2018/NHM_Components/RMNCHA/AH/guidelines/Operational_guidelines_on_School_Health_Programme_under_Ayushman_Bharat.pdf [Last accessed March, 2024].
3. Ross DA, Hinton R, Melles-Brewer M, Engel D, Zeck W, Fagan L, et al. Adolescent well-being: A definition and conceptual framework. J Adolesc Health. 2020;67(4):472-6.
4. UNESCO, UNICEF, WHO, the World Bank, Education International. (2002). FRESH: A comprehensive school health approach to achieve EFA. [online] Available from https://unesdoc.unesco.org/ark:/48223/pf0000125537#:~:text=The%20FRESH%20initiative%20(Focusing%20Resources,and%20its%20effects%20on%20education [Last accessed March, 2024].
5. Vaivada T, Sharma N, Das JK, Salam RA, Lassi ZS, Bhutta ZA. Interventions for health and well-being in school-aged children and adolescents: A way forward. Pediatrics. 2022;149(Suppl 5):e2021053852.
6. World Health Organization, United Nations Educational, Scientific and Cultural Organization. (2021). Making every school a health-promoting school: Global standards and indicators for health-promoting schools and systems. [online] Available from https://iris.who.int/bitstream/handle/10665/341907/9789240025059-eng.pdf?sequence=1 [Last accessed March, 2024].

<table>
<tr><td>**2.4**</td><td>

# Interviewing a Teenager and Anticipatory Guidance Using Basic Counseling Skills

</td></tr>
</table>

*Preeti Galagali*

## INTRODUCTION

Patient-centered, effective communication and interviewing skills are essential for establishing a therapeutic relationship with adolescents. These skills build rapport and enhance bidirectional communication, thereby enabling adolescents to freely share their problems, give consent to clinical evaluation, and be receptive to therapy and counseling. For an in-depth understanding of adolescent issues, it is preferable to interview the adolescent, parents/caretakers, extended family members, teachers, and if required, even peers in private. There are many advantages of conducting a psychosocial interview that explores the multiple domains of an adolescent's life including self, parents, schools, peers, and environment **(Box 1)**.

## ADOLESCENT–PEDIATRICIAN COMMUNICATION: OPPORTUNITIES AND CHALLENGES

In adolescence, there is an increase in verbal skills and cognition that improves the ability to communicate with pediatricians, especially with those whom they know since childhood. Adolescence is characterized by autonomy bids, identity crisis, mood swings, peer affiliations and parental conflicts. It is also an age for experimentation, questioning, emotional reactivity, impulsivity, and a tendency toward sensation-seeking behavior. Adolescents may hesitate to confide in the physician, especially regarding issues of mental health, sexuality, and substance use due to the fear of being reprimanded and judged. While interviewing adolescents, clinicians should allocate adequate time for the interview, offer privacy and confidentiality (within limits), and adopt an adolescent-friendly attitude with genuine interest and respect for the clients and their families.

Adolescents do not like to be treated as children and dislike being preached, lectured, and ordered. Anticipated health problems and risky behaviors are addressed by providing guidance on how to promote good health and avoid risks. Adolescents usually respond well to a reason and strengths-based style of communication that is relevant to them and their interests, especially during a discussion regarding therapeutic options and behavior change. For example, a 13-year-old adolescent girl, worried about her school performance, could be motivated to exercise by sharing the effect of physical activity on increasing brain-derived neurotrophic factor and thereby improving neuronal proliferations and memory.

## ADOLESCENT-FRIENDLY COMMUNICATION AND COUNSELING SKILLS

Effective communication with adolescents is more of an art than science. Dr Albert Mehrabian's work has indicated that communication is largely nonverbal, to the extent of 93%. According to him, when an individual is speaking, the listener focuses only 7% on the actual words, 38% on the way the words are delivered (the tone and accent), and 55% on facial expression. A pediatrician should master the following basic communication skills **(Table 1)**.

### Verbal Skills

Verbal skills include expressive language skills and spoken words. The pediatrician should have unconditional positive regard and use the *language of respect and civility* while speaking to adolescents, even if they are indulging in risky behaviors. For example, a drug-using adolescent should not be labeled as "bad"; instead, the reasons for using drugs should be explored in detail and later should be counseled accordingly. Labeling clients interferes with the counseling process. Pediatricians should be *nonjudgmental and empathetic.* Empathy is a communicated understanding of the other person's intended emotional message. It is looking at the situation from a client's perspective. Empathy requires listening and understanding. Pediatricians should ask *open-ended questions* to facilitate bidirectional communication. They should avoid closed-ended questions (those that can be answered with a "yes" or "no") like "is your relationship with your father good?"; instead, asking open-ended

**TABLE 1:** Effective communication and counseling skills.

| *Take consent, ensure privacy, express confidentiality limits, be respectful* | |
| --- | --- |
| *Verbal* | *Nonverbal* |
| <ul><li>Address adolescent first</li><li>Keep it short and simple without scientific jargon and "you" statements</li><li>Appropriate words, tone, and pitch</li><li>*Open ended questions*</li><li>*Active listening*</li><li>Praise, validate emotions, *empathize*, address concerns, reassure, build hope</li><li>*Nonjudgmental*/nonaccusatory</li><li>Avoid moralizing, preaching, giving solutions</li></ul> | <ul><li>Eye contact</li><li>Proximity and sit at the same level</li><li>Facial expressions</li><li>Nodding</li><li>Position of hands and legs</li><li>Silence</li><li>Holding hands, patting</li></ul> |
| Listen more, talk less | |

ones like "how is your relationship with your father" will stimulate the adolescents to reveal much more about their family. Sometimes, when an adolescent gets overwhelmed and incoherent with emotions, pauses and *silence* help the communication to become calmer, productive, and purposeful. It also gives breathing space for restructuring words, putting thoughts sequentially, and understanding the exact flow of emotions. The pediatrician should validate the adolescents' emotions, discuss successful coping skills in the past, and praise the adolescents' strengths to build up their self-esteem and help them to manage stressors and difficult emotions.

### Nonverbal Skills

Nonverbal skills include eye contact, facial expression, position of hands and legs, body movement, physical proximity, and tone and accent of delivery of words. A stern tone and a frown may convey disapproval, a smirk; cynicism, lifting of eyebrows; surprise, and a pat on the hand; reassurance. A steady eye contact between the pediatrician and adolescent during a conversation indicates their collective interest in what is being shared. An adolescent looking away may indicate a loss of interest or an intention of hiding some feelings. A frightened adolescent usually responds with hostility and pediatricians who understand this defense mechanism can adjust their own communication style accordingly and become more supportive and encouraging. Similarly, a silent, noncommunicative adolescent is often hiding worry, fear, or anger and can best be reached by a warm and caring attitude. While talking to adolescents, a pediatrician should ensure that there are no distractions in the form of phone calls or pending official work.

### Active Listening

Active listening is a powerful technique for rapport building and eliciting a detailed psychosocial history. The four components are as follows:

1. *Paying attention* that includes turning the body toward the adolescents and looking at them while talking. It also entails listening to them in a quiet place where conversation is clearly audible.
2. *Use of minimal responses* that indicate to the adolescent that the pediatrician is listening. These responses may be nonverbal like nod of the head or verbal like "Ah-ha, Oh, Yes, OK, Right, I understand, Mmm, Hummm". Such responses encourage the adolescent to communicate.

3. *Use of reflection* indicates to the adolescents that the pediatrician is attending to the detail and content of their story. This includes reflection of content (paraphrasing) and reflection of feelings. For example, if a 13-year-old adolescent boy who has changed school recently says, "I have no friends. I don't like going to school." The pediatrician uses reflection and comments, "You sound really unhappy. I do understand that at your age, you need to have friends otherwise life can get boring. As you have recently joined school, you shall need to do some ice breaking—can you tell me a few statements that will be helpful to build new friendships?" This conveys to the client that he has been understood and he in turn will be eager to share his concerns and future plans.
4. *Summarizing* involves picking up the most salient points in the adolescent's description of events and reflecting these back to the adolescent. This is particularly useful if an adolescent has been troubled by multiple issues over a period of time.

A few other counseling skills that can be used during an interaction with an adolescent client include congruence, self-disclosure, leading, use of humor, transference, and countertransference. The interview techniques and structure will vary according to the person being interviewed like adolescents, young adults, parents, and teachers and will depend upon the time available, age, developmental stage, culture, presence of chronic medical or neurodevelopmental or mental disorders, or clinical setting (e.g., transition to adult care or inpatient or outpatient care).

## ■ ADOLESCENT INTERVIEW FRAMEWORK

Adolescent clients are often unsure and sometimes scared of visits to the doctor, particularly when they are brought against their wishes, by a parent. Therefore, an attempt is made to put them at ease and build a good rapport in the initial meeting. When adolescents enter the pediatrician's office, they are greeted first; next, the pediatrician gives a self-introduction and then they are asked to introduce themselves and the accompanying adults. The opening conversation could be informal, for example, about friends, hobbies, school, or strengths, to encourage the adolescent to talk freely. This will decrease the nervousness and tension and will give insights into the adolescent's personality and background. Gradually when rapport is established (maybe in the second interview session),

**TABLE 2:** HEEADSSS psychosocial history.

| Psychosocial domain | Sample questions |
| --- | --- |
| Home | • Who lives at home with you? How is your relationship with each family member? Do you have a separate room? Who gives you a bath? Do you sleep alone? Has there been a recent change in living arrangement?<br>• If I was invisible and you were having a disagreement with your parent, what would I hear? How would I see your parent disciplining you? |
| Education/ Employment | • Are you studying/ working? How is the situation at school/ work place? How has your performance been in school this year compared to last? Are you satisfied with your performance?<br>• How is your relationship with teachers and peers at school? Has anybody ever spoken to you in a way that you have not liked?<br>• Who helps you with school work? Please share details regarding your study habits. Where do you see yourself 5 years from now? |
| Eating | • Recall your dietary intake on a typical day. How often do you eat out/drink sugar sweetened beverages? How do you stay healthy? What do you think about your diet?<br>• How do you feel about your body? Do you ever feel that food controls you rather than vice versa? Has there been any change in your appetite lately? |
| Activities | • What do you do for fun? How much time do you spend in structured or unstructured outdoor/physical activity? What are your hobbies? Do you attend special hobby classes? Are you happy with your performance? Do you have friends you socialize with? Where do you and your peers hang around for fun? How is your relationship with friends?<br>• Which digital devices do you use and own? For what purpose do you use your digital devices? Are you a member of social media sites? Which ones? Do you feel the media device controls your life? Do you get into trouble with family and friends for using media excessively?<br>• For how many hours do you sleep? Do you have any sleep related problems?<br>• Are you a part of a religious community? How often do you participate in religious activities? What role does religion have in your life? Do you have personal spiritual beliefs? What aspects of spirituality or spiritual practices do you find most useful?<br>• Have you lately lost interest in activities that you enjoyed previously? If yes, since how many days or months? |
| Drugs | • What is your attitude towards drug usage? How do you feel about this issue?<br>• Do your friends smoke, drink or use drugs? Have you ever tried? If yes, which drug and how often? |
| Sexuality | • When did you attain menarche? When was your last menstrual period? What is the length of your menstrual cycle and for how long does the bleeding last? How many pads do you use in a cycle? Do you have any problems during menstruation?<br>• I ask all teenagers a few questions pertaining to sexual health which is an important component of general health. Are you ok with that? You could let me know anytime if you are uncomfortable or embarrassed.<br>• Are you in a romantic relationship? Have you been physically intimate with somebody? If yes, with whom? What do you do in intimate moments?<br>• Are you married?<br>• Do you use any contraceptive method? Have you ever been pregnant?<br>• Do you have any vaginal/penile discharge or itching? Do you have burning micturition or pain abdomen?<br>• Has anybody touched you in a way that you did not like? |
| Suicide/ Depression | • Have you ever felt hopeless, sad and a failure in life? Has there been a recent change in your mood, behavior, sleep, appetite or academic performance? For how long have you been feeling low?<br>• What do you do when you feel sad? Do you confide your problems in someone? What would make you feel better?<br>• Sometimes when young people are in unbearable pain or trouble they wish that they could end it all. Have you ever wished the same? Have you ever tried to end your life? |
| Safety | • Do you feel safe at home, school and while playing in the neighborhood?<br>• Do you drive a vehicle? If yes, which one? Do you wear a helmet and seat belt while riding in a vehicle?<br>• Have you ever got into a physical fight with anybody? Have you ever been hurt during fights? Have you ever got into trouble with law? |

difficult and "threatening" issues like drug use and sexual behavior as appropriate could be addressed. Adolescents accompanied with their parents should be first seen together with their parents and subsequently interviewed alone. Confidentiality should be assured and the limits defined to the adolescent and parents at the start of the interaction. This is a prerequisite for eliciting an accurate history. The only indications to breach confidentiality are self-harm, sexual abuse (information to police is mandatory), criminal behavior, or hospitalization. The adolescents in these cases are assured that this sensitive information would be shared with a trustworthy adult of their choice after seeking their permission.

In India, adolescents above 12 years of age can give consent for history taking and examination while those above 18 years of age can give consent for medications and medical procedures. A detailed psychosocial history [home, education/employment, eating, activities, drugs, sexuality, suicidal ideation, and safety (HEEADSSS)] is elicited using effective communication skills **(Table 2)**. A chaperone (nurse or attender) of the same sex as the patient should be present during the examination of both girls and boys. At the end, the relevant points from the interview and examination are summarized. The diagnosis and management are discussed with the client. The parents are informed on relevant medical issues only after expressed permission from the adolescent. Collaborative care in the form of partnerships with parents, educators, peers, social workers, and multidisciplinary professionals is essential. Government of India's telemedicine guidelines are to be followed for conducting online interviews with adolescents.

## ANTICIPATORY GUIDANCE

Every teen visit is an opportunity to provide anticipatory guidance regarding a healthy lifestyle, reinforce strengths, and prevent high-risk behavior. The teens are guided regarding positive coping strategies, involvement in hobbies and sports, building parental and school connectedness, and life skills. The motivational interviewing technique is used to gently persuade adolescents to a healthy behavior change. Here, the relevance, risks, and rewards of the change are highlighted and roadblocks, if any, are addressed. The components of anticipatory guidance include information on normal development, nutrition, physical activity, menstrual hygiene and fertility calendar, injury prevention including use of helmets, safety belts, speed of driving, risks of drinking and driving, handling peer pressure and bullying, media literacy and addiction, cyberbullying, responsible sexual behavior, contraceptives and protection against sexually transmitted diseases, substance-use prevention and assistance with deaddiction, cyber and narcotics laws, Protection of Children from Sexual Offences Act (POCSO), and parenting guidance. Parents need to be educated about the developmental needs of adolescents and change from directive parenting to negotiation and supporting "independence".

## KEY MESSAGES

- Effective communication skills are essential for rapport building, history taking, and eliciting strengths and aid in therapeutic management and counseling.
- Developmentally and culturally appropriate interview techniques overcome the "normative" hesitancy of adolescents to seek medical services and healthcare, especially for sensitive issues.
- Essential communication skills include verbal, nonverbal, active listening, empathy, and unconditional positive regard.
- Motivational interviewing aids in behavior change while imparting anticipatory guidance.

## RECOMMENDED READING

1. Galagali PM, Rao C, Dinakar C, Gupta P, Shah D, Chandrashekaraiah S, et al. Indian Academy of Pediatrics Consensus Guidelines for adolescent friendly health services. Indian Pediatr. 2022;59(6):477-84.
2. Kashyap V, Galagali P. Telecounselling in clinical practice. Ind J Pract Pediatr. 2022;24(3):327-31.
3. Klein DA, Goldenring JM, Adelman W. (2014). Contemporary Pediatrics. HEEADSSS 3.0: The psychosocial interview for adolescents updated for a new century fuelled by media. [online] Available from https://www.contemporarypediatrics.com/view/heeadsss-30-psychosocial-interview-adolescents-updated-new-century-fueled-media [Last accessed March, 2024].
4. Ministry of Health and Family Welfare Government of India. Participant's Handbook for Training of Medical Officers on Adolescent Friendly Health Services. Rashtriya Kishor Swasthya Karyakram (RKSK). New Delhi: Government of India; 2023.
5. Shastri D. Respectful adolescent care-A must know concept. Indian Pediatr. 2019;56:909-10.

# 2.5 Navigating the Legal Landscape: Ensuring Ethical Adolescent Care

*Sonia S Kanitkar*

## ■ INTRODUCTION

Legal and ethical considerations are most important for professionals in the practice of medicine. This chapter provides a framework for adolescent practice. It includes:

- The knowledge of legal professional conduct while dealing with these young people, for example, consent, confidentiality, assent
- The knowledge of laws in cases of child abuse/harm
- The knowledge of legal issues in physical and mental health problems in this turbulent stage of adolescence, for example, pornography, sexuality issues, food safety issues, juvenile crimes.

It is important to understand that "Law of the Land" is dynamic and this chapter is only a basic framework to help professionals in dealing with adolescents in medical practice.

## ■ BASIC RULES IN ADOLESCENT PRACTICE

- The patient is neither a child nor an adult but has the right to know, understand, and assent to treatment.
- In this practice, the adolescent is also a participant unlike a child.
- The pediatrician should be nonjudgmental.
- The young patient expects care, respect, and a supportive attitude from the professional.
- The privacy and confidentiality are primordial when dealing with this age group.
- Professional skills like good communication, relaxed attitude, positive mind, and friendly vibe are much needed.
- Anticipatory guidance is an important tool for guiding adolescents about the legal issues concerning this age group.

## WHAT LEGAL ISSUES DOES A PEDIATRICIAN NEED TO KNOW BEFORE DEALING WITH PATIENTS IN ADOLESCENT PRACTICE?

### Consent

Consent holds a pivotal role in medical practice, and its nuances become particularly relevant in adolescent care. It is crucial to distinguish between assent and consent; assent is a simple agreement with/without proper understanding of the proposal, while informed consent involves a detailed explanation of various components. Physicians must communicate these elements to patients, parents, or guardians to ensure an informed decision regarding disease management.

**Boxes 1 and 2** depict the policy statement of the American Academy of Pediatrics.

---

**BOX 1:** Elements of informed consent for medical decision-making.

- *Provision of information about the following:*
  - Nature of the illness or condition
  - Proposed diagnostic steps and/or treatments and the probability of their success
  - The potential risks, benefits, and uncertainties of the proposed and alternative treatments, including the option of no treatment other than comfort measures
- Assessment of patient and surrogate understanding and medical decision-making capacity, including assurance of time for questions by patient and surrogate
- Ensure that there is a voluntary agreement with the plan
- Help the patient achieve a developmentally appropriate awareness of the nature of his or her condition
- Tell the patient what he or she can expect with tests and treatments
- Make a clinical assessment of the patient's understanding of the situation and the factors influencing how he or she is responding (including whether there is inappropriate pressure to accept testing or therapy)
- Solicit an expression of the patient's willingness to accept the proposed care

---

**BOX 2:** Practical aspects of assent by pediatric patients for medical decision-making.

- Help the patient achieve a developmentally appropriate awareness of the nature of his or her condition
- Tell the patient what he or she can expect with tests and treatments
- Make a clinical assessment of the patient's understanding of the situation and the factors influencing how he or she is responding (including whether there is inappropriate pressure to accept testing or therapy)
- Solicit an expression of the patient's willingness to accept the proposed care

Pediatricians must gauge the educational background and mental maturity of adolescents to ensure effective communication. The language used should align with the adolescent's developmental stage. While seeking assent or consent, it is crucial to appropriately explain medical issues.

- In India, a child achieves majority at 18 years of age, allowing them to provide valid consent for medical treatment. Children below 12 years of age lack the capacity to consent; a parent/guardian must provide consent for any medical/surgical treatment or procedure. Adolescents aged 12–18 years can consent to medical examination but not treatment (Indian Majority Act, Guardian and Wards Act, and Indian Contract Act).
- In case of orphans or unknown street children, the local court is taken as a guardian. Permission is required to be taken from a court for any treatment/procedure for such adolescents.
- In emergency situations, where parents or designated guardians are unavailable immediately, the caretaker like the principal or teacher can act as a temporary guardian (loco parentis) and give consent for emergency treatment.
- An adolescent cannot give consent for blood/organ donation (Transplantation of Human Organ Act, 1994).

## ■ EXCEPTIONS TO INFORMED CONSENT

In case an adolescent presents alone with an emergency medical condition without a parent or legal guardian, then a doctor needs no consent for first aid or to save life. It includes emergency medical examination, screening procedures, and appropriate medical/surgical care.

## ■ CONFIDENTIALITY

Confidentiality means secrecy about the sensitive information given by the patient to the doctor as this information is essential to get proper care and treatment. The protection of this information is primordial to a trust-laden doctor–patient relationship.

The Medical Council of India (MCI) Regulations, 2002 and the new National Medical Commission (NMC) guidelines for Registered Medical Practitioner (RMP) Professional Conduct (August 2023) regulate the collection of personal information and disclosure of such data. Article 5 of the Charter says that "*all patients have a right to privacy, and doctors must hold information about their health condition and treatment plan in strict confidentiality*". All patient data must be kept securely physically or in digital form, such that no leakage or theft can happen. In the case of adolescents, all the information is kept confidential by the practitioner, except in situations where divulging sensitive information is in the interest of protecting others or the patient herself/himself or if it is a notifiable disease. As per Section 7.14 of the MCI Regulations, 2002 and Revised NMC Code of Conduct August 2023, there are exceptions. In the following circumstances, a doctor may have to give out the information to the concerned authority, on the orders of the presiding judge/court. The exceptions are as follows:

- Self-harm, suicidal or criminal intentions, and sexual abuse of the adolescent
- Risk of harm to the community, locally or generally
- Presence of notifiable diseases

Sometimes, as professionals, we have to take a 360° view of the circumstances and then decide to act appropriately, as depicted by the following example. HIV is a disease with societal stigma, so a doctor has to protect an infected adolescent girl and keep her information confidential, but in case when this patient wants to marry after adulthood is achieved, there is a chance of transfer of infection to the husband after marriage. In such a case, a doctor needs to break confidentiality and reveal the truth to the future husband. This is to save him from contracting the infection. Such a case was fought in the court and the court held that "*the Right to Privacy, is not absolute and may be lawfully restricted for the prevention of crime, disorder or protection of health or morals or protection of rights and freedom of others*".

## ■ LAWS GOVERNING ABUSE IN CHILD/ ADOLESCENT IN INDIA

Adolescents are the force that guides the future of a country. We need to protect and nourish their body and souls at any cost. As per statistics:

- 1 in 5 women and 1 in 13 men are reported victims of having been sexually abused as a child aged 0–17 years.
- 120 million girls and young women below the age of 20 years have faced one or the other major/minor forced sexual contact.
- As a result of this maltreatment, the adolescents grow with many physical/mental health issues. Such youths are at risk of themselves becoming perpetrators of abuse. It is important to break this cycle.

- The social, cultural, and economic health of a country is affected adversely.

Thus, India has left no stone unturned to save the children/adolescents of our nation. As pediatricians, we come across all the good and bad happenings with this age group. In fact, we are mostly the first point of contact for our adolescents as they have been trusting us since birth. So, it becomes imperative that we act wisely, within the purview of law, in keeping with the trust they behold. Let us understand the laws related to child/adolescent, so that we can handle legal issues in adolescents in the best possible manner.

## Defining a Child

- According to the Convention on the Rights of a Child (CRC Article 1), a child is every human being below the age of 18 years, unless majority is attained earlier under applicable law.
- The Juvenile Justice (JJ) (Care and Protection of Children) Act of 2015 defines a child as any person below the age of 18 years.
- The Protection of Children from Sexual Offences (POCSO) Act 2012 also states that a child is any person below the age of 18 years.
- Article 15(3) of the Constitution empowers the state to make special provisions for women and children, recognizing their unique needs and rights.

## Child/Adolescent Employability

Article 24 of the Indian Constitution expressly prohibits the employment of any child below the age of 14 years in factories, mines, or any hazardous employment.

The 42nd Amendment reinforces the protection of children and youth, emphasizing the need to provide opportunities for healthy development, ensuring conditions of freedom and dignity. It aims to safeguard childhood and youth from exploitation and moral or material abandonment.

## Major Laws for the Protection of Children/ Youth in India

Government initiatives safeguarding youth in India include crucial laws to prevent violence, abuse, and exploitation. Key legislations such as the "Right of Children to Free and Compulsory Education Act 2009", the "Beedi and Cigar Workers (Condition of Employment) Act 1966", and the "Child Labour Regulation and Prohibition Act 1986" play a pivotal role. In this chapter, two major Acts are described in detail. These Acts are of utmost importance while dealing with the adolescent age group in practice.

### *Protection of Children from Sexual Offences (POCSO) Act 2012*

This law is the first of its kind, which is victim friendly and gender neutral. It is a comprehensive law that has made justice possible for the victim within a stipulated time set by the court. The victim is not traumatized multiple times for telling the happenings. The Act makes it favorable for the victim to get counseling and financial help. It is also gender neutral as it recognizes the crimes committed against a male or a female (under 18 years of age) as equally punishable.

The POCSO Act, 2012, was granted approval by the President on June 19, 2012. It was officially announced in the Gazette of India on the following day, June 20, in the same year.

*Definition:* "Any sexual act (consensual or nonconsensual) with child below 18 years is sexual offence."

*Main Features:*
- It is an act to protect children from offences of sexual assault, sexual abuse, and pornography.
- It is an act to provide for the provision of special courts for the trial of such offenses.
- It provides that the special court proceedings should be recorded in camera and the trial should take place in the presence of parents or any other person in whom the child has trust or confidence.
- Police is designated "the Responsible Protector".
- Compensation is to be granted within 30 days, even if the accused has not been convicted.
- Minimum punishment is prescribed and can be up to life imprisonment depending upon the gravity of the crime.
- It is mandatory for any medical or nonmedical person to report a case of any form of sexual abuse. Nonreporting is punishable under the POCSO Act.
- Not providing first-aid medical treatment is a medical offense under Criminal Amendment Law Act 2013.
- Any medical establishment, big/small, needs to follow standard operating procedure (SOP).

### *The Juvenile Justice (Care and Protection of Children) Act, 2015 (JJ Act No. 2 of 2016)*

This act came into force on December 31, 2015.

*Definition:* A legislation aimed at consolidating and refining the legal framework pertaining to children accused of and identified as being in conflict with the law, as well as those requiring care and protection. The law seeks to address the fundamental needs of such children by ensuring proper care, protection, development, treatment, and social reintegration. Embracing a child-friendly approach, the Act facilitates the fair adjudication and resolution of matters in the best interest of children, emphasizing their rehabilitation through established processes, institutions, and bodies. It encompasses related matters and addresses incidental concerns connected therewith.

WHEREAS the provisions of the Constitution confer powers and impose duties, under clause (3) of article 15, clauses (e) and (f) of article 39, article 45, and article 47, on the State to ensure that all the needs of children are met and that their basic human rights are fully protected.

AND WHEREAS, the Government of India has acceded on the December 11, 1992 to the Convention on the Rights of the Child, adopted by the General Assembly of the United Nations, which has prescribed a set of standards to be adhered to by all State parties in securing the best interest of the child;

AND WHEREAS, it is expedient to re-enact the Juvenile Justice (Care and Protection of Children) Act, 2000 (56 of 2,000) to make comprehensive provisions for children alleged and found to be in conflict with law and children in need of care and protection, taking into consideration the standards prescribed in the Convention on the Rights of the Child, the United Nations Standard Minimum Rules for the Administration of Juvenile Justice, 1985 (the Beijing Rules), the United Nations Rules for the Protection of Juveniles Deprived of their Liberty (1990), the Hague Convention on Protection of Children and Co-operation in Respect of Inter-country Adoption (1993), and other related international instruments.

## Miscellaneous Laws and Projects by Government of India

The Government of India has undertaken numerous initiatives to foster the development of a robust and law-abiding youth. These endeavors include a strong emphasis on protecting children from various forms of abuse. Several projects and treaties have been instituted to address these objectives. Some of the projects are as follows:

- The 24/7 child helpline, known as 1098, serves as the initial recourse for round-the-clock assistance, dedicated to rescuing and aiding children and adolescents in need.
- Active participation in international treaties, such as the UNCRC, underscores the commitment to global child-welfare standards.
- The establishment of the National Policy for Children in 1974 reflects a foundational framework for shaping comprehensive policies that prioritize the welfare of children.
- Promoting data collection, research, and action, exemplified by the "Study on Child Abuse 2007", highlights the government's proactive stance in addressing and understanding child-abuse issues.
- The formation of the National Commission for Protection of Child Rights in 2007 further solidifies the commitment to safeguarding the rights and well-being of children.
- The *Rashtriya Kishore Swasthya Kalyan Yojana* (RKSK) exemplifies a collaborative effort, bringing together both public and private stakeholders to enhance the overall health and well-being of the youth.

## Additional Legal Considerations

When dealing with the age group of 9–18 years, pediatricians must be attuned to various legal issues crucial to their practice. While this chapter touches on a few points, a comprehensive understanding of each of the following is vital for effective adolescent care:

- Road traffic accidents
- Suicides and mental disorders
- Substance abuse
- *Porn-related issues:* Every second 372 people are typing the word "adult" into search engines.
- Live-in relationships
- *Sexuality issues:* Homosexuality, lesbian, gay, bisexual, transgender, and questioning (or queer) (LGBTQ), etc.
- *Food safety issues:* Food Safety and Standards Act, 2006 (FSSAI)
- Legalities in immunization.

## ■ CONCLUSION

It is clear that adolescent medicine is different and more complex than pediatrics in general. The medicolegal angle has to be understood and followed in all aspects, while dealing with this group of patients. Also the adolescent practitioner needs to be updated regularly about the changes in the dynamic Laws of the respective country. With the advent of internet, this group of patients are well aware of their rights. Thus a doctor of medicine needs to have better knowledge of both disease and law.

## KEY MESSAGES

- Adolescents have specific rights and legal considerations that healthcare professionals must navigate for ethical practice.
- Clear communication, respect for privacy, and adherence to legal frameworks are essential for effective adolescent care.
- Laws like POCSO and the JJ Act play a crucial role in protecting children and ensuring justice.
- Pediatricians act as crucial advocates in recognizing and addressing the physical and mental health issues resulting from abuse.
- Government initiatives and international collaborations underline a commitment to the holistic well-being of children and youth.

## RECOMMENDED READING


1. Foreman DM. The family rule: A framework for obtaining ethical consent for medical interventions from children. J Med Ethics. 1999;25(6): 491-6.
2. India Code. (2015). The Juvenile Justice (Care and Protection of Children) Act, 2015. [online] Available from https://www.indiacode.nic.in/bitstream/123456789/8864/1/201602.juvenile2015pdf.pdf [Last accessed March, 2024].
3. Katz AL, Macauley RC, Mercurio MR, Moon MR, Okul AL, Opel DJ, et al.; AAP Committee on Bioethics. Policy Statement. Informed consent in decision-making in pediatric practice. Pediatrics. 2016;138(2):e20161484.
4. Sharma RK. Consent. In: Sharma RK (Ed). Legal Aspects of Patient Care. New Delhi: Modern Publishers; 2000. pp. 3-6.
5. Sobti PC, Biswas G, Sobti BS. Medicolegal issues in adolescent health care. In: Bhave SY, Parthasarathy A, Bhave SY, Nair MKC, Menon PKC, Greydanus DE (Eds). Bhave's Textbook of Adolescent Medicine. New Delhi: Jaypee Brothers Medical Publishers (P) Ltd; 2006. pp. 42-59.
6. The Indian Medical Council. (2002). (Professional Conduct, Etiquette, and Ethics) Regulations, 2002. [online] Available from https://www.mciindia.org/documents/rulesAndRegulations/Ethics%20Regulations-2002.pdf [Last accessed March, 2024].
7. Yadav M. Age of consent in medical profession: A food for thought. J Indian Academy Forensic Med. 2007;29:80-5.


<table>
<tr><td>**2.6**</td><td># Common Questionnaires and Formats for History Taking</td></tr>
</table>

*Sandeep Kavade*

## INTRODUCTION

In the dynamic field of adolescent medicine, effective history taking is the cornerstone of providing patient-centered care. Adolescent healthcare professionals must navigate a landscape of profound physical, emotional, and social changes. Mastery of the art of history taking is crucial to meet the multifaceted needs of this diverse age group, enabling the delivery of personalized care that aligns with their evolving needs and values.

## ADOLESCENT INTERVIEW PROCESS

- *Introduction:* Begin by introducing yourself to both the adolescent and their parents, setting a comfortable stage for the conversation.
- *Confidentiality understanding:* Ask either the parents or the adolescent to express their understanding of confidentiality in healthcare.
- *Confidentiality statement:* After hearing their perspectives, provide a brief overview of confidentiality, emphasizing its importance and the exceptions, which only apply in cases of physical risk or legal matters.
- *Trust building:* Clarify that the interview's objective is to support the adolescent in facing their situation. Stress the paramount importance of confidentiality unless extreme circumstances necessitate exceptions.

Doctors now recognize unique challenges posed by adolescent patients, leading to the evolution of various history-taking formats. These assist physicians in understanding an adolescent's life, emphasizing their social environment, school experiences, and peer relationships to uncover underlying mental health concerns.

Dealing with adolescents reveals significant variability within the same age group in maturity levels, physical development, and diverse social and familial contexts. Standardized formats provide a foundation but must be adapted to each specific adolescent.

In the Indian context, where social dynamics vary widely, tailoring history-taking approaches is crucial. Indian adolescents often have less autonomy and financial independence, requiring a more individualized approach. In the Indian context, the role of parents and extended family has to be taken into account during history taking. Healthcare professionals adjust emphasis based on age, social background, parental situation, and economic circumstances. Effective adolescent history taking is a nuanced process acknowledging diverse needs in various cultural contexts.

## HEEADSSS FORMAT

The home, education/employment, eating, activities, drugs, sexuality, suicide/depression, and safety (HEEADSSS) format, developed in the late 1980s by Dr John Goldenring, is a valuable tool for healthcare providers to gather crucial information about adolescents systematically and nonthreateningly. It has evolved to include new aspects of adolescent health, like technology and social media usage. The HEEADSSS mnemonic is a useful tool for taking a social history from adolescents.

**Table 1** summarizes the key domains and the specific inquiries to consider when engaging with adolescents on various aspects of their lives.

Salient features of the HEEADSSS format are as follows:
- Addresses various aspects of a young person's life
- Encourages open-ended questions and active listening
- Promotes a nonjudgmental and confidential environment
- Covers a wide range of adolescent concerns, including mental health, substance use, and relationships.

Utilizing the HEEADSSS framework in adolescent history taking goes beyond data collection. It is crucial to explore factors associated with each heading, which can impact adolescent health positively or pose risks.

The primary goal of HEEADSSS is to address immediate health concerns and guide adolescents in harnessing strengths to become self-reliant. Healthcare providers actively help identify coping mechanisms, resilience, and personal resources, empowering adolescents to manage their well-being proactively.

A comprehensive history-taking process is pivotal for providing tailored anticipatory guidance and preparing adolescents for potential future challenges. This includes discussions on sexual health, substance use, mental well-being, and safety.

Investing time in obtaining a detailed history builds trust between healthcare providers and adolescents, fostering openness. Genuine interest and nonjudgmental care encourage adolescents to disclose hidden or sensitive issues **(Table 2)**.

## SSHADESS SCREENING: A STRENGTH-BASED PSYCHOSOCIAL ASSESSMENT

SSHADESS, derived from the HEADSSS format, focuses on emotional and mental well-being in adolescent history taking, reflecting the increasing importance of addressing mental health issues. SSHADESS, is an acronym for Safety, Sexuality, Home environment, Alcohol and drug use, Depression and emotional well-being, Education and employment, Suicide risk, Safety from injury.

Salient features of the SSHADESS format are as follows:
- Provides a comprehensive overview of an adolescent's life, like HEADSSS
- Emphasizes emotional and mental health aspects

**TABLE 1:** Key domains and inquiries to consider when engaging with adolescents.

| Domain | Inquiry |
|---|---|
| Home | Living situation, relationships with family/friends, and significant stressors in life |
| Education/employment | School/work life and academic/vocational challenges faced |
| Eating and exercise | Diet, exercise habits, and concerns about eating disorders |
| Activities | Hobbies, extracurricular activities, and social relationships |
| Drugs and alcohol | Alcohol, tobacco, and drug use |
| Depression and suicide | Mood, suicidal thoughts, and history of self-harm |
| Sexuality | Sexual orientation, sexual activity, and concerns about sexual health |
| Safety | Safety at home, school, and in the community |

**TABLE 2:** Examples of a few helpful and detrimental factors to be considered in each domain of HEEDSSS. This list may vary as per individual case.

| Assessment | Helpful | Detrimental |
|---|---|---|
| Home | Positive parent relationship, good communication, and trusted adult | Conflicts with parents, problematic parenting, and poor communication |
| Education/employment | Positive attitude about school and trust and communication with teachers | School avoidance, discrimination beliefs, extreme academic expectations, failure, or absenteeism |
| Eating/exercise | Positive attitude about regular physical activity, exercise, involvement in sports. Balanced and nutritious diet | Poor physical activity. Over or undernutrition. Junk food habits, food fads |
| Activities | Extracurricular involvement, and religious/spiritual practice | Lack of supervision, risky behaviors, overscheduling, and inadequate nutrition/sleep |
| Drugs | No substance abuse by peers/family, negative attitude toward substances, and past use but now abstinent | Substance use by peers/family and early/consistent involvement |
| Sexuality | Intention to abstain, not currently sexually active, or using reliable protection | Unprotected sex, pregnancy/STI history, and sexual assault/abuse history |
| Suicide/depression/self-image | Caring adult support, peer network, healthy coping skills, and positive self-esteem | Depression, isolation, suicidal ideation, attempt history, and trauma |
| Safety | Good problem-solving skills and nonviolent conflict resolution | Easy weapon access and victimization through violence/bullying |

(STI: sexually transmitted infections)

- Aids in identifying potential issues like self-harm, suicidal thoughts, or emotional distress
- Encourages healthcare providers to delve deeper into the emotional state of the adolescent.

*Rationale for the modified approach:*
- *Emphasis on strengths:* Acknowledges the strengths of the youth, avoiding a singular focus on risks and reducing associated shame
- *Sequential approach to school and home:* Addresses school-related matters before discussing the home environment, considering the sensitivity of home-related issues
- *Comprehensive emotional screening:* Expands emotional screening beyond depression and suicidal thoughts to capture a range of emotions, ensuring a nuanced understanding of adolescent mental and emotional well-being.

Structured interviews, emphasizing sensitivity and trust-building, are vital. A doctor must take care about the following:
- *Sequential progression:* Start with general topics, progressing gradually to more personal ones, facilitated by the SSHADESS screening.
- *Impersonal to intimate questions:* Begin with impersonal questions within sensitive topics to ease into more personal details.

- *Neutral reaction:* Maintain a nonjudgmental stance to avoid disrupting disclosure. Minimize quick positive reactions.
- *Early praise:* Offer process-focused praise, avoiding summative praise early in the interview.
- *Open-ended questions:* Avoid yes-or-no questions to encourage depth of responses, especially when trust is being established.
- *Rapid disclosure does not decide risk:* Be cautious as rapid disclosure does not necessarily indicate low risk; it could signal a need for bonding or emotional regulation.
- *Postinterview permission:* After the interview, seek permission to address any concerns, enhancing receptiveness to guidance and suggestions.

## ■ SUMMARY OF INTERVIEW

At the end of an adolescent healthcare interview, it is vital for healthcare professionals to provide a concise summary. This summary serves as a point of alignment, ensuring a shared understanding of the healthcare plan. It should outline identified health concerns, pending tests or interventions, and the treatment plan. Addressing any unresolved issues encourages ongoing communication and problem-solving, enhancing transparency and fostering shared responsibility in the adolescent's care.

## CONCLUSION

In summary, effective adolescent history taking involves creating a comfortable environment, clarifying confidentiality, and building trust. By adapting to diverse challenges, using open-ended questions, and empowering adolescents, we can support their well-being. Providing guidance on sensitive topics and using screening tools like HEADSSS/SSHADESS help identify issues. Prioritizing trust, empathy, and empowerment fosters better communication and health outcomes for adolescents.

## KEY MESSAGES

- *Establish a comfortable introduction:* Begin by introducing yourself to create a comfortable environment for conversation.
- *Clarify confidentiality:* Discuss confidentiality and its exceptions, ensuring clarity for both the adolescents and their parents.
- *Build trust:* Emphasize on the interview's aim to support the adolescent while stressing the importance of confidentiality.
- *Adapt to diverse adolescent challenges:* Tailor history-taking approaches to suit individual needs, considering cultural and social differences.
- *Utilize open-ended, nonjudgmental approach:* Employ open-ended questions and a nonjudgmental approach to understanding various adolescent concerns.
- *Empower through history taking:* Identify coping mechanisms and empower adolescents to manage their well-being actively.
- *Provide anticipatory guidance:* Discuss potential future challenges such as sexual health, substance use, and safety.
- *Focus on trust building:* Invest time in building trust to encourage open communication and disclosure of sensitive issues.
- *Assess helpful and detrimental factors:* Understand factors impacting adolescent health within the domains of HEEADSSS.
- *Implement HEEADSSS/SSHADESS screening:* Use tools to get detailed history while giving emphasis to emotional well-being and identify potential issues like self-harm or emotional distress.

## RECOMMENDED READING

1. American Academy of Pediatrics. (2011). HEADSSS assessment: Risk and protective factors. [online] Available from https://www.heardalliance.org/wp-content/uploads/2011/04/HEADSS.pdf [Last accessed March, 2024].
2. Bhave SY, Mehta R. History taking and approach to an adolescent client. In: Bhave SY, Parthasarathy A, Bhave SY, Nair MKC, Menon PKC, Greydanus DE (Eds). Bhave's Textbook of Adolescent Medicine. New Delhi: Jaypee Brothers Medical Publishers (P) Ltd; 2006. (Chapter 1.3)
3. Ginsburg KR. The SSHADES Screening: A strength-based psychosocial assessment. [online] Available from //www.aap.org/contentassets/0e45de0366d54ec38fbfcb72382a0c6c/rt2e_ch32_sahm.pdf [Last accessed March, 2024].
4. Goldenring JM, Cohen E. Getting into adolescent heads. Contemp Pediatr. 1988;5:75.
5. Goldenring JM, Rosen DS. Getting into adolescent heads: An essential update. Contemp Pediatr. 2004;21:64.

# 2.7 | Referrals in Adolescent Practice

*Neeti Soni*

## INTRODUCTION

Adolescence is a challenging time as teenagers face a lot of complexities (due to peer pressure, academic stressors, changing body structure, discordant family, etc.), which require a thorough evaluation by an adolescent-health consultant and when needed by a specialist to help them sort out their problems. The goal of adolescent health practice is that an adolescent gets healthcare that is uninterrupted, coordinated, developmentally appropriate, and psychologically sound before and throughout the transfer of child to youth and into adult system.

Many adolescents and young adults, both male and female, grapple with a range of complex issues, such as mental health challenges, eating disorders, gynecological problems, and substance abuse. It is important to note that more than 50% of adult mental health issues first emerge during adolescence. Additionally, as obesity becomes more prevalent, an increasing number of adolescents are seeking assistance for related health problems.

In order to effectively address these issues, it is crucial to develop referral practices that foster an environment in which teenagers feel comfortable expressing themselves fully and do not fear judgment from their healthcare providers. Adolescents may feel uneasy if issues related to confidentiality, an unfriendly atmosphere, or social stigma are present in the healthcare setting. To promote the well-being of young people, it is essential to consider their potential struggles with treatment adherence and their level of satisfaction with their healthcare provider when making referrals.

Utilizing a multidisciplinary approach to patient care can significantly enhance patient management. This approach allows various experts to leverage their experience and skills in treating the patient at hand. Referrals may be necessary in a variety of fields, including psychiatry, psychology, endocrinology, dermatology, gynecology, and internal medicine.

Traditionally, a referring clinician obtains input from a specialist by either sending patient for in-person referrals or through "curbside consultations", that is, conversation that occurred between two physicians about the patient wherever they met or telephonically. Curbside consultations are initiated for a variety of reasons, including perceived reliability of expert opinion, urgency, cost, timelessness, accessibility, convenience, fear of malpractice litigation, reassurance, desire for academic discussion, and autonomy.

The teenager has fostered enough courage to put forth the problem in front of an adolescent-health consultant, and getting referred to another consultant from there is a matter of disappointment for them. Hence, while referring, it is important to take the child in confidence and discuss the referral process in detail.

- Clearly explain the need for the referral.
- Emphasize the effectiveness of psychopharmacological treatments and address concerns about addiction.
- Alleviate worries about the stigma associated with seeing a psychiatrist and taking psychotropic medications.
- Reassure the patient that the referral does not mean they are being abandoned; the relationship and follow-up care will continue.
- Set up the referral appointment and ensure the adolescent reaches the clinic. In emergencies, ensure a parent or guardian accompanies the patient and understands the seriousness of the situation.
- Provide a comprehensive referral note, addressing any shortcomings in the referral process.

*An ideal referral note should include:*
- Service/specialty clinic to be referred
- Reason for referral
- If the referral is urgent or routine
- International Classification of Diseases, Tenth Revision (ICD-10) diagnosis (if referral is for mental health problem)
- All relevant clinical documents should be sent along with:
  - Most recent heart rate and blood pressure
  - Clinic notes
  - Medication history
  - Growth charts
  - Laboratory reports
  - Diagnostic imaging reports [e.g., ultrasound, computed tomography (CT) scan, and magnetic resonance imaging (MRI)]
  - Previous specialty evaluations
- Patient's full name, date of birth, sex, address, and guardian's contact information
- Referral provider's name, phone number, and email address so that they can be contacted for additional information, if need be.

Other than infections, the major causes of morbidity and mortality experienced by adolescents can be attributed to preventable causes, including sexually transmitted infections (STIs), suicide, unintended pregnancy, accidents, and obesity. The common conditions when there is a need for referral/urgent referrals are given in the following text.

## ■ PSYCHIATRIST

Adolescents are great "minimizers" and "deniers". Every piece of information has to be immediately translated into useful knowledge in practice. Home, education/employment, peer group activities, drugs, sexuality, suicide/depression, and safety (HEADSSS) assessment is the standard protocol used by all adolescent health consultants while evaluating a patient with suspected mental health issue. Commonly seen disorders in clinical practice are: Major depression, manic episode, schizophrenia, substance abuse, eating disorders, conduct disorder, and anxiety disorders, namely panic attacks, phobias, post-traumatic stress disorder (PTSD), obsessive–compulsive disorder (OCD), etc.

These patients in moderate-to-severe cases require pharmacotherapy, psychotherapy in form of cognitive behavior therapy (CBT), and at times interventions in the form of admission, electroconvulsive therapy, etc. A primary physician can manage uncomplicated cases if they have adequate training, experience, and consultative support. However, complicated cases with comorbid conditions [attention-deficit hyperactivity disorder (ADHD) or substance abuse], bipolarity, suicide attempts, psychosis, multiple episodes of depression, or treatment-resistant cases are best handled by a child psychiatrist.

*Indications for urgent referral to a psychiatrist:*
- *Suicidal adolescent with:*
  - History of recent attempt
  - History of previous attempt
  - Family history of suicide
  - Under the state of severe agitation/panic
  - Having a suicidal plan
  - Means of suicide easily reachable
  - No social support
- Acute psychosis
- Episode of severe anger/aggression/violent behavior with threat to safety of self/others
- Overdose of addictive substance.

## GYNECOLOGIST

Certain gynecological conditions which are best to be seen by an adolescent gynecologist are:
- Painful or irregular periods
- Teen pregnancy
- Ovarian masses, cysts, and tumors
- Fertility and reproductive health
- Polycystic ovarian syndrome (PCOS)
- Pubertal aberration
- Various surgical/nonsurgical gynecological conditions

*Indications for urgent referral to a gynecologist:*
- Ruptured ectopic pregnancy
- Ruptured hemorrhagic ovarian cyst
- Ruptured tubo-ovarian abscess
- Acute abdominal pain with abnormal vaginal bleeding
- Sexual abuse

## ENDOCRINOLOGIST

Common endocrinological problems in practice are as follows:
- Height of adolescent <3rd percentile or >95th percentile for age
- Signs of precocious puberty (before 8 years for girls and 9 years for boys) or delayed puberty (no signs after 13 years for girls and 14 years for boys)
- PCOS
- Metabolic syndrome
- *Thyroid disorders:* High or low thyroid-stimulating hormone (TSH)
- High blood sugar or diabetes mellitus—type 1 or type 2
- Ambiguous genitalia
- Pituitary disorders
- Adrenal disorders

*Indications for urgent referral to an endocrinologist:*
- Thyroid storm
- Myxedema coma
- Diabetic ketoacidosis (DKA)
- Adrenal crisis

## DERMATOLOGIST

Acne, warts, molluscum, urticaria, eczema, and atopic dermatitis are common dermatological issues seen in pediatric clinics.

Few emergency situations needing urgent referrals are angioedema, Steven–Johnson syndrome, toxic epidermal necrolysis, necrotizing fasciitis, and rarely Staphylococcal scalded skin syndrome seen in immunocompromised teenagers.

## KEY MESSAGES

- Adolescent health practice aims at providing healthcare that is coordinated, uninterrupted, developmentally appropriate, and psychologically sound.
- Multidisciplinary approach is needed for enhanced management, and hence referrals may be needed.
- Curbside consultations have a lot of merit in adolescent healthcare.
- Taking the child in confidence is vital before referral.
- The referral process must be followed meticulously to alleviate worries and anxiety.
- Understanding indications to various specialists (psychiatrist, gynecologist, endocrinologist, dermatologist, etc.) is important and especially the urgent referrals.
- A detailed referral note with all the relevant information is absolutely mandatory.

## ■ RECOMMENDED READING


1. Bhave SY, Nair MKC, Parthasarathy A, Menon PSN, Greydanus DE (Eds). Bhave's Textbook of Adolescent Medicine. New Delhi: Jaypee Brothers Medical Publishers (P) Ltd; 2006.
2. De Sanctis V, Soliman AT, Fiscina B, Elsedfy H, Elalaily R, Yassin M, et al. Endocrine check-up in adolescents and indications for referral: A guide for health care providers. Indian J Endocrinol Metab. 2014;18(Suppl 1):S26-38.
3. Kansra AR, Lakkunarajah S, Jay MS. Childhood and adolescent obesity: A review. Front Pediatr. 2021;8:581461.
4. Kershnar R, Hooper C, Gold M, Norwitz ER, Illuzzi JL. Adolescent medicine: Attitudes, training, and experience of pediatric, family medicine, and obstetric-gynecology residents. Yale J Biol Med. 2009;82(4):129-41.
5. Michaud PA, Fombonne E. Common mental health problems. BMJ. 2005;330(7495):835-8.
6. Parthasarathy A, Menon PSN, Nair MKC (Eds). IAP Textbook of Pediatrics. New Delhi: Jaypee Brothers Medical Publishers (P) Ltd; 2019.
7. Peck GM, Roberson FA, Feldman SR. Why do patients in the United States seek care from dermatologists? Dermatol Ther (Heidelb). 2022;12(4):1065-72.

**Section Editors:** *Sushma Desai, Swati Ghate*


## Part A: General Mental Health


**Sub-section Editors:** *Swati Ghate, Sushma Desai*


## 3A.1 | Introduction to Adolescent Mental Health


*Chinmay Kinjawadekar, Upendra Kinjawadekar*


### ■ INTRODUCTION

As per the census of 2011, there are more than 250 million adolescents in India. This means that every fifth person one comes across is likely to be aged between 10 and 19 years. Our country also boasts of the highest adolescent population in the world. What does this signify? As we understand, the working population of a country plays an important role in its economic growth and prosperity. With the highest number of working population in the years to come, our adolescent population of today is instrumental in driving the country forward.

For any individual to be able to function to the best of their ability, their physical and mental health needs to be functioning optimally. This responsibility rests with the healthcare system to attend to the physical and mental health needs.

As a nation, we have made progressive strides in terms of looking after our children's and adolescents' physical health—improving nutrition and reducing under-5 mortality in terms of both quality of healthcare and national policies. The mental healthcare standards, however, have not realized their full potential.

Moreover, the cost of providing adequate care for mental illness places an economic burden on the family which further hampers mental health recovery.

Adolescence can be described as a physiological stage of development occurring between childhood and adulthood. In this phase, there are simultaneous developments occuring across physical, biochemical, and functional aspects in the brain.

The central nervous system compromises of certain areas like the prefrontal cortex, limbic system, ventral striatum, and parts of the midbrain which form a part of an individual's psyche. The neural connections from these areas along with its various neurotransmitters influence the cognitive, emotional, social, and behavioral aspect of an individual. These developments in an individual's psyche tend to become less receptive to change as a person ages. This suggests that adolescence is an influential period in an individual's life. Impressions that are formed during this period tend to have lasting consequences and contribute toward shaping up an individual's personality in the years to come.

### ■ EPIDEMIOLOGY

The National Mental Health Survey in 2016 reported a 7.3% prevalence rate for mental illness in adolescents aged between 13 and 17 years. This number increases if you include the prevalence of substance-use disorders. The distribution of mental illnesses among boys and girls was relatively similar. India being a vast country naturally shows disparity in the prevalence rates of certain illness across different regions. In addition, the numbers derived from community samples differ from school samples with higher observed cases in school-derived data.

Overall, there are estimated to be over 60 million children and adolescents suffering from a mental illness at any given time. The common mental disorders reported were depressive disorders, intellectual disabilities, anxiety disorders, and developmental disorders with behavioral difficulties. Sociocultural factors highlight differences in mental health concerns in different regions. Some states in India show an overall higher incidence of alcohol (15%) and tobacco-use disorder (7%) among adolescents as compared to depressive disorder.

Under-reporting of mental illnesses is a common shortcoming observed during data analysis. This could be attributed due to various factors; most notably, lack of appropriate information, the social stigma associated with mentally ill, and cultural beliefs and practices. The prevalence rates across certain urban areas in India were twice the rural regions. This disparity could partly be attributed to increased availability of healthcare resources in urban areas leading to more reporting of cases in cities.

## Adolescents and Suicide

Death by suicide is one of the leading causes of death among adolescents in India. The national suicide rate as of 2021 was approximately 12% and over 1.5 lakh Indians died by suicide in that year. Amongst these, a large proportion were students between 10 and 19 years of age. As per the National Crime Bureau reports in 2015, one student dies by suicide every hour in this country. The prevalence rate across boys is slightly higher than for girls.

Death by suicide is an unnatural form of death that can be prevented each time with timely identification and delivery of resources to the individual. Misconceptions about suicide, victim, blaming, and considering suicide as an act of weakness are some of the barriers the society faces in its attempts to educate people.

Recognising symptoms of stress in a teenager experiencing mental health difficulties can be done best by the people around them; hence, it is important to empower the parents and caregivers with appropriate knowledge. Sudden or marked changes in behavior, expressing passive death wishes or engaging in risk-taking activities, alterations in sleeping and eating habits, lethargy, and lack of motivation are often pointers toward underlying stress that the brain is experiencing.

## Adolescence and Internet

The digital revolution in recent times has modified the environment in which an adolescent grows up today. The adaptive nature of a young brain can be observed as children and teenagers seem to possess an increased capacity to absorb technology and keep up with the advancements. More than 90% of adolescents use the internet in some way or the other. Social media has incorporated itself into the life of an individual. Faster and easier communication, access to information from across the globe, and advancements in academic learning methods are some of the benefits of these digital times. On the other hand, behavioral addictions are on the rise. Cyberbullying and online abuse/hate have become a source of stress. Internet addiction and gaming addiction are now being medically recognized as disorders requiring medical and psychosocial interventions.

## ■ PSYCHOPATHOLOGY

The epidemiological triad of any infectious disease typically consists of interaction between the host, the environment, and the pathogen.

Mental illness similarly could be described as an interaction between biological, psychological, and social forces in an individual's life. These interactions are complex in nature, and multiple determinants have an impact on the severity, the manifestation, and the prognosis of any mental illness.

From the point of view of trying to understand this model of mental illness, adolescent mental health can be viewed from the point of view of its basic determinants—the individual (host), the socioeconomic influences (environment), and the stressors in the life of an adolescent (pathogen).

## Individual (Host)

Erik Erikson, one of the pioneers in the field of psychology, described the life of any individual in stages that centered around psychosocial development.

According to Erikson, adolescence is a stage where an individual is trying to establish a sense of self-identity for one's self. The development of a healthy ego identity, i.e., a conscious sense of self that we develop through our interactions in society, is the central theme in this period. Success in this stage of life leads to an ability to stay true to yourself and enables healthy development. Any conflicts during this stage of development cause more confusion in self-identity and can have long-lasting consequences on one's personality. While this development is physiological in nature, it highlights the importance of understanding the mental stage of development of the individual as most mental illnesses have been observed to have their onset in the adolescent period.

Individual characteristics and personality traits ensure variability in the manifestation of a similar mental illness across different individuals.

## Socioeconomic Factor (Environment)

The surroundings in which a child and adolescent grow naturally influence the thought process of that individual. The nature of relationships that the adolescent experiences with family members and friends and socioeconomic standard of living influence the basic mental state. The surroundings at school, influence of teachers and the academic responsibilities are additional factors affecting the mood of an individual.

A burden on any of these factors mentioned is bound to exert pressure on the growing adolescent brain. Few variables increase the likelihood of an adolescent developing psychopathology. These are called risk factors.

Environmental risk factors like poverty, social injustice, recent sociocultural changes, poor neighborhoods, substance abuse, and violence negatively impact an adolescent's mental health.

Individuals living in poverty and neglected neighborhoods are vulnerable to suffering from mental illness. They become more susceptible to acts of crime, violence, substance use, and sexual abuse.

On the other side good family support, stable living conditions, good friends/social relations, healthy lifestyle habits, crime-free neighborhood, and lack of substance use are some of the environmental factors that exert a positive effect on the developing brain.

The use of the internet and social media has increased significantly in the last decade. During the adolescent phase, the variety of unsupervised information and increased accessibility toward age-inappropriate content put the individual at risk of being misinformed. Social media has also influenced the way individuals perceive themselves in reality and in terms of their online personality. These challenges threaten to cause confusion in establishing a secure sense of self-identity, emphasizing the importance of the social environment in psychopathology.

## Stressors (Pathogen)

In the context of a mental illness, stress can be described as a qualitative force that directly impacts the individual. Stress is also unique in nature as it could be perceived differently in two different individuals in a similar situation. While the level of a certain stressor is difficult to measure, it can be observed in terms of its biological impact on the brain and the psychosocial consequences on the life of an individual.

Academic performances and social interactions are perceived to be central aspects in an adolescent's life. Academic achievements are seen to be associated with providing a sense of worth to an individual. Similarly, a healthy relationship with friends and participation in other activities—sports, art, music, etc.—provide an environment conducive to growth.

During these years, managing academics at schools and tuition, difficulties in learning, and volatile nature of friendships/relationships during teenage years are some of the challenges an individual goes through. Results and achievements are assumed to be associated with a sense of self-worth. The gap in the expectations from oneself and others around widens. During these times, a stressful event like failing an exam could trigger the onset of a chain of reactions eventually damaging the mental health. Internet bullying is becoming increasingly common and has added to the already existent burden of bullying present in schools and colleges. A recent example of a 10th standard state topper who was at the receiving end of internet trolling and abuse for her appearance indicates toxic effects of being viral on the internet.

A stressor or a stressful event is believed to trigger the onset of a cascade within the brain which involves the interplay of biological mechanisms, psychological defenses of an individual, and social environment. This cumulative effect leads to the emergence of clinical symptoms of mental illness.

## Adolescent Lifestyle after COVID Pandemic

In the 21st century and more so after the coronavirus disease 19 (COVID-19) pandemic, there has been a major shift in the lifestyle of all human beings across the globe.

The rapid shift in the market forces across all industries—education, media, health, and nutrition along with the rise of consumerism—could pose a threat to the adolescent lifestyle trends in the coming future.

The availability of fast and affordable internet coupled with the rise of social media has led to increased dependency on smartphones and devices. Increasing screen time, especially at night, is seen to negatively impact the sleep schedule and quality.

A generally reduced attention span is observed as one of the consequences of increased screen use and the type of content consumed (shorts, reels).

Online mode of teaching during the pandemic and shifting back to classroom environments have been difficult for the students to adjust to. This coupled with reduced attention span has posed further learning challenges in schools and tuitions.

There is a plethora of unhealthy food choices available in the market. The accessibility toward unhealthy food choices in the market has increased. It has become easier to procure unhealthy food at affordable prices. The consumption of ultra-processed food and sugar has increased susceptibility to obesity, diabetes at an early age, and various kinds of eating disorders. These lifestyle modifications and the current social environment are significant as they highlight the role the caregiver plays in implementing a healthier environment around the teenager. Every individual adapts to an environment and lifestyle in a unique way as per their understanding and it is imperative to consider these lifestyle changes in the current day and age before determining any teenager's behavior as problematic or pathological.

## ■ MANAGEMENT

### What are the Current Barriers in the Delivery of Mental Health Services?

The frequent barrier that makes it difficult for people to access healthcare is the lack of adequate and appropriate information about mental health.

There are myths, misinformation about psychotropic medications, and certain cultural beliefs that are prevalent in our society concerning mental health. The stigma associated with a person, if he suffers from a "mental" illness in society, is concerning and a major deterrent in consulting a mental health professional. The vast nature of our country also ensures regional variation in the beliefs and attitudes toward mental health.

Certain behavioral patterns which may be acceptable in some communities may not be acceptable in others. Standard of education, intellectual capacity, and socioeconomic conditions also influence an individual's ability to understand their mental health.

Lack of community-based interventions and trained mental health care professionals in terms of demand result in below-par delivery of mental health services.

These factors result in a delay for an individual seeking mental health care and worsen the prognosis of the illness.

### What should be the Approach to Treating a Mental Illness?

Since the origin and the manifestation of any mental illness are multifactorial, the treatment is proven to be most effective when it is managed on a biological, psychological, and social level together.

These include medical interventions using psychotropics for moderate-to-severe cases of depression, behavioral concerns associated with intellectual difficulties, substance addictions, and psychotic symptoms.

Therapy, counseling from trained mental health professionals, and community-based interventions like support groups are able to provide support for the psychological development of the individual. Delivery of adequate healthcare services requires coordination and development along all these aspects.

The number of mental health care professionals to serve the required population is low compared to the burden of mental illness. This emphasizes the need for increased sensitization among other medical professionals concerning mental health. Identifying mental disorders early or timely referral to the nearest accessible mental health clinic could provide benefits in some cases and reduce the economic burden on the family in the long run.

A crucial aspect of managing mental illness involves being able to give adequate information in a way that is understandable to the parents/caregivers. The communication between the doctor and the patient at this initial junction could determine the individual's and family's attitude toward mental health. This is an important step as destigmatizing mental illness and clearing certain myths around it are as important as treating mental illness. Good family support is a positive prognostic factor in all mental health conditions.

The nature of the social environment influences the recovery in certain cases. A teenager with substance addiction is more likely to worsen if they are blamed or shamed for their behaviors and habits. Teachers in schools and colleges are important figures in an adolescent's journey. Their recognition of an adolescent's learning difficulties or observing changes in behavior could guide a parent toward giving the required attention to their child.

Awareness among parents and teachers within institutions concerning bullying on campus and online bullying are additional responsibilities that the caretakers need to be aware of.

This inevitably boils down to the awareness and information people receive regarding mental health. General physicians, pediatricians, and surgeons are often the first point of contact for many people in healthcare. Their role in providing adequate information or addressing general concerns becomes instrumental in determining the attitude an individual and a family develops toward mental health care.

## KEY MESSAGES

- Mental illness is to be looked at holistically from a point of biological, environmental, and social factors.
- Adolescence is an influential period of development where the brain is susceptible to forming strong impressions that contribute to personality development.
- Mental illness during adolescence has an increased likelihood of developing psychiatric comorbidities during adulthood.

- Current lifestyle modifications and behavioral patterns should be considered before labeling any adolescent behavior as problematic or pathological.
- Destigmatizing mental illness is as important as managing the illness.

## RECOMMENDED READING


1. American Psychiatric Association. Diagnostic and Statistics Manual of Psychiatry (DSM-5). [online] Available from https://www.psychiatry.org/psychiatrists/practice/dsm [Last accessed March, 2024].
2. Casey P, Kelly B. Fish's Clinical Psychopathology: Signs and Symptoms in Psychiatry. Scotland: RCPsych Publications; 2019.
3. Erikson EH. Identity and the life cycle. WW Norton; 1994.
4. IACAPAP (International Association for Child and Adolescent Psychiatry and Allied Professions). Textbook of Child and Adolescent Mental Health. [online] Available from https://iacapap.org/resources/e-textbook.html [Last accessed March, 2024].
5. Thapar A, Pine DS, Leckman JF, Scott S, Snowling MJ, Taylor MJ. Rutter's Child and Adolescent Psychiatry, 6th edition. New York: Wiley-Blackwell; 2015.


<table>
<tr><td>3A.2</td><td><h1>Doing What Matters in Times of Stress</h1></td></tr>
</table>

C P Bansal

## WHAT IS STRESS?

Stress is a physical and emotional reaction to the challenges in life. Occasional stress is a normal coping mechanism of the body, but long-term stress or chronic stress may contribute to or worsen a range of physical and mental health issues and that is why it is a major underlying cause of a variety of health issues of present-day life.

## STRESS IN ADOLESCENTS

Adolescence is a period of storm and stress as they have heightened stress response. 45–80% of teens described themselves as "often or always feeling stressed." 89% of the Indian population is suffering from stress; yet, do not feel comfortable talking to medical professionals **(Fig. 1)**.

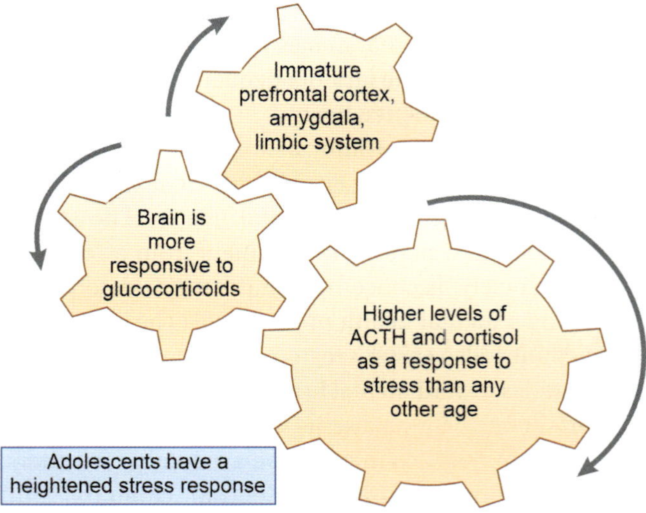


**Fig. 1:** Physiology of adolescent stress. (ACTH: adrenocorticotropic hormone)

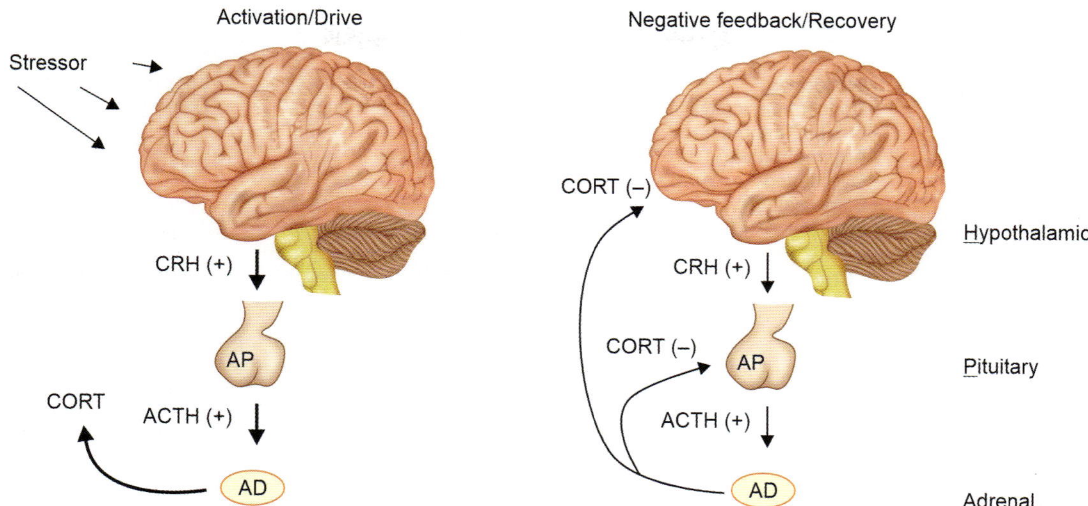

**Fig. 2:** Normal stress response. (ACTH: adrenocorticotropic hormone; AD: adrenal gland; AP: anterior pituitary; CORT: corticosterone; CRH: corticotrophin-releasing hormone)

## NORMAL STRESS RESPONSE

The body reacts by releasing hormones that produce the "fight-or-flight" response.

Stress-induced activation of the hypothalamic–pituitary–adrenal (HPA) axis as well as the negative feedback of the HPA axis recovers back to baseline following termination of a stressor **(Fig. 2)**.

## SYMPTOMS OF STRESS

"Stress" means feeling troubled or threatened by life. Everyone experiences stress at times. A little bit of stress is not a problem. But very high stress often affects the body. Many people get unpleasant feelings and many of us think a lot about bad things from the past or bad things we fear in the future. These powerful thoughts and feelings are a natural part of stress but problem is when we get "hooked" by them. It pulls us away from our "values". When hooked, our behavior changes. We often start doing things that make our lives worse. We call these behaviors "away moves" as we are moving away from our values **(Figs. 3 and 4)**.

## CAUSES OF STRESS

There are many causes of stress, including personal difficulties (e.g., conflict with loved ones, being alone, lack of income, and worries about the future), problems at work (e.g., conflict with colleagues and an extremely demanding or insecure job), or major threats in your community (e.g., violence, disease, and lack of economic opportunity).

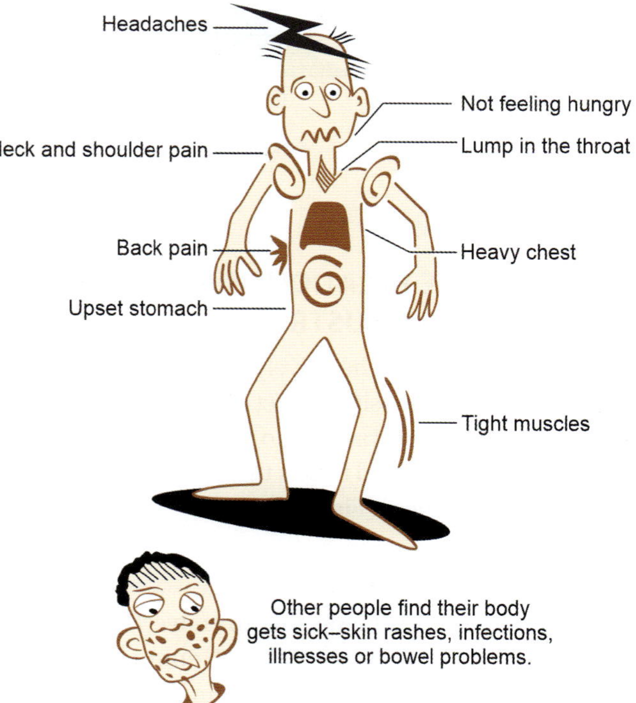


**Fig. 3:** Symptoms of stress.

If you are experiencing stress, you are not alone. Right now, there are many other people in your community and all around the world who are also struggling with stress.

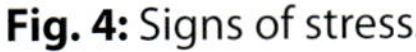



**Fig. 4:** Signs of stress.

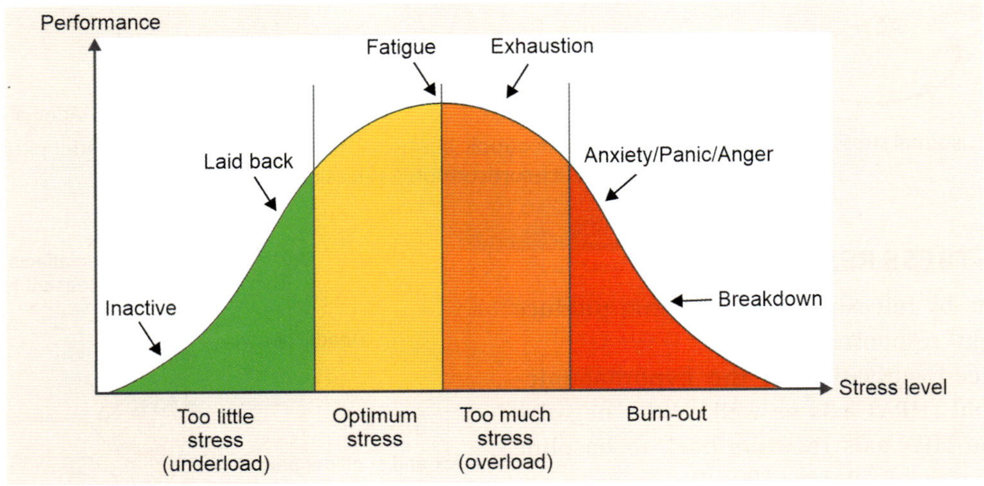



**Fig. 5:** Levels of stress.

## WHAT IS THE RELATIONSHIP BETWEEN DISTRESS AND EUSTRESS?

Distress is the stress that negatively affects you, and eustress is the stress that has positive effect on you. Eustress is what energizes us and motivates us to make a change. It gives us a positive outlook and makes us capable of overcoming obstacles and sickness **(Fig. 5)**.

## DEALING WITH STRESS

Dealing with stress is being able to convert distress into eustress or optimal stress. **Table 1** enumerates some common unproductive ways of dealing with stress. The adolescents should be educated and guided against finding solace using the above mentioned methods.

**If it is distress, what can we do (Box 1)?**

First, you learn how to focus, engage, and pay attention better.

There are many ways to practice engaging in life or focusing on what you are doing.

**TABLE 1:** Unproductive way of dealing with stress.

| Addictions | Unproductive ways |
| --- | --- |
| Alcohol | Trying not to think about |
| Tobacco | Avoiding people, places, or situations |
| Internet use | Isolating yourself—staying in bed |
| Gaming | Starting arguments |
| Drugs | Blaming and criticizing oneself |

**BOX 1:** Ways to manage stress.

- Stress management tools for adolescents
- Healthy life-style
- Role of caregivers and adults
- Relaxation techniques
- Various available resources

We have to practice with five tools for *Doing What Matters in Times of Stress* to help ourselves to relieve the stress **(Box 2)**.

<table>
<tr><td>

**BOX 2:** Stress management tools.

- Grounding
- Unhooking
- Acting on values
- Being kind
- Making room

</td><td>

**BOX 3:** Approaches to any difficult situation.

*Remember that there are three approaches to any difficult situation:*
1. Leave
2. Change what can be changed, accept the pain that cannot be changed, and live by your values
3. Give up and move away from your values

</td></tr>
</table>

## Tool 1: Grounding

*Ground yourself* during emotional storms by *Noticing* your thoughts and feelings, *Slowing Down* and *Connecting* with your body by slowly pushing your feet into the floor, stretching, and breathing, and then *Refocusing* and *Engaging* with the world around you. What can you see, hear, touch, taste, and smell? Pay attention with curiosity to what is in front of you. Notice where you are, who is with you, and what you are doing.

## Tool 2: Unhooking

*Unhook yourself* with these three steps: (1) *Notice* that a difficult thought or feeling has hooked you. Realize that you are distracted by a difficult thought or feeling, and notice it with curiosity; (2) Then silently *Name* the difficult thought or feeling; (3) Then, *Refocus* on what you are doing. Pay full attention to whoever is with you and whatever you are doing.

## Tool 3: Acting On Your Values

Choose the values that are most important to you. For example: (1) Being kind and caring; (2) being helpful; (3) being brave; and (4) being hardworking. You get to decide which values are most important to you! Then pick one small way that you can act according to these values in the next week. What will you do? What will you say? Even tiny actions matter!

## Tool 4: Being Kind

Notice pain in yourself and others and respond with kindness. Unhook from unkind thoughts by *Noticing* and *Naming* them. Then, try speaking to yourself kindly. If you are kind to yourself, you will have more energy to help others and more motivation to be kind to others, so everyone benefits.

## Tool 5: Making Room

Trying to push away difficult thoughts and feelings often does not work very well, so instead, *Make Room* for them: (1) *Notice* the difficult thought or feeling with curiosity. Focus your attention on it. Imagine the painful feeling as an object, and notice its size, shape, color, and temperature. (2) *Name* the difficult thought or feeling. (3) Allow the painful feeling or thought to come and go like the weather **(Box 3)**. As you breathe, imagine your breath flowing into and around your pain to make room for it. Instead of fighting with the thought or feeling, allow it to move through you, just like the weather moves through the sky. If you are not fighting with the weather, then you will have more time and energy to engage with the world around you and do things that are important to you.

You may know different ways like Yoga and Meditation to keep you stress-free. This brief guide based on the World Health Organization (WHO) manual makes this learning simpler for using these tools. We must strive to make all this a part of our life.

"Doing What Matters in Times of Stress" is a WHO stress management guide for coping with adversity. I highly recommend reading and following it.

### ■ KEY MESSAGES

- Stress is a physical and emotional reaction to the challenges in life.
- Occasional stress is a normal coping mechanism of the body.
- Eustress makes us motivated and capable of overcoming obstacles.
- Adolescents have heightened stress response, and it is a period of storm and stress.
- There are many unproductive ways to deal with stress but one can learn to use five tools given in "Doing what matters in stress."

### ■ RECOMMENDED READING


1. WHO. (2020). Doing What Matters in Times of Stress. [online] Available from https://www.who.int/publications/i/item/9789240003927 [Last accessed March, 2024].

# 3A.3   Relaxation Techniques for Adolescents (Yoga, Meditation, and Mindfulness)

*Pukhraj Bafna (Padmashri)*

## ■ RELAXATION TECHNIQUES

Adolescence is a period of rapid physical and biological changes that may lead to turbulence, turmoil, tension, confusion, frustration, and feelings of insecurity. It is said to be a period of storm and strife, stress, and strain due to restlessness and disturbances because of the nature of development that takes place during this period. Adolescence is a crucial period where one attains maturity—physically, emotionally, intellectually, sexually, and socially. The problems during the adolescent period may predispose to certain disorders for which the adolescent may need relaxation.

Relaxation techniques are the ways to help adolescents with stress management. It is not only about peace of mind or enjoying a hobby but a process that decreases the stress effects on mind and body. It can help in coping with everyday stress in adolescents.

## Different Types of Relaxation Techniques

Generally, relaxation techniques involve refocusing attention on something calming and increasing awareness of the body.

*Types of relaxation techniques include:*

- *Autogenic relaxation:* Autogenic means something that comes from within. Here adolescents can use both visual imagery and body awareness to reduce stress.

    One should repeat words or suggestions in mind that may help relax and reduce muscle tension. One may imagine a peaceful setting. After this one should focus on relaxing breathing, slowing heart rate, or feeling different physical sensations, such as relaxing each arm or leg one by one.

- *Progressive muscle relaxation:* Here one should focus on slowly tensing and then relaxing each muscle group.

    This can help the adolescent focus on the difference between muscle tension and relaxation. One can become more aware of physical sensations.

One can tense muscles for about 5 seconds and then relax for 30 seconds, and repeat, from head to toe or reverse.

- *Visualization:* In this relaxation technique, adolescent may form mental images to take a visual journey to a peaceful, calming place or situation.

    In visualization techniques, adolescent should try to include as many senses as they can, such as sight, smell, sound, and touch.

    Adolescent should close their eyes, sit in a quiet spot, loosen any tight clothing, and focus on breathing. The aim should be to focus on the present and have positive thoughts.

*A few other relaxation techniques include:*

- Yoga
- Meditation
- Deep breathing
- Massage
- Biofeedback
- Music and art therapy
- Aroma therapy
- Hydrotherapy

## Benefits of Relaxation Techniques

There are many benefits which can give a quality life while practicing relaxation techniques regularly, such as:

- Reducing activity of stress hormones
- Increasing blood flow to major muscles
- Reducing muscle tension and chronic pain
- Slowing heart rate
- Lowering blood pressure
- Slowing breathing rate
- Improving digestion
- Controlling blood sugar levels
- Reducing fatigue
- Improving mood and focus
- Improving quality of sleep
- Reducing frustration and anger
- Boosting confidence in handling problems.

Adolescents should use relaxation techniques along with other positive coping methods to get the most benefit, such as:

- Exercising regularly
- Eating a healthy diet
- Getting enough sleep
- Managing time and priorities
- Thinking positively
- Finding humor
- Problem-solving
- Spending time outside
- Supporting family and friends.

## YOGA FOR ADOLESCENTS

An old Indian rich heritage Yoga is the art and science of life and is concerned with the evolution of body and mind. Yoga is a technique for total personality development at physical, mental, emotional, and spiritual level. It is an internal technique through slowing down the system, calming down the mind, silencing the mind, and resting the system. Yoga increases the capacity to face frustrations and problems of life. Yoga is based on four disciplines—Asana, Pranayama, Pratyahara, and Dhyana.

Pranayama or breathing techniques supply fresh oxygen, strengthen the lungs, and have a direct effect on brain and emotions. Thus, the adolescent gets mental and creative energies in a constructive way and exhibits more self-confidence, self-awareness, and self-control.

Pratyahara or relaxation by withdrawing the awareness from the external environment lessens the stress of daily life. It gives physical and mental relaxation to adolescents; Dhyana or sustained concentration is important for stilling the turbulent mind and channeling focused mental energy creativity.

### Physical Aspects of Yoga

*Supportive systems:* The adolescent should be encouraged to maintain erect posture without tension and strain. Flexibility, agility, and correct postures are very important benefits for young bodies.

*Control systems:* Here is the role of pineal gland, which is seat of wisdom and intuition; it is closely linked with Agya chakra in yoga. A disruptive behavior is often evinced at this age such as anger, resentment or violence, much of which can be directly or indirectly attributed to hormonal changes. The imbalance of hormones may result in withdrawal, depression, anxiety, and lethargy. Adolescent may lack dynamism and cannot transform his mental energy to creative action. Yoga balances the mental component of mind (manas shakti) and the vital component of bioenergy (prana shakti). Yoga also maintains a balance between sympathetic (Pingla) and parasympathetic (Ida) nervous systems.

*Metabolic systems:* Adolescents are encouraged to practice many forms of breathing techniques, e.g., Nadi shodhana, alternate nostril breathing to balance the two hemispheres of brain. Yogic pranayama and abdominal breathing are the two important examples for achieving efficiency in respiration; thus, increasing the lung capacity, cardiovascular efficiency, and mental state.

*Emotional/behavioral aspects:* Yoga automatically brings sobriety through balance between mental component and vital component of the body.

*Mental aspects:* The ability to concentrate, remember, reason, involving conscious, subconscious, and unconscious mind with systemic stimulation of both hemispheres are included in the mental aspects of yoga. Yoga practice has been shown to significantly improve the accuracy of visual perception. Yoga also facilitates auditory perception with changes at thalamocortical level.

*Creative aspects:* In adolescents, imagination, visualization, vocalization, and cultivation of one's own personality give them creative aspects of life through yoga. Yoga has been shown to influence certain higher brain functions.

The practice of yoga helps to keep the young body strong and supple and incorporates mental activities and disciplines that help to develop attention and concentration.

*Yoga as preventive medicine:* A few simple practices starting from early adolescent age will help to balance the mental and vital energies and preserve the pineal gland, thus delaying sexual maturation and preventing needless psycho-emotional distress. The adolescent can be taught "Surya namaskar", a dynamic exercise involving 12 different movements. Stretching and relaxation are provided by yoga, thus enabling the body to rebalance the energy. Alternate nostril breathing—"Nadi shodhana Pranayama"—teaches the adolescent how to induce calmness within himself. The total practice period should not take >30 minutes a day.

## Techniques of Yoga Practice

The place of yoga practice should be calm and quiet, clean, well ventilated, and insect free, and should be carpeted if possible. Early morning is the best time of yoga practice. It should not immediately follow a meal. There should be a gap of 2 hours between eating and starting yoga practice. Asanas should be practiced first, then pranayama, ending with relaxation or concentration. One should always breathe through the nose unless instructed otherwise. Asana practice without awareness of the body is not yoga. Body awareness induces relaxation while in posture. Asana with tension may have opposite effect. The bowels should be evacuated and bladder should be empty before asana practice.

## Some Important Asanas

*Sukhasana (Easy pose):* Sit with legs stretched in front of the body, bend the right leg and place the foot under the left thigh. Then bend the left leg and place the foot under the right thigh. Place the hands on the knees and keep the spine, neck, and head in a straight line as shown in **Figure 1**.

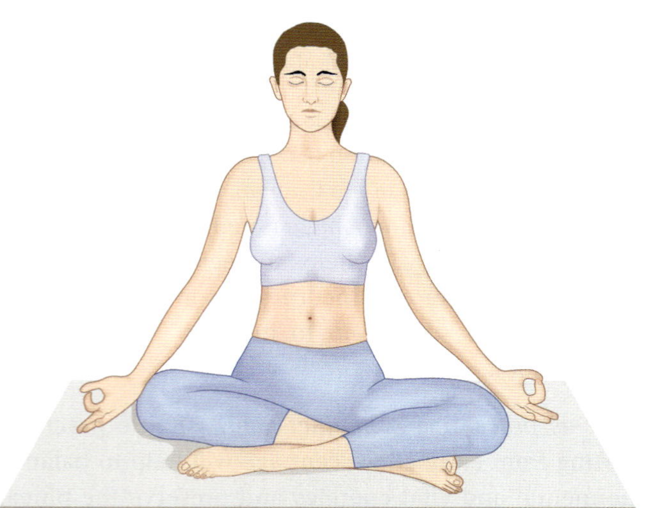

**Fig. 1:** Sukhasana (Easy pose).

*Shavasana (Corpse pose):* One should lie on the back with feet comfortably apart, spinal column straight but not rigid, and the arms rest on the floor about 15 cm away from the body with palms up. Head is in line with spine and eyes and mouth are closed. One should not move any part of the body. Become aware of the breath and let it become rhythmic and natural **(Fig. 2)**. This is the best asana for relaxation.

*Shashank asana (Hare pose):* One should seat with folded knees and soles below the buttocks (vajrasana) and place the hands on the knees, keep the spine and head straight. Now slowly inhale and raise the arms above the head synchronizing the movement of arms and breath. Keep the arms and shoulder wide apart. Exhale slowly and bend the trunk forward bringing the chest to rest on the thighs and forehead to the floor in front of the knees. The arms remain outstretched in front of the body and the palms and elbows are resting on the floor. Breathe normally holding posture for 10 seconds. Inhale while returning slowly back to upright position with arms stretched over the head. After inhaling and returning to upright position, exhale and bring the hands back to rest on knees **(Fig. 3)**. This posture is effective for toning pelvic muscles, relaxing the sciatic nerves, and regulating the functioning of adrenal glands. It helps relieve constipation, sciatica, and anger.

*Surya namaskar (Salutation to the Sun):* This yoga practice has 12 positions (Asanas) as described in **Figures 4 to 10**. Position 4 is Pranayama asana (Prayer pose), which establishes a state of concentration, calmness, and awareness of practice. Position 5 is hasta uttanasana (raised arm pose), which stretches all the abdominal organs fully, exercises the arms and shoulder, tones the spinal cord, and opens up the lungs. Position 6 is Padahastasana (hand to foot pose). It reduces surplus abdominal fat, improves digestion and circulation, and eliminates constipation. Position 7 is Ashwa sanchalanasana (equestrian pose). It tones abdominal muscles, strengthens the muscles of thighs and legs, and induces balance in nervous system. Position 8 is Parvatasana (mountain pose), which strengthens the nerves and muscles of the arms and legs and exercises

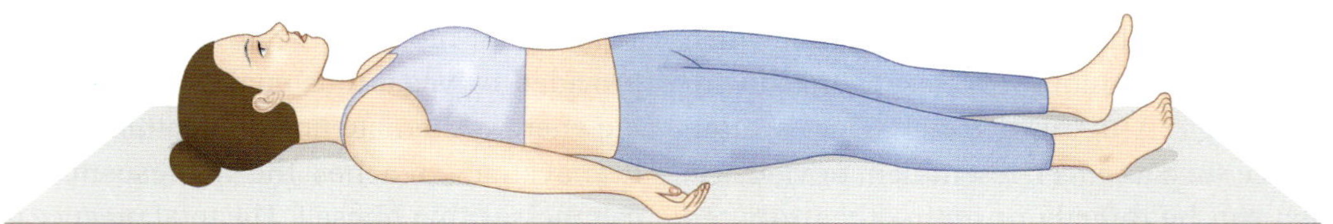

**Fig. 2:** Shavasana (Corpse pose).

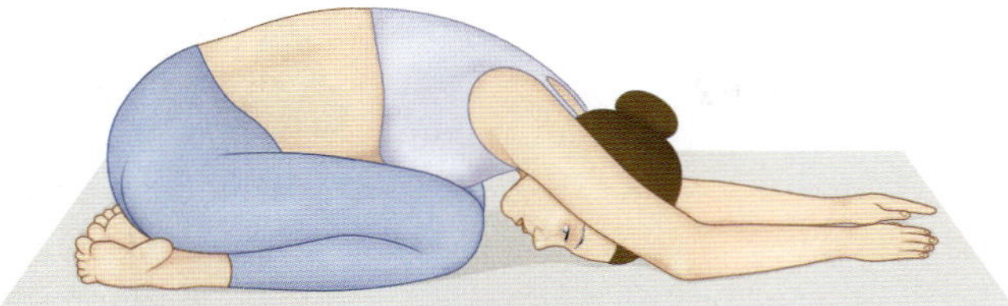

**Fig. 3:** Shashank asana (Hare pose).

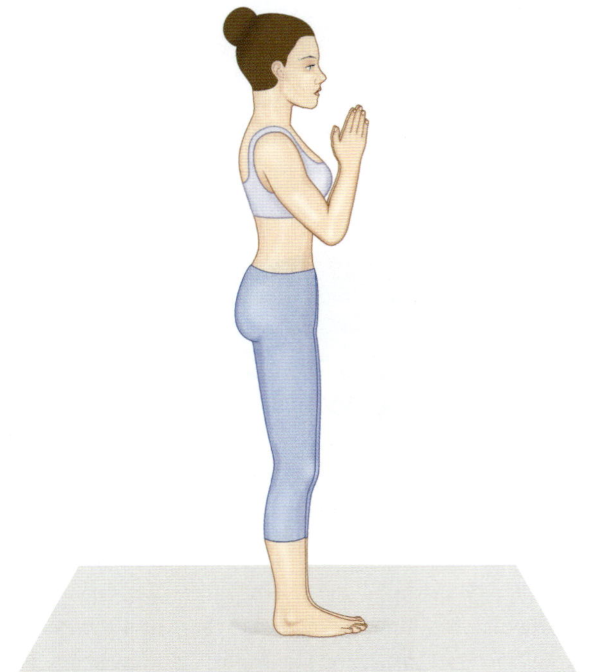

**Fig. 4:** Pranayama asana (Prayer pose).

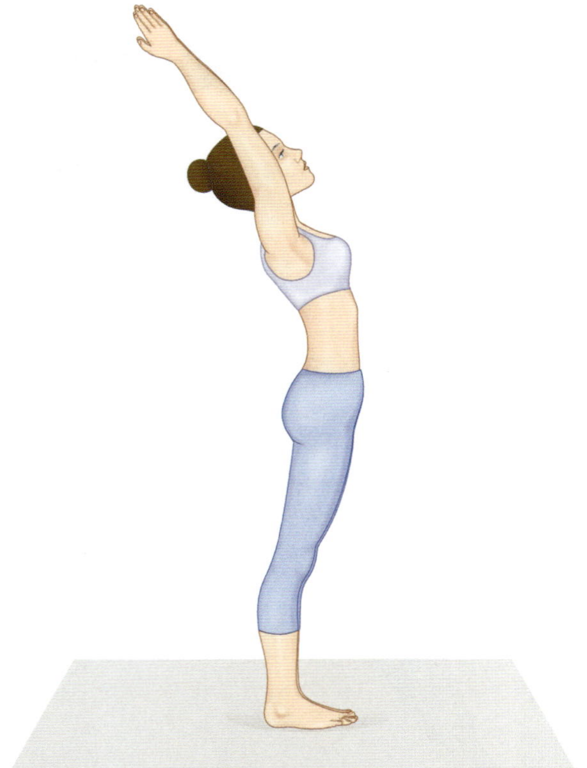

**Fig. 5:** Hasta uttanasana (raised arm pose).

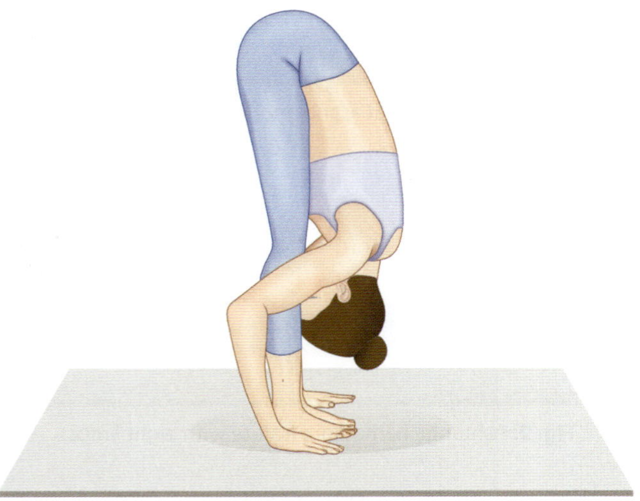

**Fig. 6:** Pada hastasana (hand to foot pose).

the spine. Position 9 is Ashtanga namaskara (salute with 8 limbs); it tones the shoulders and neck muscles, strengthens legs and arm muscles and develops the chest. Position 10 is Bhujangasana (Cobra pose), useful for all stomach ailments, improves circulation, revitalizes spinal nerves, and has a balancing effect on many hormones.

These seven asanas are repeated from back to forward like Position 10 to Position 4. Surya namaskara is an ideal yoga practice for adolescents with only a limited amount of time to devote to practices of asana and pranayama. It also influences pineal gland and hypothalamus. This balances the transition period between childhood and adolescence.

## Some Important Pranayamas

*Nadi shodhana pranayama (Alternate Nostril Breathing):* One should sit in any of the comfortable asanas, ensuring spine in erect and both knees are resting on the floor. Close the eyes, place left hand on left knee, and right hand is used to close the nostril. The index and middle fingers are placed in the center of eyebrow and remain in this position throughout the practice. The thumb is used to close the right nostril and the ring figure is used to close the left nostril. The breathing is alternated by closing one and

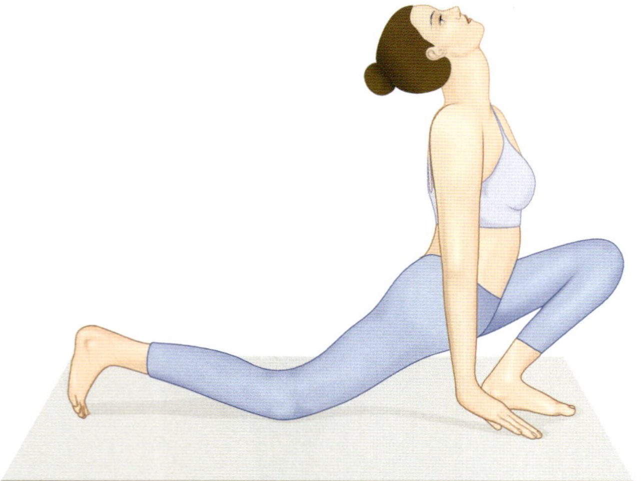

**Fig. 7:** Ashwa sanchalanasana (equestrian pose).

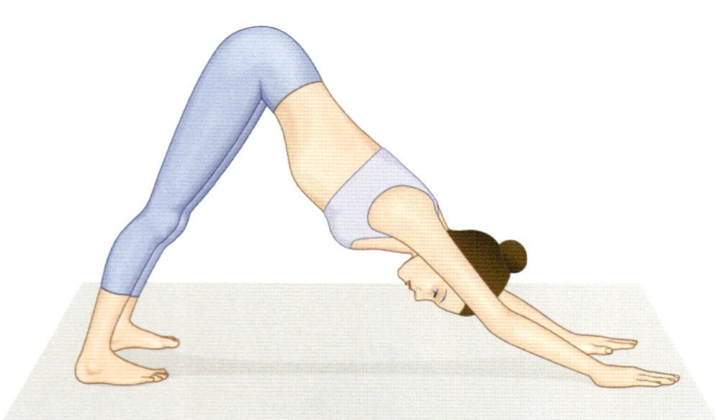

**Fig. 8:** Parvat asana (mountain pose).

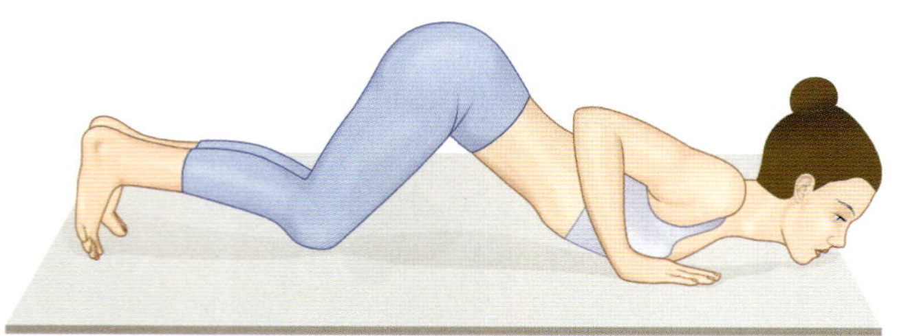

**Fig. 9:** Ashtanga namaskara (salute with eight limbs).

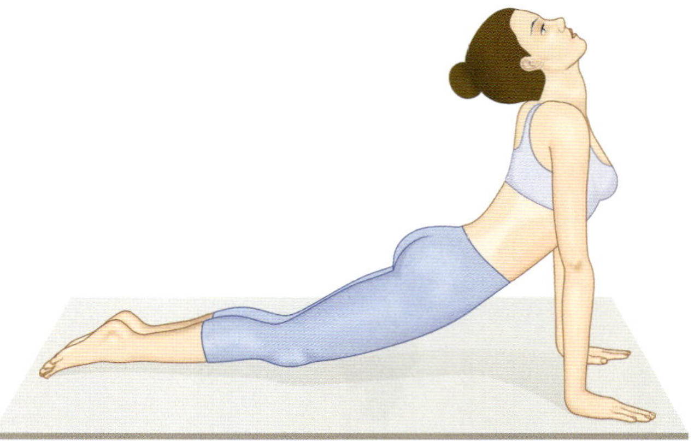

**Fig. 10:** Bhujangasana (Cobra pose).

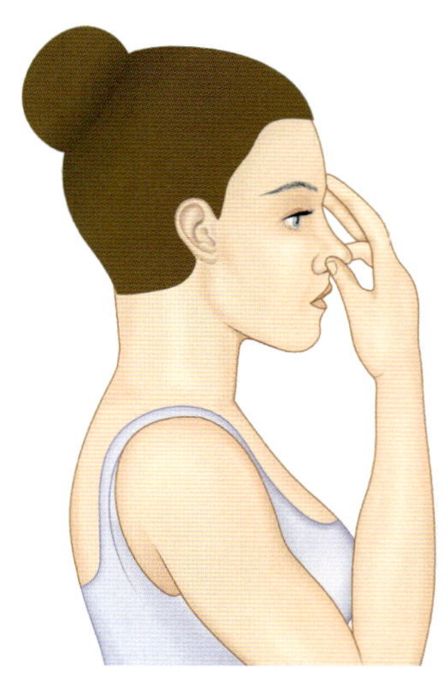

**Fig. 11:** Nadi shodhana pranayama (Alternate Nostril Breathing).

keeping the other open **(Fig. 11)**. This breathing exercise induces tranquility, clarity of thoughts, and concentration.

*Bhramari pranayama (Humming Bee Breath):* One should in any comfortable asana with spine erect, head straight, and both knees resting on the floor. One has to simply close the eyes and relax the whole body for some time. Inhale fully through both nostrils. Now plug the ears with index fingers with the teeth apart and mouth closed. Exhale completely while producing humming sound like that of a bee. Exhalation should be slow and steady and concentrate on the humming sound **(Fig. 12)**. This pranayama will not be performed lying down. This pranayama alleviates tension caused by anger and anxiety. It helps to relieve headaches and sleeplessness. It increases memory power.

*A few more important asanas:* Sampadasana, Tadasana, Pada hastasana, and Trikonasana are beneficial for this age as shown in **Figures 13 to 16**.

## Yoga Therapy in Different Ailments

*Yoga for release of tension (Tannav mukti):* Tadasana, Surya namaskara, Yognidra (relaxation without sleeping), Shavasana, and Bhramari pranayama are the real remedies for tension.

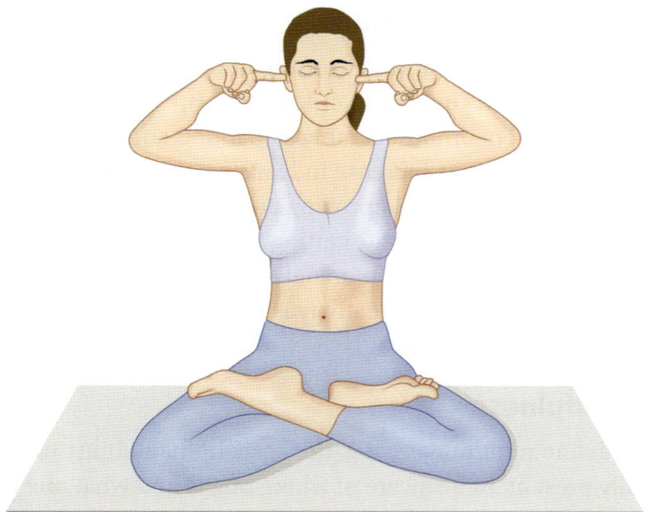

**Fig. 12:** Bhramari pranayama (Humming Bee Breath).

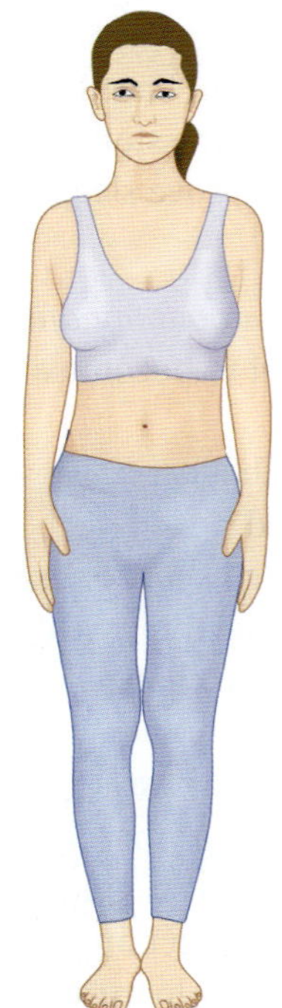

**Fig. 13:** Sampadasana.

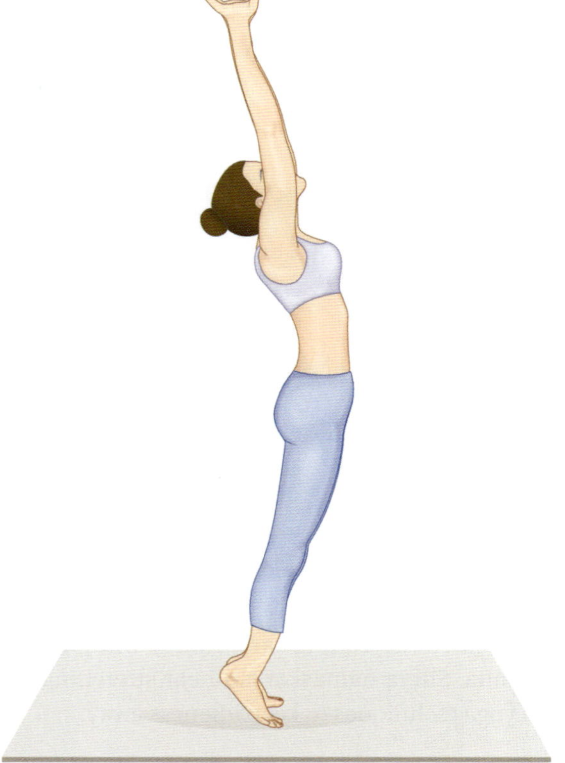

**Fig. 14:** Tadasana.

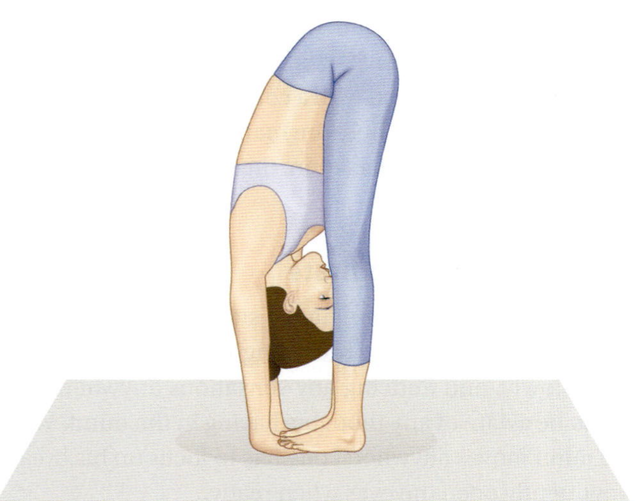

**Fig. 15:** Pada hastasana.

*Yoga for addiction (Nasha mukti):* Practices of Preksha meditation and kayotsarga have been observed to make young people free of addiction (Acharya Mahapragya).

*Yoga to enhance memory power:* Bhramari pranayama, Sarvangasana (shoulder stand or candle pose), and Shashank asana (pose of the hare) may help in activating dormant areas of brain and significant increase in visual, audio, verbal, and audiovisual memory.

*Yoga for headache:* Eye movements, Shavasana, Yognidra, and Kayotsarga are helpful in relieving different types of headaches.

*Yoga for anger:* Shashank asana, Yoga mudra, Yognidra, Bhramari pranayama, and deep breathing exercises diminish anger and make the adolescent calm.

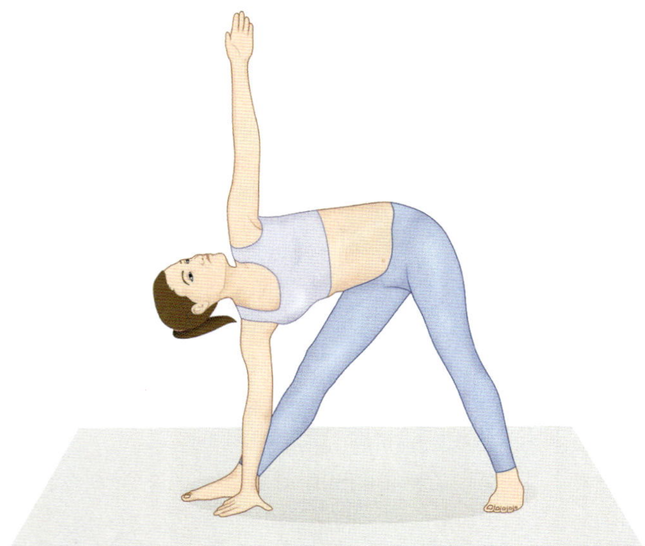

**Fig. 16:** Trikonasana.

*Yoga for idleness:* Namaskar mudra, Bhujang asana, Matsyasana, Surya namaskar, and ear stretching are the proved yoga techniques to keep idleness away.

## ■ MEDITATION FOR RELAXATION

Meditation is a powerful process of yoga that provides profound rest to the system, which allows the mind to calm down to its normal states. It is a practice that focuses and clears adolescents mind with a combination of mental and physical techniques. There are many ways of meditations; one can meditate for relaxation, thus reducing anxiety and stress.

### Simple Steps to Meditate

To meditate honestly one has to sit upright comfortably, closing the eyes gently, breathing deeply, scanning the body slowly, and noticing any sensations anywhere. One has to be aware of any thoughts having in the mind. When the mind moves anywhere, one has to focus on his breath. Now, gently open the eyes when ready.

Meditation is a solution to reduce stress of adolescent in the midst of busy academic activities and lifestyle.

A few popular types of meditation practice include Mindfulness, Spiritual, Focused, Transcendental, Movement meditation, Meditation with Mantras, Progressive relaxation, visualization meditation, etc.

Every type of meditation practice may not be right for everyone. Different skills and mindsets are required for different people; one has to choose the befitting one.

## Benefits of Meditation

Daily practice of meditation for about 15–20 minutes morning and evening cultivates the energy and cultures it. The mind becomes expanded and awareness increases. There is increase in learning ability, in solving problems accurately, improving academic performances, improving relations, and getting clear and undisturbed thoughts. The stress and anxiety are decreased; there is relief from insomnia; creativity is increased and provides balanced and stable health.

## Mindfulness

To define mindfulness, it is the basic human ability to be fully present, to be aware of where one is and what one is doing, not very reactive or overwhelmed by what is going on around. Mindfulness is something everyone naturally possesses. If we practice regularly, it is more readily available to us.

Mindfulness treatment based on mindfulness reduces anxiety, stress, and depression. Mindfulness can lower blood pressure and improve sleep and help to cope with pain.

*Some points to ponder about mindfulness:*
- It has the potential to become a transformative social phenomenon.
- It is how to live with life.
- It is evidence based.
- Mindfulness is not obscure or exotic.
- It is not a very special thing we do.
- One does not need to change.
- It is easy to do.
- It is innovative in many ways.

One should remember that Mindfulness is a state of mind and state of calmness, gratitude, and compassion, which has a profound effect on adolescents. To practice mindfulness, one has to learn breathing methods and guided imagery and other practices for relaxation of mind to reduce stress.

## ■ KEY MESSAGES

- Relaxations are need-based and problem-oriented techniques for physical and mental problems, such as stress and anxiety. There are different types of relaxation techniques; the choice depends from person to person according to need, time, and situation.
- Yoga can prove to be an excellent edition as a part of lifestyle and routine practice for adolescents.

- Yoga can be an essential tool in total personality building of young adolescents. It has the power of solving all sensitive problems of this age.
- Yoga can be of great help in preventing and curing many illnesses if practiced properly and timely under some expert's supervision.
- Meditation is essential as daily practice which gives peace of mind and concentration among adolescents.
- Mindfulness is the need of the day for all ages, particularly adolescents who keep them busy for their academics, career, and jobs.
- All the above relaxation techniques cost nothing but regularity and timely involvement.

## ■ RECOMMENDED READING


1. Bafna P. Yoga for adolescents. In: A Parthasarathy, Swati Y Bhave, MKC Nair, PSN Menon, Donald E Greydanus (Eds). Bhave's Textbook of Adolescent Medicine. New Delhi: Jaypee Brothers Medical Publishers; 2006. p. 860.
2. Bertone HJ. (2021). Which Type of Meditation Is Right for Me? [online] Available from https://www.healthline.com/health/mental-health/types-of-meditation#What-meditation-is-all-about [Last accessed March, 2024].
3. KS Vashundhara, R Nagratna, HR Nagendra. Effect of Yoga on Creativity in Children. Bangalore: Yoga Sudha, Swami Yoganand Prakashan; 2002. XVIII (9);25.
4. Mahapragya A. Amrit Pitak. Ladnun: Jain Vishwa Bharti; 1985.
5. Mayo Clinic. Relaxation techniques: Try these steps to lower stress. [online] Available from https://www.mayoclinic.org/healthy-lifestyle/stress-management/in-depth/relaxation-technique/art-20045368 [Last accessed March, 2024].
6. Mindful. (2020). What is Mindfulness? [online] Available from https://www.mindful.org/what-is-mindfulness/[Last accessed March, 2024].
7. Nowakowska C, Fellmann B, Pasek T, Hauser J, Słuzewska A. Evaluation of the effect of relaxation and concentration exercises based on yoga. Psychiatr Pol. 1982;16(5-6): 365-70.
8. Platania-Solazzo A, Field TM, Blank J, Seligman F, Kuhn C, Schanberg S, et al. Relaxation therapy reduces anxiety in adolescents. Acta Paedopsychiatr. 1992;55(2):115-20.
9. Saraswati S. Yoga Education for Children. Munger, Bihar, India; Yoga Publication Trust. Bihar School of Yoga; 1990. pp. 01-5.
10. Shannahoff-Khalsa DS, Boyle MR, Buebel ME. The effect of unilateral forced nostril breathing on cognitive performance. Int J Neurosci. 1993;73(1-2):61-8.
11. Study of effect of Preksha Meditation and Yoga on Adolescents—A thesis for Phd and science of living. Ladnun: Jain Vishwa Bharti Institute 2004.


# 3A.4    Emotional Intelligence

*Vaishali Deshmukh*

## ■ WHAT IS EMOTIONAL INTELLIGENCE?

In 1990, John Mayer and Peter Salovey put forth the theory of emotional intelligence (EI). This theory was further developed and made popular by Daniel Goleman.

*Emotional intelligence is defined as:* The ability to monitor one's own and other's feelings and emotions, to discriminate among them, and to use this information to guide one's thinking and action.

People with high EI have certain characteristics. These include:
- They can anticipate and adapt to the situations better.
- They can be more empathetic.
- They do not overreact.
- They can take rational, effective, and safer decisions.
- They are good at maintaining friendships and relationships.
- Can handle, and bounce back from failures.
- Can cope with the stresses and negative emotions.
- They are more realistic about themselves and have higher self-confidence.
- They are more popular and more likely to be successful.

Emotional intelligence can be measured as emotional quotient (EQ) by certain available tools, such as The Mayer-Salovey-Caruso Emotional Intelligence Test (MSCEIT) and The Emotional Quotient Inventory (Bar-On). Unlike IQ, EI can be learnt. Adolescence, being a period of heightened emotionality, can benefit greatly by nurturing the EI.

## ADVANTAGES OF HIGH EMOTIONAL INTELLIGENCE

Better EI means a person is better oriented toward their own emotional state and that of others. Such persons are more likely to be:

- Academically successful
- Have better and lasting relationships
- Make good career choices
- Become good team members or team leaders
- Be happier
- Have a better mental and social health
- More likely to become successful, satisfied, and well known.

## DISADVANTAGES OF HIGH EMOTIONAL INTELLIGENCE

Yes, highly emotionally intelligent people can have some drawbacks too!

- They may have poor creativity. This happens because they anticipate obstacles very strongly and that can prevent them from exploring multiple options.
- They tend to take decisions themselves by underestimating others. This may restrict others from being creative. Consequently, they can be less popular.
- They are also more likely to manipulate others.

## EMOTIONS DURING ADOLESCENCE

As we are well aware, the adolescent brain is undergoing major reforms, one of them is the emotional domain. There are extensive neurobiological changes which include myelination, pruning, maturation of the frontal and prefrontal cortex, etc. The limbic system is in overdrive. Hence, the emotions are vivid and strong. The frontal and prefrontal cortexes, which control emotions by rational thoughts, are still immature. This leads to difficulties in emotional regulation.

This holds particular significance in adolescents, because they are going through a stressful period of their lives owing to major life changes. And that exposes them to a range of emotional challenges. Additionally, new strange emotions such as romantic attraction dominate their thinking.

Another factor is the majorly concrete thinking. Adolescents are yet to develop their abstract thinking. So, their interest is in the short-term, immediate outcome. They are incapable of considering the long-term consequences.

The emotional turmoil is the result of both, the internal and biological changes, as well as the external stressors, which is why G Stanley Hall described this phase as Sturm und Drang, i.e., storm and stress.

With time, cognitive maturity improves and this results in better emotional regulation. Those with higher EI are at an advantage here.

### Need for Emotional Intelligence during Adolescence

Adolescents are changing in three spheres: the body, brain, and emotions. The abovementioned characteristics of adolescents make them vulnerable to high-risk behaviors. According to Eric Ericson's theory, each stage of life has certain tasks to fulfil. The task for adolescence is identity formation. The development of identity is in multiple areas such as personal, sexual, social, and political. Naturally, there is a tug-of-war between this psychological developmental urge and social expectations. Since they are at the crossroads of life, a lot of important decisions await them, such as decisions regarding their career, relationships, independence, value system, sexuality, and more.

The dramatic physical changes make them extremely body image-conscious. The peer influence is at its peak. The tussle between the immature thought process and the wish for independence leads to impulsivity, experimentation, and risk-taking behavior.

All these factors underline the need for better EI during this stormy phase, so as to facilitate development, and decision-making, and to avoid lasting damage.

### Methods to Teach Emotional Intelligence to Adolescents

- Emotional intelligence training can be a part of school curriculum that includes self-awareness, self-regulation, social awareness, relationship skills, responsible decision making, etc. Teachers can be trained to conduct these sessions.
- World Health Organization (WHO)-recommended life skills can be used as a starting point. Various case scenarios can be enacted, and movie clips can be discussed.
- Schools and student groups can have poster competitions to highlight the importance of emotions in our lives.

- *Emotional literacy:* This involves teaching children the names of various emotions, and discussions regarding appropriate and inappropriate emotions. For this purpose, the *Plutchik model of emotions* can be used. Psychologist Robert Plutchik created the emotion wheel, where eight basic emotions (joy, trust, fear, surprise, sadness, anticipation, anger, and disgust) are organized in a wheel. By using various combinations and intensities of emotions, we can teach adolescents to identify, classify, and find the purpose of each emotion **(Fig. 1)**.

  Relationship between gender and emotions, the myths and misconceptions such as boys do not cry and girls do not show rage, can also be addressed during these trainings. This enables children to express and respect all emotions.

- *Parental education about EQ:*
  - Parents benefit in their own lives and relationships from being aware of EQ.
  - They can be more enlightened parents.
  - They can be good role models for identifying, expressing, and managing emotions.
  - They can teach children how to manage emotions during day-to-day life situations.

## Present and Future Impact of Emotional Intelligence on Adolescents

Emotionally intelligent adolescents will be better aware of their present volatile emotional state, and their inability to control emotions, and will be empowered to handle the explosion of emotions during stressful situations.

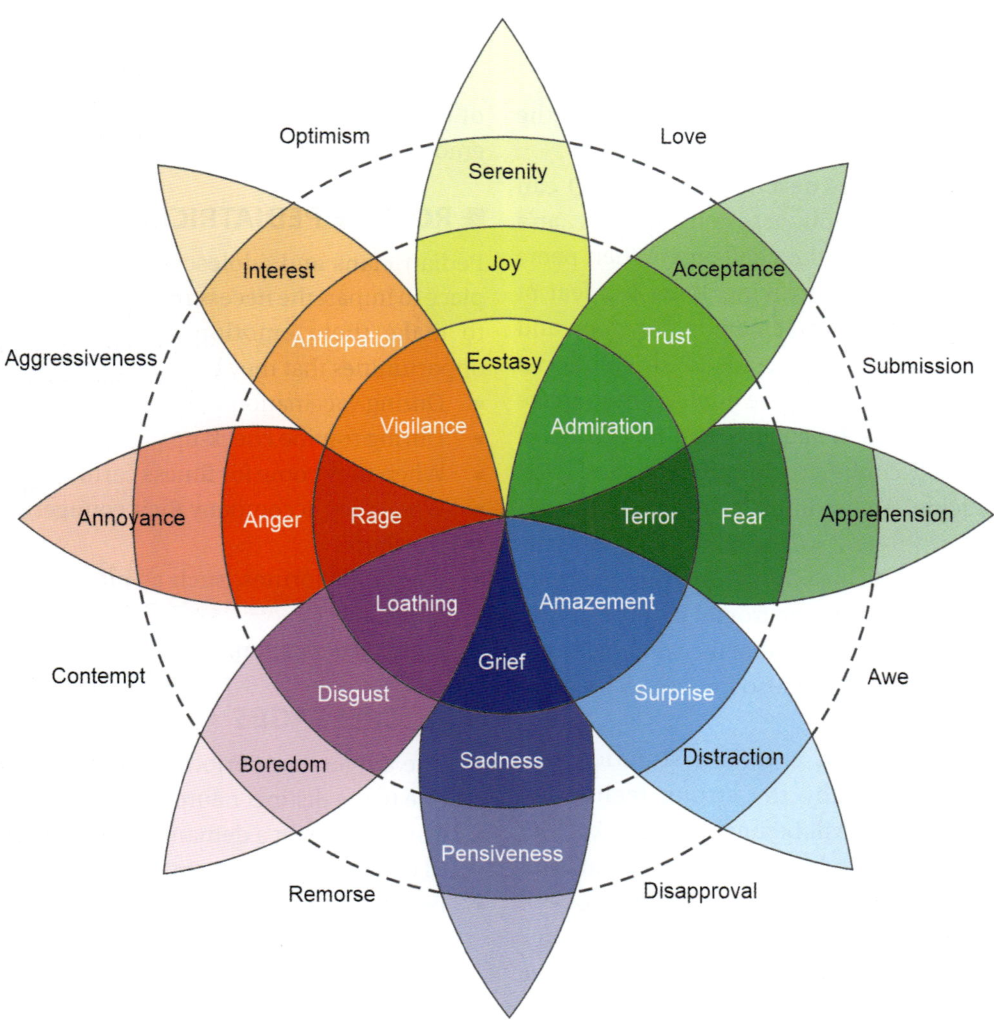


**Fig. 1:** Plutchik's emotion wheel.

**TABLE 1:** Application of EI in adolescents.

| Situation | Emotions | Effects | How EQ helps |
|---|---|---|---|
| Peer pressure | FOMO, anger, disappointment, and anxiety | High-risk behavior and experimentation | Decision-making and rational thinking |
| Drunken driving | Thrill and stress | Accidents | Impulse control |
| Sexual experimentation | Attraction, desire, fear, and pleasure | STIs, pregnancy and its complications, and emotional trauma | Risk assessment |
| Crime/violence | Contempt, anger, disgust, and fear | Injuries and unlawful activities | Coping with urges |
| Anger outbursts | Anger, frustration, and sadness | Crime, violence, broken relationships, and losses | Coping with emotions |
| Scholastic deterioration | Anxiety, sadness, fear, and shame due to abuse | Lost educational and vocational opportunities | Identifying the roadblock |
| Academic failure | Shame, embarrassment, and guilt | Depression, self-harm, and unhealthy coping (addictions, etc.) | Coping with failure and stress |
| Romantic relationships and break-ups | Pain, anger, sadness, despair, and rejection | Self-harm, trust issues, and lost self-confidence | Handling frustration |
| Risky online behavior | Love/attraction, FOMO, anxiety, and loneliness | Blackmail, digital bullying, and dangerous liaisons | Critical thinking and media literacy |

(EI: emotional intelligence; EQ: emotional quotient; FOMO: fear of missing out; STIs: sexually transmitted infections)

Emotional intelligence will be advantageous in the situations mentioned in **Table 1**.

In each of the situations described earlier, EQ can help identify the real emotion, assess its severity, and find the best way to manage the challenge. When peers insist on things such as rule-breaking, there is a fear of missing out (FOMO), an urge to remain in the group and a lack of abstract thinking. This leads to an emotional rush, which makes it difficult for the adolescent to make safe and correct decisions. It can also lead to feelings of isolation, reduced self-confidence, depression, and even self-harm and suicide. An emotionally aware adolescent will be able to realize this and will be able to give himself/herself time to reflect, during which time the emotions will calm down somewhat and the frontal cortex can take over. Here, there are more chances that the adolescent will avoid unnecessary risks and will also be able to preserve the friendship.

An adolescent caught in a violent situation will probably be so overcome by the strong feelings of revenge, anger, etc. that he will be unable to think about the consequences of harm to himself or others, unlawful behavior, punishment, impact on career, and loss of friendship. This can have a far-reaching impact on him/her and their future. Adolescents with EI will be able to see through the acute strong emotions, will realize that it may affect his/her present and future negatively, and will think of alternative ways to express and handle these violent emotions.

## ■ ROLE OF PEDIATRICIANS

Pediatricians and adolescent physicians are at an ideal place to impart the necessary education to our adolescents to make them emotionally intelligent. Some of the opportunities that they have are as follows:

- During vaccination visits
- During routine check-up
- When they come for fitness certificates
- When they accompany their younger siblings
- In schools
- On public forums, such as public talks, newspapers, radio, and TV
- Parental education.

## ■ KEY MESSAGES

- The adolescent period has a volatile emotional state due to the distinct neurobiological changes.
- They also are at a demanding developmental phase.
- EI can be acquired by training.
- Better EI will definitely be advantageous to adolescents to effectively manage their extreme emotions, for correct decision-making in the acute situations in their lives, and also to avert long-term negative consequences.

- Pediatricians and adolescent physicians can play an active role in this process, as well as the parents and teachers.

## ■ RECOMMENDED READING


1. Karibeeran S, Mohanty S. Emotional Intelligence Among Adolescents. Hum Soc Sci. 2019;7(3):121-4.
2. McLaughlin KA, Garrad MC, Somerville LH. What develops during emotional development? A component process approach to identifying sources of psychopathology risk in adolescence. Dialogues Clin Neurosci. 2015;17(4):403-10.
3. Plutchik's Wheel of Emotions: Exploring the Emotion Wheel. [online] Available from https://www.6seconds.org/2022/03/13/plutchik-wheel-emotions [Last accessed March, 2024].
4. Salovey P, Mayer JD. Emotional intelligence. Imagination, Cognition and Personality. 1990;9:185-211.


# 3A.5 | Relationships during Adolescence

*Ashok Banga*

## ■ INTRODUCTION

Teenage relationships can sometimes be complex and challenging, and therefore, it is important to discuss this issue.

## ■ WHAT IS RELATIONSHIP DEVELOPMENT?

This is the action of causing the repetitive connection and evolution toward accomplishing the common purposes of two or more people in the family, friends, in dating, marriage, and business or profession.

## ■ WHY DOES THE DEVELOPMENT OF RELATIONSHIPS MATTER?

This is the process of development of close connections with adults in the family and society, and peers that help young people cultivate their abilities to shape their own lives, build resilience, and thrive. Through this, children learn how to think, understand, communicate, behave, and express emotions and develop social skills.

## ■ WHAT IS THE CHANGE?

Impulsive actions as a form of risk-taking behavior peak during early adolescence (a consequence of asynchronous limbic-prefrontal cortex maturation).

Impulsive choice declines from childhood to adulthood, reflecting the trend of increasing, prefrontal regulated executive functions throughout adolescence. Because of an increase in reasoning and decision-making skills, they gradually go through less conflict with others.

They show more independence from their parents. They develop a deeper capacity for caring and sharing and for developing more intimate relationships.

*Relationships that influence an adolescent:*

- *Parents:* Parents influence their child's values and future choices. A strong relationship may lead to the child seeking their parent's guidance.
- *Peers:* Peers help adolescents understand personalities. Adolescents look toward peers for guidance and direction.
- *Community and society:* Society can influence adolescents in many ways.
- *Teachers:* Teachers can help adolescents develop a balanced personality. They teach life skills and promote positive attitudes.
- *Romantic partners:* Romantic relationships can contribute to identity formation, emotional and behavioral adjustments, and changes in family and peer relationships.

## ■ RELATIONSHIP DEVELOPMENT IN THE FAMILY

Parent–child relationships are among the most important relationships for adolescents and these are often reorganized during puberty.

One of the developmental tasks of adolescence is to separate from one's family as one becomes an independent young adult. A part of this process is coming to terms with specific feelings about one's family. Teens want more independence and more emotional distance between them and their parents. They begin to realize that their parents and authority figures in the family do not know everything or have solutions to all types of struggles. Some teen rebellion against parents is common and normal.

Over time, disagreements often decrease.

## RELATIONSHIP DEVELOPMENT AMONG PEERS

Adolescents spend more time with their peers than they did as children. They have friends of either sex, in small groups or large. Peers and friends might influence an adolescent's behavior, interests, appearance, self-esteem, choices, and ways of working. Teens tend to gravitate toward peer groups with whom they share common interests and activities, similar cultural backgrounds, and/or similar outlooks on life.

Developing stronger peer attachments has been associated with better psychological well-being.

*Relationships are important, because relationships help teens to:*

- Learn social and emotional skills, such as empathy, cooperation, problem-solving, and build relationship skills
- Develop self-confidence and personal identity
- Find independence from parents
- Encourage healthy behavior, like positive academic engagement and the confidence to take positive risks
- Develop positive social skills, such as cooperation, communication, conflict resolution, and resisting negative peer pressure.

*Peer relationships can also have some negative effects:*

- Bullying, exclusion, deviant peer processes, and negative peer pressure
- Body dissatisfaction and low self-esteem
- Overdependence on peers.

## DEVELOPING RELATIONSHIPS AMONG TEENS

Changes in a teen's physical and thinking development come with big changes in their relationships with family and friends. A teen's focus often shifts to social interactions and friendships. Sexual maturity triggers interest in dating and sexual relationships.

### Changes in Relationship with Self

During the teen years, a new understanding of one's self occurs. This may include changes in these self-concepts:

- *Independence:* It means making decisions for one's self and acting on one's thought processes and judgment. By this, they start to face new responsibilities and enjoy their thoughts and actions. Teens also begin to have thoughts and fantasies about their future and adult life.
- *Identity:* This is a sense of self or one's personality. One of the important tasks of adolescence is to reach a sense of personal identity and a secure sense of self. A teen gets comfortable with and accepts a more mature physical body. Trouble occurs when a teen cannot resolve struggles about who they are as a physical, sexual, and independent person.
- *Self-esteem:* This is how you feel about yourself. In adolescence, a decrease in self-esteem is somewhat common due to the many body changes, new thoughts, and new ways of thinking about things as they are more thoughtful about who they are and who they want to be. Self-esteem increases as teens develop a better sense of who they are.

### Changes in Peer Relationships

Teens spend more time with friends and feel more understood and accepted by their friends.

Close friendships tend to develop between teens with similar interests, social class, and ethnic backgrounds and expand to include similarities in attitudes, values, shared activities, and educational interests. In the case of girls, close, intimate, self-disclosing conversations with friends help to explore identities and define one's sense of self. Conversations with friends also help teens explore their sexuality and how they feel about it.

### Changes in Different Sex (Romantic) Relationships

The male–female and sexual relationships are influenced by sexual interest and by social and cultural influences and expectations. In adolescence, developmental tasks include struggles to gain control over sexual and aggressive urges. Discovering possible love relationships also occurs. Sexual behaviors in this period may include impulsive behavior, a wide range of experimental interactions of mutual exploring, and eventually intercourse.

## TEN STAGES OF RELATIONAL DEVELOPMENT

*Stages when relationships come together:*

- Initiating
- Experimenting
- Intensifying

- Integrating
- Bonding

*Stages when relationships come apart:*
- Differentiating
- Circumscribing
- Stagnating
- Avoiding
- Terminating.

Each of these stages varies in length and intensity. At each stage, thoughts and feelings are guiding you about what to do and when to do it.

## COMMON RELATIONSHIP ISSUES AMONG ADOLESCENTS

- Immaturity
- Insecurities
- Communication issues
- Trust issues
- Disapproval from parents
- Jealousy
- One-sided love
- Unexpected bouts of anger
- Taunting or bullying, monitoring and/or controlling
- Embarrassment
- Intimidation
- Physical hurting.

## WHAT MAKES A RELATIONSHIP HEALTHY?

Being in a relationship can be exciting and should make one feel happy. A healthy relationship is when everyone feels respected, trusted, and valued for who they are. When they can talk openly about things without feeling scared of what might happen, or being judged for what has been said.

## ARE TEENAGE RELATIONSHIPS GOOD OR BAD?

Teenage love and romantic relationships are impossible to classify as either "good" or "bad" for their development. They are an integral part of a teenager's social and emotional development. The relationships created during teenage years may prepare teens for adult romantic relationships. There are both, benefits and risks, and it is not unusual for the two to coexist.

*Positive outcomes of teenage relationships include:*
- Developing interpersonal skills and additional emotional support
- Experience for future relationships

- Enhanced self-esteem and increased feelings of self-worth

*Potential negative outcomes can be:*
- Distraction from schoolwork and isolation from friends' circles
- Increased vulnerability to depressive symptoms
- Increased risk of emotional strain conflict and partner violence
- Sexual health risks and unplanned pregnancies.

## SIGNS OF PROBLEMATIC RELATIONSHIPS

Most teenagers in love often experience infatuation, heightened emotions, and plenty of ups and downs. If it appears that a teen has more lows than highs with the partner and there seems to be an unhealthy relationship, these are some of the signs to identify toxic teenage relationships:
- Possessiveness, signs of extreme jealousy or controlling tendencies in the partner
- Treats poorly in front of parents or their friends
- Partner invading teen's privacy
- Teen found to have unexplained injuries
- Changing habits of teens
- Feeling the need to check in with their partner frequently.

## ARE UNHEALTHY RELATIONSHIPS COMMON?

As teenagers in love do not always have the experience or wisdom to spot red flags or recognize unhealthy patterns, unhealthy or abusive relationships are common. A US national survey found that almost 1 in 3 teens reported being verbally or psychologically abused, and 1 in 10 had been the victims of physical dating violence within the past year.

## HOW TO TEACH ADOLESCENTS ABOUT HEALTHY RELATIONSHIPS?

Teens do not have the life experience to know how a healthy relationship functions. The best way for them to learn this is to see it modelled by their parents. They learn by witnessing how their father and mother treat their spouse, friends, and family with kindness, respect, open communication, loyalty, and honesty.

*Parenting and care when a teen is dating:*

- Establish reasonable boundaries and rules
- Keep the lines of communication open
- Always meet who they are dating
- Keep a watch on their social media use
- Discuss any age gaps in relationships
- Talk about consent.

It is not always easy to talk to your teenage daughter or son about relationships, but this is always needed and helps both, you and your child.

*Advice for healthy relationships:*

- Good communication
- Talking about what is important to you
- Do not keep feelings bottled up
- Get to know each other well
- Talking about values, beliefs, life goals, and dreams.

## PARENTS' ROLE IN ADOLESCENT RELATIONSHIP

### Before Relationships Build

Be close to your adolescent from the beginning. Have conversations in the family about feelings, friendships, and relationships early on. The relationship between the parent and child should be so strong that the adolescent will disclose everything in his/her life to his parents, whom he trusts. Discuss the changes that will happen in adolescents and the subsequent behaviors, which include physical, mental, social, and hormonal ones. Also, discuss the errors that can happen in the judgments and decisions of teens as well as adults. Your children must understand what constitutes a healthy relationship and the thin line between friendship and romance. Set limits on dating time, mobile use, and internet etiquette like not disclosing identity.

They must take care as sometimes it is difficult to judge the other's true character during a relationship, as both will try to be on their best behavior.

Most teenagers may experiment with sexual behavior at some stage. Let them have clear information on consent, mutual respect, contraception, safe sex, and sexually transmitted infections (STIs). Guide them, on how to deal with unwanted sexual and peer pressure. Also, let them know the basics of the POCSO (Protection of Children from Sexual Offences) Act.

### Once the Relationship has been Established

Once parents come to know about the relationship, they should deal with it calmly and not get angry. They should respond, not react. A violent outburst or criticism is always unwelcome.

Let them understand that the people most concerned about their well-being will always be their parents.

Help them eat good food, celebrate success, watch movies together, play together, spend time together in nature, exercise, meditation, etc. Reinforce the bond, show that you love them, and hug them. Reminding them about family values and moral values may help, but a prudent approach is to help the adolescent think and tackle the issue in a logical way.

Parents must explore, why the teen wants this relationship. Think about whether this relationship will help them attain their life goals positively, or is it consuming their time and decreasing their performance in studies and activities. Better recommend them to wait a few years before making a decision whose consequences are for a lifetime.

Encourage the friend to come home regularly. Parents may discuss the issue with both together and separately. A person in a true relationship will find it positive. The parents also will come to know the real intentions and behavior in such a way. It is always good to know the person well, the positivity in a relationship, the social and economic consequences, whether the person nurtures you, allows growth and respect, stands up for you, and considers a lifetime relationship—is it really worth it.

An open discussion between the parents of both adolescents may be of help in sharing the concerns. Then both the parents can talk to both adolescents and discuss pros and cons, set the priorities straight, and find a working solution. They can write down the pros and cons themselves as a chart. Once clarity sets in, teens must be appreciated for their decision and must be offered the support needed.

It is like waiting on the orange light, neither red nor green, making them consider the consequences.

### Follow Them Up: What Ultimately Happens?

It is also important to follow up on their relationships as there are different outcomes. They may healthily continue as friends or may try to maintain their relations despite interventions, some may reach the stage of marriage and some may break up. Some may go into depression after a break-up, while others may feel liberated.

At any time if the parents or caretakers feel that professional help is needed, they may resort to it without inhibition.

## ■ RELATIONSHIP ISSUES AFTER MARRIAGE

### Stages of a Relationship Every Couple Goes Through

- Merge
- Doubt and denial
- Disillusionment
- Decision
- Wholehearted love.

Every single relationship moves through these five stages many times.

### Most Common Relationship Problems

Here is the list of the most common relationship problems among adolescents and adults, most often among couples:

- Significant differences in core values and beliefs
- Lack of communication about important matters
- Life stages—having "outgrown" each other or have "changed" significantly for whatever reason
- Bored in or with your relationship
- Knowing you should not have got married in the first place!
- Dealing with a jealous partner
- Affairs/infidelity/cheating
- Sexual issues
- Traumatic and/or life-changing events causing change in relationship dynamics
- Responses to prolonged periods of stress, such as work-related stress, long-term illness, mental health issues, financial problems, problems with children, infertility, and many more
- Domestic violence—verbal as well as physical abuse: This is the most serious relationship problem
- Lack of responsibility regarding finances, children, health, and many other issues
- Unrealistic expectations from each other. Poor division of labor and/or one-sided lack of responsibility for chores and tasks
- Perceived lack of concern, care, and consideration/attentiveness from the partner
- Addictions—substance abuse
- Excessive reliance on social media at the cost of the relationship
- Lack of support during difficult times from people that matter
- Having "blended" family issues

- Overinvolvement in your relationships with family or friends
- Long-term depression or other mental health issues suffered by one partner or both
- Significant differences in opinion on how to discipline/deal with the children and/or parents/in-laws.

## ■ HOW DO YOU, AS AN ADULT (DOCTOR), BUILD AUTHENTIC RELATIONSHIPS WITH ADOLESCENTS?

- Listen
- Show your human side
- Set boundaries if needed
- Consider their resistance as protection
- Learn basic counseling skills
- Practice self-care.

## ■ KEY MESSAGES

- The process of development of close connections (relationships) with persons around is the basic essential of everyone's life.
- Most important is the relationship with parents, peers, and society.
- Healthy relationships make life happy.
- Some of the relationships may turn out to be toxic. One can come out of it.
- Teach the adolescents about healthy relationships as they do not have life experience to know. Observe and guide them.

## ■ RECOMMENDED READING

1. Bhave SY (Ed). Bhave's Textbook of Adolescent Medicine, 2nd edition. New Delhi: Peepee Publishers; 2016.
2. Healthy Relationships in Adolescence. [online] Available from https://opa.hhs.gov/adolescent-health/healthy-relationships-adolescence [Last accessed March, 2024].
3. Nair MKC (Ed). Adolescent Counseling, 1st edition. New Delhi: Jaypee Brothers Medical Publishers; 2016.
4. Prior E. (2022). How to fix these 25 common relationship problems and prevent a relationship breakdown. [online] Available from http://www.professional-counselling.com/common-relationship-problems.html [Last accessed March, 2024].
5. Teens: Relationship Development. [online] Available from https://www.stanfordchildrens.org/en/topic/default?id=relationship-development-90-P01642 [Last accessed March, 2024].

# 3A.6 — Anger Management

*Piyali Bhattacharya*

## INTRODUCTION

*"Anger and intolerance are the enemies of correct understanding."*

—Gandhi

Adolescence is a period of profound change and growth, characterized by physical, emotional, and social transformations. During this time, teenagers often experience heightened emotions, including anger, which can be challenging to manage. Anger management in adolescence is a critical aspect of healthy development, as poorly controlled anger can have detrimental consequences for both the individual and those around them. Therefore, it becomes imperative to explore the significance, causes, consequences, and strategies for effective management of anger management in adolescence.

## DEFINITION OF ANGER

According to Charles Spielberger, a psychologist who specializes in the study of anger, "Anger is an emotional state that varies in intensity from mild irritation to intense fury and rage." It is a natural, adaptive response to threats and it provokes powerful, aggressive, feelings, and behaviors which allow us to fight and to defend ourselves when we are attacked.

## SIGNIFICANCE OF ANGER MANAGEMENT IN ADOLESCENCE

Anger is a natural emotion that everyone experiences. In adolescence, however, the intensity and frequency of anger can escalate due to various factors, such as hormonal changes, peer pressure, academic stress, and a developing sense of independence. When left unmanaged, anger can lead to aggressive behaviors, conflicts, and even physical violence. Adolescents who struggle to control their anger are at risk of harming their relationships, physical and mental well-being, and future prospects. Effective anger management is crucial for the well-being and success of teenagers during this crucial phase of their lives. The role of a pediatrician is early identification, providing anticipatory guidance to the children. Parental training and referral for

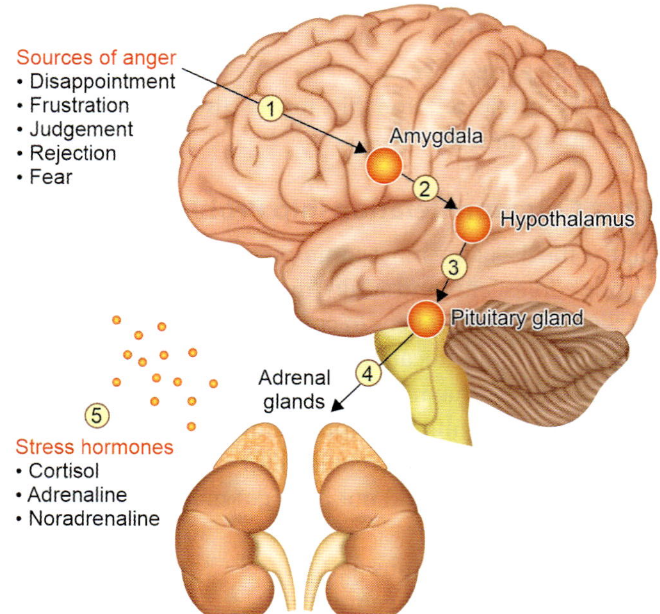


**Fig. 1:** Anger pathway.

the underlying neurobehavioral or psychiatric problem are present.

Anger is accompanied by physiological and biological changes. The hypothalamus stimulates pituitary gland which releases adrenocorticotropic hormone (ACTH) into blood. ACTH stimulates adrenal glands to secrete further chemicals that affect other organ systems, e.g., cortisol, adrenaline, and noradrenaline, which cause an increase in heart rate and blood pressure, rapid breathing, sweating, and increased blood sugars **(Fig. 1)**.

## EFFECTS OF ANGER

- *Physical health:* Anger makes one more susceptible to heart disease, diabetes, insomnia, weakening of the immune system, and high blood pressure.
- *Mental health:* It clouds your thinking and leads to stress, depression, and other mental health problems.
- *Relationships:* Anger alienates! It causes lasting scars on your loved ones and destroys way of friendships and relationships. Explosive anger is especially damaging as it makes it hard for others to trust you, speak honestly, or feel comfortable in your presence.

## CAUSES OF ANGER IN ADOLESCENCE

Anger can be caused by both external and internal events. External stressor may be major life events, e.g., moving from one place to another, death of a family member or friend, divorce of parents, financial pressures, meeting deadlines, arguments, or even lack of sleep.

Internal stressors also play a role; for example, values and beliefs, faith, goals, self-image, expectations of self or others significantly contribute to anger in adolescents.

Several factors contribute to the heightened levels of anger in adolescents:

- *Hormonal changes:* Puberty brings significant hormonal fluctuations, which can impact mood regulation and emotional responses.
- *Peer pressure:* Adolescents often face peer pressure, leading to frustration and anger when they feel compelled to conform to social norms.
- *Academic stress:* The pressure to excel academically, prepare for standardized tests, and make important educational decisions can be overwhelming.
- *Identity development:* Adolescents are exploring their identities and may become angry when they face resistance or judgment from peers, family, or society.
- *Parent–child conflict:* As teens seek independence, conflicts with parents over rules and boundaries can lead to anger.

## CONSEQUENCES OF POOR ANGER MANAGEMENT

Failure to manage anger effectively can result in numerous negative consequences for adolescents:

- *Damaged relationships:* Frequent anger outbursts can strain relationships with peers, family, and romantic partners, leading to isolation and social difficulties.
- *Mental health issues:* Uncontrolled anger is linked to mental health problems, including depression and anxiety.
- *Academic challenges:* Anger can disrupt concentration and motivation, affecting academic performance.
- *Legal issues:* Physical violence or aggressive behaviors may lead to legal consequences.
- *Physical health problems:* Chronic anger can manifest physically, contributing to stress-related health issues like high blood pressure.

## OTHER CAUSES

- *Neurobehavioral causes:* These include attention-deficit/hyperactivity disorder (ADHD), learning disability, oppositional defiant disorder (ODD), conduct disorder, mood disorder, disruptive mood dysregulation disorder (DMDD), etc.
- *Psychiatric causes:* Bipolar disorder, schizophrenia, depression, panic disorders, post-traumatic stress disorder (PTSD)
- *Medical causes:* Epilepsy and mental retardation, brain damage (Injury), Tourette syndrome, anemia, B12 deficiency, thyroid dysfunction, etc.

## STRATEGIES FOR ANGER MANAGEMENT IN ADOLESCENCE

The goal of anger management is to reduce both your emotional feelings and the physiological arousal that anger causes. The three main approaches to help adolescents manage their anger effectively are expressing, suppressing, and calming. Be aware of anger signs. Knowing the triggers, identifying anger cues, knowing your own anger style, and modifying it in a constructive way are ways of handling anger.

- *Identifying their feelings:* Admit that you are angry! Adolescents should be educated about recognizing and understanding their emotions, including anger and the physiological responses associated with it. Explore what is really behind your anger.

  Question yourself as to "Why am I angry?" Is it a feeling of embarrassment, disappointment, jealousy, fear, helpless, sadness, or being left out?
- *Identifying aggressive acts by self or others:* For example, throwing or breaking things, hitting others, calling names, ganging up, or spreading rumors. Use the anger meter to rate your anger **(Fig. 2)**.

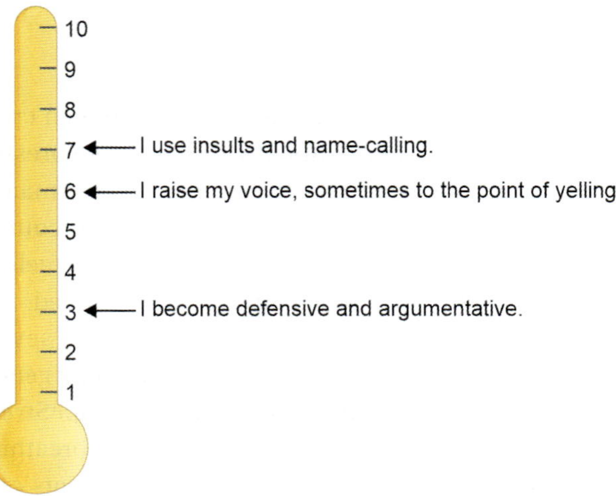


**Fig. 2:** Anger thermometer.

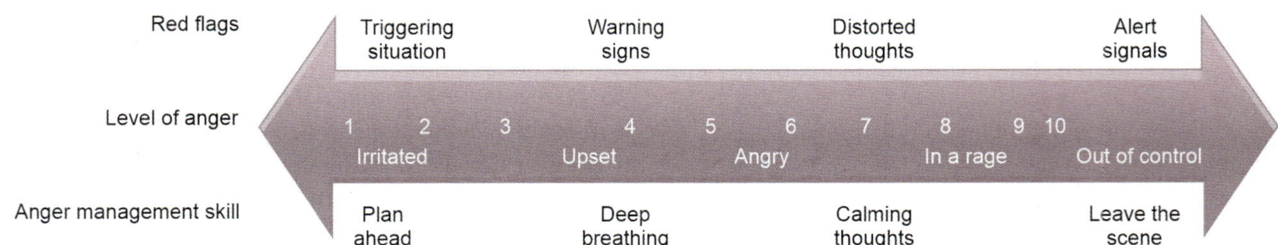

**Fig. 3:** Anger management skills.

- *Identifying self-destructive behavior:* For example, negative self-talk, blaming others, overeating, overdrinking, reckless driving/taking drugs, looking for fights, or just feeling outraged.
- *Identify potential harm or consequences to others or self:* Adolescents who are constantly putting others down, criticizing everything, and making cynical comments have not learned how to constructively express their anger. Developing an awareness of the effect our actions have on others and understanding possible consequences are important aspects of managing anger. Am I getting a bad reputation? Am I causing physical harm to self or others? Is there destruction of property? Is my act going to land me in jail?
- *Cognitive restructuring:* (Changing the way we think) Believe you can control your anger! Calm down! Replacing emotionally charged thoughts with more rational ones, using positive words, and self-talk has a huge influence on our feelings. Create positive self-talk phrases....

*It is okay to feel angry.*
*The more I learn to take care of my anger the more powerful I become.*
*I learn how to express my anger in helpful ways.*
*I use fair words.*

- *Communication skills:* Unexpressed anger can create problems. Express yourself assertively! Expressing angry feelings in an assertive, nonaggressive manner is the healthiest way to express anger. Encourage open and healthy communication to express feelings, resolve conflicts, and seek support when needed.
  - *Stress-reduction techniques:* Practicing several relaxation techniques to help improve our general feeling of positivity and well-being. Stress-management strategies, such as deep breathing, meditation, and exercise, help adolescents cope with anger triggers. Advice the adolescent to do a countdown, breathe deeply, visualize a relaxing experience, go for a walk, chant a mantra, play some music, or maintain a journal. Creating a thought record can be used to record events and situations that cause us to feel angry, stressed, or anxious and learn to overcome them.
  - *Problem-solving skills (life skills):* Every problem has a solution. Decide how to solve the problem. Teach problem-solving techniques and coping mechanisms to address the underlying issues causing their anger and express anger without loss of control **(Fig. 3)**.
- Spiritual or religious affiliations
- *Role modeling:* Be a positive role model, demonstrating how to handle anger constructively in real-life situations.
- *Seek professional help:* If anger is really out of control and have an impact on relationships and important parts of life, it may be necessary to involve mental health professionals to provide therapy (cognitive–behavioral therapy) and support for adolescents struggling with anger issues. A psychotherapeutic program can help the adolescent to prevent and control anger.

Various validated self-reporting anger scales in children and adolescents help in evaluation and management of anger. For example,
- Children's Inventory of Anger (ChIA)
- Anger Expression Scale for Children (AESC)
- Clinical Anger Scale
- Aggression Questionnaire
- State Trait Anger Expression Inventory (STAXI).

## ■ CONCLUSION

Anger management is a critical aspect of adolescent development. Anger management is not about learning to suppress your anger. The true goal of anger management is to understand the emotion and express it in a healthy way without losing control.

During this period of transformation and self-discovery, teenagers need the skills and support to navigate their emotions, including anger, in a healthy and constructive manner. By addressing the causes and consequences of anger in adolescence and implementing effective strategies for managing it, we can help teenagers transition into adulthood with greater emotional resilience and overall well-being.

## ■ KEY MESSAGES

*Adolescents should be empowered to:*
- Be mindful about their emotions
- Focus on the present
- Respond and not react
- Be assertive
- Be willing to forgive
- Know when to let something go—agree to disagree
- Disengage if things are getting out of hand.

## ■ RECOMMENDED READING


1. Adachi T, Yamada K, Fujino H, Enomoto K, Shibata M. "Associations between anger and chronic primary pain: a systematic review and meta-analysis". Scand J Pain. 2022;22(1):1-13. https://doi.org/10.1515/sjpain-2021-0154.
2. Lerner H. The Dance of Anger: A Woman's Guide to Changing the Patterns of Intimate Relationships. New York: William Morrow; 2014.
3. Lohmann RC. The Anger Workbook for Teens: Activities to Help You Deal with Anger and Frustration. Oakland, CA: New Harbinger; 2009.
4. Ong JG, Lim-Ashworth NS, Ooi YP, Boon JS, Ang RP, Goh DH. An Interactive Mobile App Game to Address Aggression (RegnaTales): Pilot Quantitative Study. J MIR Serious Games. 2019; 7(2):e13242. Published online 2019 May 8. doi: 10.2196/13242.
5. Scheff L, Edmiston S. The Cow in the Parking Lot: A Zen Approach to Overcoming Anger. New York: Workman Publishing; 2010.


<table>
<tr><td>3A.7</td><td><h1>Identification of Adolescent at Risk<br>(For Mental Health Issues)</h1></td></tr>
</table>

*Sunita Manchanda*

## ■ INTRODUCTION

Globally, one in seven 10–19-year-olds experiences a mental disorder, accounting for 13% of the global burden of disease in this age group. Adolescents in India are particularly vulnerable to mental health problems like anxiety disorders and depression.

The National Mental Health Survey (2015–2016) reported a 7% prevalence of psychiatric disorders in 13–17 years which was nearly equal among both the genders. A meta-analysis reports that 6.5% of the community and 23.3% of school children and adolescents in India have psychiatric disorders.

Mental health issues and disorders are underreported because awareness about these issues is lacking. Parents are hesitant to seek help (due to stigma attached to it), and a teen's desire and expectation of self-reliant also make it unaddressed. Insufficient prioritization of mental health concerns in the policy framework is also a deterrent to identifying mental issues at the earliest. Mental illness is preventable. However, in most cases, parents are quite late in seeking help even though issues have been going on for months. *Most parents remain in denial and think that "It can't happen to my child."* If mental health issues are not addressed in time, it will impact future physical and mental health of youth and limit their opportunities to lead fulfilling lives as adults.

To identify adolescents at risk of mental health issues, it is important to know risk factors (which make an adolescent vulnerable) and red flag signs. Different stakeholders should come together and work in collaboration for identification and early intervention.

## ■ RISK FACTORS

Risk factors which can predispose a teenager to develop mental health difficulties can be discussed in the following domains and are enumerated in **Box 1**: (1) Individual, (2) family, (3) school, and (4) community.

## ■ RED FLAG SIGNS

There are various signs which can alert a physician, teacher, and parent that the teenager is facing mental

---

**BOX 1:** Risk factors which predispose adolescents to mental health issues.

- *Individual factors:*
  - Female gender
  - Genetic predisposition
  - Perinatal insult
  - History of birth asphyxia and hospitalization
  - Head injury
  - Conduct problems
  - Behavioral issues
  - Developmental disorders (ADHD, autism)
  - Chronic diseases
  - Low self-esteem
  - Insecure attachment
  - Poor social and communication skills
  - Early substance use
- *Family factors:*
  - Poverty
  - Family dysfunction
  - Domestic violence
  - Parent–child conflict
  - Inconsistent discipline style
  - Negative family environment
  - Child abuse/maltreatment
  - Single-parent family
  - Divorce
  - Marital conflict
  - Family conflict
  - Parent with mental health issues
  - Parental drug/alcohol use
  - Parental unemployment
  - Lack of adult supervision
  - Poor attachment with parent
- *School factors:*
  - Academic pressure
  - School-level stressful or traumatic events
  - School violence
  - Peer rejection
  - Peer pressure
  - Bullying
  - Poor student–teacher relationship
  - Breakdown or lack of positive friendship
- *Community factors:*
  - Socioeconomic disadvantage
  - Homelessness
  - Discrimination
  - Disaster, war survivors
  - Lack of access to support system

---

**BOX 2:** Red flag signs of mental health concerns.

- Notable changes in sleep pattern, eating habits, or other everyday patterns
- Loss of interest in the things they usually enjoy doing
- Withdrawing from friends, family, and community and prefer to sit alone
- Sudden fall in grades or academic performance
- Continuously worrying about something
- Recent inclination to new friends
- Obsession with a certain goal, with the thought that they cannot achieve this
- Signs of drug, alcohol, or other substance use
- Signs of self-harm, e.g., cuts, bruises
- New or more intense interest in sexual activity

## ROLE OF DIFFERENT STAKEHOLDERS IN IDENTIFICATION OF "ADOLESCENTS AT RISK"

Identification of an adolescent at risk involves a multisectoral approach. Different stakeholders work at various levels as mentioned below to identify an adolescent in need and help in planning early intervention **(Table 1)**:

- Primary care physician level
- School level
- Government level
- Community/social media level

### Primary Care Physician Level

A primary care physician, especially a pediatrician, is one of the important persons to identify adolescents at risk. Their familiarity with the child's medical history and his family puts him at ease to get information even from the child. But to make it effective, it is important that every pediatrician, in fact every doctor, be aware of adolescent issues and red flags of mental health issues so that timely referral to an adolescent pediatrician or psychologist and timely intervention can be taken. They can keep few screening questionnaires at their clinic like Trivandrum Screening Questionnaire (TSQ-T) (2011):

- Empower themselves by learning "How to Get into Adolescent Mind"
- Make themselves aware of red flag signs as described above.

### School Level

Schools have tremendous potential as platforms for public mental health interventions, which can secure positive effects on mental health and guide the implementation of

health difficulties and thus encourage them to seek help. Biological changes including hormonal changes can affect their child's mood, school performance, and more **(Box 2)**.

**TABLE 1:** Levels of identification of at-risk adolescents.

| Level | Intervention |
|---|---|
| Primary care physician level | • Equip themselves with basic knowledge about adolescent mental health issue<br>• Empower themselves by learning "How to Get Into Adolescent Mind"<br>• Make themselves aware of red flag signs as described above<br>• Should be able to provide anticipatory guidance to every teenager and parents<br>• Timely referral to mental health professional if needed |
| School level | • Every school should have "Trained School Counselor" if possible<br>• Teachers training to be "Teachers as Counselors"<br>• Sincere contribution in implementing various national health policies<br>• Organize Adolescent Health Awareness Sensitization workshop for parents, teachers, and adolescents<br>• Able to recognize red flags signs<br>• Timely referral to a mental health professional if needed |
| Government level | • Implementation of various health policies at school/hospital/community level<br>• Rashtriya Kishor Swasthya Karyakram (RKSK) program—establishing Adolescent Friendly Health Services (AFHS) and ensure their proper functioning<br>• Conducting National Mental Health Survey for identifying adolescent at risk and plan timely interventional strategies involving health professionals |
| Social media level | Prepare informative and encourage and encourage adolescents to seek help if needed, e.g., Adolescent Job Aid App |

strategies to promote, protect, and restore mental health among their students.

## Government Level

The government should continue to make the improvement of school environments and ensure inclusion of mental health issues also a priority along with addressing health concerns like malnutrition and anemia.

## Community or Social Media Level

Awareness at community level can be done by involving nongovernmental organizations (NGOs), clubs, etc., as today's adolescents are tech-savvy and use social media. Various apps can be developed using IT team and we can encourage them to use these apps effectively.

With the present burden and effect of mental health disorders among adolescents, it is necessary to identify an adolescent at risk of mental health issues and plan early interventions. Thus, now is the time to explore the paradigm of mental health awareness as a means for combating stigma, enhancing prevention, ensuring early recognition, and planning simple and practical interventions within the community.

## ■ KEY MESSAGES

- Early identification of adolescents at potential risk of mental health issues is crucial for timely intervention and providing support.
- Healthcare professionals involved in care of children should be aware of known risk factors (which makes an adolescent vulnerable) and red flag signs to identify them early.
- School teachers and counselors should get training for identifying teens at risk and taking appropriate measures.
- Schools should be utilized as a platform to promote, protect, and restore mental health among their students.
- Different stakeholders, e.g., government, corporates, policy makers, and health care professionals, should come together and work in collaboration for identification and early intervention.

## ■ RECOMMENDED READING


1. Bansal CP, Tuteja JS, Kanikar A, Galgali P. Mission Kishore Uday. Gwalior: Indian Academy of Pediatrics; 2013.
2. Malhotra S, Patra BN. Prevalence of child and adolescent psychiatric disorders in India: a systematic review and meta-analysis. Child Adolesc Psychiatry Ment Health. 2014; 8:22.
3. Mehra D, Lakiang T, Kathuria N, Kumar M, Mehra S, Sharma S. Mental health interventions among adolescents in India: a scoping review. Healthcare (Basel). 2022;10(2): 337.
4. World Health Organization. Key facts: Mental health of adolescents. [online] Available from https://www.who.int/news-room/fact-sheets/detail/adolescent-mental-health. [Last accessed March, 2024].

# Part B: Mental Health Disorders

*Sub-section Editors:* Swati Ghate, Sushma Desai

## 3B.1 | Body Image Distortion

*Swati Ghate*

### INTRODUCTION

Every individual carries a mental framework of his body and its functionality in his mind, which could be realistic or otherwise. This self-perception of his body is an important part of his self-identity and casts a significant effect on his psychosocial well-being. Body image acquires a very crucial place in the life of an adolescent because adolescence is a period of rapid bodily changes, egocentrism, and heightened emotionality. Distortion of this image is likely to affect his mental health considerably.

### WHAT IS BODY IMAGE?

Body image is a multidimensional construct, a mental picture, which combines the individual's perception of his body regarding its physical appearance, competence, and biological integrity. It has four dimensions:
1. *Perceptual:* Mental picture on sensory domains like visual images, tactile, proprioceptive, and interoceptive inputs coming from the body
2. *Cognitive:* Thoughts and beliefs regarding the body
3. *Affective:* Feelings and emotions that arise in the context of the body
4. *Behavioral:* Actions with reference to the body like exercising, eating mindfully, caring, grooming, etc.

### DEVELOPMENT OF BODY IMAGE

Around the age of 2 years, a child starts recognizing himself as a separate individual, beyond being merely an extension or part of the mother–child duo. He knows and identifies himself as a separate entity with an independent physique, name, likes, dislikes, and actions.

By 4 years of age, the child gets the capacity to compare and look for similarities and differences. He then starts comparing his body with those of others around him. Major comparing points are outward and conspicuous like clothing and hair. By 5 years of age, the concept of size emerges, and the child knows big and small. He then gets fascinated by "big" figures around him and wants himself to be sizable and larger than what he is. By 6 years of age, socio–cultural factors have sown their seeds in the young mind through parental comments, media influence, and toys. He absorbs a lot of information from the surroundings and is surprised to find himself a lot more different than what he sees. This sets in the roots of body dissatisfaction in his psyche.

During the adolescence, identity formation is a major task to be accomplished. Body image is an important and integral part of this process. The adolescent starts looking at his body more intently and gives deeper thoughts to its good and not-so-good qualities. The "on stage phenomenon", which makes the adolescent believe that he is constantly being watched by the world around, makes him highly conscious about his looks and style. Peer acceptance is very important for an adolescent and he desires a body that will fit him in his group. He is exposed to increasing media influence, body shaming, and bullying, and his high emotionality makes him feel low about his shortcomings, even though the world finds them trivial.

Thus, body image is about perception and not the factual way of looking at the body in different contexts.

"Body appreciation" is a state where one accepts, respects, and loves his body and rejects unrealistic ideals.

### BODY IMAGE DISTORTIONS

All of us possess something in our body that we do not approve of. But when the dissatisfaction causes either or all of the following, then it is called body image distortion.
- Becomes a cause of persistent worry
- Makes one unable to focus on his responsibilities at work/home or academics
- Significantly affects the daily routine and/or inter-personal relationships.

There are other terminologies denoting this condition like altered body image perception, body image misperception, body image disturbance, negative body image, altered body image, body dissatisfaction, etc.

## NEUROCOGNITIVE BACKGROUND

Since body image is an integration of multiple sensory inputs, a deficit in the working of brain areas related to body awareness, visual information, and sensory integration is postulated to cause this issue. The somatosensory cortex for the collection of biased and misinterpreted information in visual, tactile, proprioceptive, and interoceptive domains, the parietal cortex for sensory integration, and the insula for integrating the body sensations, emotions, and cognition are the brain areas supposed to be working atypically in individuals suffering from body image distortion.

## INCIDENCE AND GENDER DIFFERENCES

Globally, studies have shown that a significant number of individuals suffer from body dissatisfaction. Various studies quote figures from 40 to 70% in adolescents. Females outnumber males with the incidence ranging from 35 to 81% for girls, whereas it is 16 to 55% among boys. In the young adult group, 45% females and 25% males are seen to harbor significant body image issues.

In the United States, 80% women and 34% men have been found to have body image concerns.

53% of 13-year-old US girls are unhappy with their bodies and the figure rises to 78% for girls who are 17 years old. A 2019 UK study found that 20% of its adults were ashamed of their bodies, 34% felt low, whereas 19% felt disgusted.

Studies on college-going girls have observed an incidence of 81% and 77.6% in a North Indian and a South Indian study, respectively. The incidence is higher if the body mass index (BMI) is on the higher side and in those belonging to higher socioeconomic strata.

Body parts for which females are bothered are obviously different from those of boys' concerns. Girls are seen to be more worried about their weight, complexion, breasts, buttocks, excessive hair, nose, skin, belly, teeth, and thighs in decreasing order of frequency. Boys, on the other hand, are bothered about their body build, muscularity, height, genitalia, and thinning of hair. Girls respond to these issues and show social anxiety, depressive behavior, and eating disorders, while boys go on a workout spree or indulge in substance abuse.

## HIGH-RISK FACTORS

Female gender and a high BMI are the two most prominent high-risk factors for body dissatisfaction. Media consumption and body image issues go hand in hand. Studies have proven that time spent on social media sites like Facebook and watching (morphed) photos of peers are directly proportional to body image distortions.

Misuse of sites like pro-anorexia sites or fitness applications on smartphones has emerged as a cause of concern for the same.

Lack of physical activities is also an important predisposing factor. Personality traits like poor self-esteem, perfectionism, and introversion increase the risk. Family influences like poor parental attachment, body size attitudes of parents, their modeling, and eating patterns cast effect on the body image of adolescents. Negative cultural and peer influences promote body dissatisfaction.

Adverse childhood experiences and ongoing traumatizing adversities lead to the same. Adolescents with dysmorphism, disfigurement, growth and puberty problems, chronic illnesses, congenital malformations, and disabilities are more likely to suffer.

## SYMPTOMATOLOGY

Negative outcomes of body image distortion could be physical and/or psychosocial.

Low self-esteem, low mood, irritability, low motivation, and low confidence are commonly seen. Stage fear, poor socialization, school refusal, academic underperformance, and interpersonal conflicts often ensue. Negative sexual experiences are reported by people with body dissatisfaction.

Adolescents sometimes openly express their dislike about their body parts or weight with their parents and use negative expressions such as "I feel ugly" or "I wish I had a better body". But more often, it is their behavioral or emotional pattern that points indirectly to their concerns. Some common red flag signs are as follows:

- Always looking for "imperfections" in the mirror
- Covering face/using excessive cosmetics
- Wearing bulky clothes, scarfs, and caps to mask the body
- Seeking cosmetic changes/surgery
- Seeking reassurance for their looks from others

- Avoiding social situations
- Counting calories and crash diets
- Unhealthy weight control behaviors (fasting, dieting, and obsessive exercising)
- High protein/steroids intake
- Completely ignoring their obesity.

## BODY IMAGE ISSUES AND PSYCHOPATHOLOGIES

Psychopathologies have a cause-and-effect relationship with body image issues.

There are umpteen studies that prove a significant role of body dissatisfaction as being a precursor of major psychopathologies. Important among them are:
- Body dysmorphic disorder
- *Eating disorders:* Anorexia nervosa and bulimia
- Depression
- Anxiety disorder
- Suicidality
- Substance abuse
- Personality disorders.

Most of these disorders have very high morbidity and mortality, therefore making timely addressal of body image issues is very important.

## MANAGEMENT

### In-office Practice

Pediatricians should always keep in mind that though body dissatisfaction is rampant in adolescents, it is often missed. All adolescents should be screened for the same during every visit. This can be best done during the routine HEEADSSS (home, education/employment, eating, activities, drugs, sexuality, suicidal ideation, and safety) psychosocial history taking. The open-ended questions one can ask could be:
- How do you feel when you look in the mirror?
- Can you describe your thoughts and feelings about your body?
- What do you not like about your appearance?
- How much time do you spend per day thinking about your appearance?
- How much distress do these appearance concerns cause you?
- How much does it interfere in your life?

One should strictly avoid asking closed-ended questions like: Are you worried about your increasing weight?

Adolescents with high risk should be screened more meticulously.

Validated screening tools like Body Image Questionnaire—Child and Adolescent version (Schneider), Body Shape Questionnaire (BSQ) (Cooper), and Adolescent Body Image Satisfaction Scale (ABISS) may be used for objective evaluation.

Ruling out comorbidities like eating disorders, depression, and substance-use disorder is very important.

### Treatment

The goal of the therapy is to resize the defect.
- *Cognitive behavioral therapy (CBT):* It helps in identifying and evaluating the negative thoughts and cognitive errors. It teaches the reconstruction of thoughts so that they are less distressing.
- Socialization training is given through systematic desensitization of threatening social situations starting from a safe setting.
- *Mirror therapy:* Here, the aim is to develop a more holistic view of self-appearance.

The strategies followed in this therapy are:
- *Positive focus:* Describing only the good parts of body
- Focusing on objectively (vs. negatively) describing body
- Describing the negatively viewed body parts using neutral words
- *Pharmacotherapy:* In severe cases, selective serotonin reuptake inhibitors (SSRIs) like fluoxetine may be considered
- Timely referrals made to mental health professionals should be made for severe/resistant cases and adolescents with associated significant psychopathologies.

### Preventive Measures

#### Empowerment of Adolescents

Schools/clubs are good platforms to conduct group sessions for:
- Providing psychoeducation related to body image
- Routine anticipatory guidance about pubertal growth
- Life skill training
- Promoting self-esteem
- Teaching media literacy and media resistance
- *Positive stress management:* Breathing exercises, games, and hobbies
- Promoting physical fitness and healthy eating.

*Anticipatory Guidance to the Parents*

Parents should be advised to:

- Develop and maintain body satisfaction for themselves.
- Focus on the functionality of body parts rather than the looks.
- Address and not neglect concerns that the child raises for his body/looks.
- Avoid comparison, especially about their looks.
- Avoid casual comments on body/body parts.
- Appreciate qualities such as kindness, helpful nature, or talents of the children.
- Communicate with other family members/friends to stop commenting on body image.
- Model and encourage healthy eating and physical activity.

## KEY MESSAGES

- Body image issues are very common among adolescents and are often missed.
- Family, society, and media are major contributors.
- They are closely associated with major psychiatric disorders.
- Prevention through awareness and empowerment should be undertaken.

- Primary pediatrician should screen, pick up early, and assess for severity and comorbidities.
- Management involves various psychotherapeutic techniques and pharmaceutical agents, if needed.

## RECOMMENDED READING


1. Aroor AR, Galagali P. Body image issues during adolescence. In: Pemde HK, Kumari R, Galagali PM, Velmurugan SL (Eds). Adolescent Friendly Pediatric Practice, 1st edition. New Delhi: Jaypee Brothers Medical Publishers (P) Ltd; 2023.
2. Grover S, Raju VV, Sharma A, Shah R. Depression in Children and Adolescents: A Review of Indian studies. Indian J Psychol Med. 2019;41(3):216-27.
3. Hosseini SA, Padhy RK. Body Image Distortion. In: StatPearls [Internet]. Treasure Island (FL): StatPearls Publishing; 2024. [online] Available from https://www.ncbi.nlm.nih.gov/books/NBK546582/ [Last accessed March, 2024].
4. Nivedita N, Sreenivasa G, Sathyanarayana Rao TS, Malini SS. Eating disorders: Prevalence in the student population of Mysore, South India. Indian J Psychiatry. 2018;60(4):433-7.
5. Slade PD, Brodie D. Body-image distortion and eating disorder: a reconceptualization based on the recent literature. Eur Eat Disord Rev. 2006;2(1):32-46.


---

## 3B.2 Somatic Symptom Disorder and Malingering

*Somashekar AR, Amruthvarshini Inamadar*

### SOMATIC SYMPTOM DISORDER

#### INTRODUCTION

When a bodily symptom is not consistent with a definite physical sickness, the patient is said to have a psychosomatic disorder. Psychosomatic presentations have a high incidence and they are typically benign events that occur during childhood and adolescence. However, psychological somatization becomes a disorder when symptoms significantly impair the patient's emotional behavior and functionality. Patients with somatization most frequently describe pain as a symptom.

The National Mental Health Survey of India 2021–2022 indicates that between 10% and 25% of children and adolescents report having psychosomatic problems.

#### DEFINITION AND DIAGNOSTIC CRITERIA

According to the Diagnostic and Statistical Manual of Mental Disorders, Fifth Edition (DSM-5), somatic symptom disorder (SSD) is defined as a condition in which a patient reports subjectively experiencing physical symptoms that are distressing, interfere with their day-to-day functioning, and result in ideas, emotions, and actions that are out of proportion to the symptoms, for a prolonged period.

It falls under the group somatic symptom and related disorder. It is characterized by excessive thoughts, feelings, or behaviors related to the somatic symptoms or associated health concerns as manifested by at least one of the following:

- Disproportionate and persistent thoughts about the seriousness of one's symptoms

- Persistently high level of anxiety about health or symptoms
- Excessive time and energy devoted to these symptoms or health concerns
- Although any one somatic symptom may not be continuously present, the state of being symptomatic is persistent (typically >6 months)
- One or more somatic symptoms that are distressing or result in significant disruption of daily life.

Somatic symptom disorder could be mild, moderate, or severe, depending on the presence and severity of the symptoms.

## ETIOPATHOGENESIS

In psychosomatic disorders, the individual brings out underlying stress through somatic complaints and maybe associated with secondary gains. Hence, psychosomatic disorders have a complex etiology that contributes to perception and manhandling of stress. Numerous elements, including genetic, environmental, biochemical, and psychological aspects, are contributory to the pathophysiology of psychosomatic illnesses. Chronic physical illnesses and mental subnormalities are common predisposing factors in adolescents.

Broken family, mental health issues in parents, unhealthy parenting styles (permissive or neglectful), stressors in the school (like bullying, academic difficulties, and conflicts with peers) and children with psycho-pathologies like anxiety, depression, and substance abuse are found to have more incidence of psychosomatic disorder.

Somatic syndrome disorder appears to present owing to hyperresponsiveness to stress. Any external or internal stimulus that arouses the sympathetic nervous system and the hypothalamic–pituitary–adrenal (HPA) axis and alters physiology is considered as a stressor. The HPA axis is the main regulator of the neuroendocrine response to stress. HPA-axis dysregulation is more commonly seen in children with functional somatic symptoms.

## CLINICAL FEATURES

- Although psychosomatic pain can occur anywhere in the body, it is most frequently described as headache or stomach discomfort.
- It could show up in multiple body parts at once, or it could move over time.
- Usually, it starts as sporadic discomfort that gets worse over time and becomes a daily presence, eventually

making it harder for the person to go about their daily lives.

- It persists for months or even years without a helpful therapy.
- Adjuvants like gabapentin and neuroleptics, as well as common analgesics like opioids, are ineffectual.
- It is frequently accompanied by noticeable fatigue.

Psychosomatic illnesses can cause the following symptoms in their sufferers:

- Unease, light-headedness, altered appetite, insomnia, muscle aches, agitation or rage, constipation, and elevated blood pressure
- Gastrointestinal problems, dizziness, poor concentration, tachycardia, chest discomfort, confusion, sweating, stomach issues, and mood fluctuations.

Most of the times, excessive attention is being paid to the symptoms by the caretakers. Even after getting all the investigations normal, they insist on re-evaluation and are hailbound to get some concrete cause for the symptoms. They end up doing doctor shopping for the same and miss out on seeing a mental health professional.

### Differential Diagnosis

This includes factitious disorder, hypochondriasis, generalized anxiety disorder, and mood disorders.

## APPROACH FOR DIAGNOSIS

Instead of being perceived as exclusive, somatization and SSD should be seen as a part of a cluster of psychiatric comorbidities or significant stressors.

A detailed history indicative of the following supports the diagnosis of SSD:

- Female gender
- Presence of a previously diagnosed chronic disease
- Adolescent age
- Mild intellectual disability
- History of violence, abuse, or life adversities during childhood
- High conflictual level within the family
- Familiarity with psychiatric disorders
- History of chronic school absenteeism or bullying and victimization
- High family or social expectations regarding the subject.

To the pediatrician, they usually bring a noteworthy medical dossier that compiles the results of their examinations and assessments. These characteristics should be regarded as strongly suggestive of SSD. One should keenly look for anxiety and depression, which are commonly associated. Having been diagnosed with a chronic disorder does not disqualify but further substantiates the diagnosis. Physical examinations of these patients are typically unremarkable.

## MANAGEMENT

If left undiagnosed and untreated, psychosomatic disorders can be extremely debilitating. It might have a negative effect on adolescence and result in a functional disability.

The pediatrician should first become skilled at actively questioning patients and their families to draw attention to the amnestic features that may point to psychosomatic disorders. This includes learning to recognize discrepancies between physical examination results and reported symptoms, as well as significant functional limitations brought on by symptoms that are accompanied by social disengagement and chronic absence from school.

Families often support their children's inappropriate medicalization and doctor shopping, which these patients frequently experience. Surprisingly, the pediatrician should be strong enough to refuse an improper request for more research and only recommend additional diagnostic tests when they are clearly needed. With the assistance of a child psychiatrist, pediatricians must positively convey the diagnosis in accordance with DSM-5 criteria. Their words can reassure patients and their families, relieving them of the worry that they may have an unknown illness.

To coordinate the care of these patients, a multidisciplinary approach involving all the professionals who work with children is required, including child psychologists, educators, sports trainers, child psychiatrists, occupational therapists, etc. In moderate cases, assurance might be sufficient. However, physicians should also take into account the possibility that patients' families will find it difficult to accept this diagnosis. A consultation with a pediatric psychologist or psychiatrist may be beneficial.

The goals of psychotherapy are to refocus attention away from symptoms and restore social functioning, identifying potential triggers, and acquiring the coping mechanisms required to manage this illness. The patient's degree of impairment increases with the severity of the case. In severe cases, hospitalization is essential to initiate a multidisciplinary care approach with child psychiatrists, physiotherapists, pediatricians, child psychologists, and nurses to clarify the diagnosis and begin functional rehabilitation.

For these patients, pharmaceutical treatment is not recommended, with the exception of psychiatric comorbidities. Therefore, only after a thorough psychiatric evaluation should pharmaceutical therapies be prescribed. Adjuvants and major opioids, as well as most common analgesics, are usually ineffective in treating psychosomatic pain. As a result, using them is not advised. To help with their symptoms, the patient might also be prescribed digital therapy and distraction techniques. Play therapy (for younger patients), family therapy, cognitive behavioral therapy (CBT), and relaxation techniques should be employed in the treatment.

*If untreated, SSD may lead to:*
- Chronic absenteeism at school
- Unable to pursue hobbies
- Unable to practice sports
- Poor socialization skills/poor peer connect
- Use of medical aids such as crutches or wheelchairs, or incongruous medicalization can cause children to develop a real disability.
- These patients' functional impairment can have a detrimental effect on the whole family, with parents having to spend a lot of time and money attending to their kids' symptoms.
- Significantly higher adverse life events and lower self-esteem were reported by patients with functional somatic complaints, which include hyperventilation syndrome, limb pain, chest pain, and recurrent abdominal pain.

## PREVENTION

- Psychosomatic illness is difficult to treat, but it can be prevented or controlled to some degree.
- *Self-care:* It is critical to preserving health and minimizing psychosomatic illness symptoms. A healthy diet, positive self-talk, staying hydrated, exercising frequently, getting enough sleep at night, practicing meditation on a regular basis, talking to friends and family about stressing issues, keeping a journal, engaging in enjoyable activities, such as viewing films or listening to tunes and music are some tips that could be shared with the adolescents.

*Additional strategies for coping with psychosomatic illnesses include:*
- Being nice and helpful to others
- Reducing alcohol and tobacco use

- Reducing intake of caffeine and sugar
- Taking part in entertaining activities
- Being part of a support group
- Having a break from taxing tasks
- Letting go of negative thought patterns and grudges
- Realizing what one can and cannot control.

## MALINGERING

### INTRODUCTION

Malingering is the falsification or profound exaggeration of illness (physical or mental) to gain external benefits. In the case of adolescents, it could be in the form of school absenteeism, exam concession, exemption from laborious work or sports, empathy and leniency in problematic behavior trials, procurement of substance for abuse, etc.

### ETIOPATHOGENESIS

The etiology of malingering is unknown; however, socioeconomic factors are among its causes. It is frequently reported by homeless people hoping for financial assistance or rations, workers avoiding work, students skipping school, and prisoners avoiding trial. Drug addicts frequently fabricate illnesses, agonizing ailments, or sleeplessness to obtain illicit drugs. It is closely linked to both the histrionic personality trait and antisocial personality disorder.

In order to obtain a secondary benefit from outside sources, the person may pretend to be ill, either physically or psychologically. The patient knowingly lies about his condition; once this benefit is obtained, he ceases to complain. Malingerers cannot be cured by medication or other therapies. A detailed history drives the deceiver to exhaust all excuses and give up.

### DIAGNOSTIC CRITERIA

Malingering is not a psychiatric illness according to DSM-5 but is a "V" code condition.

According to the DSM-5, malingering should be taken into consideration if a patient exhibits any combination of the following four complaints:

1. The presentation's medicolegal context, such as a lawyer referring a client for assessment or a patient presenting with a disease while on trial
2. A marked disparity between the person's "objective finding and observation" and their "claimed stress or disability"

3. Noncompliance with the course of treatment, follow-up care, and diagnostic evaluation
4. Presence of antisocial personality disorder.

### CLINICAL APPROACH

To rule out malingering, a thorough history must be taken.

- As you take a thorough, extended history, pay close attention to any behavioral inconsistencies.
- Examine the patient's personality in great detail (histrionic traits, antisocial personality disorder).
- Learn about the patient's legal situation.
- Pose quick questions and check for logical gaps in the responses.
- Pose a leading, open-ended question. (A positive response may also be obtained by posing questions concerning symptoms unrelated to the "illness faked by the patient".) The patient could answer "yes" to any question because they do not know much about the presumed illness.
- Keep an eye out for the exaggeration of mental symptoms, such as delusions and hallucinations.

### MENTAL STATUS EXAMINATION

- *Behavior and appearance:* Could come across as messy, with unbrushed hair, unkempt clothes, no eye contact, and a lack of rapport-building; angry and hostile actions.
- *Mood:* Responses are either depressed or joyful, never typical euthymic; unable to simulate ineffectiveness or anhedonia.
- *Thoughts:* People suffering from schizophrenia or psychosis may have irrational delusions and steadfast beliefs. Exaggerated delusions are sometimes mistaken for actual psychiatric thought disorders, but they cannot imitate formal thought disorders like schizophrenia.
- *Perception:* Exaggerated auditory and visual hallucinations.
- *Knowledge:* Possess a solid understanding of the illness; nearly always admit to having the illness they pretend to have.
- *Cognition:* Sometimes difficult to evaluate accurately due to patient noncompliance and lying.

It is recommended to conduct multiple examinations and record any inconsistencies in the results. Patients are given different tasks, and their performance is recorded on various occasions. When the same task is completed more than once, the inconsistent score suggests that someone is lying.

*Additional domains to be examined consist of:*

- Hospitalization and medication history
- Medication history currently taken
- Family history
- Social history

## ◼ DIFFERENTIAL DIAGNOSIS

- *Organic disorder:* Before considering malingering, any physical illness must be ruled out
- *Conversion disorder:* Unintentional production of neurological symptoms with the belief that the illness is "real"
- *Factitious disorders:* Munchausen syndrome, deliberately assuming "patient's role", for sympathy or support
- Thought disorders such as schizophrenia and psychosis
- Somatic symptom disorder (SSD)
- Hypochondriasis
- Mania and depression
- Disorders of dissociation.

## ◼ MANAGEMENT

The history, physical examination, and psychological testing are used to diagnose malingering. There are no available diagnostic laboratory tests to identify deception. Nonetheless, laboratory tests are helpful in ruling out organic causes and determining the validity of an illness. These laboratory investigations may consist of the following:

- The complete blood count (CBC) and serum electrolytes, renal functions, liver function tests, blood alcohol content, urine and blood toxicology screen (to rule out drug abusers who are seeking opioids by lying).
- To rule out organic brain disorders, brain magnetic resonance imaging (MRI) or computed tomography (CT) scanning should be taken into consideration.
- *Psychological tests include the following:* The F-scale, the Rey 15-item test, the temporal memory sequence test, the Minnesota multiphasic personality inventory (MMPI), the test of memory malingering, the negative impression management scale, and the symptom and disposition interview (SDI).

## Practical Points to Remember

Avoid having direct conversations with the patient. Never challenge the patient's beliefs. Refrain from accusing the patient of making up their illness. Violence, a lawsuit against the physician, and patient–doctor disputes could happen. Instead, address the patient subtly. Provide a rational scientific explanation without refuting the patient's beliefs. Avoiding invasive diagnostics and interventions is advised because the risks outweigh the benefits. The doctor can assist through motivation.

## Treatment Modalities

- Behavioral therapy
- Psychotherapy
- Counseling

## ◼ PROGNOSIS

The prognosis is uncertain. The malingerer typically does not stop until his motivation or desired outcome is achieved.

## ◼ PREVENTION

Malingering is an extremely challenging disorder to identify and manage. An interprofessional team comprising a psychotherapist, psychiatrist, and mental health nurse is best suited to manage the disorder. If their demands are not fulfilled, these patients have the potential to be combative and even file lawsuits. For the most part, these patients have a cautious prognosis. Most of them eventually have legal issues stemming from their mental illness.

## ◼ KEY MESSAGES

- Stress is an important precursor of psychosomatic disorders.
- Organic causes must be ruled out before diagnosing psychosomatic disorders.
- Comorbid psychopathologies should be looked for.
- Multidisciplinary care involving pediatricians, educators, child psychiatrists, psychologists, nurses, and physiotherapists is necessary for patients.
- Only after a thorough mental assessment is pharmacological treatment prescribed.
- Antisocial personality disorder is linked to malingering.
- Diagnosis to be made using DSM-5.
- It is important to perform mental status examination.
- Present a scientific explanation while respecting the patient's beliefs.

medication) or another medical condition (e.g., hyperthyroidism).

Anxiety disorders in adolescence present clinical features, epidemiology, and therapeutic approaches specific to adolescence.

Adolescence sees both bodily and mental changes, owing to the transition of a child into adulthood.

Many clinical presentations in anxiety could be directly related to these physical and mental rearrangements.

The uniqueness of anxiety disorders of adolescents makes it necessary to consider clinical features related to their prognosis as well as draw up specific considerations relevant to the therapy.

## ■ EPIDEMIOLOGY

### Global

Epidemiological studies have estimated that the prevalence of anxiety disorders in early adolescence ranges from 10 to 20%.

In the community adolescent populations, prior anxiety symptoms are strong and consistent predictors of later anxiety symptoms.

Further, an anxiety disorder diagnosis in adolescence is a strong predictor of later diagnosis for the same or another anxiety disorder, and untreated anxiety symptoms in childhood and adolescence often persist into adulthood.

### India

The pooled prevalence of anxiety disorder among adolescents in India is found to be 0.41% or 41% [confidence interval (CI) 0.14–0.96] for studies with more than low risk and 0.29% or 29% (CI 0.11–0.46) for studies with low risk. This is from a meta-analysis of nearly 13 studies in India. The patient populations had heterogeneity in the associated risk factors. Hence, two different sets of data were drawn up.

Anxiety disorders with the highest burden are found in both male and female adolescents and young adults.

*The most frequently encountered anxiety disorders during adolescence are:*
- Generalized anxiety disorder
- Separation anxiety disorder
- Social anxiety disorder.
  *In contrast in adulthood, the most common clinical disorders concern specific phobias.*

## ■ CLINICAL FEATURES

### Diagnostic and Statistical Manual of Mental Disorders, Fifth Edition Criteria

#### For Generalized Anxiety Disorder

- Excessive worrying about events and activities such as school performance
- Difficulties controlling the worries
- Restlessness, fatigue, difficulties with concentration, irritability, and sleep problems.

#### For Separation Anxiety Disorder

- Developmentally inappropriate and excessive fear of separation
- Worries about losing significant attachment figures
- Persistent fear of being alone
- Difficulties going to sleep alone without being near an attachment figure.

#### For Social Anxiety Disorder

- Fear or anxiety in social situations such as social interactions and being observed or performing in front of others
- The individual fears humiliation, and the social situations provoke anxiety and cause significant distress.

## ■ DIAGNOSTIC SCREENING TOOLS

Several validated scales are freely available:
- Screen for Child Anxiety-Related Emotional Disorders (SCARED)
- Spence Children's Anxiety Scale (SCAS)
- Preschool Anxiety Scale (PAS)
- General Anxiety Disorder-7 (GAD-7)

The symptoms are often mixed and blend with each other such that separating among them is both not practical and often not even necessary.

## ■ CORRELATES AND RISK FACTORS

Studies have shown the influence of some of the following:
- Demographic variables
- Temperament and personality—in particular, behavioral inhibition as a risk for social anxiety in adolescence
- Comorbidities
- Environmental and developmental factors—including the impact of different events of life or early life for example death in a family.

- Influence of familial, social, and academic environment and neurobiological factors
- Genetic factors and heritability
- Subgroups of individuals who exhibit different patterns of depressive and anxiety disorders over the course of adolescence and young adulthood anxiety
- Gender
- Familial loading of psychopathology and childhood abuse.

## Relationship with Body Dysmorphic Disorder

Literature showed that body image is significantly correlated with self-esteem and depression, anxiety, social phobia, and obsessive–compulsive symptoms.

## ■ MANAGEMENT AND TREATMENT

It is evident that an adolescent with anxiety disorders is at an increased risk of worsening with subsequent depression, substance abuse, or dependence, as well as educational underachievement in the young adult state.

Early assessment and treatment are essential.

## Treatment Strategies

- Psychotherapy
- Medications
- Combinations of interventions in a *multidisciplinary approach* will be the mainstay of therapy.

### Psychotherapy

It needs to incorporate:

- *Cognitive behavioral therapy (CBT):* CBT is a talking therapy that can help you manage your problems by changing the way you think and behave.
- *Psychodynamic approach:* The goals of psychodynamic therapy are the client's self-awareness and understanding of the influence of the past on present behavior.
- Parent–child and family interventions, with particular emphasis on the importance of comprehensive care.

### Medications

- *Selective serotonin reuptake inhibitors (SSRIs):* For anxiety disorder symptoms are moderate or severe, but when impairment makes participation in psychotherapy difficult, or when psychotherapy results in a partial response, SSRIs are used.
- Medications other than SSRIs still need to be further studied.

However, noradrenergic antidepressants, buspirone, and benzodiazepines have been suggested as alternatives to be used alone or in combination with SSRIs.

Comorbid conditions strongly influence the selection of medication.

## Prognosis

The prognosis for anxiety disorders in children depends on the severity, availability of competent treatment, and the child's resilience.

Many children struggle with anxiety symptoms into adulthood.

However, with early treatment, many children learn how to control their anxiety.

## Follow-up

Repeat administration of the *GAD-7 every 4 weeks* to monitor symptoms.

Follow-up for a minimum period of 12 or 6 months of consistent symptomatic improvement. Yearly follow-up for 5 years thereafter is considered an appropriate assessment of how the individual sustains himself/herself through various challenges.

## ■ KEY MESSAGES

- Classification of teenage anxiety disorders is well and truly necessary as per DSM-5 criteria.
- The most common manifestation of an anxiety disorder may be school refusal; most children couch their discomfort in terms of somatic complaints.
- Consider anxiety as a disorder in children only when anxiety becomes so exaggerated that it greatly impairs functioning or causes severe distress and/or avoidance.
- The physical symptoms that anxiety can cause in children can complicate the evaluation.
- Behavioral therapy (using principles of exposure and response prevention) is most effective when done by an experienced therapist who is knowledgeable of child development and who tailors these principles to the child.
- When cases are more severe or when access to an experienced child behavior therapist is limited, medications may be needed.

## RECOMMENDED READING

1. Achenbach TM, Howell CT, McConaughy SH, Stanger C. Six-year predictors of problems in a national sample: IV. Young adult signs of disturbance. J Am Acad Child Adolesc Psychiatry. 1998;37(7):718-27.
2. Copeland WE, Shanahan L, Costello EJ, Angold A. Childhood and adolescent psychiatric disorders as predictors of young adult disorders. Arch Gen Psychiatry. 2009;66(7):764-72.
3. Costello EJ, Mustillo S, Erkanli A, Keeler G, Angold A. Prevalence and development of psychiatric disorders in childhood and adolescence. Arch Gen Psychiatry. 2003;60(8):837-44.
4. Ferdinand RF, Dieleman G, Ormel J, Verhulst FC. Homotypic versus heterotypic continuity of anxiety symptoms in young adolescents: Evidence for distinctions between DSM-IV subtypes. J Abnorm Child Psychol. 2007;35(3):325-33.
5. Ferdinand RF, Verhulst FC. Psychopathology from adolescence into young adulthood: An 8-year follow-up study. Am J Psychiatry. 1995;152(11):1586-94.
6. Lewinsohn PM, Holm-Denoma JM, Small JW, Seeley JR, Joiner TE Jr. Separation anxiety disorder in childhood as a risk factor for future mental illness. J Am Acad Adolesc Psychiatry. 2008;47(5):548-55.
7. Morris RJ, Kratochwill TR. Childhood fears and phobias. In: Kratochwill TR, Morris RJ (Eds). The Practice of Child Therapy, 2nd edition. New York: Pergamon; 1991. pp. 76-114.
8. Muris P, Merckelbach H, Mayer B, Meesters C. Common fears and their relationship to anxiety disorders symptomatology in normal children. Pers Individ Diff. 1998;24(4):575-8.
9. Pal D, Sahu DP, Maji S, Taywade M. Prevalence of Anxiety Disorder in Adolescents in India: A Systematic Review and Meta-Analysis. Cureus. 2022;14(8):e28084.
10. Shaffer D, Fisher P, Dulcan MK, Davies M, Piacentini J, Schwab-Stone ME, et al. The NIMH diagnostic interview schedule for children version 2.3 (DISC-2.3): Description, acceptability, prevalence rates, and performance in the MECA study. Methods for the Epidemiology of Child and Adolescent Mental Disorders Study. J Am Acad Child Adolesc Psychiatry. 1996;35(7):865-77.

---

# 3B.4 Eating Disorders

*Newton Luiz, Jayant Pandharikar*

## INTRODUCTION

Eating disorders (EDs) are complex mental health disorders that manifest as highly abnormal eating behaviors, caused by an irrational concept of beauty as having a morbidly thin figure (the "thin ideal"). A valuation of self-worth based on perceived weight and body shape and a distorted perception of one's own body image result in intense dissatisfaction with oneself and extreme attempts to attain the desired thinness. This has significant consequences on the physical health, the emotional status, and the social interactions of the individual, which are often overlooked but are potentially life-threatening if untreated. In developed countries, EDs rank third among the major common chronic mental illnesses in adolescent females.

## TYPES OF EATING DISORDERS

- *Anorexia nervosa (AN):* The patient (typically a female adolescent) is convinced that she is obese, and she drastically reduces her food intake until she becomes severely undernourished. Yet, she continues to insist that she is overweight, and in extreme cases, she may starve herself to death. The severity of this psychiatric disease is assessed by the degree of malnutrition, i.e., whether mild, moderate, severe, or extreme. An occasional patient who was obese to start with may rapidly lose weight and present with a normal weight ("atypical AN").

  *There are two variants:* (1) Restricting type, who attains weight loss by a highly restricted food intake and/or excessive exercise, and (2) binge-eating/purging type, who additionally indulges in recurrent secretive episodes of binge eating and purging. Binge eating refers to episodes of uncontrolled and excessive food intake, unrelated to the taste of the food, often eaten rapidly and with a perceived loss of ability to control one's food intake, so the person continues to eat even while feeling excessively full until she is forced to stop due to nausea and abdominal pain. Purging often follows on its heels; the person immediately attempts to get rid of the extra calories by self-induced vomiting and/or by the misuse of laxatives, diuretics, and enemas.

- *Bulimia nervosa (BN):* It is characterized primarily by very frequent episodes of binge eating in association with compensatory weight-loss maneuvers like purging, fasting, or excessive exercise, occurring over a period of at least 3 months. There are two variants of BN: (1) Purging type, engaged primarily in induced vomiting or misuse of laxatives and enemas, and (2) nonpurging type, engaged more in fasting and excessive exercise. It manifests in girls who are extremely fearful of gaining weight. As weight loss is often mild or absent, the condition is difficult to diagnose. Severity is assessed by the frequency of inappropriate compensatory strategies, which occur on average 1–3 times a week in mild cases, 4–7 times if moderate, 8–13 times if severe, and 14 or more times in extreme cases.

- *Binge-eating disorder (BED):* This is characterized by frequent binge eating, with infrequent compensatory purging behavior and intense shame and guilt about bingeing. People having BED are often overweight, and concerned about it, but they are less concerned about their body image than in BN and do not routinely overestimate their weight. Persons who binge regularly at least once a week for 3 months are labeled as having BED.

- *Other specified feeding and eating disorder (OSFED):* This refers to other inappropriate attitudes toward eating such as night eating syndrome (where a person often wakes up unexpectedly in the middle of the night and raids the refrigerator before going back to bed) or purging without bingeing. They are sometimes termed "disordered eating", and the concern is that they are more likely to develop a full-blown ED in the future.

  It is presumed that the above conditions represent the same psychopathology of body image distortion, and the patient may shuttle between the different diagnostic states over a period of time (diagnostic crossover).

- *Avoidant/restrictive food intake disorder (ARFID):* It is a condition characterized by the person avoiding or restricting certain foods or types of food, because of adverse eating experiences or the sensory quality of the food, resulting in significant unintended weight loss or nutritional deficiencies.

In the Diagnostic and Statistical Manual of Mental Disorders, Fifth Edition (DSM-5), EDs are placed in the section on feeding and EDs, which additionally includes pica and rumination disorders.

## ◼ EPIDEMIOLOGY

In developed nations, AN, BN, and BED affect approximately 0.5–1%, 2.0%, and 4% of adolescent girls, respectively. Girls are affected 5–10 times more commonly than boys in AN, while BN and BED are at least twice as common in girls as in boys. This gender difference is probably due to the greater concern of females about their body shape and weight. The prevalence of EDs has increased in recent decades side by side with the rapid rise in the prevalence of obesity and overweight.

A beautiful woman is conceptualized as a tall and unusually thin girl with big breasts (recall Barbie, the adolescent doll). The adolescent does not realize that the slim and trim figures sported by models and influencers on Instagram are the result of intense daily exercise and strict diet control. Female adult models are expected to have a body mass index (BMI) in the 15–18 range, which is below the medically recommended range of 18.5–25. EDs are more common in professions that demand thinness, such as models, dancers, and gymnasts.

The family has a significant influence on the development of EDs. This is believed to be primarily due to genetic factors, like a proneness to anxiety, depression, or obsessive–compulsive behaviors, and environmental factors, like the food habits of the family and its attitude toward physical activity. EDs are frequently comorbid with depression, anxiety, and obsessive–compulsive disorder. Parental and sibling teasing or criticism for being overweight are important factors, but their role has been exaggerated in the past. While poor family dynamics can precipitate or aggravate any psychiatric illness, they are unlikely to be causative.

Indian publications report negligible numbers of EDs. This is not unexpected in Asian and African countries, where thinness is socially associated not with beauty but with poverty or tuberculosis or even human immunodeficiency virus (HIV). There is some evidence that EDs increase as countries make economic progress.

A comprehensive review in 2019 of all studies on EDs published in India in the previous 5 decades uncovered only 39 articles (15 studies and 24 case reports or case series). Most of the cases were adolescent females with restrictive AN. Of the five cases of BN, only two cases were typical. No cases of BED were reported. Mammen et al. from CMC Vellore reported that between 2000 and 2005, their Child and Adolescent Psychiatry Unit diagnosed only six cases of AN. There are no population studies from developing countries, and the 15 articles were mostly convenience samples of medical or nursing schools or school-based studies. The conclusion was that severe EDs were quite rare, but disordered eating was common. As per the National Institute of Mental Health and Neurosciences (NIMHANS) survey (2015), 2% of the Indian population suffers from EDs.

## ETIOLOGICAL FACTORS

The onset of EDs in adolescents may be related to their pubertal changes, sexuality, concern about body image, and increasing autonomy and cognitive ability. Genetic factors, hormonal changes (especially in girls), inappropriate dietary practices, and the influence of the media and advertising may contribute. EDs are more prevalent in adolescents who have experienced physical/emotional/sexual abuse or suffer from anxiety, mood disorders, other mental health illnesses, and addiction to alcohol or drugs. AN typically affects adolescent girls in early-to-middle adolescence who tend to be perfectionistic, anxiety-prone, and above average in intelligence and socioeconomic status. BN tends to occur in late adolescence and is commonly associated with depressive symptoms.

## DIFFERENTIAL DIAGNOSIS

Differentiating EDs from organic illness is generally not difficult, so long as the possibility is considered. While there are many illnesses that are associated with chronic weight loss and/or anorexia, *in organic illnesses the patient is extremely unhappy about weight loss and loss of appetite*. In addition, erythrocyte sedimentation rate (ESR) is high in inflammatory diseases like systemic lupus erythematosus (SLE) and in malignancies, while hormone tests rule out diabetes mellitus, thyroid diseases, and adrenal insufficiency. Nevertheless, chronic drug use may be missed. Brain tumors like craniopharyngioma that damage the hypothalamic appetite center tend to cause chronic anorexia and severe weight loss without symptoms of hunger, and symptoms of raised intracranial tension appear late **(Box 1)**.

## EATING BEHAVIORS

### Anorexia Nervosa

The patient consistently takes very little food at every meal or takes a normal volume of low-calorie food like salads, fruits, and vegetables, resulting in steady weight loss. She strictly avoids calorie-rich food, totally avoids snacks,

**BOX 1:** Differential diagnosis.

- Substance abuse
- Malignancy
- Inflammatory disorders like SLE
- Hyperthyroidism
- Hypothyroidism
- Inflammatory bowel disease
- Diabetes mellitus
- Adrenal insufficiency
- Brain tumors (craniopharyngioma)

(SLE: systemic lupus erythematosus)

and may become a pure vegetarian and drink a lot of water. She may count her calories obsessively. If she eats more than usual, she feels guilty and tends to do vigorous exercise and diet strictly. She may exercise compulsively, and increasingly, and may excel in long-distance running. She may occasionally chew food and then spit it out. In the binge-purge variant, she may eat a moderately larger amount than she had planned and then vomit it. She may use laxatives to relieve the constipation brought about by inadequate food intake.

It may not be possible to differentiate between AN and an intelligent and planned dietary program until weight loss becomes excessive. The patient may justify her behavior by pointing to the benefits of exercise, the desire to be successful in sports, and the fact that a close relative has high cholesterol levels or had a heart attack.

### Bulimia Nervosa

Binge eating is the essential feature, and it is often secretive and associated with guilt. She goes on binges when unhappy, angry, or lonely, but at other times, her calorie intake is often normal, or she may diet. During binges, she tends to eat calorie-rich food that she normally avoids; at other times, she mostly eats the usual food. She usually vomits after a binge, and sometimes after a normal meal, but as the binge is often prolonged, the vomiting has limited efficacy as most of the calories have already passed down into the small intestine. She uses laxatives to wash out the food that she has consumed, but it is ineffective as laxatives act only on the large bowel, while absorption occurs in the small intestine. Though they are ineffective as weight-loss strategies, she persists with vomiting and laxative use as they are a form of self-punishment and relieve her guilt. She snacks sometimes, and this often precipitates a binge. She is not strict about counting calories. She claims that she is too weak to follow a strict diet, and her dieting is often impulsive, brief, and erratic.

## CLINICAL FEATURES

### Anorexia Nervosa

She feels fat even when extremely emaciated, may complain that her abdomen is too prominent or her thighs are not slim, and is fanatically concerned about thinness. Depression, anxiety, and obsessive–compulsive symptoms are common. When emaciated, she may feel cold, tired, and weak all the time, she may have faints or palpitations, her hands may feel cold, she may have scalp hair loss while lanugo-type hair grows on her face, and she may have constipation.

### Bulimia Nervosa

Forceful vomiting may result in acid erosion of the lingual side of the teeth, subconjunctival bleeds, loss of gag reflex, and calluses over the proximal joints of the dominant hand due to recurrent incisor bites. There may be abdominal discomfort after a binge and cramps from laxative use. The parotids may enlarge. She may have depressive symptoms and self-injurious behavior and may rarely be suicidal. Unless the diagnosis is kept in mind, it is likely to be missed, as most of the patients present only when features of complications have already set in.

**Box 2** mentions the major complications of eating disorders.

## INVESTIGATIONS

There is no confirmatory laboratory test. Complete blood count (CBC) and ESR are normal or may show anemia. There may be nonspecific changes like low serum potassium and chloride, mildly elevated liver enzymes and cortisol, and low glucose and gonadotropin levels. Blood urea nitrogen (BUN) may be elevated. Electrocardiogram (ECG) may show low voltage and may detect bradycardia or arrhythmia.

## MANAGEMENT

Therapy is multidisciplinary and requires the combined efforts of a pediatrician, a psychiatrist, a nutritionist, and often an exercise therapist, an occupational therapist, and a social worker. A nurturant authoritative approach is most useful in dealing with EDs. The primary goal should be not only attaining and maintaining weight but also improving the overall health.

*Counseling:* The clinician should explain the diagnosis but agree that the patient may have difficulty accepting both the diagnosis and the treatment. The instinctive desire to point out that the patient is too thin is counterproductive; one should accept that she feels fat and gently point out that symptoms and signs suggest that she is too thin for her own good. Emphasize that troublesome symptoms like tiredness and insomnia will be relieved by modest weight gain.

The clinician should describe the illness as a coping mechanism to stress rather than as the stubborn behavior of the patient. One should state that treatment requires time and effort. One should identify troublesome symptoms of excessive weight loss that interfere with the functioning of the patient, such as feeling tired or lacking energy and concentration, and explain how they can be overcome only by adequate food intake. One should avoid criticism and compliment the patient on her progress in health and appearance with treatment and her efforts to reduce weight by exercise.

*Family-based treatment* is very important. The parents are highly stressed by what they conceive as deliberate starvation and need proper guidance by the clinician. They are necessarily the primary caretakers for these chronic disorders. *Group therapy* can be more beneficial but requires a skilled clinician.

*Nutritional correction* requires expertise to prevent refeeding syndrome. Food should be described as the fuel needed for improving energy. It should be 15–20% from proteins, 55% from carbohydrates, and 25–30% (or less) from fats. Multiple small feeds are preferred. There should be a structured meal plan, with at least three main meals a day (especially breakfast) and snacks 1–3 times a day. Food may be increased by 200 calories twice weekly, and the long-term goal is to increase weight by 1–2 kg a month. Calcium should be supplemented to provide 1,300 mg.

---

**BOX 2:** Complications of eating disorders (EDs).

- EDs are chronic health disorders, so no organ is spared from its harmful effects
- Depression is common, and suicide is the most common cause of death
- Amenorrhea is common in females and erectile dysfunction in males
- Osteoporosis is common and may be irreversible if osteopenia occurs during the critical growth period of postpubertal bone accretion
- Starvation can result in bradycardia, hypotension, cold peripheries, and rarely fatal ventricular arrhythmias
- Refeeding syndrome during treatment may be fatal

Vitamin D supplementation is also required. If purging is suspected, the bathroom should be locked for 2 hours after each meal. Constipation may be temporarily treated with stool softeners but never with laxatives and will be rectified when food intake increases.

Psychotherapeutic treatment modalities like cognitive behavior therapy are effective and must focus on restructuring "thinking errors." Simultaneous care of comorbid conditions is important. They are often combined with pharmacotherapy, for which evidence is lacking in AN, though selective serotonin reuptake inhibitors (SSRIs) like fluoxetine in high doses do help in BN. Comorbidities like depression should be treated simultaneously.

*Exercise* improves mood and compliance but should be restricted to a single 30-minute period daily. A daily record of weight, food intake, exercise, and mood helps. Weight should be recorded every morning on awakening after emptying the bladder.

Inpatient care is needed for patients with AN with weight <80% of the expected weight for height, suicidal intent, coexisting psychiatric disorders, dehydration, hypothermia, bradycardia, hypotension, postural hypotension and fainting, arrhythmias, low serum potassium or glucose, or hepatic/renal/cardiac complications.

## PREVENTION

- Create awareness among adolescents and their caretakers about body image issues and EDs.
- During routine HEEADSSS (home, education/employment, eating, activities, drugs, sexuality, suicidal ideation, and safety) screening, enquire about present weight, recent gain or loss, ask "what would you like your weight to be?" and body image concerns. Ask about usual diet, eating habits, whether they have ever been on a diet, bingeing and purging, and exercise to the adolescent and the family. Praise mature attitudes.
- Media literacy about how misleading social media is and the wise use of apps for monitoring calories in the food we eat.
- Lifestyle and life skill training.
- Management of psychiatric illnesses.

## PROGNOSIS

Eating disorders persist because the patient actively resists treatment and denies ill health, as punitive behaviors like purging, fasting, and exercising cause relief from guilt obtained and result in a feeling of self-control. Most persons with EDs do not seek therapy until they have suffered in secret for many years, often due to shame or denial of illness. They prefer to seek help for weight reduction rather than their ED. When they do seek care, they do not stay on the course due to the cost and the prolonged therapy required.

For females aged 15–24 years, the mortality rate from AN is 12 times the baseline rate and double in BN but is not significantly different in BED. 70% of AN recover eventually, of whom one-third recover in 3 years, one-third in 6 years, and one-third in 12 years. The overall mortality is <4%. Recovery should be not only physical (normal weight and health parameters) but also behavioral (no more food restriction, bingeing, purging) and psychological.

## KEY MESSAGES

- EDs are psychiatric disorders that manifest in adolescence as highly abnormal eating behaviors.
- They are caused by an irrational concept of beauty as extreme thinness, and a distorted perception of oneself as overweight, resulting in very low self-esteem.
- They are more prevalent in adolescents who have experienced adverse childhood events, especially sexual abuse, or suffer from mental health illnesses or addiction to alcohol or drugs.
- AN typically affects girls in early adolescence, who severely restrict their diet, and may even starve to death.
- BN typically occurs in older adolescents, who are often depressed, and is characterized by uncontrolled binge eating followed usually by purging.
- BED is milder and more common, and the patient is usually mildly overweight and does not purge after bingeing.
- The differential diagnosis includes a large variety of organic conditions, but in most of them, the patient is quite upset about anorexia and weight loss.
- EDs are most common in countries where being overweight is common, and thinness is, therefore, idealized. They are an emerging threat in developing countries.
- Management is multidisciplinary and involves counseling, nutritional rehabilitation, family therapy, psychotherapy, and pharmacotherapy.
- Counseling requires a nurturant authoritative approach that accepts the patient's self-perception and focuses on removing the troublesome adverse effects of the ED.

## ■ RECOMMENDED READING

1. American Psychiatric Association. (2023). What are Eating Disorders? [online] Available from https://www.psychiatry.org/patients-families/eating-disorders/what-are-eating-disorders [Last accessed March, 2024].
2. Feeding and eating disorders. In. Sadock BJ, Sadock VA, Ruiz P (Eds). Kaplan and Sadock's Comprehensive Textbook of Psychiatry, 10th edition. Philadelphia: Wolters Kluwer; 2017.
3. Hay P. Current approach to eating disorders: a clinical update. Intern Med J. 2020;50(1):24-9.
4. Health Canada. (2022). A Report on Mental Illnesses in Canada. [online] Available from https://www.phac-aspc.gc.ca/publicat/miic-mmac/pdf/chap6e.pdf [Last accessed March, 2024].
5. Mammen P, Russell S, Russell PS. Prevalence of eating disorders and psychiatric comorbidity among children and adolescents. Indian Pediatr. 2007;44:357-9.
6. Prasad KE, Rajan RJ, Basker MM, Mammen PM, Reshmi YS. Clinical profile of adolescent onset of Anorexia Nervosa at a tertiary care centre. Indian Pediatr. 2021;58(8):726-8.
7. Shah M. Eating disorders in India: A systematic review. Acta Neurophysiol. 2023;4(3):180022.
8. Vaidyanathan S, Kuppili PP, Menon V. Eating disorders: An overview of Indian research. Indian J Psychol Med. 2019;41(4):311-7.

---

# 3B.5 | Disruptive Mood Dysregulation Disorder

*Poonam Bhatia*

## ■ INTRODUCTION

Since past many years, mental health professionals encountered challenges in accurately diagnosing children and adolescents displaying severe and chronically irritable behavior. This difficulty stemmed from the fact that chronic irritability is one of the diagnostic criteria for various mood, anxiety, and disruptive disorders outlined in the Diagnostic and Statistical Manual of Mental Disorders, 4th edition, Text Revision (DSM-IV-TR), such as oppositional defiant disorder (ODD), major depressive disorder (MDD), intermittent explosive disorder (IED), and generalized anxiety disorder. Often, these young individuals did not fully meet all the criteria outlined for these specific mental health conditions and were being overly and inaccurately diagnosed and treated as having bipolar disorder (BD).

To address this issue, in May 2013, the Diagnostic and Statistical Manual of mental disorders, 5th edition (DSM-5), introduced a new diagnostic category of mental illness known as Disruptive Mood Dysregulation Disorder (DMDD). The DSM is a manual published by the American Psychiatric Association (APA), to diagnose all categories of mental health disorders for both adults and children. The National Institute of Mental Health (NIMH) identifies DMDD as a childhood mood disorder with "extreme irritability, anger, and frequent, intense temper outbursts". Many a times, the disease is confused with simply "being in a bad mood", but the striking difference is that while most of the children overcome bad mood quite quickly and easily children with DMDD cannot.

The disease causes children to experience unstable emotions, which they cannot regulate like extreme outbursts of anger. These outbursts often occur in response to trivial stimuli like giving a bath, brushing hair, or visiting a doctor. These children are susceptible to developing other mood disorders as well.

## ■ PREVALENCE

Prevalence of DMDD among children and adolescents is estimated to be 2–5% (APA, 2013).

## CRITERIA FOR DIAGNOSING DISRUPTIVE MOOD DYSREGULATION DISORDER

As per DSM-5, in order to meet diagnosis of DMDD, a child must meet the criteria given in **Box 1**.

## CAUSES OF DISRUPTIVE MOOD DYSREGULATION DISORDER

The research till date indicates that some environmental and biological factors could be responsible for the development of DMDD.

- Recurrent or persistent migraine in some children/adolescents causes increased irritability leading to aggressive behavior, which when persists leads to diagnosis of DMDD.

**BOX 1:** DSM-5 Diagnostic criteria for DMDD.

1. Severe recurrent temper outbursts manifested verbally (e.g., foul language and disregarding elders) and/or behaviorally (e.g., physical aggression toward others or damaging property) that are grossly out of proportion in intensity or duration to the situation or provocation
2. The temper outbursts occurring three or more times per week and are inconsistent with developmental level
3. The mood between such outbursts is constantly irritable or angry most of the time of day, almost every day, and is observable by others (e.g., family members, schoolteachers, and peers)
4. Above 3 criteria should have been present for 12 months or more. Throughout that time, the individual has not had a period lasting 3 or more consecutive months without all of the above symptoms
5. All these symptoms are present in at least two of the three settings (i.e., at home, at school, and with peers) and are severe in at least one of these
6. The diagnosis should not be made for the first time before the age of 6 years or after the age of 18 years
7. By history or observation, the age of onset of criteria 1–5 is before 10 years
8. There has never been a clear period lasting more than 1 day when complete manifestation apart from duration, for a manic or hypomanic episode, has been met
    *Note:* The mood elevation which occurs in anticipation or context of an event should not be considered a symptom of mania or hypomania
9. Such behaviors do not occur only during an episode of major depressive disorder and are not explained by another mental disorder (e.g., ASD, PTSD, separational anxiety disorder, or persistent depressive disorder)
10. The symptoms are not attributable to the physiological effects of a substance or to another medical or neurological condition

(ASD: autism spectrum disorder; DMDD: disruptive mood dysregulation disorder; PTSD: post-traumatic stress disorder)

- Early childhood trauma of any form like physical, emotional, or sexual abuse.
- Recent parental divorce, change of residence, or death in the family.
- Lack of certain nutrition or vitamin deficiency has also been found to contribute to the development of DMDD.
- Children of parents with mental illness or substance abuse are at a higher risk of developing DMDD.

## ■ PATHOPHYSIOLOGY

Underactivity of amygdala (part of the brain that is responsible for interpretation and expression of emotions) is the root cause of impaired learning from rewards and consequences. These children face difficulty in processing negative social experiences and negative emotional stimuli, which cause frustration culminating into symptoms like persistent aggression and irritability.

Evolutionarily, the primitive brain was tuned to work quickly without thinking (as thinking brain developed slowly). In cases of *mood disorders,* functional neuroimaging studies show poor connection between the lower (hindbrain—the primitive brain) and higher (prefrontal cortex) parts of the brain. Functional magnetic resonance imaging (fMRI) also showed that under stressful conditions, like in the middle of tantrum, heated argument, etc., increased activity in the lower parts of the brain was seen. Hence, in these children, minor provocations like refusing their demands or a simple "No" are perceived as an attack or severe threat resulting in a fight-or-flight response.

In a study on facial affect recognition task (fMRI), participants with DMDD showed marked amygdala activity across all emotions like joyful, angry, and fearful faces, but children with BD showed increased amygdala activity only for fearful faces.

## ■ SYMPTOMS OF DISRUPTIVE MOOD DYSREGULATION DISORDER

Most children become irritable in response to frustration, but irritability and outbursts are out of proportion to the situation for children with DMDD. Irritability is defined as a decreased threshold to frustration or else it is a heightened proneness to anger **(Flowchart 1)**.

- *Physical symptoms:* Increased heart rate and blood pressure and stiffness of muscles like clenching fists and teeth during temper outbursts
- *Cognitive symptoms:* Difficulty in self-regulation, managing and expressing emotions
- *Psychosocial symptoms:* Extreme irritability, verbal aggression, and highly unpredictable mood.

Participating in team sports and engaging in social gatherings is a challenging task for such children/adolescents. Poor emotional expression seems to be a major hurdle in maintaining healthy relationships with family or peers.

With time, as children grow, they learn to cope up with disappointment and frustration, and the symptoms of DMDD may change. For example, an adolescent or a young adult with DMDD might experience fewer episodes

**Flowchart 1:** Approach to an irritable adolescent.

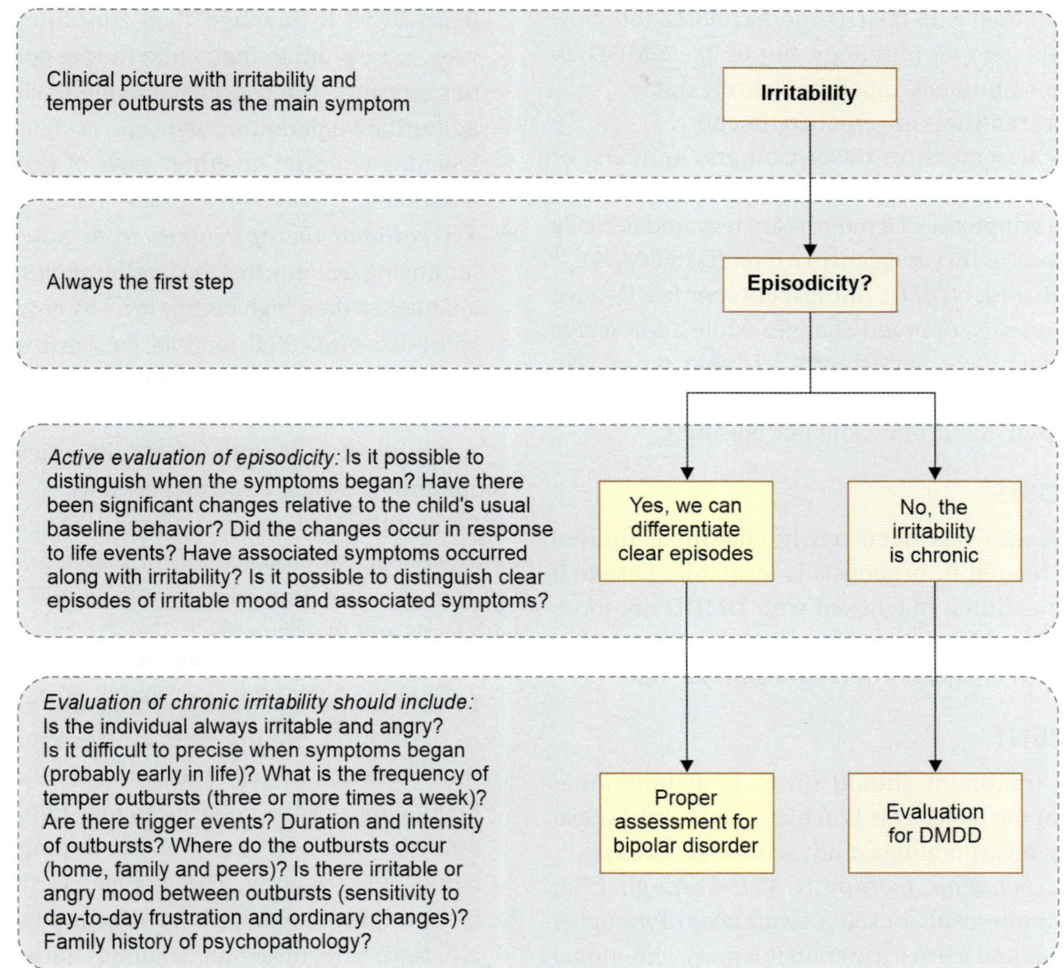


(DMDD: disruptive mood dysregulation disorder)
*Source:* Krieger FV, Leibenluft E, Stringaris A, Polanczyk GV. Irritability in children and adolescents: Past concepts, current debates, and future opportunities. Braz J Psychiatry. 2013;35 Suppl 1(0 1):S32-9.

of tantrums, but symptoms of depression or anxiety begin to appear.

## SCREENING TOOLS

Although there is no validated screening tool for DMDD, the NIMH research group uses versions of the Kiddie Schedule for Affective Disorders and Schizophrenia for school-aged children to diagnose DMDD.

## DIFFERENTIAL DIAGNOSIS

Because of various biopsychosocial changes, teens experience new thoughts and emotions. Moreover, adolescence is also the period of heightened affective reactivity leading to excessive sensitivity to both rewarding and aversive stimuli (caused by differential brain development and upsurging hormones.). All these lead to frequent moodiness or irritability, which is considered a normative part of adolescence. But constantly escalating moodiness, inability to cope up with day-to-day challenges or showing aggression with minimal or perceived discomfort are all red flags which clinicians as well as parents should not ignore.

The diseases that have overlapping symptoms but with variable management and hence need to be differentiated are given in the following text:

- *Oppositional defiant disorder (ODD):* An adolescent with ODD routinely defies rules and argues with authority figures. He/she is vindictive and hurts people and animals purposefully.

- *Intermittent explosive disorder (IED):*
  - Like children with DMDD, these children too show episodic temper outbursts, but unlike DMDD, in between outbursts, mood is relatively stable.
  - Temper tantrums or verbal arguments
  - Physical aggression toward others, animals, or property
  - Active symptoms of 3 months are required to make diagnosis of IED as against 12 months in DMDD.
- *Bipolar disorder (BD):* Adolescents with BD have *discrete* episodes of mood changes while adolescents with DMDD have persistently irritable mood. No child can be diagnosed with DMDD if he/she has ever suffered from manic or hypomanic episodes.

## PROGNOSIS

Since the disease has been newly classified, limited information related to prognosis is available. Research suggests that children diagnosed with DMDD are more likely to develop depression or anxiety disorders during adulthood. Their chances of developing BD are rare.

## TREATMENT

The goal of treatment should be to treat functional impairment of the child. This is achieved by psychosocial interventions, incorporating family, school, and friends.

- *Cognitive behavior therapy (CBT):* Through CBT, children/adolescents develop awareness of thoughts and feelings and learn frustration tolerance, emotional coping, and communication skills. Psychotherapy helps children and adolescents to recognize their angry/irritable mood and they implement the appropriate skill to de-escalate themselves/the situation, or they learn to tolerate uncomfortable feelings.
- *Dialectical behavior therapy (DBT):* This therapy helps children learn to regulate their emotions, thereby avoiding extreme or prolonged outbursts. In DBT-C, the children learn skills (with the help of a counselor) that help in regulating their moods and emotions. During treatment, the therapist repeatedly exposes them to events that cause irritability or anger through which these children are trained in various methods for increasing their tolerance levels.

  Combining CBT with DBT and family therapy is likely to create a compounding effect in improving overall symptoms.
- *Parenteral therapy:* Family therapy sessions are needed as this condition significantly disturbs the family dynamics. Through therapy, family members learn ways to manage their emotions and better ways to respond to their child during episodes of his/her tantrum. The conducive home environment and authoritative parenting style play a significant role in teaching children healthier ways of expressing their emotions.
- *Recreational therapy:* Apart from talk therapy and improving dynamics of the family, adolescents need to channelize their high energy level by engaging in team sports like basketball, football, etc. Participating in gym is an alternative for teens who are not comfortable in group games.

A combination of all the above therapies will create a compounding effect in treatment results.

Some other treatment options like real-time fMRI neurofeedback and pulsed electromagnetic field (PEMF) that are showing promising results should be discussed with teens and their parents.

- *Neurofeedback:* The basic deficits in children with DMDD are poor reward learning and poor response to frustration. Neurofeedback treatment uses real-time feedback to train and aid in rewiring the brain. Reinforcing positive behavior by rewarding the children optimizes the likelihood of developing the desired habits subsequently. The changes in the activity of brain improve a patient's feelings and behavior. They also learn to regulate their emotions, thereby managing intense mood swings. Hence, neurofeedback is particularly useful for developing emotional regulation skills, especially when using methods focusing on specific brain areas.
- *Pulsed electromagnetic field therapy:* It is a noninvasive scientifically proven therapy which reduces inflammation and stress level and improves mental wellness. This therapy uses gentle brain massage with the help of electromagnetic pulses, which stimulate the natural healing ability of the brain. This treatment helps in alleviating emotional dysregulation, thereby improving mood and reducing irritability.

### Medications

No specific medications are approved for treating DMDD. But with symptomatic treatment, especially drugs which work for hyperactivity, these adolescents can be managed well.

- *Stimulants:* Medicines like methylphenidate help to decrease the frequency and intensity of irritability.
- *Antidepressants:* Selective serotonin reuptake inhibitors (SSRIs) and serotonin and norepinephrine reuptake inhibitors (SNRIs) tackle negative or low mood.
- *Antipsychotics:* Risperidone, aripiprazole, and quetiapine help in reducing aggression and irritability.
- *Anticonvulsants:* Lithium, valproate, and carbamazepine act as mood stabilizers and decrease irritable behavior.

## CONCLUSION

Disruptive behavior of children and adolescents is due to their struggle to manage emotions which affects daily functioning of the family. When young people continue to grapple with the symptoms of DMDD, a variety of unpleasant effects are highly likely to occur. Hence, parents need to possess the right understanding and support their children so that they can thrive well **(Box 2)**. However, with effective and comprehensive treatment, many negative outcomes like poor school performance, family conflict, disturbed peer relationships, poor social development, self-harm, suicidal ideation/attempts, etc., can be prevented.

## KEY MESSAGES

- DMDD is the only diagnosis in the DSM-5 depressive disorder section that requires childhood onset.
- For making a diagnosis of DMDD, a child or adolescent should have chronic irritable, angry mood almost every day with severe temper outbursts at least 3 times a week.
- DMDD is diagnosed in children between 6 and 18 years of age.
- Child should have difficulty in functioning in multiple settings like at home, in school, and/or with friends.
- DMDD can coexist with MDD, attention-deficit/ hyperactivity disorder (ADHD), conduct disorder (CD), and substance use disorders (SUD).
- DMDD cannot coexist with ODD, IED, and BD. If the criteria for both DMDD and ODD or IED and DMDD are met, then the child will be diagnosed as a case of DMDD.
- CBT is an excellent tool which teaches adolescents to regulate their mood and increase their frustration tolerance.
- A peaceful environment at home like minimizing distractions, creating cozy spaces, and incorporating calming activities helps adolescents to manage their stormy emotions.
- As for all children, positive disciplining works best for raising these children as well.
- When moodiness or defiant behavior of teens causes frequent family conflicts, then parents must consult their pediatrician or mental health professional.

---

**BOX 2:** Tips for parents.

- *Set clear rules:* Set simple rules and expectations, provide structure and predictability for kids. It will guide them through the ups and downs of their emotions
- *Identify and encourage emotional expression:* Tracking emotional changes allows parents and children to learn about their moods, identify triggers, and identify patterns that may be present
  Healthy expression of feelings is crucial. We can teach them to use words, art, or play to communicate their feelings
- *Work on communication skills:* Parents need to fine-tune their communication skills. Active listening and empathetic responses can work wonders in understanding their child's perspective
- *Foster a calm environment:* Emotional energy is transferable; hence, parents might also feel irritable during a child's outburst. By taking a few deep breaths to calm themselves, parents can model the best behavior for their child
- *Celebrate positive behaviors:* Offering rewards or extra privileges for positive behaviors like a step toward self-regulation encourages children to work hard toward desired behavior
- Self-care is a necessity and not a luxury for parents. Adequate sleep, eating a balanced diet, and exercising along with finding time for their own hobbies help to rejuvenate
- *Safety first:* Remove things that can be thrown during a bout of physical aggression
- Identify triggers and predefine strategies to improve their reactions in the future
- The child should be aware of safe spaces where he/she can go during an outburst

---

## RECOMMENDED READING

1. American Academy of Child and Adolescent Psychiatry. (2019). Disruptive mood dysregulation disorder (DMDD). [online] Available from https://www.aacap.org/AACAP/Families_and_Youth/Facts_for_Families/FFF-Guide/Disruptive-Mood-Dysregulation-Disorder-_DMDD_-110.aspx [Last accessed March, 2024].
2. American Psychiatric Association. Diagnostic and Statistical Manual of Mental Disorders: (DSM), 5th edition. Washington, DC: APA; 2013.
3. Baweja R, Mayes SD, Hameed U, Waxmonsky JG. Disruptive mood dysregulation disorder: Current insights. Neuropsychiatr Dis Treat. 2016;12:2115-24.

4. Kahn J, Gusman M, Wintner S. Neurofeedback for pediatric emotional dysregulation. In: Oberman LM, Enticott PG (Eds). Neurotechnology and Brain Stimulation in Pediatric Psychiatric and Neurodevelopmental Disorders. Cambridge: Academic Press; 2019. pp. 277-311.

5. Krieger FV, Pheula GF, Coelho R, Zeni T, Tramontina S, Zeni CP, et al. An open-label trial of risperidone in children and adolescents with severe mood dysregulation. J Child Adolesc Psychopharmacol. 2011;21(3):237-43.

6. National Institute of Mental Health. (2022). Disruptive mood dysregulation disorder: The basics. [online] Available from https://infocenter.nimh.nih.gov/sites/default/files/2022-01/disruptive-mood-dysregulation-disorder-basics.pdf [Last accessed March, 2024].

7. Rao U. DSM-5: Disruptive mood dysregulation disorder. Asian J Psychiatr. 2014;11:119-23.

8. Roy AK, Lopes V, Klein R. Disruptive Mood Dysregulation Disorder: A new diagnostic approach to Chronic Irritability in Youth. Am J Psychiatry. 2014;171(9):918-24.

9. TMS Health. (2022). What is Disruptive Mood Dysregulation Disorder? [online] Available from https://www.tmshealthandwellness.com/what-is-disruptive-mood-dysregulation-disorder/ [Last accessed March, 2024].

# 3B.6 | Depression in Adolescents

*Harmesh Singh Bains*

## ■ INTRODUCTION

Depression in adolescents has been increasing worldwide in the past several years. It also has high recurrence rates, chances of continuation into adulthood, and poor psychosocial outcomes and academic performance. There are multiple risk factors and comorbidities; hence, it is important to identify associated risk factors and comorbidities so as to treat it early and effectively. Depression (major depressive disorder) is a common and serious disorder in adolescents. It can present with changes in mood, behavior, and physical symptoms.

The reported prevalence of depression in adolescents is 4–8%. Some of its symptoms may overlap with anxiety disorders. Almost half of the adolescents with depression are diagnosed before adult age. In the adolescent age, the male:female ratio is 1:2.

## DIAGNOSTIC AND STATISTICAL MANUAL OF MENTAL DISORDERS, FIFTH EDITION DIAGNOSTIC CRITERIA

The Diagnostic and Statistical Manual of Mental Disorders, Fifth Edition (DSM-5), outlines the following criteria to make a diagnosis of depression. There must be 5 or more symptoms during the 2-week period with at least either depressed mood or loss of interest or pleasure. There is significant distress or impairment in social, occupational, or other important areas of functioning. The symptom must persist most of the day, daily, for at least 2 weeks in a row, excluding A3 and A9.

*Class:* Depressive disorders.

There must be >5 criteria with at least A1 or A2.

- *A1:* Depressed mood—indicated by subjective report or observation by others (in children and adolescents, it can be irritable mood)
- *A2:* Loss of interest or pleasure in almost all activities—indicated by subjective report or observation by others
- *A3:* Significant (>5% in a month) unintentional weight loss/gain or decrease/increase in appetite (in children, failure to make expected weight gain)
- *A4:* Sleep disturbance (insomnia or hypersomnia)
- *A5:* Psychomotor changes (agitation or retardation) severe enough to be observable by others
- *A6:* Tiredness, fatigue, low energy, or decreased efficiency with which routine tasks are completed
- *A7:* A sense of worthlessness or excessive, inappropriate, or delusional guilt (not merely self-reproach or guilt about being sick)
- *A8:* Impaired ability to think, concentrate, or make decisions—indicated by subjective report or observation by others
- *A9:* Recurrent thoughts of death (not just fear of dying), suicidal ideation, or suicide attempts.

## ■ RISK FACTORS

- *Genetic:* Biologic risk factors include possible genetic predisposition. Twins studies demonstrate higher rates of depression in monozygotic twins as compared to dizygotic twins.

- *Familial/environmental factors:*
  - Parental depression/mental illness in a family member
  - Family discord, broken family/divorce
  - Parental substance abuse or criminality
  - Physical/sexual abuse and neglect
  - Bereavement due to the loss of a sibling or parent
  - Parenting problems
  - Comparison with peers
- *Chronic illnesses:*
  - Asthma
  - Diabetes mellitus
  - Epilepsy
  - Cancer
  - Heart disease
  - Body image issues
  - Learning disabilities/attention deficit hyperactivity disorder (ADHD)
- *Other causes:*
  - Sexually harassed teens
  - Bullying
  - Other adverse childhood experiences and trauma in childhood
  - Problems with friends or other teens at school
- *Stress:*
  - Physical/mental
  - Lack of time for extracurricular activities after school
  - Forced learning against wish/interest
  - Excess academic pressure
- *Gender and hormonal changes:* More common in girls
- Substance abuse.

## CLINICAL PRESENTATION

- School failure may be the first manifestation of depression in teens.
- Clinical picture may look similar to adults; however, there may be more behavior problems.
- Compared to children, adolescents experience more sleep and appetite disturbances and acts of impairment in functioning.
- Frequent sadness, tearfulness, and crying
- Decreased interest in activities or inability to enjoy formerly favorite activities
- Hopelessness
- Continuous feelings of boredom, weakness, tiredness, and lack of energy

- Social isolation and poor communication
- Difficulty with relationships
- Frequent headaches/pain in abdomen
- School absenteeism, scholastic deterioration, and lack of concentration
- Feeling overwhelmed easily or often
- A major change in appetite—eating much more or much less
- *Sleep disturbances:* Insomnia, oversleeping, and waking up early
- Missing from home without informing parents
- Suicidal ideations/self-harm
- Neglecting responsibilities or personal appearance
- Feeling irritable, agitated, or anxious.

## DIFFERENTIAL DIAGNOSIS

- Substance/medication-induced mood disorder
- Adjustment disorder with depressed mood
- Anxiety disorders
- Post-traumatic stress disorder
- Eating disorders
- ADHD

## MEDICAL CONDITIONS MIMICKING DEPRESSION

- Hypothyroidism
- Anemia
- Chronic fatigue syndrome
- Autoimmune diseases
- Seizure disorders
- Medications (i.e., corticosteroids, contraceptives, and stimulants).

## RED FLAGS AND NEED FOR REFERRAL

- Suicidal tendency/suspicion
- Development of psychotic symptoms
- Lack of parental supervision/support
- Problems in multiple areas—school, social, and family
- Comorbid substance abuse
- *Abuse:* Physical, sexual, emotional neglect.

## SCREENING TOOLS

- Patient Health Questionnaire-2 (PHQ-2)
- Patient Health Questionnaire-9 (PHQ-9) **(Table 1)**
  These are validated tools and are quick and easy to use/administer.
  (Refer to *Annexure* page 507)

**TABLE 1:** Patient health questionnaire-9 (PHQ-9) interpretation—severity of depression and treatment options.

| PHQ-9 Score | Severity of depression | Treatment option |
|---|---|---|
| 0–4 | None–minimal | None |
| 5–9 | Mild | Watch, repeat PHQ 9 during follow-up |
| 10–14 | Moderate | Counseling and/or pharmacotherapy |
| 15–19 | Moderate to severe | Pharmacotherapy, psychotherapy, and refer |
| 20–27 | Severe | Refer to child psychiatric |

**TABLE 2:** Pharmacotherapy of depression.

| Drug | FDA approved age | Dose | Maximum dose |
|---|---|---|---|
| Fluoxetine | >8 years | 10 mg/day initially and increase to 10 mg BID after 2 weeks | 20–60 mg |
| Escitalopram | >12 years | 10 mg/day and increase by 10 mg after 3 weeks | 20 mg/day |
| Imipramine | >6–12 years | 1.5 mg/kg/day in 3–4 divided doses and increase 1.0–1.5 mg/kg/day after 3–4 days | 5 mg/kg/day |
|  | >12 years | Start with 30–40 mg/day in 3–4 divided dosages and may increase 10–25 mg/day over 3–4 days | 100 mg/day |

(FDA: Food and Drug Administration)

## ■ TREATMENT

Treatment includes the following:

- Cognitive behavioral therapy (CBT)
- Interpersonal psychotherapy (IPT)
- Pharmacotherapy
  Effective therapies for adolescent depression include CBT and IPT. (Refer to psychotherapy chapter for the detailed information.)

Pharmacotherapy has been shown to be effective as well for the treatment of depressive disorders in children and adolescents. A combination of both CBT and pharmacotherapy is more effective in reducing and treating symptoms of depressive disorders.

### Cognitive Behavioral Therapy

Cognitive behavioral therapy is effective in the treatment of adolescent depression. It is a psychotherapy that focuses on how thoughts, feelings, and behaviors are intertwined in everyday functioning and how changes in any one domain can lead to improvement in others. Altering a person's unhelpful thinking can lead to healthier behavior and improved emotion regulation. Up to 6–16 weekly sessions of CBT may be required.

### Pharmacotherapy

The drugs used for pharmacotherapy of depression along with their recommended dosage are given in **Table 2**.

## ■ KEY MESSAGES

- Depression in adolescents is a common and serious mental health problem and has been increasing worldwide in the past several years.
- It is more common among females.
- There are biologic and familial or environmental risk factors. Chronic illnesses also pose a risk for depression.
- Adolescents may present initially with school absenteeism, scholastic deterioration, lack of concentration, behavior problems, appetite and sleep disturbances, decreased interest in activities, weakness, tiredness, and frequent headaches/pain in abdomen.
- Some medical conditions may mimic depression, for example, hypothyroidism, anemia, chronic fatigue syndrome, and seizure disorders.
- The PHQ-2 is step 1 to screen patients for depression. If it is positive, PHQ-9 is used to diagnose, monitor, and measure the severity of depression.
- Effective therapies for adolescent depression include CBT and IPT, and sometimes pharmacotherapy.

## ■ RECOMMENDED READING


1. David D, Cristea I, Hofmann SG. Why cognitive behavioral therapy is the current gold standard of psychotherapy. Front Psychiatry. 2018,9:1-4.
2. Grover S, Raju VV, Sharma A, Shah R. Depression in children and adolescents: a review of Indian studies. Indian J Psychol Med. 2019;41(3):216-27.
3. Hofmann SG, Asmundson GJ, Beck AT. The science of cognitive therapy. Behav Ther. 2013.44(2):199-212.
4. Jha KK, Singh SK, Nirala SK, Kumar C, Kumar P, Aggrawal N. Prevalence of depression among school-going adolescents

in an urban area of Bihar, India. Indian J Psychol Med. 2017,39(3):287-92.

5. John T, Cherian A. Depressive disorders in the child and adolescent population. Indian Pediatr. 2001;38:1211-6.

6. Kroenke K, Spitzer RL, Williams JB. The Patient Health Questionnaire-2: Validity of a two-item depression screener. Med Care. 2003;41(11):1284-92.

7. Kroenke K, Spitzer RL, Williams JB. The PHQ–9: Validity of a brief depression severity measure. J Gen Intern Med. 2001;16(9):606-13.

8. Sagar R, Salvakumar N. Prevalence of depression in Indian adolescents. Indian J Pediatr. 2021;88(5):427-8.

9. Shoeb SM. Depression in Indian teenagers; causes, symptoms & suggestion. IJISRT. 2019,4(6):306-8.

# 3B.7 | Adolescent Suicide

*Sushma Desai*

## GRAVITY OF THE PROBLEM

Worldwide, close to 7 lakh people die by suicide every year (Global Statistics 2021), out of which 164,033 (23.4%) suicides occurred in India only [National Crime Records Bureau (NCRB) 2021], which was 133,000 in the year 2019. The coronavirus disease 2019 (COVID-19) pandemic has led to an alarming increase in the number of adolescent suicide.

Youth suicide in India is the highest in the world. Every day, 35 students commit suicide in India. Changing trend: Alarming rise of suicide amongst girls under 18 *(in 2021, 5,607 girls under 18 died by suicide as compared to 5,075 boys) (NCRB 2021).*

The highest number of suicides occurs in the age group 15–29 years. Suicide rates in 15- to 29-year-old Indian men are twice the global average, while rates in young Indian women are nearly six times as high **(Fig. 1)** [World Health Organization (WHO) global statistics].

Underlying mental health problems (depression on the top of the list) is the leading cause of suicidality amongst adolescents and young adults. Ironically, there is a huge 87% shortage of mental health professionals in India, leading to higher chances of missing the suicidal youth having underlying mental health problems to provide them timely help.

## FACTORS PROMOTING SUICIDE IN ADOLESCENTS

In spite of the several already identified background factors, one cannot know the real reasons behind suicide,

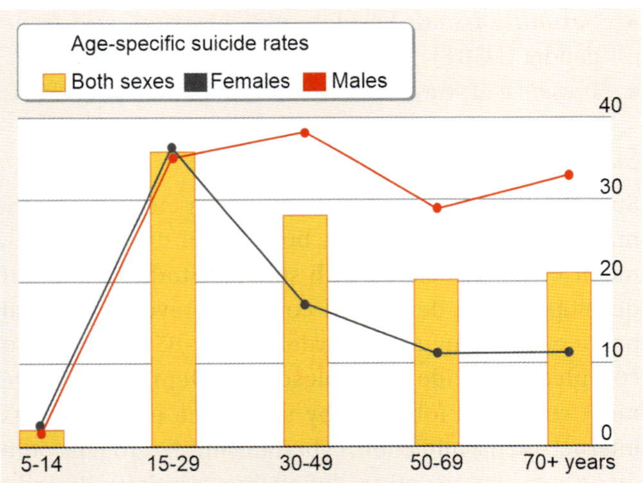


**Fig. 1:** Age-specific suicide rates in both sexes.
*Source:* Data: World Health Organization. 2012.

because suicide is multicausal and can never be traced back to one single cause.

Victims of suicide are not healthy individuals. They are harboring at least one or multiple problems like psychiatric or mental, physical or somatic, and social and cultural issues.

The most common suicide risk factor is an unidentified and untreated mental disorder.

Teen suicide is a multidimensional disorder, which results from a complex interaction of biological, genetic, psychological, sociological, and environmental factors. Poor coping skills (emotions/stress) together with characteristic impulsivity and risk-taking behavior contribute to a large extent.

The presence of one or multiple risk factors *enhances* and protective factors *reduces* the chance of suicidal behavior.

On average, every single suicide event intimately affects at least six other people. If a suicide occurs in a school or workplace, it has an impact on hundreds of people.

## Personal Factors

- Mental health problems
- Prior suicide attempt leads to an increased risk for suicidal impulses for a lifetime, with the highest risk during the first year.
- *Inappropriate media use or media influence:* Internet addiction, cyberbullying, gaming addiction, and pornography addiction
- Victim of physical/domestic/sexual abuse
- *Sexuality issues:* Lesbian, gay, bisexual, and transgender (LGBT)
- Presence of stressors coupled with poor coping skills.

### Suicide and Mental Health Disorders

Suicide is in itself not a disease, nor necessarily the manifestation of a disease, but mental disorders are a major factor associated with suicide. Studies from both developing and developed countries reveal an overall prevalence of mental disorders of 80–85% in cases of completed suicide in adolescents. Depression is the most common, followed by substance use disorders, internet/media addiction, cyberbullying, neurobehavioral disorders like attention-deficit/hyperactivity disorder (ADHD)/conduct disorder (CD)/oppositional defiant disorder (ODD)/specific learning disorder (SLD), and psychiatric comorbidities like psychosis/schizophrenia.

*Collaborating with the psychiatrist and ensuring that adequate and appropriate treatment is given is a crucial function of the pediatricians/general physicians.*

## Familial Factors

- History of psychiatric disorder and suicide in the family
- Family stressors, family discord, faulty parenting style, and loss of parent
- Substance misuse in one or both parents.

## Factors Related to School/Academics/Peer Group

- Negative school environment and lack of connectedness to school and teachers
- Negative peer pressure, bullying, and lack of supportive friends
- Poor academic performance and SLD.

## Others

- Easy availability of lethal means
- Having been exposed to suicide (family, friend, and media reporting)
- *Copycat suicide:* Young people may be susceptible to imitating the suicidal behavior of celebrities or others known to them where those deaths are glorified.

## Protective Factors

- *Strong family support:* Warm and caring environment, authoritative parenting, close family bond, and values
- Absence of/early detection and treatment of underlying mental health disorder
- Absence of addictive substance abuse (alcohol and drugs)
- Judicious media use
- Supportive peer group and school environment
- *Personality:* Academic/sports achiever, spiritual, positive mental outlook, and good coping skills/resilient
- Lack of availability/access to the means of suicide. "Safe Environment".

## ■ WARNING SIGNS

American Association of Suicidology has suggested mnemonic IS PATH WARM to suggest warning signs of suicidality.

- *I:* Ideation
- *S:* Substance abuse
- *P:* Purposelessness
- *A:* Anxiety and agitation
- *T:* Trapped feeling (like there is "No way out")
- *H:* Hopelessness and helplessness
- *W:* Withdrawal from family and friends
- *A:* Anger and rage
- *R:* Reckless/risk-taking behavior
- *M:* Moodiness—dramatic mood changes.

The following are some warning signs more specific to adolescent suicide:

- Sudden change in behavioral pattern
- Loss of interest and passion in the favorite activities
- Withdrawal from family and friends

- Change in appetite and sleep patterns (increased or decreased)
- Unusual preoccupation with death or dying (talking about suicide, posting indicative messages on social media, and searching pro-suicide websites)
- The giving away of valued personal possessions
- Signs of depression
- Moodiness, hopelessness, helplessness, and worthlessness
- Start taking addictive substances or increase the consumption.

The most common sign is a significant feeling of hopelessness, helplessness, and despair.

## Caution

- *Misleading or false improvement:* When an agitated patient suddenly appears calm, he or she may have made the decision to commit suicide and hence are feeling relaxed about getting a solution to end emotional pain.
- *Refusal or denial:* Sometimes adolescents having a strong intention of killing themselves may deliberately deny such ideas.

80% of people talk about or give hints about suicide before committing it.

## ASSESSMENT AND SCREENING FOR SUICIDALITY

A good clinical interview is one of the best assessment tools to identify the individual who is at risk of committing suicide.

How to identify the high-risk adolescent?
- There have been suicides in the family or close social circle.
- The young person has attempted suicide previously.
- There are other comorbid psychiatric disorders (e.g., mood disorders like depression, substance abuse, and internet addiction), impulsivity, and aggression.
- They have access to lethal means (e.g., firearms and pesticides) and opportunities (e.g., youth without social support).
- They have experienced negative events in the recent past (e.g., exam failure, relationship breakup, disciplinary crises, and physical or sexual abuse), which act as a trigger.

*Suicidal behavior and risk need to be carefully evaluated in every depressed young person.*

*HEEADSSS:* Psychosocial screening details the presence of risk factors, triggers, warning signs, and ideation/ plan.

*Assessment of the risk (suicide-related screening questionnaire):* It is important to ask some more questions to assess the frequency and severity of the ideas. Such questions are to be asked:

**How to ask?**

It is not easy to ask patients about their suicidal ideas. It is helpful to lead into the topic gradually. A sequence of useful questions is:
- Do you feel unhappy and helpless?
- Do you feel desperate?
- Do you feel unable to face each day?
- Do you feel life is a burden?
- Do you feel life is not worth living?
- Do you feel like committing suicide?

**When to ask?**
- After a good rapport has been established
- When the adolescent feels calm and comfortable about expressing his or her feelings
- When the patient is ready to discuss his or her negative feelings

*The probe questions are:*
- Sometimes when things get difficult, young people think of death and hurting/killing themselves. Have you had any such thoughts?
- If yes, ask, have you actually tried hurting/killing yourself anytime?
- If no, enquire about coping and stress management skills and praise the adolescent for his/her resilience.

*Risk assessment: If suicide screen is positive:*
- Identify the warning signs ("IS PATH WARM")
- Assess severity and immediacy of risk
- Short nonjudgmental questions are asked to assess intent, thoughts, and plan for suicide.

*Various assessment tools are:*
- *C-SSRS (Columbia Suicide Severity Rating Scale):* It is designed to distinguish between suicidal ideation and suicidal behavior. Different forms of this scale have been developed, including versions for children. It is translated in more than 100 languages. Forms are available on the C-SSRS website. Administration time is only a few minutes. Intensive training is recommended before clinical implementation.

- *Ask Suicide Screening Questions (ASQ)—NIMH Suicide Risk Screening Tool:* It helps assess the immediacy of suicide risk.
- *Assessment tools to identify or rule out underlying mental health problems:* Teenage Screening Questionnaire for Mental Health (TSQ-M), Patient Health Questionnaire 2 (PHQ-2), PHQ-9, Beck Depression Inventory and Beck Suicide Ideation Scale, Screen for Child Anxiety Related Disorders (SCARED) (Child as well as Parent versions) for anxiety disorders, S2BI (SBIRT), and CRAFFT questionnaire for the substance use disorder.

## MANAGEMENT OF SUICIDAL ADOLESCENTS AND YOUNG ADULTS

All the teens with suicidality should be referred to psychiatrist. The adolescent and the caregivers should be explained the reason for the referral, and the physician should try to ally the anxiety and the stigma related to the psychiatric referral.

- If a patient is emotionally disturbed, with vague suicidal thoughts, the opportunity to ventilate thoughts and feelings to a physician who shows concern may be sufficient.
- *Mental Health First Aid (MHFA) is very effective in handling suicidal adolescents in crisis.*
- It is very important for the pediatrician/physician to stay connected with the youth as a nodal person, even after the referral to psychiatric care.

*Identifying and enlisting the reasons for living:* Suicidal individuals are usually ambivalent about wanting to live and wanting to die. Assessing the reasons for living, such as social and familial responsibilities, moral or spiritual objections to suicide, and life goals inculcates hope for life in them.

### Identifying and Mobilizing Support

The physician should assess the available support systems, identify a relative, friend, acquaintance, or other person who would be supportive of the patient, and solicit that person's help. A supportive peer group and/or a warm and caring environment at home has a great role to play. It is very important to keep suicidal adolescents under constant observation.

### Reducing Access to Lethal Means

The parents and other caregivers should be specifically counseled regarding making the surroundings safe to prevent easy access to lethal means like medicines, pesticides, rope, guns, and knives. Often suicidal impulse dies out if the weapon is not readily available.

### Contracting

Entering into a "no suicide" contract *or* providing a *safety plan* is a useful technique in suicide prevention. Other people close to the patient can be included in negotiating the contract. The negotiation of the contract can promote discussion of various relevant issues including the strengths or positive aspects of the youth's personality, a list of warning signs specific to the youth, contact details of supporting persons/physician/psychiatrist as well as local Mental Health Help Line Numbers.

Contracting is appropriate only when patients are not under suicide impulse and have control over their actions.

### Treatment of Underlying Mental Health Problems

Problem-specific pharmacotherapy along with counseling sessions (cognitive behavioral therapy, dialectical therapy and interpersonal therapy) is highly effective. The family counseling sessions are useful.

Regular follow-up with the treating pediatrician or physician helps in maintaining compliance with the psychiatric treatment.

Empowering the youth with coping skills, life skill education, and healthy lifestyle are effective modalities for the treatment as well as prevention of youth suicide **(Table 1)**.

## STEPS TO PREVENT SUICIDE IN ADOLESCENTS (FIG. 2)

- Identification of at-risk adolescents to provide timely help
- Early identification and timely intervention for mental health problems
- Empowering the youth with stress management techniques and essential life skills to handle life stressors
- Spreading awareness regarding stressors, and warning signs, as suicide prevention measures amongst the stakeholders (parents, teachers, social workers, and doctors) and in the community
- Making the environment safe by restricting access to the means of suicide
- Responsible media reporting of suicide events

**TABLE 1:** Proposed management plan by the World Health Organization (WHO).

| Suicide risk | Symptom | Assessment | Action |
| --- | --- | --- | --- |
| *Suicide risk: Identification, assessment, and plan of action* | | | |
| 0 | No distress | - | - |
| 1 | Emotionally disturbed | Enquire about suicidal thoughts | Listen with empathy |
| 2 | Vague ideas of death | Enquire about suicidal thoughts | Listen with empathy |
| 3 | Vague suicidal thoughts | Assess the intent (plan and method) | Explore possibilities Identity support |
| 4 | Suicidal ideas, but no psychiatric disorder | Assess the intent (plan and method) | Explore possibilities Identity support |
| 5 | Suicidal ideas and psychiatric disorder or severe life stressors | Assess the intent (plan and method) Make a contract | Refer to psychiatrist |
| 6 | Suicidal ideas and psychiatric disorder or severe life stressors or agitation and previous attempt | Stay with the patient (to prevent access to means) | Hospitalize |

- Training of health workers and medical professionals regarding how to handle suicidal adolescents
- Taking care of vulnerable adolescents when there is a recent suicide in school/home/community.

## KEY MESSAGES

- Globally, the highest number of suicides takes place in the age group 15–29 years (both sexes).
- Neurobiological development, hormonal serge, constant exposure to intrinsic as well as extrinsic stressors coupled with poor coping skills and characteristic high-risk behavioral patterns make adolescents more vulnerable to mental health problems and suicidality.
- Factors leading to suicide are multidimensional. Suicide is the end result of a complex interaction between various biopsychosocial and environmental factors.

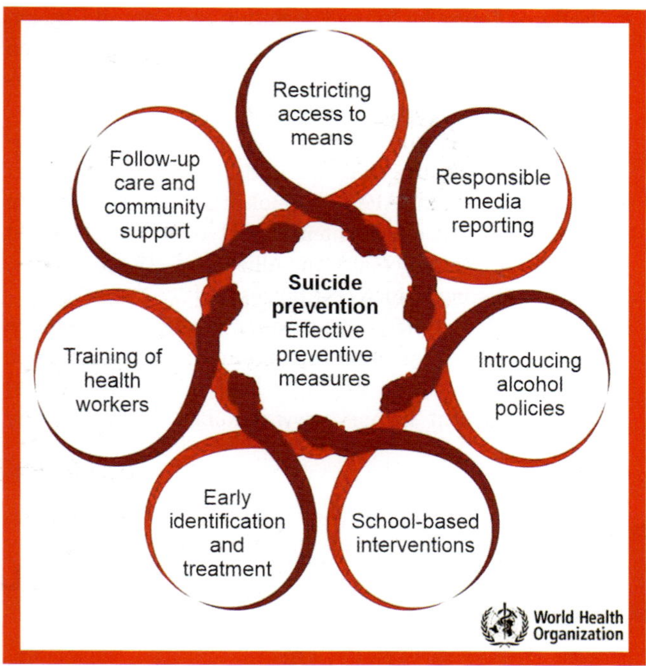


**Fig. 2:** "SUPRE" Suicide Prevention Program, proposed by the World Health Organization (WHO).

- 80% of people show some warning signs before attempting suicide.
- The most common risk factor is undetected and/or untreated mental health problems.
- A detailed HEEADSSS psychosocial analysis provides information regarding the adolescent's personal, social, and environmental aspects including risk and protective factors, warning signs, recent triggering events, and suicide ideation/plan/history of a suicide attempt.
- Various office-friendly tools are available to detect underlying mental health problems.
- Suicide is preventable with the help of early detection of at-risk adolescents and treatment of mental health problems, responsible media reporting, making the environment safe from probable means of suicide, and spreading awareness regarding various aspects of adolescent suicide amongst the stakeholders.

## RECOMMENDED READING


1. IASP (International Association for Suicide Prevention) & Department of Mental Health and Substance Abuse World Health Organization guidelines for the Physicians.
2. Kalmár S. The possibilities of suicide prevention in adolescents. A holistic approach to protective and risk factors. Neuropsychopharmacol Hung. 2013;15(1):27-39.

3. National Centre for Injury Prevention and Control Division of Violence Prevention, CDC. The Relationship between Bullying and Suicide: What we know and what it means for school. [online] Available from https://www.cdc.gov/violenceprevention/pdf/yv/bullying-suicide-translation-final-a.pdf [Last accessed March, 2024].

4. Palacio JD (Ed). IACAPAP Textbook of Child and Adolescent Mental Health. Geneva: International Association for Child and Adolescent Psychiatry and Allied Professions; 2015.

5. Suicide-Getting Help: NHS Choices files

6. WHO. (2016). WHO Surveillance guidelines: Practice manual for establishing and maintaining surveillance systems for suicide attempts and self-harm [online] Available from https://www.who.int/publications/i/item/practice-manual-for-establishing-and-maintaining-surveillance-systems-for-suicide-attempts-and-self-harm [Last accessed March, 2024].

7. WHO. mhGAP Intervention Guide for mental, neurological, and substance use disorders in non-specialized health settings under the WHO Mental Health Gap Action Program. (Version 1). 2010.

8. WHO. Preventing Suicide: A Resource for General Physicians Mental and Behavioural Disorders Department of Mental Health World Health Organization (part of SUPRE, the WHO worldwide initiative for the prevention of suicide). [online] https://www.who.int/publications/i/item/preventing-suicide-a-resource-series [Last accessed March, 2024].

# 3B.8   Thought Disorders

*Hiral Kotadia, Ayushi Soni*

## ■ INTRODUCTION

Thought disorder is a disorganized way of thinking, leading to abnormal ways of expressing language (speech and written sample). Although thought disorders are the primary symptoms of schizophrenia spectrum and other psychotic disorders, they may also be present in other disorders, such as manic and depressive disorders. The schizophrenia spectrum and psychotic disorders include schizophrenia, delusional disorder, brief psychotic disorder, schizophreniform disorder, schizoaffective disorder, substance/medication-induced psychotic disorder, and psychotic disorder due to another medical condition. This chapter focuses on schizophrenia in adolescence.

## ■ ASSESSMENT OF THOUGHT

Thinking is divided into: (1) Undirected fantasy (dereistic) or autistic thinking which goes past rationality and possibility; (2) Imaginative thinking is a kind of fantasy thinking, but it does not go beyond the possible and the rationale; (3) Rational or conceptual thinking which is used for reasoning and problem solving. Thought of an individual is assessed on the following parameters—flow/stream, form/process, content, and possession.

- *Flow:* Speed of thought. It is assessed by rate of speech (e.g., thought retardation, flight of ideas, etc.).
- *Form/process of thought:* It is the manner in which an individual's thoughts are formulated, organized, and expressed, i.e., the connections between the ideas. Normal thought process/form is linear (unidirectional), organized (the ideas are connected and logical), and goal directed. For inferring the form of thought, assess the following in a speech/written sample: (1) Whether the individual idea/thought is meaningful; (2) Whether the ideas are logically interconnected; (3) Whether the individual reaches the desired goal (in terms of context) eventually (e.g., poverty of thought, tangentiality, neologism, word salad, and thought block).
- *Content of thought:* It is the theme of the individual's thought or idea. It is inferred by speech/written sample which the individual expresses spontaneously or in response to specific questions (e.g., delusion, obsession, ideas of worthlessness, hopelessness, helplessness, and suicidal ideas).
- *Possession of thought:* Normally, an individual experiences a sense of control over one's own thoughts. In certain psychiatric disorders, an individual loses this sense of control, i.e., he/she feels that an external entity controls his thoughts (e.g., thought alienation).

## ■ AGE-APPROPRIATE DEVELOPMENT OF THOUGHT

Preschool years (age 3–6) are characterized by imaginary and fantasy thinking, which may also be present in early school years. Children in preschool and early school years may also have an imaginary companion. However, this imaginary thinking and imaginary companion are replaced by logical and abstract thinking in adolescent period. Disordered thoughts, delusions, and hallucinations can occur normally in healthy nonpsychotic children of preschool age group. Persistence of these thought disturbances in preadolescent and adolescent years may be indicative of a mental illness. The understanding of developmental age appropriateness is an important factor in evaluation of a thought disorder and the same has to be kept in mind.

## ■ EPIDEMIOLOGY

Transient psychotic experiences like occasional hallucinations and delusions are common in childhood and adolescence. The prevalence of psychotic symptoms in children and adolescents varies from 10 to 20%, which is higher than the adults. Early-onset psychosis (EOP) is defined as onset of psychotic symptoms before 18 years of age. Early-onset schizophrenia (EOS) is defined as schizophrenia spectrum disorder with onset of symptoms before 18 years of age, and childhood-onset schizophrenia (COS) is defined as schizophrenia with onset before 13 years of age. COS is a less common entity affecting less than 1 in 40,000 children. The onset of schizophrenia prior to 5 years of age is rare. However, the prevalence of schizophrenia in adolescents increases by 50 times. It is more common in a male child as compared to a female child with an estimated ratio of 1.67:1. Boys are generally identified earlier than girls. The prevalence of schizophrenia in parents of children having EOS is 8%. This is almost twice the prevalence among parents of individuals having schizophrenia, which has onset in adulthood. National Mental Health Survey of India 2015–2016 found that the prevalence of various psychotic disorders in adolescents to be 1.3%.

## ■ ETIOLOGY

Early-onset schizophrenia and EOP are considered to be a neurodevelopmental disorder in which various gene environment interactions lead to aberrant brain development and abnormal connectivity between different regions of brain. This aberrant connectivity in brain regions is presumed to be a contributing factor in the development of various psychotic symptoms along with cognitive deficits. Various possible factors contributing to development of EOS spectrum disorders are enlisted in **Table 1**.

**TABLE 1:** Etiological factors of EOS and EOP.

| | |
|---|---|
| Genetic factors | • Monozygotic twins have 50% concordance rate for schizophrenia<br>• Dizygotic twins have a concordance rate of about 10%<br>• Genetic factors do not account fully for the emergence of schizophrenia spectrum disorders<br>• Environmental factors also play an essential role |
| Endophenotype markers for childhood-onset schizophrenia/early-onset schizophrenia | • Currently, there is no reliable method to identify persons at the highest risk for schizophrenia<br>• However, the following are noted in childhood of individuals who later develop schizophrenia:<br>  – Neurodevelopmental abnormalities<br>  – More neurological soft signs<br>  – Impairment in attention, working memory, and information processing<br>  – Lower premorbid IQ |
| Neurochemistry | • Almost all of the major neurotransmitter systems are affected in schizophrenia<br>• *Most common:* Aberrations in the dopaminergic system (striatal presynaptic dopamine synthetic capacity is increased)<br>• *Other neurotransmitters:* Glutamate/GABA abnormalities which leads to cognitive dysfunction in schizophrenia (excess of glutamate in the medial prefrontal cortex is noted in early stages of schizophrenia) |
| Environmental factors | • Fetal malnutrition, birth hypoxia, and prenatal infections<br>• Trauma, stress, social adversity, and isolation |

An individual's sensitivity to adverse environmental events may be affected by gene—environment interactions

(EOP: early-onset psychosis; EOS: early-onset schizophrenia; GABA: gamma-aminobutyric acid; IQ: intelligence quotient)

## ■ CLINICAL FEATURES AND DIAGNOSIS

The symptoms of schizophrenia can be divided into: (1) Positive, (2) negative, (3) disorganization, and (4) cognitive.

- *Positive symptoms*: Symptoms that are present persistently and usually observable. These are different and in excess to normal behaviors. They include hallucinations and delusions. Hallucinations are abnormal perceptual disturbances that the adolescent may experience in various sensory modalities with or without a real perception. To establish an inference of the perceptual experience as a hallucination, the perceptual experience should be vivid (clear, not blurred or clouded), in outer objective space (not in imagination, fantasy thinking or in mind), and not under one's control. The adolescent might find them to be disturbing and try to control and stop them but would not succeed. Various types of hallucinations are auditory, visual, tactile, olfactory, kinesthetic, functional, and elementary. Adolescents seldom are forthcoming to discuss their hallucinations, and the parents of the adolescents are mostly oblivious. Delusions are fixed, firm, and false beliefs/thoughts of an individual which either do not match the sociocultural beliefs or are not scientifically explained. Being a product of internal morbid process, the delusion is unamenable to external influences. Though they are false, the individual does not have insight into the falsity. These abovementioned features must be established before interpreting the thought as a delusion. These delusions may not be fixed or systematized prior to middle adolescence.

- *Negative or deficit symptoms*: These are defined as those thought, mood, or behavior which should be normally present but are absent in the illness. Negative symptoms seen in psychotic disorders are the absence of affect (blunted affect), the absence of thought, the absence of motivation (avolition), the absence of pleasure (anhedonia), and the absence of expressive functions (alogia). Negative symptoms mostly persist with the course of illness.
- Disorganization symptoms are characterized by disintegration of thought process (formal thought disorder), bizarre behavior, catatonia, and bizarre or disorganized observable mood. Adolescents may giggle inappropriately or cry without being able to explain the reason. Illogical thinking, loss of connections between the thoughts, and poverty of thinking are common features among youth with schizophrenia. The process of assessment of the thought disorders has been mentioned under "form/process of thought" in earlier part of the chapter.
- *Cognitive symptoms*—impairments in normal cognitive functions. These are the impairments of attention, working memory, and executive functioning. Cognitive and motor/sensory and social functioning

| **TABLE 2:** Key features of EOS and EOP. | |
| --- | --- |
| Epidemiology | • COS is a less common entity affecting less than 1 in 40,000 children. Prevalence in adolescents increases by 50 times<br>• Male:Female ratio of 1.67:1 |
| Onset | Insidious, gradual over a period of 3–4 years |
| Clinical features | • Delusions—not well systematized or fixed<br>• Hallucinations—may be present in many modalities beyond auditory hallucinations. Requires direct evaluation by the assessor as the adolescent himself or herself may not report it<br>• Negative symptoms—over 60% of children and adolescents with EOP experience negative symptoms as compared to 30–40% of individuals with an adult-onset first episode of psychosis<br>Children and adolescents with EOP have more frequent negative symptoms. Earlier age at onset is associated with more and severe negative symptoms<br>The assessment and management of negative symptoms in children and adolescents with EOP should be prioritized |
| Course and outcome | • Chronic, unremitting course<br>• Most of the individuals have a guarded prognosis<br>• Certain symptoms persist in adulthood<br>• The course becomes static over a period of few years, i.e., it does not worsen but does not remit either |

(COS: childhood-onset schizophrenia; EOP: early-onset psychosis; EOS: early-onset schizophrenia)

are deteriorated and comparatively more severe than adults.

The abovementioned symptoms occur in EOS, EOP, and adult-onset schizophrenia and psychotic disorders. The developmental level of the individual significantly influences the presentation of the symptoms. The presentation of above symptoms in EOP and EOS is different from adult-onset psychotic disorders. The key features in terms of symptom presentations, course, and outcome of EOS and EOP as compared to its adult-onset counterparts are highlighted in **Table 2**.

The diagnostic criteria for schizophrenia spectrum and psychotic disorders as per the Diagnostic and Statistical Manual of Mental Disorders 5 (DSM-5) include:

- The individual must have experienced at least two of the following symptoms: Delusions, hallucinations, disorganized speech, disorganized or catatonic behavior, and negative symptoms.

At least one of the symptoms must be the presence of delusions, hallucinations, or disorganized speech.

- Continuous signs of the disturbance must persist for at least 6 months, during which the patient must experience at least 1 month of active symptoms (or less if successfully treated), with social or occupational deterioration problems occurring over a significant amount of time.
- For a significant portion of time since the onset of the disturbance, level of functioning in one or more major areas, such as work, interpersonal relations, or self-care is markedly below the level achieved prior to the onset (or when the onset is in childhood or adolescence, there is a failure to achieve expected level of interpersonal, academic, or occupational functioning).
- These problems must not be attributable to another condition.

## ■ PSYCHIATRY COMORBIDITIES

Individuals with EOS have frequent comorbidities, including attention deficit hyperactivity disorder, oppositional defiant disorder, and major depressive disorder.

## ■ DIFFERENTIAL DIAGNOSIS

A major concerning factor is the misdiagnosis of EOS, which may be due to multiple factors such as a child's difficulty describing a symptom that may be outside their normal experience, overinterpretation of these symptoms, and an overall higher occurrence of positive psychotic symptoms in various child psychiatric disorders apart from EOS. While evaluating a child or adolescent presenting with psychotic symptoms, the child or adolescent must be interviewed separately from their guardians. The focus should be to clarify the development, functioning, temperament, experiences, and trauma faced by them. A detailed workup of family history and any prevalent psychiatric illness must be considered. The various disorders from which it should be differentiated are as follows:

- *Major depressive disorder with psychotic features:* Although older adolescents with depression can clearly describe their low mood, those suffering from EOS exhibit through their behavior, their emotional numbing which reflects their state of negative symptoms.

- *Bipolar affective disorder with psychotic features:* The major differentiating feature between the two disorders is the presence of hypersexuality and decreased need for sleep in children with bipolar mood disorder when compared to the EOS, which has predominant negative symptoms.
- *Substance-induced psychosis:* This is mostly accompanied by a recent history of substance use, intoxication, or withdrawal. Although a comorbid substance use as a means of self-medication may be used by many adolescents, a history suggestive of prior onset of psychotic symptoms is not indicative of substance-induced psychosis.
- *Autism spectrum disorder:* The two disorders may be distinguished on the basis of developmental course, their progression, and presence/severity of psychotic symptoms. The extreme concrete and rigid thinking along with a difficulty in expression of formal thought disorder is a distinguishing feature of autism from EOS. EOS usually has a rare onset before 10 years of age.
- *Anxiety disorders and post-traumatic stress disorder (PTSD):* The presence of transient hallucinations is seen in adolescents with anxiety disorders or PTSD is observed. However, the negative symptoms and formal thought disorders are rarely present in anxiety disorders or PTSD.
- *Organic brain disorders:* It is very important to rule out various medical disorders presenting with similar symptom profile. These are: (1) Delirium, (2) central nervous system (CNS) lesions (space-occupying lesions, head trauma, and congenital malformations), (3) autoimmune disorders [anti-N-methyl-D-aspartate (NMDA) encephalitis and lupus], (4) seizure disorders, (5) metabolic disorders (endocrinopathies and Wilson's disorders), (6) toxic disorders, (7) infectious disorders [encephalitis, meningitis, and human immunodeficiency virus (HIV)-related disorders], and (8) neurodegenerative disorders (Huntington's chorea and lipid storage disorders).

## ■ ONSET, COURSE, AND PROGNOSIS

The key features of EOS and EOP in terms of onset, clinical features, course and outcome are given in **Table 2**.

Early-onset schizophrenia and EOP have a very insidious and gradual onset. It may take few years to the symptoms to develop into a disorder. Hence, during assessment of youth for EOS and EOP, it is important to ask about changes in functioning and behavior that have occurred over the past 3–4 years. Individuals with EOS have subtle symptoms that may be present throughout the childhood. Overt psychotic symptoms have gradual onset. EOS and other psychotic disorders mostly have a chronic, unremitting course. It has been observed that after few years there is no progressive decline. However, the symptoms mostly persist in adulthood. Less than 20% of individuals with EOS have good outcome with minimum impairment in adult life. Around 30–60% have poor outcome with moderate to severe impairment. A high proportion of children have chronic impairment despite being on treatment. The important predicting factors of the course and outcome of COS and EOS are premorbid level of functioning, intelligence quotient (IQ), premorbid cognitive functioning, duration of untreated psychosis, length of first psychotic episode, negative symptoms, and comorbid psychiatric disorders. Individuals with early age of onset, comorbid developmental delays, prolonged first episode, and presence of negative symptoms have guarded prognosis.

## MANAGEMENT (ASSESSMENT AND TREATMENT)

Detailed history from all possible sources, physical examination, and mental state examinations are the major aspects of assessment. If the diagnosis is in doubt, it is suggested to do serial assessments and observations before prescribing any pharmacotherapy. When in doubt of diagnosis, certain validated tools for assessment like Kiddie Schedule for Affective Disorders and Schizophrenia (K-SADS) (for ages 6–18 years), which is a semistructured interview, can be used. For unstructured interviews, certain supplementary scales may be used for diagnosis. Tools like scale for assessment of positive symptoms and scale for assessment of negative symptoms can be used at follow up for monitoring course of illness and response to treatment. The management plan is elaborated in **Flowchart 1**.

The various phases of treatment are enlisted in **Table 3**.

The risk of relapse of symptoms with discontinuation of antipsychotics is high compared to adults. If termination of treatment is considered, the dose of antipsychotics

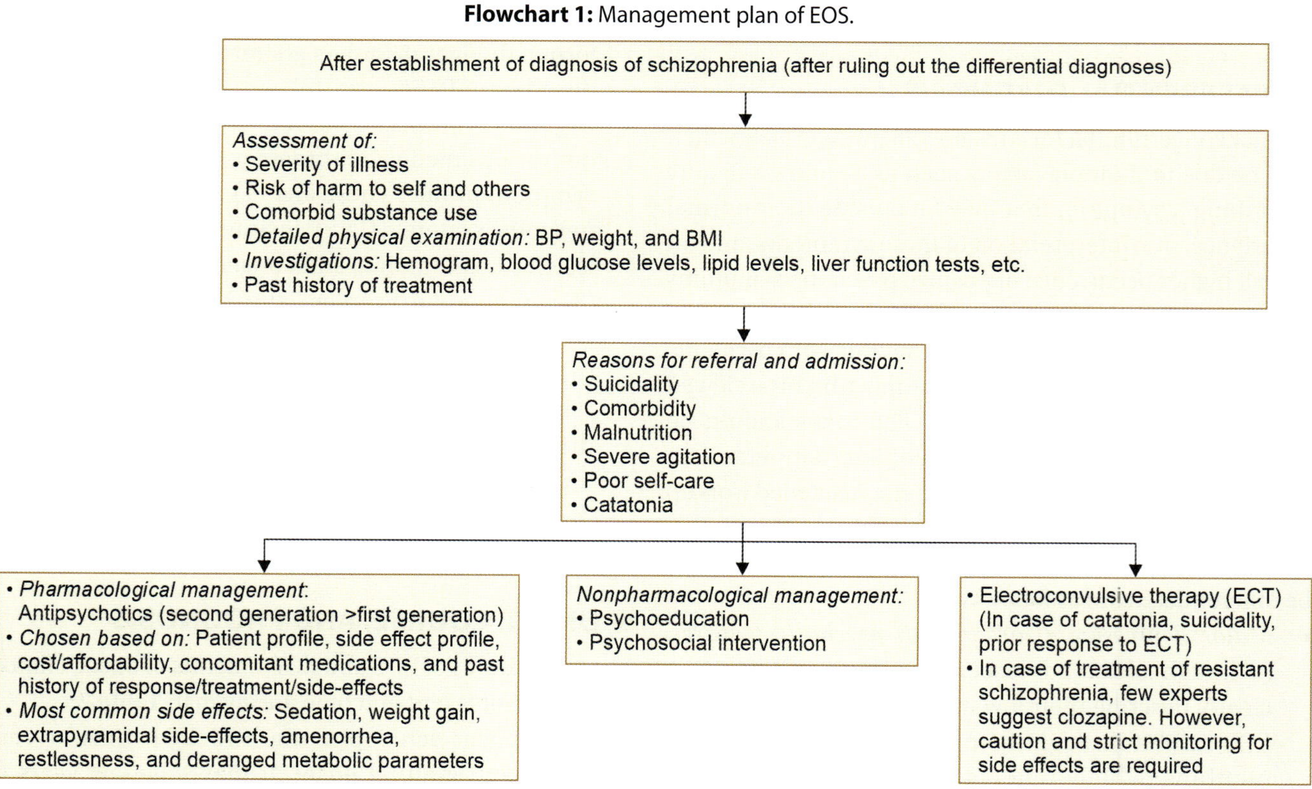

**Flowchart 1:** Management plan of EOS.



(BMI: body mass index; BP: blood pressure; EOS: early-onset schizophrenia)

**TABLE 3:** Phases of treatment.

| Phase | Duration and mode of treatment | Treatment goals |
|---|---|---|
| *Acute phase:* Patients present with florid psychotic symptoms in the form of hallucinations, thought disturbances, delusions, disorganized behavior, and severe impairment in functioning | • Start low-dose antipsychotic and gradually increase as per response and tolerability<br>• If no response for 4–6 weeks, change the antipsychotic<br>• Consider admission* | • Reduce/eliminate symptoms<br>• Ensure and promote safety<br>• Reduction of self-harm |
| *Stabilization phase:* Commences with reduction or remission of symptoms seen in the acute phase | • Usually lasts about 6–12 months<br>• Continue antipsychotics at the same dose used in acute phase to which patient responded | • Further reduction in the symptoms<br>• Consolidation of remission and prevention of early relapses |
| Stable/maintenance phase | • Dose of medications needs to be individualized based on response and side effects<br>• First episode—maintenance treatment of 1–2 years<br>• *Maintenance phase of 5 years or longer indicated in:* Multiple episodes, multiple relapses while on treatment, evidence of relapses when the medications are tapered off, history of two episodes in the last 5 years, and presence of residual psychotic symptoms | • Maintaining or improving the level of functioning<br>• Recurrence/relapse prevention<br>• Rehabilitation of the patient into society |

*As per the Mental Health Care Act 2017.

should be gradually reduced and then stop. After the withdrawal of medications, monitoring for relapse has to be monitored for at least next 2 years and any re-emergence of symptoms has to be treated.

The United States Food and Drug Administration (FDA) approved antipsychotics for treatment of schizophrenia in adolescents (≥13 years of age) are risperidone, aripiprazole, olanzapine, quetiapine, lurasidone, paliperidone, and haloperidol.

## ATTENUATED PSYCHOSIS SYNDROME AND INDIVIDUALS AT RISK FOR PSYCHOSIS

A new diagnostic category, attenuated psychosis syndrome (APS), has been included in DSM-5 as a condition for further study. This syndrome has subthreshold psychotic symptoms, which may be present in prodromal psychotic states. These symptoms must have been present at least once per week for 1 month and must have emerged or worsened in past 1 year. These symptoms cause some impairment, but the symptoms should not have progressed to full psychotic episode. Psychological intervention is the main stay of intervention of APS.

"Individuals at risk for psychosis" is an emerging concept, which identifies adolescents and young individuals who may develop psychosis at later age. Individuals with subtle disturbances of thought, speech, and perception have been considered to develop psychosis in later age. However, the current evidence regarding the reliability of these factors is insufficient.

## EARLY IDENTIFICATION IS THE KEY

- The symptoms of psychosis in adolescents and children are very subtle in the initial part of the illness.
- Awareness and vigilance help clinician in identifying the subtle and early signs.
- Brief evaluation of possibility of psychosis in adolescence and children should be a part of routine screening in child and adolescent clinics.
- In suspected cases of at-risk psychosis, a regular follow-up and serial evaluation are suggested.
- Parents need to be educated regarding identification of early signs of psychosis in children and adolescents.
- Teachers need to be trained to identify the subtle signs and changes in behavior of children and adolescents. They should also be sensitized about the skills needed for communication regarding this to parents keeping harmful psychosocial consequences in mind.
- Further research is required for developing tools that help in identifying certain specific early signs, which currently are nonspecific.

## KEY MESSAGES

- The prevalence of psychotic disorders in children and adolescents is low but increases as the age progresses.

- Fleeting hallucinations are not uncommon in healthy children. Hence, the diagnosis of psychotic disorders in children should not be made on these alone.
- The developmental age of the individual should be kept in mind while evaluating for symptoms of schizophrenia and psychotic disorders in adolescent or a child.
- Impairment in normal domains of social, educational, work, and personal care in an adolescent should be taken seriously and evaluated vigilantly for presence of psychotic disorders.
- Assessment and management of comorbidities are equally important.
- The course of EOS and EOP is usually chronic and unremitting.
- Negative symptoms are common symptoms in children and adolescents in schizophrenia and in early stages of psychosis, and are associated with poor outcomes.
- There is good evidence that early intervention may help in reduction of morbidity and mild improvement of functioning in these individuals. Hence, early recognition and early intervention are necessary.
- Multidisciplinary intervention that encompasses psychopharmacologic, psychotherapeutic, and early psychosocial interventions is recommended.
- Involvement of professionals from field of pediatrics, child and adolescent psychiatry, psychology, speech and occupational therapy, and psychosocial work is highly suggested.

## ■ RECOMMENDED READING


1. Boland R, Verdiun M, Ruiz P (Eds). Kaplan & Sadock's Synopsis of Psychiatry, 12th edition. Philadelphia: Lippincott Williams & Wilkins, Wolters Kluwer; 2022.
2. Grover S, Avasthi A. Clinical practice guidelines for the management of schizophrenia in children and adolescents. Indian J Psychiatry. 2019;61(Suppl 2):277-93.
3. Kane JM, Robinson DG, Schooler NR, Mueser KT, Penn DL, Rosenheck RA, et al. Comprehensive versus usual community care for first-episode psychosis: 2-year outcomes from the NIMH RAISE Early Treatment Program. Am J Psychiatry. 2016;173:362-72.
4. Martin A, Volkmar FR, Bloch M (Eds). Lewis's Child and Adolescent Psychiatry: A Comprehensive Textbook, 5th edition. Philadelphia: Lippincott Williams & Wilkins; 2018.
5. Rey J (Ed). IACAPAP e-textbook of child and adolescent mental health. Geneva: International Association of Child and Adolescent Psychiatry and Allied Professions; 2012.
6. Sikich L, Chandrasekhar T. Early onset psychotic disorders. In: Sadock BJ, Sadock VA, Ruiz P (Eds). Kaplan and Sadock's Comprehensive Textbook of Psychiatry, 10th edition. Philadelphia: Lippincott Williams & Wilkins, Wolters Kluwer; 2017. pp. 9369-88.
7. Sunshine A, McClellan J. Practitioner Review: Psychosis in children and adolescents. J Child Psychol Psychiatry. 2023;308-12.
8. Thapar A, Pine DS, Leckman JF, Scott S, Snowling MJ, Taylor EA (Eds). Rutter's Child and Adolescent Psychiatry, 6th edition. John Wiley & Sons; 2017.


# 3B.9 Conduct Disorder

*Prerna Kukreti, Saloni Seth*

## ■ INTRODUCTION

*Defiance in adolescents* can be defined as resistance or outright disobedience and can be considered to be an exaggerated overt expression of independence or wanting to be differentiated from the family. Adolescents exhibit a variety of disrespectful or destructive behaviors throughout their journey of growing up.

Certain psychopathologies such as attention-deficit/hyperactivity disorder (ADHD), oppositional defiant disorder (ODD), conduct disorder (CD), and substance use disorder, which exhibit similar "Externalizing behaviors" need urgent attention and intervention. Hence, differentiating between normative adolescent behavior and a problematic defiant teen is crucial, which is elaborated on later in the chapter.

Conduct disorder, the most important of these psychopathologies, is classified in the category of disruptive behavior disorders, which also includes the diagnosis of ODD. ODD usually precedes CD and leads to antisocial personality disorder (ASPD) in adulthood.

**Flowchart 1:** Environmental and dispositional risk factors for conduct disorder (CD).

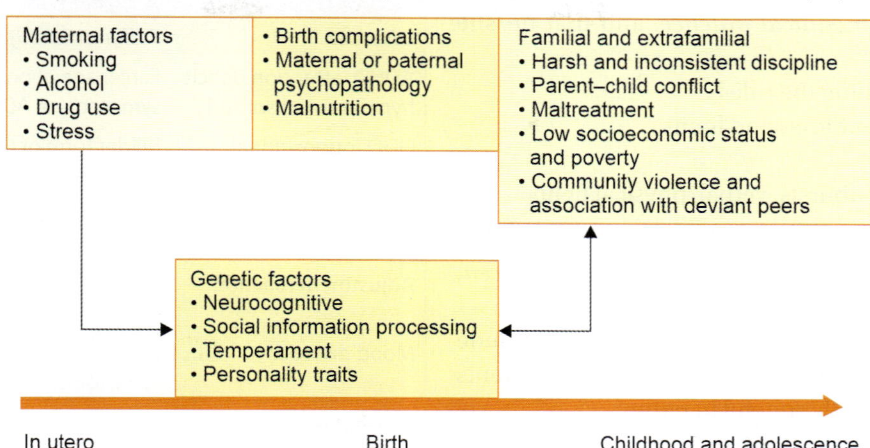



The CD is characterized by aggression and violation of the rights of others and is known to evolve. CD is comorbid with many other psychiatric conditions, including ADHD, depression, bipolar disorder, and learning disorders, and thus a thorough psychiatric evaluation is required to understand the psychopathology before initiating an appropriate treatment plan.

## EPIDEMIOLOGY

It is important to stress that occasional rebellious behavior and a tendency to be disrespectful and disobedient toward elders can present commonly during childhood and adolescent periods. For a diagnosis of CD to be made, it is, therefore, important to demonstrate a pervasive and repetitive pattern of the above behaviors, with frequent episodes of destruction of property and violation of the rights of others.

Conduct disorder is more common in boys than girls, and the ratio could range from 4:1, and this is surprisingly consistent among different race and ethnic groups. Children with CD often develop ASPD in adult life, though that should not be taken as a rule. Early onset of CD in childhood years leads to a worse prognosis of the condition. Multiple socioeconomic factors contribute to a higher incidence of CD in children and adolescents, which includes substance use disorders and a history of involvement in various criminal activities by the parents of these children **(Flowchart 1)**.

## ETIOPATHOGENESIS

- *Environmental risk factors:*
  - Environmental risk factors predisposing to CD operate at different stages and levels during the lifespan.

  - Harsh and inconsistent parenting style is more important during childhood, whereas associating with deviant peers is more likely to be important during adolescence age group.
  - Parental involvement in substance abuse and criminal activities
- *Genetic risk factors:* It is well known that parents with a defiant temperament have children with similar kind of behavioral patterns. One of the most consistent findings seen is that gene encoding the monoamine oxidase "A" (MAOA) enzyme moderates the effect of childhood maltreatment on CD. Boys carrying the low-activity variant of MAOA are more susceptible to developing CD due to the effect of maltreatment than those carrying the high-activity variant. The hypothesis behind the same is that low-activity MAOA carriers are more reactive to emotional stimuli and less capable of regulating their emotions, thereby predisposing to various behavioral problems.

## CLINICAL FEATURES

Defiant behavior, which can be a part of normal adolescent behavior, can eventually become a problem for parents or caregivers.

Clinical features of CD take several years to develop and insidious in onset. This progresses to a stage where a consistent pattern develops, which involves violation of basic rights of others. It exists on a continuum, where ODD is the least severe and ASPD is the most severe. As these behaviors are present in some children during normal development, *it is essential for the clinician to differentiate if it is a part of development process or pathological in nature.*

A *defiant teen* may exhibit the *following behaviors, which can be used in clinical practice*, and that he/she needs extra support:

- Consistently violating the rules
- Overstepping boundaries and limits
- Easily irritable
- Frequent anger outbursts, verbal/physical fights
- Makes frequent snide, rude, or sarcastic comments.

The *differences between a defiant behavior in an adolescent and ODD include:*

- The typical adolescent defiant behavior may include altercations and frequent power struggles with parents but is not purposefully spiteful in nature.
- Hostile and purposefully spiteful behavior, on the other hand, is seen in ODD, against parents and others.
- ODD has a prepubescent onset, unlike the adolescent onset of teenage defiant behavior.
- Defiant children express guilt once they calm down and take responsibility for their action, unlike children with ODD, who are purposefully hurtful or defiant and do not take accountability of their actions.

Conduct disorder symptoms develop earlier in boys than girls. The age of presentation is usually 10–12 years in boys, whereas it is 14–16 in case of girls. Individual having CD shows behavioral manifestations in the following four categories as per DSM-5:

- *Aggression to people and animals* which includes behaviors such as threatening, frequent physical fights, using weapon that can cause damage to others or showing physical cruelty to people or animals
- *Destruction of property* which includes setting of fire or deliberately destroying others property
- *Deceitfulness or theft* involves stealing or breaking into others house
- *Serious violations of rules* involve showing disobedience to parental prohibitions or truancy from school.

As per DSM-5, when at least one symptom appear before the age 10 years, then it is specified as *childhood-onset*; while no symptoms before 10 years for CD, then it is classified as *adolescent-onset type CD*. The International Classification of Diseases 10 (ICD-10) on the other hand has classified CD into three types based on setting in which behaviors are manifested: *CD confined to the family, unsocialized CD, and socialized CD.*

## ■ DIFFERENTIAL DIAGNOSIS

The most frequent comorbid psychiatric and developmental disorders in individuals with CD are ADHD,

**TABLE 1:** Differential diagnosis.

| Disorder | Differentiating features |
|---|---|
| ADHD (attention deficit hyperactive disorder) | Earlier age of onset than CD; symptoms of ADHD present on history |
| ODD (oppositional defiant disorder) | Milder form of CD; no serious violation of rules |
| ASPD (antisocial personality disorder) | Diagnosed above 18 years of age |
| Adjustment reaction | Symptoms subside after termination of stress |
| Mood disorder | Presence of low mood and other core symptoms |

(CD: conduct disorder)

ODD, developmental language disorder, dyslexia, anxiety disorders, depression, post-traumatic stress disorder, and substance use disorders **(Table 1)**.

Conduct disorder also co-occurs with ADHD, substance use disorder, and mood disorder and are associated with poor prognosis.

## ■ ASSESSMENT AND MANAGEMENT

The assessment process involves the following aspects:

- The CD symptoms, and their comorbidities
- Presence or absence of delinquent behavior
- The age of onset of CD, i.e., childhood/adolescent onset
- The syndromic diagnosis of CD, which is differentiated from ODD as described
- The nature and severity of current and past offenses or problem behaviors like violence, self-harm, fire setting, bullying, and abuse.

Following schedules are available currently for assessment:

- Diagnostic interview schedule for children (DISC-IV)
- Diagnostic interview for children and adolescents (DICA)
- The schedule for affective disorders and schizophrenia for school-age children (K-SADS)
- Child and adolescent psychiatric assessment (CAPA)
- The Achenbach's child behavior checklist has an Indian adapted version and known as childhood psychopathology measurement schedule (CPMS). It is a semistructured interview schedule having 75 items and has a cut-off score of 10.
- DISC-IV and DICA are structured interview and do not require trained professionals for administration, while

K-SADS and CAPA should be administered only by trained professionals.

- *Vanderbilt ADHD Parent Rating Scale (VADPRS)* is used to diagnose ADHD in children between the age of 6–12 years. It has a total of 55 questions, includes all 18 of the DSM criteria for ADHD and should be completed by a parent of the child. It also has a teacher-rated version available. The advantage of this scale is that it also has items for comorbidities with ADHD, including ODD, CD, anxiety/depression, and has screening items for the same.

## ■ TREATMENT

- *General principles of management:*
  - As there are numerous risk factors involved, an effective treatment plan must be multimodal in nature.
  - It should be a family-based and social systems-based approach, address multiple areas, and continue over a long period.
  - Treatment should start with psychoeducation of the patient and the family members about the disorder and the long-term consequences.
  - Various psychosocial crises must be dealt with appropriate psychological intervention at that time.
- *Practical tips for parents:*
  - Validate and *empathize with the child's feelings.*
  - Setting of clear boundaries/*limit setting*
  - *Differential reinforcement:* Positive reinforcement for desirable and negative reinforcement for undesirable behaviors
  - *Consistent parenting styles:* All parents/care givers should be on same page, otherwise the child manipulates his ways through the more lenient parent.
  - *Modelling the right behavior:* Make sure to carry out actions that one wants their child to follow, otherwise the child will think of the parent/caregiver as a hypocrite and become even more defiant.
- *Recommendations for teachers:*
  - Discuss with students while framing the rules.
  - Do not just mention the rules but *also teaching how to apply them*, to avoid them, finding "loopholes" in the same, and violating them.
  - *Provide a structure to classroom work*, as it prevents defiant child to get overwhelmed.

- *Try to ignore the student's disruptive behavior*, especially if the behavior is to gain attention.
- *Avoid intimidation and avoid reprimanding in the public* as it increases the disruptive behavior.
- *Use time-outs* when appropriate.
- *Nonpharmacological management:*
  - Nonpharmacological management has been the mainstay of treatment in managing CD.
  - In preschool children, such programs (for example, *Head Start)* have been tried, which empower parents on normal development and crisis management.
  - In the clinical setting, the interventions are targeted toward the temperamental issues of the child, the interpersonal relationship issues of the family, and enhancing the parental efficiency in dealing with the child's behavioral issues.
  - In the school-aged children, the primary target of intervention is the triad of child, family, and the school. Training of the child to improve peer relationships and social competence are therefore essential.
  - In adolescent period, there is an increased relative importance of the friends and peers; the interventions, therefore, should also be targeted toward the peer group of the child.

*Cognitive behavioral skill training:* Behavioral training is useful in children with ODD and other behavioral problems as it helps to improve the social cognitive deficit and improve problem skills of children. It teaches them the same in a stepwise manner. Therapist plays an active role in teaching the skills through modeling and role-playing techniques.

*Parent management training (PMT):* The major objective of PMT is to teach parents the skill of developing and implementing a systematic contingency management plan in home setting. This aims to improve the parent–child interaction at home and thereby help in causing a positive behavioral change in the child.

Studies on parent training programs, carried out for various behavioral and emotional problems in children, including ADHD, have demonstrated improvements in the underlying symptoms as well as in the overall impairment in children. Interestingly, parent training also improves parental functioning (e.g., decreased stress and enhanced competence).

- *Pharmacological management:*
  - *Aims at treatment of psychiatric comorbidities* with appropriate medications such as stimulants and nonstimulants for the treatment of comorbid ADHD, antidepressants for the treatment of depression, and mood stabilizers for the treatment of aggression, symptoms of mood dysregulation, and comorbid bipolar disorder.
  - Mood stabilizers include both conventional mood stabilizers like antiepileptic drugs and second-generation antipsychotics.
  - Studies, including a Cochrane review, showed *maximum evidence for risperidone.* Dose should be increased from 0.25 to 0.5 mg, depending upon the weight of the child, and was useful in reducing aggression in disruptive behavioral problems. Monitoring should be done for metabolic side effects and for extrapyramidal symptoms (tremors, rigidity, etc.).
  - *Clonidine (alpha$_2$-agonist)* has been found effective in ADHD and comorbid conditions. Low dose is initiated (starting from 0.025 to 0.50 mg, according to weight and age) and titrated as per response. Most common side effects include sedation, dizziness, headaches, and constipation that may require titration of doses accordingly.
  - *Psychostimulants* (methylphenidate and its congeners) have a good effect on reduction of aggression and is effective for use in ADHD, with or without ODD/CD and for emotional dysregulation.
  - *Mood stabilizers (lithium, valproate, and carbamazepine)* has a low evidence for use in the above disorders.

## PROGNOSIS

Prognosis is variable and depends on the presence or absence of psychiatric comorbidities and the initiation of early interventions. Low intelligence capacities and a dysfunctional family environment with history of criminality in parents predispose to a poorer prognosis. Adequate treatment of ADHD and other comorbid conditions, assistance for difficulties in learning, higher verbal intelligence, and positive parenting, on the other hand, all contribute to a better prognosis.

## KEY MESSAGES

- Defiance is resistance or outright disobedience in the adolescents for adults.
- It may be a manifestation of trying to achieve independence from parents or differentiation from the family.
- CD is a highly impairing psychiatric disorder that emerges usually in childhood or adolescence.
- Etiology is complex and is usually an interplay of genetic and environmental causes.
- Management includes parent-based or family-based psychosocial interventions, although stimulants and atypical antipsychotics are sometimes used, especially with comorbid ADHD.

## RECOMMENDED READING

1. Bansal PS, Waschbusch DA, Haas SM, Babinski DE, King S, Andrade BF, et al. Effects of Intensive Behavioral Treatment for Children with Varying Levels of Conduct Problems and Callous-Unemotional Traits. Behav Ther. 2019;50(1): 1-14.
2. Chung YE, Chen HC, Chou HL, Chen IM, Lee MS, Chuang LC, et al. Exploration of microbiota targets for major depressive disorder and mood related traits. J Psychiatr Res. 2019;111:74-82.
3. DeLisi M, Drury AJ, Elbert MJ. Do behavioral disorders render gang status spurious? New insights. Int J Law Psychiatry. 2019;62:117-24.
4. Gatej AR, Lamers A, van Domburgh L, Crone M, Ogden T, Rijo D, et al. Awareness and perceptions of clinical guidelines for the diagnostics and treatment of severe behavioral problems in children across Europe: a qualitative survey with academic experts. Eur Psychiatry. 2019;57:1-9.
5. Miranda-Mendizabal A, Castellví P, Parés-Badell O, Alayo I, Almenara J, Alonso I, et al. Gender differences in suicidal behavior in adolescents and young adults: systematic review and meta-analysis of longitudinal studies. Int J Public Health. 2019;64(2):265-83.
6. Thomson KC, Richardson CG, Gadermann AM, Emerson SD, Shoveller J, Guhn M. Association of Childhood Social-Emotional Functioning Profiles at School Entry with Early-Onset Mental Health Conditions. JAMA Netw Open. 2019;2(1):e186694.
7. Weintraub MJ, Axelson DA, Kowatch RA, Schneck CD, Miklowitz DJ. Comorbid disorders as moderators of response to family interventions among adolescents with bipolar disorder. J Affect Disord. 2019;246:754-62.

<table><tr><td>**3B.10**</td><td># Mental Health Issues in Adolescents with Special Needs</td></tr></table>

*S Sitaraman, Chitra Sankar*

## GENERAL OVERVIEW

Neurodevelopmental disorders are a group of conditions, including autism spectrum disorder (ASD), intellectual disability (ID), attention deficit hyperactivity disorder (ADHD), specific learning disability (LD), and cerebral palsy. They manifest during the early developmental period and affect various aspects of functioning, leading to academic, psychosocial, behavioral, cognitive, and emotional challenges, finally affecting the mental health of the individual. Besides these, there are various types of physical and sensory disabilities, which are lifelong conditions and have a great impact on the lives of affected individuals, causing limitations in body function or structure, mobility, activity, participation, and functioning in different life stages and situations.

They cause specific challenges with learning as in specific learning disorder (SLD), executive dysfunctions as in ADHD, global impairments as in ID, physical disability as in cerebral palsy, and sensory impairments causing disability as in vision and hearing. Frequently, more than one condition may occur together; for example, ASD may occur along with ID, and SLD and ADHD may occur together. They pose unique challenges to affected individuals during adolescence, which is a period of transition between childhood and adulthood marked by several physical, social, sexual, emotional, and cognitive demands.

Adolescence is a period of physical growth, cognitive maturation, and psychosocial transformation. It is a time during which crucial aspects of autonomy, positive identity, and individuality around gender, physical attributes, and sexuality are formed. There is a strong need for conformity to peers and peer acceptance and not seen to be "different" from peers, especially during early adolescence. Adolescents with disabilities lack the cognitive and emotional abilities to achieve these tasks satisfactorily. They are routinely excluded from most educational, social, and cultural opportunities and struggle with feelings of inadequacy, loneliness, and social isolation, which is often exacerbated by stigma, peer rejection, and societal stereotypes. They struggle to form meaningful and lasting friendships and are often bullied. Difficulties with communication and low social competence, as seen in ASDs, result in feelings of frustration and heightened levels of anxiety and stress. Adolescents with physical disabilities have difficulties in developing a positive body image of themselves and may experience shame and negative sexual body image.

Therefore, adolescents with special needs have an additional set of issues compared to the ones the average adolescent has to cope with. Coping strategies and the issues that arise as part of growing up are profoundly influenced by the underlying disabilities that the adolescent has. The psychological changes in these adolescents, superimposed by the limitations of special needs, not only pose a diagnostic problem but also have therapeutic implications.

Adverse childhood experiences (ACEs) along with parenting styles affect mental health. Some parents themselves may have a mild ID and struggle with parenting. Children of depressed mothers are reported to have more behavior problems and run a risk of psychopathology. Emotional dysregulation is exaggerated in the presence of nonoptimal parenting, increasing the risk of attempted suicide by adolescence.

## INTELLECTUAL DISABILITY

This is a heterogeneous condition of multiple etiologies with an overall prevalence of 1%. Published data by Jain et al. of 101 children (3 months to 12 years with a median age of 22 months) provided an etiological yield of 82.1% with genetic causes being the most common (61.4%) of ID, followed by perinatal acquired (20.4%), CNS malformations (12%), external prenatal (3.6%), and postnatal acquired (2.4%). Mild delay was seen in 11.7%, moderate in 21.7%, severe in 30.6%, and profound in 35.6%.

As per DSM-5 criteria, ID is characterized by:

- Deficits in intellectual functioning (reasoning, problem solving, planning, abstract thinking, judgment, memory, academic learning, learning from experience, and practical understanding). Intelligence quotient (IQ) scores are typically below 70.

- Deficits in adaptive skills and functioning in one or more areas of conceptual, social, and practical domains necessary for independent living (communication, social skills and participation, academic or occupational functioning, and personal independence and safety).
- Has its onset in the development period.

Deficits are categorized as mild, moderate, severe, or profound based on the levels of support required for adaptive functioning in the conceptual, social, and practical domains of daily life. There may be other challenges, such as coexisting physical and sensory impairments.

The challenges of adolescents with borderline intellectual functioning (BIF) (IQ of 70–85) are under-recognized. They do not have ID but have low IQs. They face academic as well as social challenges. Adolescents with BIF can be identified by the following: Limited cognitive capacity, slow learning, poor grade retention, overall poor performance in all school subjects, significant problems with arithmetic and written expression, poor reasoning, memory, decision-making, motivation, self-concept, attention deficit, poor organization skills, difficulty managing emotions and aggression, poor social skills, mood swings, low frustration tolerance, and a lack of common sense.

Repeated failures result in frustration, low self-esteem, low self-confidence, feelings of low self-worth, anxiety, and depression. They are at high risk of developing mental health disorders. Low birth weight is identified as an important risk factor for BIF, others being mothers with low education, and negative family environment. Adolescents in the category of BIF are neglected and do not receive educational concessions or social supports reserved for specific LDs or IDs.

Associated comorbid medical and psychiatric conditions are more common in adolescents with IDs and BIF than in typically developing adolescents. Epilepsy, hypothyroidism, cerebral palsy, obesity, developmental coordination disorder, ADHD, oppositional defiant disorder (ODD), ASD, sleep disorders, anxiety, obsessive-compulsive disorder (OCD), depression, and impulse control disorders are common. Maladaptive behaviors such as tantrums, meltdowns, aggressive behaviors (hitting and biting), self-injurious behaviors (head banging, self-hitting, and biting), destruction of property, noncompliance, and stereotypical behaviors

**TABLE 1:** Causes of ID.

| Genetic | Nongenetic |
|---|---|
| Chromosomal abnormalities, e.g., Trisomy 21 | Prenatal infections (TORCH and Zika), brain malformations, and congenital hypothyroidism |
| Single gene disorders like Fragile X syndrome, Rett syndrome, tuberous sclerosis, PKU, and inborn errors of metabolism (small molecule and lysosomal storage disorders) | Perinatal factors—severe birth asphyxia, infections, and extreme prematurity |
| Defects of genomic imprinting—Prader–Willi syndrome and Angelman syndrome | Environmental—traumatic brain injury, abuse, neglect, and malnutrition |
| De novo mutations | Childhood illnesses—meningitis and encephalitis |
| Deletion syndromes—Williams syndrome and DiGeorge syndrome | Toxins—fetal alcohol syndrome, lead, and other toxins |
| Undetermined | |

[ID: intellectual disability; PKU: phenylketonuria; TORCH: toxoplasmosis, others (syphilis, hepatitis B), rubella, cytomegalovirus, and herpes simplex]

are also frequently seen. However, depression may not be identified in individuals with severe ID due to problems with communication of feelings or changes in mood. Changes in appetite (increase or decrease), early morning wakening or excessive sleep, poor concentration, and anhedonia are common. The child may appear to regress or may exhibit an increase in stereotypical behavior, such as rocking, compared to baseline levels of functioning **(Table 1)**.

## ■ AUTISM SPECTRUM DISORDER

Autism spectrum disorder is a neurodevelopmental condition of diverse etiology (genetic, environmental) that is increasing in prevalence globally, manifesting as persistent and pervasive challenges in:

- Social communication and social interaction (difficulty in initiating and maintaining back and forth conversation, lack of initiation or response to social interaction, poor eye contact, nonverbal communication)
- Restricted and repetitive patterns of behavior and interests (stereotyped behaviors, insistence on sameness, highly restricted, rigid, and fixated interests, and sensory sensitivities).

An adolescent with ASD presents with a varied degree of problems, depending on whether he/she has been diagnosed earlier and has been undergoing therapies. Residual issues that compound growing up are related to sensory insensitivities, sleep, eating, and problems of inappropriate behavior, especially in relation to the opposite sex. Only 1/4 are recognized by the age of 16 years. Since social etiquette is not in concordance with age, they land up in embarrassing and dangerous situations in society. If they are diagnosed to be atypical much before they reach their age, and if anticipated, appropriate intervention can be done. They have higher rates of concurrent mental health problems.

Some of the children with scholastic difficulties consequently acquire delinquent behavior.

These adolescents would have problems of adjustment in school. If these are unrecognized and undiagnosed, they would have problems with parents and consequently develop feelings of low self-esteem, despair, anxiety, and aggression and become children with ADHD-ODD. Resolving the issue with remedial education may help them come up as productive individuals.

## ■ LEARNING DISABILITIES

Learning disabilities are educational difficulties seen in children with good intelligence manifested as intelligence performance discrepancies in the school. The three main varieties are dyslexia, dysgraphia (writing difficulty), and dyscalculia (difficulty with numerical).

Dyslexia is a condition with unexpected difficulty in reading and is the most common form of LD. In adolescents, it presents as slow or choppy reading when reading aloud. There may be a history of phonologically based reading difficulties. Some of the clues from school age would be: Mispronunciation of long words, improper language, dysfluent speech, problems in reading, choppy oral reading, disastrous spelling, and messy handwriting. In dyslexia, reading speed is more crucial than word recognition and comprehension.

Failure of the system to accommodate such students results in low self-esteem, frustration, anxiety, and depression in them since they are unable to compete with typical adolescents. Depression can further interfere with communication, memory, and auditory processing, leading to anxiety disorder, which in turn may lead to social phobia. Such youth are likely to be rejected by the peer group, and as a consequence, some adopt delinquent behavior, which serves as an alternate means of obtaining social status.

Social isolation on account of behavior of "the rebel" causes the society to be less supportive of the child.

Some of the children have language learning impairments and have difficulty sequencing ideas or have problems with pragmatics. Appropriate remedial measures (though only a few are likely to receive them), if provided in a timely manner, prevent the development of any emotional problems associated with antisocial behavior.

## ■ SENSORY IMPAIRMENTS

The literature on the impact of sensory impairments such as hearing and visual impairments on adolescents and their mental health is limited and varied. Studies of hearing-impaired children have been impaired by the lack of availability of standardized tests for assessing hearing-impaired children as many of the tests are standardized for normal hearing children. Numerous studies have concluded that deaf children of deaf parents attain better emotional and cognitive development than do deaf children of hearing parents. Due to communication difficulties, physical appearance, or the use of devices such as hearing aids or cochlear implants, children with hearing loss are at risk of low self-esteem. Adolescents with visual impairments have issues with independent identity. They are at risk of developing distorted concepts of sexuality, leading to inappropriate behavior and subsequent social isolation.

## ■ ATTENTION DEFICIT HYPERACTIVITY DISORDER

Attention deficit hyperactivity disorder is characterized by persistent patterns of inattention, hyperactivity, impulsivity, and distractibility that cause impairments in social, academic, or occupational functioning, with onset in childhood. Frequently impairments are seen in attention, executive functioning, and memory. Comorbid conditions include mood, conduct disorder, and substance use disorder increasing the risk of suicide attempts. Adolescents with ADHD have a higher prevalence of smoking and drug abuse (more than twice) over the life span. The girls have depression, anxiety, poor teacher relationships, and impaired academic performance. They report more of an external locus of control. They have frequent job changes and maladjustments. Some of these children have Tourette syndrome, which is defined as the presence of multiple vocal tics over 1 year. It has a prevalence of 0.3% in teenagers. They are associated with

OCD and ADHD. They are affected by depression (36%), anxiety (40%), and LD (80%).

## MANAGEMENT

The management strategies involve behavioral management and pharmacological intervention. Numerous drugs (e.g., methylphenidate and atomoxetin) have been successfully tried with satisfactory results. However, these interventions have to be supported at home and schools with behavioral strategies to ensure optimum results.

*Two interventions are often used:* Both interventions are targeted toward high-risk adolescents with severe unremitting mental disorders associated with child maltreatment.

1. Dialectical behavior therapy (DBT) is useful for the treatment of mood disorders, including suicidal thoughts and self-harm, and victims of sexual abuse.

   Multisystem therapy for child abuse and neglect (MSN-CAN) refers to referral behavior and key environmental risk factors.

2. Adolescents with physical disabilities or dysmorphisms are likely to have issues with body image and functionality. Their problems are compounded if there is an additional cognitive impairment. Their peer group interaction is compromised, leading to depression, anger, and social isolation. Proactive and responsive parenting will help them maintain self-confidence and become productive individuals. These adolescents should be periodically assessed by behavioral scales to recognize and prevent any psychopathology.

## PROVISIONS BY THE GOVERNMENT

### The National Trust Act in India

The National Trust Act in India, officially known as the "National Trust for the Welfare of Persons with Autism, Cerebral Palsy, Mental Retardation, and Multiple Disabilities Act, 1999," was established to provide legal support and assistance to individuals with disabilities, particularly those with autism, cerebral palsy, mental retardation, and multiple disabilities.

Key provisions of the National Trust Act in India include:

- The National Trust Act provides a mechanism for appointing legal guardians for person with disability (PwD) who are unable to take care of themselves to ensure their well-being and protection.
- It outlines the rights and entitlements of PwD.

- Training and research initiatives related to the welfare of PwD.
- Provides funding, assistance, and support for various programs, services, and activities designed to benefit PwD.
- Promotes awareness and advocacy for the rights and well-being of PwD to reduce stigma and discrimination. The National Trust Act provides several important schemes designed to support individuals with disabilities under the act.
- DISHA (Early Intervention and School Readiness Scheme) provides day-care facilities with age-specific activities, therapies by physiotherapists, occupational therapists, counsellors, and early intervention therapists.
- VIKAAS (Day Care) is designed to provide day-care facilities with age-specific activities for at least 6 hours a day for 21 days a month for PwDs who are transitioning to higher age groups, providing interpersonal and vocational skills and helps in supporting family members of the PwDs to get some time during the day to fulfill other responsibilities.
- *Nirmaya scheme:* It provides health insurance to PwD with health insurance coverage of 10 lakhs, covering outpatient treatment, medicines, diagnostic tests, surgeries, ongoing therapies, alternative medicine, and transportation costs.
- Other schemes are Sahyogi scheme to train caregivers; Gyan Prabha to provide educational and vocational courses, leading to employment or self-employment providing financial support, fees, transportation, books, and other expenses; Prerna for Marketing Assistance; Sambhav for Aids and Assisted devices; and Badhte Kadam for community awareness and community interaction.

### Concessions Extended by CBSE Boards for Classes X and XII

- Candidates with disabilities as defined in The Rights of Persons With Disabilities Act 2016 are permitted to use a scribe or allowed compensatory time or both.
- Exemption from the study of a third language.
- Flexibility in choosing subjects.
- Alternate questions/separate questions are provided in place of questions having visual inputs for visually impaired candidates in the subject of social science.
- Separate question paper and questions in lieu of practical component containing multiple choice

questions in lieu of practicals in the subjects of Physics, Chemistry, and Biology.

- To facilitate easy access, a few selected schools are made examination centers for special students.
- Registration and examination fee for classes IX, X, XI, and XII will not be charged from visually impaired students.

General concessions and exemptions are provided based on medical certificates issued by the designated institutions of central and state governments.

*CBSE board mandates that:*

- No child with special needs is denied admission in mainstream education.
- Schools are to provide support through assistive devices, availability of trained teachers, and physical infrastructure to make the premises disabled friendly.
- Availability of study material for the disabled such as Talking Text Books, Reading Machines, and computers with speech software.

## National Institute of Open Schooling

National Institute of Open Schooling (NIOS) is an "Open School" to cater to the needs of a heterogeneous group of learners up to the predegree level. At the secondary and senior secondary levels, NIOS provides flexibility in the choice of subjects/courses, pace of learning, and transfer of credits from CBSE, some Board of School Education, and State Open Schools to enable learner's continuation. A learner is extended as many as nine chances to appear in public examinations spread over a period of 5 years.

## ■ KEY MESSAGES

- Neurodiverse adolescents and those with special needs have higher chances of emotional and social problems.
- They also have academic difficulties and vocational challenges.
- They require help from a multidisciplinary team including therapists and educators.
- Parents should be made aware of various government schemes and concessions that help adolescents with special needs.

## ■ RECOMMENDED READING


1. Allington-Smith P. Mental health of children with learning disabilities. Adv Psychiatr Treat. 2006;12(2):130-8.
2. American Psychiatric Association. (2022). Intellectual Disabilities in Diagnostic and Statistical Manual of Mental Disorders, 5th edition. [online] Available from chrome-extension://efaidnbmnnnibpcajpcglclefindmkaj/https://www.psychiatry.org/File%20Library/Psychiatrists/Practice/DSM/APA_DSM-5-Intellectual-Disability.pdf [Last accessed March, 2024].
3. Dube SR, Anda RF, Felitti VJ, Chapman DP, Williamson DF, Giles WH. Childhood abuse, household dysfunction, and the risk of attempted suicide throughout the life span: findings from the Adverse Childhood Experiences Study. JAMA. 2001;286(24):3089-96.
4. Goodman S, Gotlieb I. Risk of psychopathology in children of depressed mother. Psychol Rev. 1999;60:458-90.
5. Jain S, Chowdhury V, Juneja M, Kabra M, Pandey S, Singh A, et al. Intellectual Disability in Indian Children: Experience with a Stratified Approach for Etiological Diagnosis. Indian Pediatr. 2013;50(12):1125-30.
6. Joshi G, Petty C, Wozniak J, Henin A, Fried R, Galdo M, et al. The heavy burden of psychiatric comorbidity in youth with autism spectrum disorders: a large comparative study of a psychiatrically referred population. J Autism Dev Disord. 2010;40(11):1361-70.
7. Juneja M, Gupta A, Sairam S, Jain R, Sharma M, Thadani A, et al. Diagnosis and Management of Global Development Delay: Consensus Guidelines of Growth, Development and Behavioral Pediatrics Chapter, Neurology Chapter, and Neurodevelopment Pediatrics Chapter of the Indian Academy of Pediatrics. Indian Pediatr. 2022;59(5): 401-15.
8. Ruesse RL. Language impairment and psychiatric morbity. PCNA. 2007;54523-2.
9. Sandler A. Tics and tourette syndrome. In: Voight RG (Ed). AAP Developmental and Behavioral Pediatrics, 2nd edition. p. 301.
10. Timmer SG, Urquiza AJ. Specialized behavioral therapies for children with special needs. Pediatr Clin North Am. 2016;63(5):873-85.
11. van Steensel FJ, Bögels SM, Perrin S. Anxiety disorders in children and adolescents with autistic spectrum disorders: a meta-analysis. Clin Child Fam Psychol Rev. 2011;14(3):302-17.

# Part C: Therapeutic Interventions for Mental Health Concerns

***Sub-section Editors:*** *Swati Ghate, Sushma Desai*

## 3C.1 | Self-counseling

*MKC Nair, Gurmeet Kaur*

### ■ INTRODUCTION

Globally, 1 in 7, 10–19 year-olds experiences a mental disorder, accounting for 13% of the global burden of disease in this age group.

Depression, anxiety, and behavioral disorders are among the leading causes of illness and disability among adolescents. Suicide is the 4th leading cause of death among 15–29-year-olds.

The consequences of failing to address adolescent mental health conditions extend to adulthood, impairing both physical and mental health and limiting opportunities to lead fulfilling lives as adults.

This suggests that there is a huge demand for psychological services, but very few clinical psychologists/counselors/child and adolescent psychiatrists are there. It is in this context that we need to think about self-counseling as an alternative community strategy for at least the large majority with only mild symptoms. It also helps to take more control of oneself and address one's anger, anxiety, and addictive habits.

Self-counseling is a practice of self-analysis and self-awareness examining one's own behavior by using psychoanalytic methods of free thinking and free association. Self-therapy requires self-training to take more effective control of emotions in everyday situations. When we can master reading, writing, and arithmetic, why cannot we master our own psychological makeup too?

Self-counseling is to achieve clarity of thoughts by the practice of cross-examining oneself and learning self-acceptance, motivation, and determination leading to a change of thoughts and actions. *It is learning to listen to oneself with an open heart, ask for clarification from oneself, and look for options and answers from oneself.* It is all based on top psychotherapy approaches like person-centered therapy and rational emotive behavioral therapy. The prerequisites for effective self-counseling would be: (1) Self-awareness, (2) self-motivation, and (3) self-screening.

### ■ SELF-AWARENESS

Self-awareness means being aware of different aspects of the self, including mental, physical, aesthetic, sexual, spiritual, and social aspects, and more. In this, the person is focusing on oneself and not trying to look outside.

#### Emotional Self-awareness

Emotional self-awareness is an inherent ability to understand one's own emotions and their effects on one's day-to-day life and performance. One can "self-talk" to enquire about one's feelings and know one's emotional strengths.

- Expressing emotion is easy for me.
- Know what causes my mood change and be aware of inner emotions.
- Think about ways to make oneself feel better.
- One's thinking, feelings, and behavior match.

#### Social Self-awareness

Social self-awareness focuses on recognizing and understanding others' feelings and how they perceive us. It is practicing stepping back (in one's mind) to examine oneself to recognize one's social competencies.

- Care a lot about how I present myself to others
- Easy for me to mingle with others/strangers
- Reasonably concerned about what others think of me
- Do not feel nervous speaking and working in front of a group
- Enjoy family time/outings with family.

## Sexual Self-awareness

Sexual self-awareness is the understanding of the totality of oneself as a sexual being, including the positive and negative concepts and feelings.

- Do not feel uncomfortable discussing sex/sexuality
- Readily accept sexuality-related changes within me
- Positively conscious about how attractive I look
- Can handle sexual thoughts and feelings
- Self-stimulation/masturbation does happen
- Firm believer of commitment in relationship
- Aware of sexual orientation (homo-, hetero-, and bisexual).

## Spiritual Self-awareness

Spiritual self-awareness is the soul's intelligence or intelligence of the "whole/total awareness" of oneself.

- Believe in religious activities and experiences
- Use religion and faith to face life problems
- Believe that God has sent me here with a purpose
- My religious belief has an impact on my behavior
- Believe in prayers, religious practices, and religious basic concepts
- Have tolerance for other religions and their beliefs *(such as the Creator of the world, the concept of soul, and life after death).*

## ■ SELF-MOTIVATION

Self-motivation is the ability to push oneself to take initiative and stretch one's mind to its limits in a voluntary effort to accomplish something difficult and worthwhile. It is an inner drive to act, create, achieve goals, and complete tasks. There are many techniques that one can follow to improve self-motivation:

- *Believe in yourself that you can do it:* This is probably the first step in gaining self-confidence. Do not get held back by the stumbling blocks; know that you have the ability to accomplish your goals.
- *Finish what has been started:* It is important to finish off the work that has been started, to accomplish our goals and improve self-esteem.
- *Get out of your comfort zone:* Do not be afraid to make mistakes. Wisdom helps us avoid making mistakes and comes from making a million of them. "It is only those who work beyond their comfort zone are able to achieve and transform."
- *Never give up when you are frustrated:* Keep going and focus on the end goal of your true potential. Visualizing what one wants to accomplish and moving forward can help in self-motivation.

- *You have to want it:* All of the above aspects can significantly contribute to self-motivation, but remember the basic rule is the desire for self-motivation.

## ■ SELF-SCREENING

There are mental health self-check screening tools available; when using them, one can grade one's changes in mood, thinking and attitude, behavior, performance, physical changes, and addictive behaviors. One can score oneself as healthy, reacting, injured, or ill by using these screening tools. It helps adolescents to reflect on and enhance their mental health by self-counseling or seeking expert help.

## ■ MKC'S 10 COMMANDMENTS OF SELF-COUNSELING

1. *Do not bluff to yourself, though you may have to bluff to others sometimes:* It is important that we are true to ourselves, accepting our good and bad in true spirit. The theoretical underpinning behind this is probably Rogers' theory of self-concept which consists of three dimensions:
   i. *Self-image:* How we perceive ourselves
   ii. *Self-esteem:* How much value we place on ourselves
   iii. *Ideal self:* How we wish we were really like.
   Self-concept, when congruent or aligned with reality, helps us battle the challenges of life.

2. *You are not God and are likely to make mistakes; hence, take precaution always:* However much we think great of ourselves, at some point in time, we realize that we are vulnerable to make mistakes. The theoretical underpinning behind this is probably Elkind's personal fable theory, suggesting that adolescent egocentrism stems from two phenomena: (1) Belief of an imaginary audience who is interested in their lives and (2) personal fable, i.e., the idea that the adolescent is special, and different from others, hence should be the center of attention. These two phenomena may give rise to a delusion of grandeur, where adolescents believe that they are omnipotent and may indulge in impulsive, high-risk activities. It is essential that we learn about the limitations of our capabilities, while nurturing a positive outlook toward life, and plan, organize, and strategize.

3. *Do not think others have to like you always; indulge in self-love:* Is it not unfortunate that many youngsters crave "likes" on social media from mostly unknown people, ignoring to love and trust themselves? The theoretical background behind this is probably Grieger's theory of

self-acceptance, which proposed that unconditional self-acceptance is independent from their actions and qualities and having good self-esteem.

4. *Caring and not love:* Love can be a craving, the intensity of which may come down with time, but caring and affection only can increase with time if well reciprocated. This is based on Sternberg's triangular theory of love in which love has been graded as intimacy, passion, and commitment. Companionate love is often found in marriages where the passion has faded out, but intimacy and commitment are strong even though consummate love, where all three elements are equally present, can be considered as the ideal type.

5. *Refuse to take insults; then nobody can hurt you and you will always be happy:* The theoretical basis can be probably explained by Coon and Mitterer that suggested that one of the most common reasons people take offense is insecurity about the self, which the offending statement may be challenging. A person with a strong self-concept is less likely to take offense.

6. *Do not keep a grudge; it eats you up emotionally:* It is well known that moving on and forgiveness are associated with improved health and peace of mind, less anxiety, stress, hostility, and depression, but it is also true that it is not easy to forget and forgive. Grudges also often feature persistent rumination about the person and/or incident at the center of your ill will.

7. *Disarm your perceived enemy by caring when they really need it:* The best way to disarm the perceived enemy is by giving a helping hand when he/she needs it badly. Affiliative responses like relationship repair or reconciliation may promote physiological downregulation and homeostasis after incidences of incivility or rude–unsociable speech or behavior.

8. *Do not think that others are lesser than you; you are also lesser than someone else:* We must understand and learn to accept, respect, and value people, focusing on their strengths and scaffolding their weaknesses. As per Adam's equity theory, one's motivation is driven largely by one's sense of equity or fairness of others toward them. At times, least competent persons in a certain subject area overestimate their skills the most and most competent people think less of their own talents and vice versa (Dunning–Kruger effect).

9. *Think of other person's point of view; be a third party when analyzing yourself:* Perspective taking is a multidimensional modality that helps us understand our own and other's assessment and perception of an event or personal reaction. Although there are many theoretical concepts involved, the main theoretical base is the *uncertainty reduction theory*, which asserts the notion that, when interacting, people need information about the other party to reduce their uncertainty leading to inappropriate reactions.

10. *Do not hurt others, if possible; do not hurt yourself ever:* The theoretical underpinning behind this concept is probably *social exchange theory*, according to which "give and take" forms the basis of almost all relationships though their proportions might vary as per the intensity of the relationship. In a relationship, every adolescent has expectations from his/her friend, and a relationship without expectations is meaningless.

Let us take an example of self-counseling. Here, the client is the self and the self is an inner counselor.

*Client (Adolescent):* I have an anger issue. I seem to be angry all the time which is ruining my relationship at home and in school (self-awareness).

*Inner Counselor:* What I am hearing is that anger is ruining your relationship everywhere and you cannot stand yourself. Is that correct?

*Client (Adolescent):* That is right, I have arguments at home with my Mom and in school with my peers.

*Inner Counselor:* What was the trigger at home that caused you to argue and lose your temper?

*Client (Adolescent):* My mom keeps shouting at home telling me to study all the time and not to play games on my phone.

*Inner Counselor:* You judged that your mom was being disrespectful, then you reacted with anger, but how would you do it differently?

*Client (Adolescent):* I guess that I could have taken a breath, calmed myself, and explained to my mom that I was taking a break from my studies.

*Inner Counselor:* This is wonderful learning; I am going to learn how to change my negative emotions and appreciate myself for this learning.

## ◼ CONCLUSION

The stress among young adults is increasing day by day, and hence, we need a biopsychosociospiritual approach to tackle the same at the community level. The effectiveness of self-counselling as an alternative strategy has been shown and the same is awaiting publication.

## KEY MESSAGES

- There is a huge demand for psychological services but very few clinical psychologists/counselors/child and adolescent psychiatrists. It is in this context that we need to think about self-counseling.
- It helps to take more control of oneself and address one's anger, anxiety, and addictive habits.
- Self-counseling is a practice of self-analysis and self-awareness, examining one's own behavior by using psychoanalytic methods of free thinking and free association.
- It is learning to listen to oneself with an open heart, ask for clarification from oneself, and look for options and answers from oneself. It is all based on top psychotherapy approaches like person-centered therapy and rational emotive behavioral therapy.
- Self-motivation is the ability to push oneself to take initiative and stretch one's mind to its limits in a voluntary effort to accomplish something difficult and worthwhile.
- Self-screening tools are mental health self-check screening tools; by using them, one can grade one's changes in mood, thinking and attitude, behavior, performance, physical changes, and changes in addictive behaviors.

## RECOMMENDED READING


1. Chen SP, Chang WP, Stuart H. Self-reflection and screening mental health on Canadian campuses: Validation of the mental health continuum model. BMC Psychol. 2020;8(1):76.
2. Nair MKC, George B, Neethu C. Adolescent anxiety disorders. In: Nair MKC, George B, Sumaraj L (Eds). Adolescent Pediatrics, 2nd edition. Delhi: Noble Vision (Medical Book Publishers); 2023. pp. 110-8.
3. Nair MKC, George B, Sunitha RM. Adolescents needing supportive counselling. In: Nair MKC, George B, Sumaraj L (Eds). Adolescent Pediatrics, 2nd edition. Delhi: Noble Vision (Medical Book Publishers); 2023. pp. 97-109.
4. Nair MKC, Kumar S, Lukose R, Girish CS, Binod D, Sreejith S. Self-counselling. Pediatr Companion. 2022;1:16-20.
5. TSW Training. (2023). How can Adams' equity theory boost your team's motivation. [online] Available from https://www.tsw.co.uk/blog/leadership-and-management/adams-equity-theory/ [Last accessed March, 2024].
6. Vanbuskirk S. (2023). The mental health effects of holding a grudge. [online] Available from https://www.verywellmind.com/the-mental-health-effects-of-holding-a-grudge-5176186 [Last accessed March, 2024].


<br>

# 3C.2 — Psychotherapy in Adolescents

*Harmesh Singh Bains*

## INTRODUCTION

Psychotherapy is a type of treatment involving the interaction of the therapist with the adolescent and/or family. The adolescent and his/her family are helped to understand the nature of the problem and change the teen's behavior in a positive direction. Depending upon the approach used, psychotherapy may be classified into different types. Sometimes, we need to combine different types of psychotherapy and/or pharmacotherapy to make it more effective. It is more important to understand the difference between guidance, counselling and psychotherapy **(Table 1)**.

## TYPES OF PSYCHOTHERAPY

- Cognitive behavior therapy (CBT)
- Interpersonal psychotherapy (IPT)
- Parent–child interaction therapy (PCIT)
- Family therapy
- Dialectical behavior therapy (DBT)
- Play therapy
- Group therapy

## SETTINGS OF PSYCHOTHERAPY SESSIONS

- Psychotherapy for children and adolescents can be done in the outpatient department (OPD) and inpatient department (IPD).
- History and clinical assessment of the teen from a psycho-therapeutic point of view should be completed first.
- Long waiting period should be avoided so that a teen does not become uncooperative and irritable during the interview.
- The clinics should have an attractive appearance and fulfill the requirements of an adolescent-friendly clinic.

**TABLE 1:** Difference between guidance, counseling, and psychotherapy.

| *Guidance* | *Counseling* | *Psychotherapy* |
|---|---|---|
| Guidance is advice given by an elder or superior/expert | Counseling is professional advice provided by a counselor | Psychotherapy is provided by a therapist |
| It helps the teen in the selection of suitable option | • Counseling focuses on the present<br>• It is short term and geared toward solutions<br>• It is preventive | • It tends to be long term and focuses on problems; past concerns are often explored<br>• It is remedial and curative |
| Education and career-related issues | Personal and sociopsychological issues | Psychological issues |
| Open and less private | Confidential | Confidential |
| One to one or one to many | One to one and provided only in an outpatient setting | To one/or family and provided in both inpatient and outpatient settings |

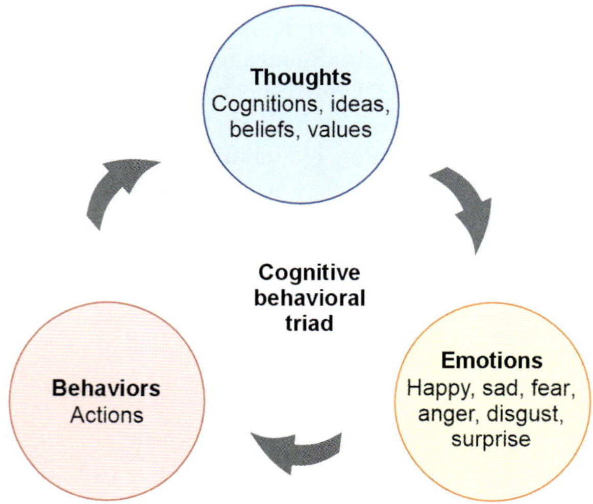


**Fig. 1:** Interrelations between thoughts, emotions, and actions.

- It is better to have one of the parents so that the child remains comfortable.
- Maintain privacy and confidentiality.
- Avoid very long sessions.

## Cognitive Behavior Therapy

- CBT is designed to change both maladaptive cognitions and behavior.
- The teen is made clear about the interrelation between thoughts, emotions, and actions **(Fig. 1)**.
- The basic aim of CBT is to develop better communication skills, problem-solving skills, and anger management.
- It can control their feelings by differentiating between their feelings and thoughts. It might also address behavior patterns that contribute to withdrawal and lack of enjoyment with strategies such as helping adolescents identify activities they have enjoyed in the past and planning to engage in them regularly.

- Parents will be educated about the underlying cause of depression so that their teens can identify and modify the negative thinking and behavior. Treatment begins with the therapist educating the adolescent, often with their parent/guardian, on how thoughts, feelings, and behaviors interact with one another. The therapist explains that there are ways in which the adolescent can modify their thinking and behavioral patterns that would benefit them emotionally and behaviorally.
- Adolescents are asked to complete a "mood diary" outside of the session, which will bring out the situation triggering the thoughts that then influenced the way they felt and behaved in that situation. For example, an adolescent fails in an examination (*situation*) and jumps to the conclusion, "I will be dismissed from school" (*automatic thought*). He might then withdraw socially due to perceiving himself as unsuccessful (*behavior*), leading to a sad and depressed mood (*feeling*). The adolescent works with the therapist to identify triggering situations in the diary to begin to identify and address the unhelpful thinking and behavior patterns. After identifying common triggers, the adolescent will be encouraged to apply the behavioral component of CBT by identifying activities that they used to enjoy (like playing or hanging out with peers) and then incorporate these into a schedule of pleasant activities. CBT helps to change the mood and behavior of the child and also reduces anxiety by exploring abnormal thinking patterns. There is evidence that CBT is a very effective therapy for depression and anxiety in adolescents.

Cognitive behavioral therapy can be helpful in the following problems of adolescents:

- Depression
- Anxiety/worry/trauma
- Phobias
- Obsessive–compulsive disorder (OCD)
- Low mood
- Eating disorders

## Interpersonal Psychotherapy

- IPT is a brief, specially developed, and well-established treatment for depressed adolescents. It may be useful in various other clinical conditions. The focus of IPT is on helping adolescents understand and address common teen relationship problems with their family members and friends, including romantic relationships. The need is to concentrate on how interpersonal issues affect an adolescent's emotional state. IPT is active, is structured, and includes a big psychoeducational component. It is usually conducted in an individual therapy format, where the therapist works one on one with the adolescent and his or her family. In this, teens learn skills for better communicating their feelings and expectations and also develop skills to handle conflicts. It is usually a 12–16-week therapy; parents are also asked to participate in some of the sessions.
- The basic concept of IPT revolves around the type of interpersonal relationships as these can be a cause as well as can act as a buffer against depression. IPT acts by improving interpersonal relationships, thus preventing or minimizing depression. It educates teens about the connection between their mood and problems in relationships and teaches them how enhancing interpersonal interaction skills and addressing those interpersonal issues can help them get rid of depression.
- As therapy progresses, the adolescent gains more control over their relationship with parents and develops a greater problem-solving capability.
- IPT works by addressing interpersonal issues and strengthening the individual by increasing both independence and interdependence.
- IPT improves autonomy and helps the individuation of the child, thereby making the treatment more desirable to them.

## Parent–Child Interaction Therapy

Parent–child interaction therapy is useful for parents and children having problems with behavioral issues. In this, the therapist guides the parents to have a positive interaction while interacting with their children.

## Family Therapy

Family therapy is indicated in overt and disturbing conflicts among family members, with or besides symptomatic behaviors in one or more members. The pattern of communication in the family is explored first. Education and support are provided so that the family develops a positive and constructive way of communication. In these sessions, parents, teens, siblings, and grandparents can be included so that the whole family learns the way of positive communication. In case of marital problems, parents are educated about positive communication and avoid creating odd situations in the presence of children.

*Caution:* Family therapy is to be avoided in explosive family problems, and where one or more of the participants are severely destabilized requiring hospitalization.

## Dialectical Behavior Therapy

Dialectical behavior therapy is helpful in older adolescents with chronic suicidal ideation and self-harmful behaviors. It helps the teen in exploring the method of his/her dealing with the negative emotions and conflict.

## Group Therapy

In group therapy, there are more than one patient in a session. In this, the principle of group dynamics and interaction among peers is used. It helps them understand mental health issues and also improves their social skills.

## Play Therapy

Play therapy is tried in younger children. It involves the use of toys, blocks, dolls, puppets, drawings, and games to help the child recognize, identify, and verbalize feelings. The child is closely observed while playing and using toys to understand the basic problem and its pattern.

## ■ KEY MESSAGES

- Psychotherapy plays a very important role in dealing with depression and other mental health issues in adolescents.

**BOX 1:** Do's and don'ts of psychotherapy.

*Do's*
- Be open
- Be flexible
- Be trustworthy
- Be approachable
- Be understanding
- Be patient
- Show respect
- Good nonharmful humor

*Don'ts*
- No interrogation mode
- No imposing of your values
- No blaming attitude
- Inadequate time/showing hurry
- Not being hasty
- No technical jargons
- Not to be judgmental
- Do not influence values, attitudes, beliefs, interests, and decisions

- Various types of psychotherapy include CBT, IPT, PCIT, family therapy, DBT, play therapy, and group therapy.
- One should keep in mind the do's and don'ts of psychotherapy **(Box 1)**.

## ■ RECOMMENDED READING

1. Bhide K, Chakraborty K. General principles for psychotherapeutic interventions in children and adolescents. Indian J Psychiatry. 2020;62(Suppl 2): S299-318.
2. David D, Cristea I, Hofmann SG. Why cognitive behavioral therapy is the current gold standard of psychotherapy. Front Psychiatry. 2018;9:1-4.
3. Hofmann SG, Asmundson GJ, Beck AT. The science of cognitive therapy. Behav Ther. 2013;44(2):199-212.

# 3C.3 — Rational Emotive Behavior Therapy: An Introduction

*Atul Kanikar*

## ■ INTRODUCTION

Most of our emotional disturbances emerge out of a "deranged" triad of thinking, feeling, and behaving for which we are likely to *regret later*, because we tend to overgeneralize an event, a person's behavior, or experiences with the person or similar ones in the past. This chaos not only affects our inner peace and growth but also reflects on our relationships, daily routine, and personal growth. Removing irrational beliefs causing emotional disturbances and changing the "self-sabotaging patterns" of thinking around practical problems is the chief purpose of rational emotive behavior therapy (REBT).

Albert Ellis in 1955 coined the term REBT (a version of cognitive behavioral therapy) after "amalgamating" most of the contemporary theories of psychology. Ellis agrees that REBT's integrative aspect borrows and employs all the relevant concepts of Freud's unconscious motives and defense systems, the unconditional positive regard, and full acceptance of the client as suggested by Carl Rogers, Skinner's homework assignments and operant conditioning, Alfred Adler's theory of the *vital role of cognition* in beliefs and emotions, and experimental and feeling methods of Gestalt along with Piaget's constructive view of the human tendency to rise above the adversities (natural or manmade).

However, the roots of REBT go back to Epictetus (Greek Stoic philosopher) who believed that "People are disturbed not by things, but by the view which they take of them" and Lord Buddha's saying that "Nobody but ourselves define our destiny and to conquer oneself is a greater task than conquering others." Ellis states that we are *born* to be rational and irrational. These innate tendencies are later aggravated by family and cultural values along with the child's upbringing methods deployed by parents. We have a biological and cultural tendency to think crookedly and to needlessly disturb ourselves. We *construct* problems even if there are none. We are self-talking, self-evaluating, and self-sustaining humans and our *self-talk* causes emotional disturbances, especially when we convert our desires into grandiose demands. However, we have a priceless capacity to change the way we feel, think, and behavior since *all three are interconnected*.

The crux of this therapy is to help clients achieve *their* potential goals when unhealthy emotions and behavioral reactions impede goal attainment. The error lies in the cognition (thought process) of the disturbed person. Through a fruitful counseling process a client feels *concerned* and not anxious (e.g., examination stress), *sad* and not depressed (e.g., loss of job or broken heart), *regretful* and not guilty (e.g., harming someone), *disappointed* without sorrow (e.g., missing out on some vital task), and *jealous* and *angry* in a constructive way without harm to others (competing positively). The principal aim of the therapist is to convert unhealthy emotions to healthy ones, because *healthy negative emotions are essential for existence and personal growth.* For example, having concern (healthy negative emotion) and not anxiety (unhealthy negative emotion) is essential for a student to excel in academics.

Rational emotive behavior therapy has a psycho-educational, multimodal, didactic (educational), problem and problem-solving approach, which makes it a teenage-friendly therapy and acts like a *dart,* because the intelligence is at its peak during teenage and youth. As mentioned by Epictetus and seconded by many other great thinkers, our view (beliefs) will decide how a particular event or adversity will affect us. The same adversity can thus have multiple outcomes (consequences) for people with different perspectives as depicted below. Our personality, culture, parenting styles, peer group influence, expectations, desires, past experiences, and mainly *self-talk* will shape our belief systems.

Imagine a situation during coronavirus disease (COVID) pandemic. How communities have reacted differently? Those who blamed the people responsible for the "making" and spread of the virus became *angry.* Those who worried about their children and high-risk adults at home became *anxious.* Those who brought the infection home felt *guilty.* Those who lost their near and dear ones and their jobs became *sad.* And those owning a pharmaceutical company, vaccine production industry or intensive care earned a fortune and felt *happy.* In short, the *same* adversity of a pandemic brought out *different* emotional and behavioral consequences from different people. Thus, we can conclude that it is *not* the adversity but our perspective along with our readiness to mend, that matters. In other words, Adversity (A) does not directly cause Consequences (C); it just triggers our thoughts, emotions, and behaviors. All this is depicted in **Figure 1**.

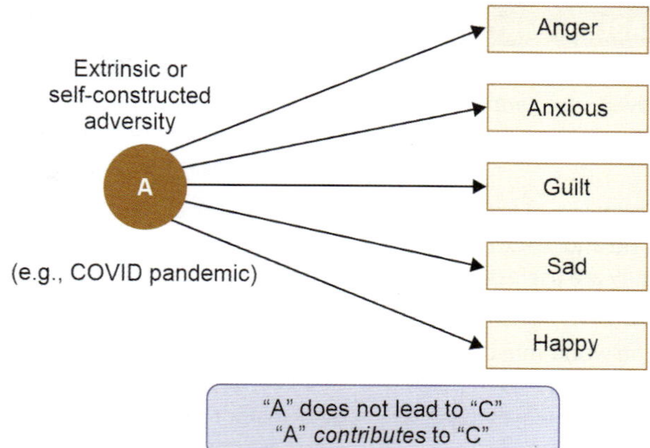


**Fig. 1:** Various emotional outcomes of same event. (COVID: coronavirus disease)

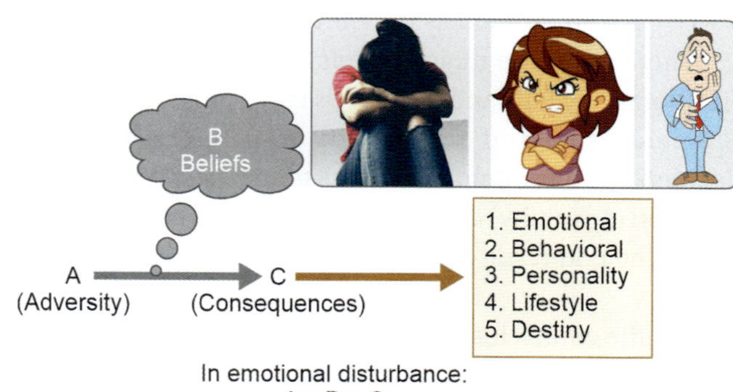


**Fig. 2:** The typical model of rational emotive behavior therapy (REBT).

We can apply this illustration to any other adversities in life. Hence, it is *our own perspective* governed by our belief system with self-talk and *not* the adversity that decides our emotional, cognitive, and behavioral outcomes. Ellis states that in emotional disturbance the belief (B) system *blows up* the emotional and behavioral consequences (C) triggered by the adversity (A) **(Fig. 2)**.

Rational emotive behavior therapy uses following abbreviations:

- A: *Adversities* in life (external or self-created)
- B: *Belief* system principally governed and nurtured by our self-talk after the adversity.
- C: *Consequences* secondary to faulty thinking, emotions, and behavioral processes.
- D: *Disputation* by the therapist aiming at converting unhealthy negative emotions to healthy ones.
- E: *Effective* new philosophy that the client perceives and inculcates resulting in better outcomes.

**TABLE 1:** Outcomes of irrational beliefs.

| | |
|---|---|
| I must be perfect and be loved, else I am useless | • Anxious, self-evaluating<br>• People pleasers, depressed<br>• Compromisers, blind followers<br>• Sensitive, easily humiliated |
| Others must be perfect, kind and just to me, else they are useless | • Angry, rebellious, dominating<br>• Poor interpersonal relations<br>• Ruminate anger and settle scores<br>• Dictate terms to the weak |
| The world must make things easy for me, else life is not worth living | • Low frustration tolerance<br>• Self pity, always grumbling<br>• Seek instant pleasures, gamble<br>• Good beginners, poor finishers |

- F: A new set of *feelings* of being molded and down to earth, rational to self and others.
- G: *Goal* attainment as per the client's preferences.

There are three major beliefs which are described as "irrational" by Ellis and most of us carry those. Our nature, temperament, and personality and interactions are decided by our principle belief system displayed in a given situation (adversity) as shown in **Table 1**. The right column shows the end result and characteristics of person's belief system.

It is the counselor's task to identify which belief system is carried and depicted by the client in a given adversity. The counselor also *visualizes client's self-talk* that led to the emotional turmoil and deranged thought process resulting in behavioral consequences. Albert Ellis has categorized the irrational beliefs as follows:

- *Rigid demands:* "I must", "you ought to", "everybody should", "it has to be", etc.
- *Awfulizing beliefs:* "It is terrible", "you are horrible", "it is the end of the world", etc.
- *Low frustration tolerance (LFT):* "I can't take it", "this is intolerable", "life is excruciating", etc.
- *Depreciation beliefs:* "I am no good", "you are hopeless", "The world has gone to the dogs", etc.

After this is done, then the counselor informs the client about the list of irrational beliefs and "absolutistic" musts in the self-talk. Once educated, the client can self-detect his/her irrational beliefs to prevent a relapse during future adversities. The client also learns to successfully convert the grandiose demands into *nondogmatic preferences,* which diminish his/her stress to a manageable level. This will enhance his/her efforts and reflect on the ultimate outcome positively. In short, the irrational beliefs are rigid and extreme, inconsistent with reality, illogical, and nonsensical, lead to dysfunctional triad of thinking, feeling, and behaving. As a result these beliefs impede goal attainment and spoil productivity and relationships.

In addition to the basic counseling skills like empathy, privacy, confidentiality, and maximum use of nonverbal communication and open-ended questions, the therapeutic process in REBT primarily includes the following vital tools:

- *Cognitive tools:*
  - Disputation: (See later)
  - Referencing: This is similar to the cost–benefit analysis realized by the client with the help of counselor. For example, if a teenage girl mentions that physical intimacies will help me to win emotional support from many boys. *(The counselor can ask "who will be at risk and how?")*
  - Self-therapy: Asking oneself about the type of belief system that has been employed in a given adversity and "relearning" unconditional acceptance.
  - Bibliography: Recommending reading relevant books, and watching movies/drama relating the issue at hand
  - Teaching REBT to others: This boosts the client's rationality and self-confidence through revisions.
- *Behavioral tools:*
  - Paradoxical interventions: In this, the client is suggested to do the very thing that he/she is afraid of. For example, a teenager who is afraid to enter the dark room is encouraged to do so for a short while only to realize that nothing happen to him/her.
  - Time-out procedures: This is nothing but "self-discipline" where the client voluntarily gives a penalty to self by taking a time out for some time which leads to self-realization and the errors are not repeated. For example, a teenager who has smoked but now regrets will avoid consuming his/her favorite ice cream for a week or will not meet their best friend for a few days.
  - Systemic desensitization: This works very well for specific phobias. For example, a teenager with a severe phobia of dogs is shown a picture of a puppy, followed by a dog toy, followed by a cartoon movie clip of a dog, followed by a movie clip of a very friendly dog, followed by a showing of a sweet little puppy, which is quite playful, followed by a live adult yet friendly dog, and followed by a gentle touch to a cute puppy. Over the period, the phobia dilutes significantly.

- *Emotive tools:*
  - Shame attacking exercises: These are difficult to initiate, e.g., public speaking or diminishing stage fear. However, over the period and with patience, persistence, and practice the client eventually overcomes the hurdles and even masters the art.
  - Rational emotive imagery: The client visualizes the success and feels better and more confident to deal with the adversity at hand, e.g., academic stress.
  - Strong coping self-statements: The client goes to a quiet room or washroom and says loudly something like, "I will be happy. I can and will help myself. This problem will soon be resolved. Life will become better and tolerable."
  - Reverse role-playing: In this process, the client and the counselor exchange their roles through which the client gets a new perspective of the situation at hand.

The most crucial and difficult step in bringing the change in the client's deranged triad is the *disputation (D)* of irrational beliefs. The process of disputation along with other tools could be shaped as per the client's age and issue at hand. For example, if a teenager *demands* that she *must* get admission to *the best* medical college in India; else her *life* will be ruined *forever*. Disputation can be this way:

- *Empirical/realistic:* For example, "Where is it mentioned that all the students from the said medical college become good doctors?"
- *Logical:* For example, "You are my patient since you were born. I am not a student from the said medical college but still, you have been keeping quite healthy. What do you say?"
- *Functional/practical:* For example, "What will happen to your studies and exam performance if you keep on thinking about getting admission to the so-called best college *all the time?*"
- *Philosophical:* "Is it a medical college or student's efforts that decide the "LIFE" of a student?"

The modified statement after successful disputation could be: "I *prefer* to obtain admission to a *reasonably good* medical college and will do my best to achieve this. If not, I will do my best to learn well and serve my patients so as to *feel satisfied as a professional.*"

Thus, stress is less and *resilience is more* if we convert our *demands* into *preferences*. All that decides client's destiny is *unconditional acceptance of self* (I may not be perfect *all* the time), *others* (they can commit mistakes too), *and the world* (I have limitations to change things out of my control).

The earlier we learn and practice this, the better for self and others since we are fallible human beings but with an immense capacity to change. We can achieve what are capable of. And this remains the duty of an authentic counselor. A majority of emotionally "disturbed" adolescents can be eased out of their troubles by REBT although a few mentally "disordered" teens will warrant a psychiatrist's reference. **Flowchart 1** depicts the entire cycle of adversity causing an emotional disturbance and the outcome of timely interventions.

**Flowchart 2**: sums up the typical therapeutic process.

Thus, REBT is like passive and active immunization. Clients not only *feel* better, they *get* better to achieve their

**Flowchart 1:** Role of rational emotive behavior therapy (REBT) in troubled teens.

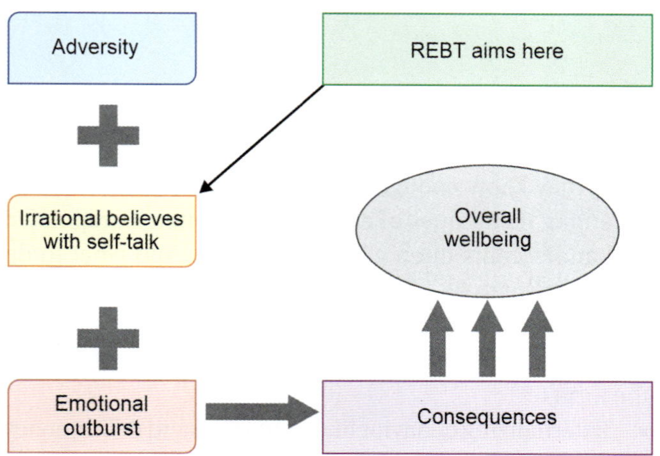


**Flowchart 2:** Flow of rational emotive behavior therapy (REBT).

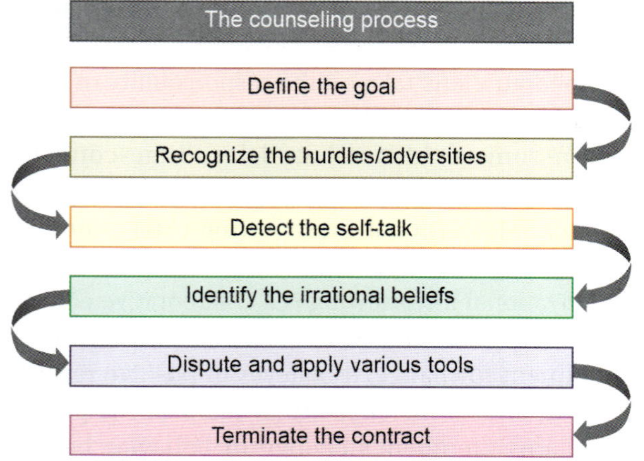

full potentials so as live a reasonably happy, creative, and *less* disturbed life.

## KEY MESSAGES

- The core philosophies and belief systems shape our emotions and behaviors.
- REBT works for emotionally disturbed teenagers with practical problems.
- Disputation and other tools can change the way we feel.
- The principal aim of the therapy is to make the client realize the defective pattern of thinking, feeling, and behavior and achieve the goal.

## RECOMMENDED READING

1. Dryden W, Neenan M, DiGiuseppe R (Eds). A Primer on Rational Emotive Behavior Therapy, 3rd edition. Research Press; 2010.
2. Ellis A (Ed). How to Make Yourself Happy and Remarkably Less Disturbance. Impact Publishers; 1999.
3. Ellis A, Harper RA (Ed). A Guide To Rational Living. Prentice-Hall; 1975.
4. Ellis A, Maclaren C (Eds). Rational Emotive Behavior Therapy—A Therapist's Guide, 2nd edition. Impact Publishers; 2005.

# 3C.4 Motivational Interviewing

*Shamik Ghosh*

## INTRODUCTION

Adolescents are often in a transitional stage wherein they think they know enough and do not need to be schooled. Parenting techniques of childhood are often extrapolated and adolescents often get tired of being told what to do and what not to do.

This potentiates the inherent proneness of the adolescents to behavioral and mental health problems in the form of:

- Externalizing behavior like aggression and delinquency
- Internalizing behavior like anxiety, depression, and substance use.

Globally 1 in 7 adolescents (14.3%) experience mental health issues. Indian figures from a variety of studies quote around 20–29%.

As pediatricians take on the responsibility of helping these adolescents and their families, pediatricians need to learn some evidence-based less time-consuming counseling techniques that are useful in a variety of problems. Motivational interviewing (MI) is one such powerful tool.

Motivational interviewing is a collaborative conversation to strengthen a person's own motivation for and commitment to change. It believes in positive regard for the client and in his capacity to manage his problem. It facilitates the client's change in behavior by gently assisting him in reaching his goals through empathy and in a nonjudgmental way.

## THE PROCESS OF MOTIVATIONAL INTERVIEWING

When an adolescent is brought to the pediatrician for bringing out some behavioral change, the first question that needs to be answered in these situations is:

- Is the child prepared to even listen?
- Is the child in any way contemplating change?

This brings us to elaborate on the various *stages of patient readiness* for change:

- *Precontemplation:* Adolescent not even realizing what is wrong with his behavior
- *Contemplation:* The individual is giving thought to bringing out a change but is not sure.
  (Needs to be shown how the behavior is coming in between his goals)
- *Preparation:* Ready to change, figuring out the plan.
  (A plan needs to be negotiated)
- *Action:* Plunges into action as per the plan.
  (The commitment to change has to be reaffirmed and proper follow-up ensured)
- *Maintenance:* Continues with the plan.
  (Active problem-solving has to be encouraged)

- *Relapse:* Goes back to the previous unhealthy behavior. (Need assistance in coping and restart with action)
- *Termination:* Confidently handles maintenance and relapse, if any.
  (A mutually agreed end of treatment with an avenue to follow up if required)

## PRINCIPLES OF MOTIVATIONAL INTERVIEWING

The concepts of Carl Roger's person-centered therapy are to promote positive change. Here are the four main underlying principles of MI:

1. *Expressing empathy:* It is a *collaborative therapy* with the therapist showing empathy toward the child rather than displaying criticism or being judgmental. This is crucial for the relationship as the client is usually expecting negative judgments for their behavior.
2. *Developing discrepancy:* The contrast between *current behavior* and the *desired behavior* is emphasized. *Specific individual goals* for the individual have to be elicited and an understanding is needed of how their current behavior will not help them achieve those goals. This helps to *motivate them for the change.*
3. *Rolling with resistance:* In MI, the therapist accepts, rather than fights, the client's resistance. The more you try to tell a client that he is wrong, the more he will become obstinate and unwilling to change. The goal then is to help him figure out on his own that change is to his benefit, rather than trying to force him into adaptive behavior. He is given the liberty to bring about change whenever he is willing and in a way he likes.
4. *Support self-efficacy:* Self-efficacy is all about boosting and reposing faith in the adolescent's self-confidence that he can change for the better. When an individual thinks he can stop smoking, he is said to have self-efficacy for that. Counsellor's job is to believe in the client's capacity and uncover the feeling that, "I can do it!".

## MOTIVATIONAL INTERVIEWING TECHNIQUES

Therapists who employ MI use the following techniques exemplified by the acronym OARS:

- *Open-ended questions:* These questions encourage to speak more openly and descriptively about what is on their mind. They are insightful into the mind of the patient and give us clues to elicit a therapeutic line. They generally are framed as "What do you think about...., tell me something about...., how will you describe your....., etc." In contrast, close questions usually end in yes or no, and are best avoided. For example, rather than asking, "Do you want to quit smoking?", one should ask, "What do you think about your smoking?"
- *Affirmations:* Therapists use affirmations to help boost the confidence of clients in moments of self-doubt, so that there are concrete efforts toward change. Being positive with clients is one of the cornerstones of motivational counseling. Affirmations like:
  "I am happy to that you have tried to go to the gym in the past."
- *Reflections:* Reflection, put simply, is reflecting back on what the adolescent has said. This technique lets the client know that the therapist understands what he is putting across and allows him to continue thinking and speaking about important topics. Ultimately, it shows that the therapist is empathizing with the client.
- Summaries take reflection one step further. The therapist is asked to filter the meaning of what the client is saying and summarize the main points. This builds the confidence of the client that the therapist grasps their meaning and allows them to clarify any parts that the therapist may have misunderstood. The therapist may also use the summary to frame a client's goals.

## ADVANTAGES OF MOTIVATIONAL INTERVIEWING

- Motivational interviewing is a particularly effective intervention for those who are not interested in change (precontemplation) but also has its utility in the other stages of readiness.
- It is useful in wide problem areas, like substance abuse, obesity, defiance, high-risk behaviors, depression, and anxiety.
- It is useful for those who are rather passive and would not like commitments and assignments required for other therapies like cognitive behavior therapy (CBT) and rational emotive behavior therapy (REBT).
- It takes less time than other therapies and hence is brief and cost-effective.
- It can be delivered by the primary pediatrician in his office after undergoing training.

- It is useful for increasing patient compliance with medical problems.
- It can be used in other settings like schools where adolescents' behaviors are a pressing concern.
- It can be used in groups for adolescents facing similar behavioral issues.

## ■ ILLUSTRATIVE EXAMPLE

Mr X, 17 year old, is a known case of bronchial asthma, and has smoking as a substance use disorder.

*Doctor:* Hello, Mr X, glad to see you today. How are you feeling?

*Patient:* Well, my asthma is acting up again. I might need a different medicine.

*Doctor:* You are thinking maybe a new medication would help? (Reflection)

Let us put that on the list of possibilities. (Avoiding premature focus, agenda setting)

First, let me listen to your breathing.

Okay, I hear the trouble you are having. (Providing information)

I would like to spend about 5 minutes talking about your asthma broadly before we decide together on the best approach to manage it. (Agenda setting, collaborative spirit)

How does that sound? (Open question)

*Patient:* OK, that sounds good.

*Doctor:* Tell me what concerns you most about your asthma. (Open question)

*Patient:* Well, it is really scary when I have an attack.

I am afraid I could die from this. But even on a regular day, I have less energy, and I feel older due to it.

*Doctor:* So, attacks make you worry you might die, and they are truly scary. (Reflection)

But even on a daily basis, your life is diminished due to asthma. (Complex reflection)

*Patient:* Exactly. It is such a handicap! I wish I could get rid of it.

*Doctor:* I bet you have thought about how you could lessen your symptoms and reduce the impact of asthma on your life. (Affirmation)

*Patient:* Yes, I have. I think the first thing I should do is quit smoking.

*Doctor:* You are clearly aware that smoking is making things worse, and you think you should quit. (Affirmation, Reflection)

*Patient:* Yes, and I have already cut way back. I do not smoke in the house or car anymore, and I am down to half a pack, where I was smoking a pack a day.

*Doctor:* You have already made a serious dent in the number of cigarettes per day. (Affirmation, reflection)

How has that gone for you? (Open question)

*Patient:* Well, I made up my mind, and am keeping track of my smoking. I have a chart and I check off when I have a cigarette, and I stretch out the time between them.

*Doctor:* You are really taking it seriously. (Affirmation)

You are already doing some of the things that experts recommend to make quitting work for you. (Providing information)

What else have you thought about trying? (Open question)

*Patient:* Well, I heard there were some new medicines to help you quit. But I figured I have to be more ready.

Can you tell me about the newer options?

*Doctor:* You are not sure you are totally ready. (Reflection)

I see you are already committed to what you are doing. (Reflection)

Maybe considering a medication to quit smoking might be the next step to be even more ready. (Affirmation)

I would be happy to review with you some of the information regarding the new medications. (Providing information)

And then we can talk further about what the next best steps are for you. (Summarize)

Till then, I am sure, you will continue further your efforts on cutting smoking. (Supporting self-efficacy)

*Patient:* No, I want to try out the medicines now!

*Doctor:* Fine, let me gather all the relevant information. (Rolling with resistance)

## ■ KEY MESSAGES

- Behavioral issues in adolescents are a key component of adolescent health.
- Most adolescents are brought to the doctors in the precontemplation stage of behavioral change.
- MI is a proven and reliable intervention to motivate adolescents to make correctional behavioral changes.

- Empathy is the key to eliciting a partnership with the client.
- Avoiding confrontation helps in honing our listening skills and gives the client an appreciation of the open-mindedness of the therapist.
- Boosting the adolescents self-confidence gives them a concrete platform to make meaningful changes in their behavior.
- The OARS technique remains the unique method in MI.

## ■ RECOMMENDED READING

1. Erickson SJ, Gerstle M, Feldstein SW. Brief interventions and motivational interviewing with children, adolescents, and their parents in pediatric health care settings: a review. Arch Pediatr Adolesc Med. 2005;159:1173-80.
2. Ingersoll K. Substance use disorders: Motivational interviewing. [online] Available from https://www.uptidate.com/contents/substance-use-disorder-motivational-interviewing [Last accessed March, 2024].
3. Miller WR, Rollnick S (Eds). Motivational Interviewing: Preparing People for Change, 2nd edition. New York, NY: Guilford Press; 2002.
4. Motivational Interviewing: Resources for Clinicians, Researchers, and Trainers. [online] Available from www.motivationalinterview.org. [Last accessed March, 2024]. This Website lists workshops and motivational interviewing network trainers across the U.S. and worldwide, and other resources.
5. Prochaska JO, DiClemente CC. Stages and processes of self-change of smoking: toward an integrative model of change. J Consult Clin Psychol. 1983;51:390-5.
6. Rollnick S, Miller WR. What is Motivational Interviewing? Behav Cogn Psychother. 1995;23:325-34.

# 3C.5 | Psychopharmacology for Adolescents

*Arun B Nair*

## ■ INTRODUCTION

This chapter tries to provide a practical overview regarding the use of psychopharmacology for behavioral problems in children and adolescents. The acceptance of education use in child psychiatry has enhanced significantly following the results of several double-blind placebo-controlled trials, which have categorically documented the safety and efficacy of drug treatments for disorders including attention deficit hyperactivity disorder (ADHD), depression, anxiety disorders, obsessive–compulsive disorder, psychosis, and enuresis. This article tries to focus on the judicious selection and use of psychopharmacology evaluating the risk–benefit ratio in the given situation.

## ■ BACKGROUND

Mental health conditions account for 16% of the global burden of disease and injury in persons between 10 and 19 years. The recent National Mental Health Survey has identified that 7.3% of children and adolescents between 13 and 17 years suffer from mental health conditions. Overall 8–13% of children are in need of mental health services.

Common mental health problems in children requiring pharmacological intervention include neurodevelopmental disorders including ADHD, externalizing disorders including conduct disorders, and internalizing disorders including depressive disorder, anxiety disorders, obsessive–compulsive disorder, and psychosis. Pharmacological intervention may be necessary to contain aggressive and self-injurious behavior in children with intellectual developmental disorders and autism spectrum disorders as well.

## PHARMACOTHERAPY OF ATTENTION DEFICIT HYPERACTIVITY DISORDER

Attention deficit hyperactivity disorder is the most common behavioral disorder in school-going children. Studies say that 5–7% of school-going children suffer from ADHD requiring intervention. The pharmacotherapy of ADHD includes both stimulant and nonstimulant medications. Commonly used stimulant medications include methylphenidate and dextroamphetamine. Out of these, methylphenidate is the only one which is available in India. The nonstimulant medications available for the treatment of ADHD include atomoxetine, modafinil, and clonidine. In severe cases which are not responding to the abovementioned medications, low doses of antipsychotics and mood stabilizers can be used as second-line treatment.

Methylphenidate, which is regarded as the drug of choice for the treatment of ADHD, improves all the three symptom domains of the condition including inattention hyperactivity, and impulsivity. The mechanism of action of this drug is to enhance the level of dopamine in the prefrontal cortex as well as to improve the coordination of the functioning of both cerebral hemispheres. Methylphenidate is available as both, a plain formulation and a sustained-release formulation. Plain formulation has duration of action of around 4 hours, while the sustained release formulation may act up to 8–12 hours. The plain formulation is available as 5 and 10 mg tablets, while the sustained-release formulation is available at doses 18 mg, 36 mg, and 54 mg. The daily dose of methylphenidate is 1 mg/kg. Starting at the lowest possible dose with plain formulation only in the morning is always better. Depending upon response, the drug dose may be titrated up to 60 mg/day. The most common adverse effects of methylphenidate include lack of appetite, growth retardation, and physical fatigue. Rarely cardiac conduction abnormalities and renal abnormalities can also surface. Before starting a child on methylphenidate, it is better to do all the baseline evaluations including electrocardiography (ECG) and renal function tests. If a child is unable to tolerate methylphenidate, it is always wise to substitute it with a nonstimulant medication.

Among the nonstimulant medications, atomoxetine is the most popular one. It is available as 10, 18, 25, and 40 mg tablets, which are best administered daily in the morning after food. It improves the level of norepinephrine and dopamine in the brain thus enhancing attention span. Poor appetite is the most common adverse effect seen with atomoxetine as well. Sometimes the adolescent may present with mood swings, including rare emergence of depressive thoughts or even suicidal ideas. Atomoxetine should be discontinued in such cases.

Modafinil is another drug that is used especially in children with inattention prominent type ADHD. It is available as 100 and 200 mg tablets. The starting dose is 50 mg daily morning after food, as is gradually titrated to 200 mg once daily. Adverse effects include insomnia, headache, rashes, and mood instability.

Clonidine is an alpha-adrenergic agent used to control ADHD in small kids. It is available as 100 µg tablets. The drug is started at a dose of one-fourth of a tablet thrice daily and is gradually hiked as per clinical requirements. Adverse effects include hypotension and rebound hypertension, especially on sudden stoppage of the drug without tapering the dose.

## ANTIDEPRESSANTS

Antidepressants are used for varied indications including depressive disorder, obsessive–compulsive disorder, and anxiety disorders in children and adolescents. Commonly used antidepressants include selective serotonin reuptake inhibitors (SSRIs) and serotonin-norepinephrine reuptake inhibitors (SNRIs). Some other medications including tricyclic antidepressants (TCA) and norepinephrine and specific serotoninergic antidepressants (NASSA) are also used for specific indications. *Among SNRI, fluoxetine, escitalopram, and fluvoxamine are approved for use in children and adolescents for depressive disorder and obsessive–compulsive disorder.*

Fluoxetine is available in 10, 20, 40, and 60 mg tablets and in liquid formulations with content of 20 mg in 5 mL. The dose for depression is 10–20 mg/day but in OCD a higher dose up to 60 mg/day may be necessary, especially in adolescents.

Escitalopram is available in 5, 10, and 20 mg tablets. The dose for depression is 5–20 mg/day, but in OCD a higher dose up to 30 mg may be necessary, especially among adolescents.

Fluvoxamine is available as tablets 25, 50, 100 mg and extended-release tablets of 150 mg. In depression, the dose is 50–100 mg/day, but in OCD a higher dose of up to 300 mg/day may be indicated.

The common adverse effects of SSRIs include nausea, vomiting, diarrhea, headache, insomnia, anxiety, and agitation. In persons with susceptibility to bipolar mood disorders, the use of SSRIs may sometimes lead to a switch to mania, which is characterized by over-talkativeness, excess energy, excess happiness, or even violent behavior.

Tricyclic antidepressants are used more commonly for conditions like nocturnal enuresis and obsessive–compulsive disorder. Imipramine, a TCA, is considered to be the drug of choice for nocturnal enuresis. It is administered at a dose of 10 and 25 mg at night. Amitriptyline is another TCA which is also used in resistant cases of nocturnal enuresis in the same dose. The common adverse effects of TCAs include anticholinergic adverse effects like dryness of mouth, constipation, sedation, worsening of glaucoma, and cardiac conduction defects.

They may also lead to cognitive impairment, especially if used on a long-term basis.

Selective serotonin reuptake inhibitors are commonly used in cases of resistant depressive disorder as well as for anxiety disorders with prominent somatic symptoms. The commonly used drugs in this group include venlafaxine, desvenlafaxine, duloxetine, milnacipran, and levomilnacipran. Out of these, venlafaxine and desvenlafaxine are the most commonly used ones. Venlafaxine is used at a dose between 37.5 and 150 mg/day. Desvenlafaxine is used at a dose between 50 and 100 mg/day. The common adverse effects include hypertension, nausea, vomiting, and gastrointestinal upset. Another major problem with this group of drugs is the discontinuation symptoms like headache, a feeling of electric shock in parts of the body, and sweating. Because of this phenomenon, SNRI should never be stopped suddenly; they should be tapered slowly before stopping.

## ANTIPSYCHOTICS (BEST AVOIDED AS A PRESCRIPTION DRUG BY PEDIATRICIANS)

Antipsychotics are a group of medicines which are used for the treatment of psychotic disorders. These are essentially mental health problems in which the patient is unlikely to have an insight about his own condition. Disorders in this group include schizophrenia and delusional disorder.

In pediatric practice, low-dose antipsychotics are also used for conditions including tic disorders, Tourette's syndrome, ADHD, and for controlling the behavioral problems in children with mental retardation and autism.

The commonly used antipsychotics in pediatric practice include risperidone, aripiprazole, and haloperidol. The dose in which these medicines are used is much lower than the dose used in adult clinical practice. Risperidone is used at a dose ranging from 0.5 to 2 mg/day. Haloperidol is used in a dose ranging from 0.25 to 3 mg/day, and aripiprazole from 2 to 5 mg/day. The most common adverse effects include extrapyramidal side effects, including acute dystonia, akathisia, drug-induced parkinsonism, and tardive dyskinesia. In small children, major adverse effects including oculogyric crisis and laryngeal dystonia may be a cause of concern while using antipsychotics. Using the lowest dose for the shortest period of time is generally advised while prescribing antipsychotics for pediatric practice. Medicines like risperidone and haloperidol can produce elevated levels of prolactin in adolescence leading to clinical manifestations like amenorrhea and galactorrhea in females and sexual dysfunction among male adolescents. Aripiprazole, which is considered as a dopamine serotonin system stabilizer, actually reduces prolactin levels and hence does not produce any amenorrhea or galactorrhea in adolescent girls. However, there are case reports of polymorphous in females and hypersexual behavior among boys taking aripiprazole **(Table 1)**.

## MOOD STABILIZERS

Bipolar mood disorders are seen among adolescents and may require treatment with a class of medicines termed as mood stabilizers. Commonly used mood stabilizers include lithium, sodium valproate, carbamazepine, oxcarbazepine, and lamotrigine. Lithium is the first discovered mood stabilizer and is equally efficacious in mania and depression alike. Sodium valproate, carbamazepine, and lamotrigine are more effective in mania while lamotrigine is more effective in depression. But these molecules also have adverse effects which may be of concern unless prescribed judiciously.

For example, lithium, which is the first discovered mood stabilizer, is a drug with excellent antisuicidal properties and hence may be of great benefit in bipolar disorder among adolescents with suicidal tendencies. However, lithium is a drug with a narrow therapeutic window of between 0.6 and 1.2 mEq/L. While prescribing lithium it is essential to do baseline investigations including renal function tests and ECG. Lithium should be best avoided in people with cardiac conduction defects or renal failure. Periodic estimation of serum lithium levels should be done to ensure that the serum level of the medicine is within the therapeutic window and does not go into toxicity levels. Lithium toxicity which is essentially considered as a serum level of above 1.5 mEq/L is a medical emergency that requires immediate management. Symptoms of this condition may include confusion, irritability, cardiac conduction defects, diabetes insipidus, seizures, and even delirium. Immediate withholding of lithium and supportive treatment with intravenous fluids is necessary at this point of time. If serum lithium level goes beyond 4 mEq/L, hemodialysis is indicated. Quite a lot of cosmetic adverse effects including acne and skin lesions are possible in adolescents put on lithium. The usual dose of lithium in children and adolescents may reach from 300 to 900 mg/day in divided doses.

**TABLE 1:** Etiology of gynecomastia

| | |
|---|---|
| Estrogen excess | Testicular tumor (Leydig or Sertoli cell tumor), feminizing adrenocortical tumors, obesity, hCG-secreting tumors, exogenous estrogen |
| Androgen deficiency | Klinefelter syndrome, anorchia or hypogonadism due to trauma/radiation, androgen insensitivity syndrome, defects in testosterone synthesis |
| Drugs | Anabolic steroids, ketoconazole, flutamide, bicalutamide, spironolactone, cyproterone, phenytoin, methyldopa, cimetidine, ranitidine, isoniazid, amiodarone, antidepressants, antipsychotics, antiretroviral therapy, 5 alpha reductase inhibitors (finasteride), GH, GnRH analogs, estrogens, phytoestrogens, estrogen-containing substances, e.g., lavender and tea tree oils |
| Others | Ovotesticular DSD, hyperthyroidism, liver disease, renal failure and dialysis, starvation, and refeeding |

(DSD: disorders of sexual development)

regrowth of breast tissue. The most common technique is subareolar resection with or without liposuction and tissue sent for histopathology.

## ETIOLOGY

The etiology of gynecomastia is given in **Table 1**.

## RECOMMENDED READING


1. Braunstein GD. Gynecomastia. N Engl J Med. 2007;357: 1229-37.
2. Carlson HE. Approach to the patient with gynecomastia. J Clin Endocrinol Metab. 2011;96:15-21.
3. Cuhaci N, Polat SB, Evranos B, Ersoy R, Cakir B. Gynecomastia: Clinical evaluation and management. Indian J Endocrinol Metab. 2014;18(2):150-8.
4. Soliman AT, De Sanctis V, Yassin M. Management of adolescent gynecomastia: an update. Acta Biomed. 2017;88(2):204-13.


# 4A.3 Polycystic Ovary Syndrome

*Diksha Shirodkar, Shaila S Bhattacharyya*

## INTRODUCTION

Polycystic ovary syndrome (PCOS) is a significant public health issue with endocrine, reproductive, cardiometabolic, dermatologic and psychological features. The diagnosis and treatment of PCOS remain challenging and controversial during adolescence due to the physiological changes, marked clinical heterogeneity and ethnic differences. This culminates in delayed diagnosis and dissatisfaction with care.

## EPIDEMIOLOGY

Polycystic ovary syndrome is one of the most common conditions, affecting around 10% (8–13%) of reproductive-aged women worldwide (including India). The cumulative prevalence of PCOS was about 10% using Rotterdam's and Androgen Excess Society's (AES) criteria, while it was 5.8% using National Institute of Health (NIH) criteria. There has been an increase in the incidence of PCOS in adolescence due to lifestyle changes and early diagnosis.

## DEFINITION

There have been several consensus to define PCOS as stated in **Table 1**. The most recent was the first International Evidence-based Guideline for the Assessment and Management of PCOS ("the Guideline") by Pena et al in 2020, describing the criteria specific to adolescents. The aim of this guideline was to accurately diagnose PCOS in adolescence, provide optimal care, prevent complications, and address psychological issues arising and improve patient health outcomes.

## PATHOPHYSIOLOGY OF POLYCYSTIC OVARY SYNDROME (FIG. 1 AND FLOWCHART 1)

Puberty is initiated with the maturation of the hypothalamic–pituitary–ovarian (HPO) axis and the release of gonadotrophin-releasing hormone (GnRH) pulses, which is quiescent during childhood. Varying GnRH pulses trigger the release of luteinizing hormone (LH) and follicle-stimulating hormone (FSH) from the anterior pituitary, which in turn stimulate ovarian theca

**TABLE 1:** Consensus for defining PCOS over the years.

| | *Menstrual cycle* | *Hyperandrogenism* | | *Ultrasound finding* |
| --- | --- | --- | --- | --- |
| PCOS diagnostic criteria | Oligomenorrhea (<6–9 menses per year) or oligo-ovulation | Clinical hyperandrogenism (Ferriman–Gallwey score ≥8) or biochemical hyperandrogenism (elevated total/free testosterone) | | Polycystic ovaries on ultrasound (≥12 antral follicles in one ovary or ovarian volume ≥10 cm$^3$) |
| NICHD (1990) | Yes | Yes | | No |
| Rotterdam (2003/2006) | Yes | Yes | | Yes |
| *For the above consensus:* 2/3 criteria were required to be satisfied | | | | |
| AE-PCOS Society (2009) | Yes | Yes | Yes | |
| *For the above consensus:* Androgen excess +1/2 criteria were needed | | | | |
| NIH 2012 | Yes | Yes | Yes | |
| *For the above consensus:* 2/3 criteria were required to be satisfied | | | | |
| First international guidelines on Adolescent PCOS 2020 Pena et al. | Yes (as per the **Table 2**) | Yes | | No |

(AE-PCOS: androgen excess and polycystic ovary syndrome; NICHD: Eunice Kennedy Shriver National Institute of Child Health and Human Development; NIH: National Institute of Health)

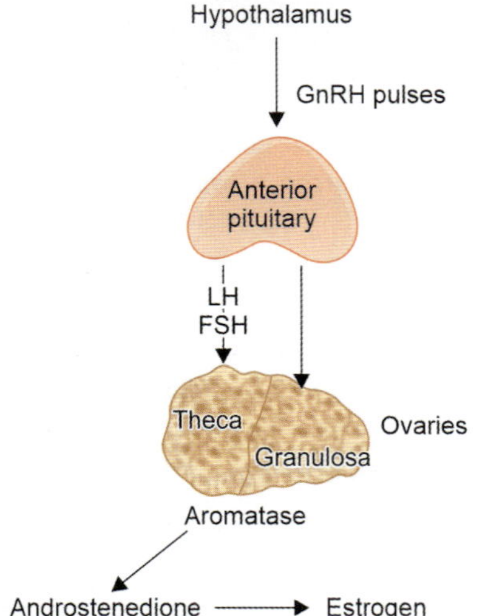


**Fig. 1:** Pathophysiology of normal puberty. (FSH: follicle-stimulating hormone; GnRH: gonadotropin-releasing hormone; LH: luteinizing hormone)

and granulosa cells, respectively. Theca cells produce androstenedione which aromatizes into estradiol.

The resulting changes during puberty include breast and uterine development, bone growth, and adiposity. The adrenal gland also releases androgens like dehydroepiandrosterone (DHEA) and DHEA sulfate (DHEAS), which are responsible for the pubarche.

The exact etiology of PCOS remains elusive and is multifactorial involving an interaction of hormonal, environment, genetic, and epigenetic factors. However, the core problem is elevated androgen levels. Hyperandrogenism, ovulatory dysfunction, and abnormal GnRH pulses resulting in abnormal gonadotropin secretion complemented with insulin resistance have been implicated in the pathophysiology of PCOS. This aberrant GnRH pulse frequency increases LH secretion which in turn stimulates the ovarian theca cells to produce more androgens. The relative decrease in FSH secretion leads to less aromatization of androgens to estradiol and impaired follicular development, resulting in oligomenorrhea that is characteristic of PCOS. Hyperinsulinemia (common in healthy adolescents) and insulin resistance are exaggerated in PCOS. Insulin resistance promotes release of nonesterified fatty acids from the liver and adipose tissue due to decreased lipoprotein lipase activity, causing dyslipidemia that is associated with PCOS. Insulin also stimulates ovarian theca cell synthesis of androgens and inhibits hepatic production of sex hormone-binding globulin, thus increasing free androgen levels, accentuating the underlying pathophysiology of PCOS.

## CLINICAL FEATURES AND HISTORY TAKING

Teens seek evaluation when the menstrual irregularities become worrisome, and they have to battle acne or hirsutism due to peer-related criticism. As with all

**Flowchart 1:** Pathophysiology of PCOS.

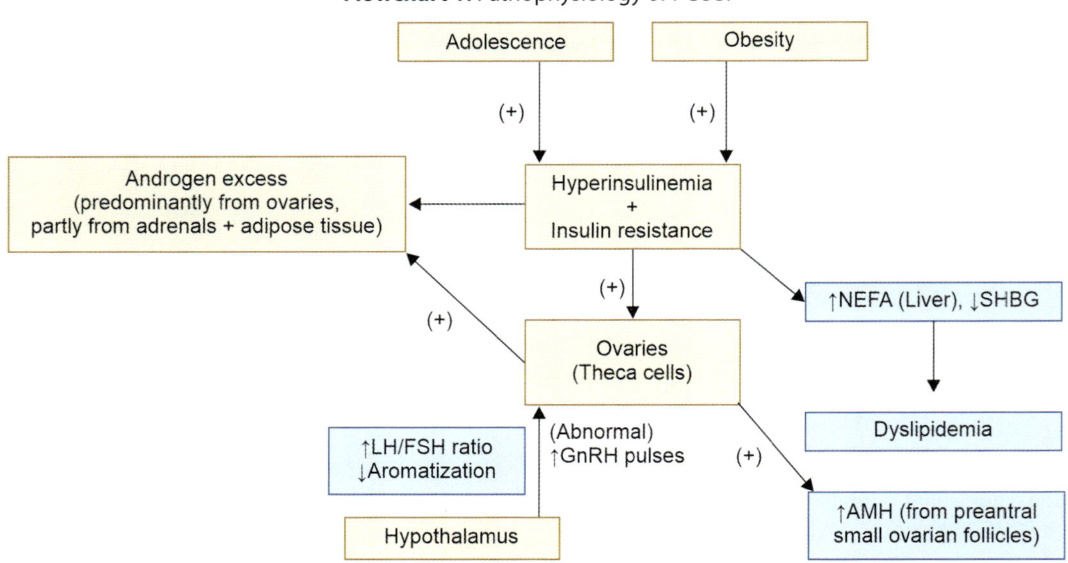



(AMH: anti-Müllerian hormone; FSH: follicle-stimulating hormone; GnRH: gonadotropin-releasing hormone; LH: luteinizing hormone; NEFA: nonesterified fatty acid, PCOS: polycystic ovary syndrome; SHBG: sex hormone-binding globulin)

adolescent visits, a detailed, patient-centered session is critical, which includes an assessment of present illness, pubertal history, menstrual history, social history (including sexual behaviors and pregnancy), and drug use (contraceptives, antiseizure medications, and anabolic steroids). A detailed systemic examination (to look for weight gain, hair-loss, skin changes, acanthosis nigricans, presence of a goiter, headache and galactorrhea) is of prime importance to differentiate PCOS from other systemic causes as mentioned in the differential diagnosis of PCOS. Tanner staging and examination of the external genitalia to assess for virilization are important.

## DIAGNOSTIC EVALUATION

- *Irregular menstrual cycles and ovulatory dysfunction (Table 2):* Adolescence is one of the stages in life with higher variability in the menstrual cycle, which decreases with age and time, with majority of girls achieving regular menstrual cycles from 3–5 years postmenarche. The menstrual irregularities are categorized as mentioned in **Table 2**, which should alert the physician.
- *Hyperandrogenism:*
  - *Biochemical:* Since androgen levels in adolescence reach adult values at menarche, calculated free testosterone, free androgen index, or bioavailable testosterone is favorable to assess biochemical

**TABLE 2:** Defining menstrual irregularity in adolescents as per gynecological age.

| Gynecological age | Definition of irregular menstrual cycles |
|---|---|
| <1 year following menarche | Irregular menstrual cycles are normal |
| >1 to <3 years following menarche | <21 day cycle or >45 days cycle |
| >3 years following menarche | • <21 day cycle or<br>• >35 day cycle or<br>• <8 cycles/year |
| >1 year following menarche | • >90 days for any one cycle<br>• Primary amenorrhea by the age of 15 years or >3 years postthelarche |

*Note:* Gynecological age: Number of years postmenarche

hyperandrogenism. Androstenedione and DHEAS are useful in diagnosing androgen-secreting tumors and nonclassical congenital adrenal hyperplasia (CAH), if highly elevated. Important practice points include avoiding the assessment of biochemical hyperandrogenism in women on hormonal contraception (a drug withdrawal of 3 months is recommended). Careful interpretation of androgen levels is needed as the reference ranges are age dependent and pubertal-stage specific **(Table 3)**.

- *Clinical hyperandrogenism (**Figs. 2A and B**):* Alongside the evidence of biochemical hyperandrogenism is a comprehensive history and physical examination to look for severe acne and hirsutism. Mild acne is common in adolescent girls but moderate or severe acne (i.e., 10 or more comedonal lesions) in early puberty or moderate-severe inflammatory acne during the perimenarcheal years is uncommon and is related to clinical hyperandrogenism. The predictors of severe acne in adolescent girls apart from androgen excess and menstrual abnormalities include family history, race, early-onset acne, higher body mass index, and environmental factors. Modified Ferriman–Gallwey (mFG) scale **(Fig. 3)** evaluates terminal hair, which can be used to assess hirsutism. However, this scale is ethnicity and self-treatment dependent.

## ■ LABORATORY EVALUATION

The goals of laboratory assessment are to support the diagnosis of PCOS, exclude other causes of clinical hyperandrogenism and menstrual irregularities, and manage the associated comorbidities, e.g., obesity, diabetes, hypertension, and dyslipidemia. **Box 1** illustrates the desirable workup to diagnose PCOS only after ruling out pregnancy.

## DIFFERENTIAL DIAGNOSIS/ EXCLUSION CRITERIA

The diagnosis of PCOS is a diagnosis of exclusion—all other etiologies that can cause menstrual irregularities and/or hyperandrogenism must be excluded although less common in teens.

- Pregnancy
- Primary gonadotropin deficiency, e.g., hypothalamic amenorrhea
- Hyperandrogenism secondary to nonclassic congenital adrenal hyperplasia (NCAH), characterized by a marked elevation of androgen levels secondary to 21-hydroxylase deficiency. Diagnosis of NCAH is

**TABLE 3:** Normal references for testosterone, free testosterone, DHEA, and DHEAS in adolescent females.

| Biochemical parameter | Normal reference range | PCOS |
|---|---|---|
| LH/FSH ratio | <2 | >2 (but usually not very specific/sensitive) |
| Testosterone | 35–72 ng/dL | <150 ng/dL (>200 indicates an adrenal tumor) |
| Free testosterone | 0.7–3.6 pg/mL | Usually >3 pg/mL |
| Androstenedione | 22–225 ng/dL | Usually >300 ng/dL |
| Free androgen index (total testosterone/SHBG) | 0.18–7.07 | >5 |
| SHBG (sex hormone-binding globulin) | 18–144 nmol/L | Low levels are associated with PCOS |
| DHEAS | 35–400 µg/dL | <800 µg/dL (>800 µg/dL indicates adrenal tumor) |

(DHEAS: dehydroepiandrosterone sulfate; FSH: follicle-stimulating hormone; LH: luteinizing hormone; PCOS: polycystic ovary syndrome)

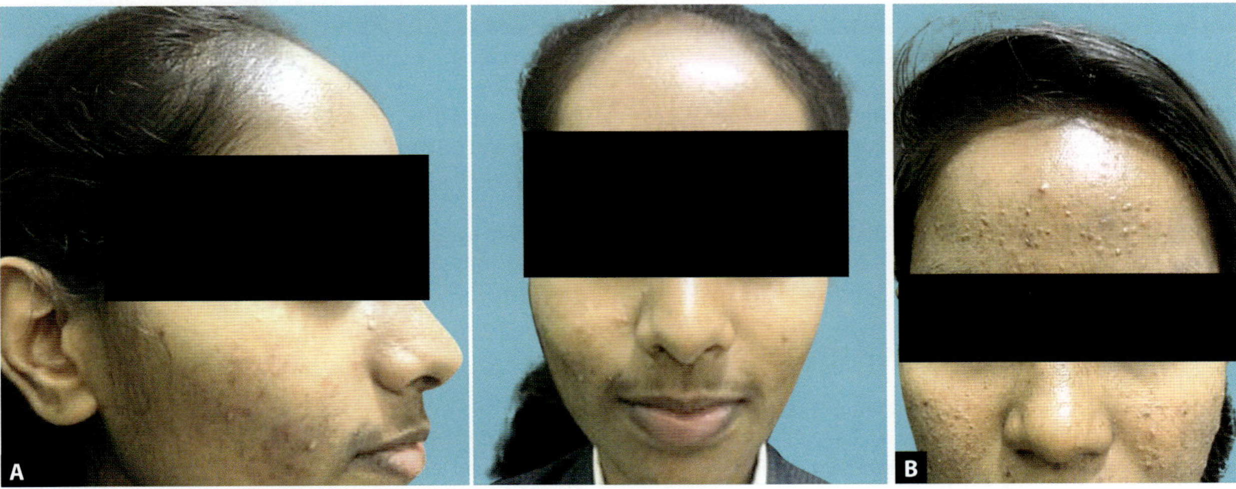

**Figs. 2A and B:** Clinical hyperandrogenism seen in adolescents with polycystic ovary syndrome (PCOS). A 17-year-old with evidence of clinical hyperandrogenism: (A) Hirsutism and acne; (B) Acne and a patchy area of alopecia.

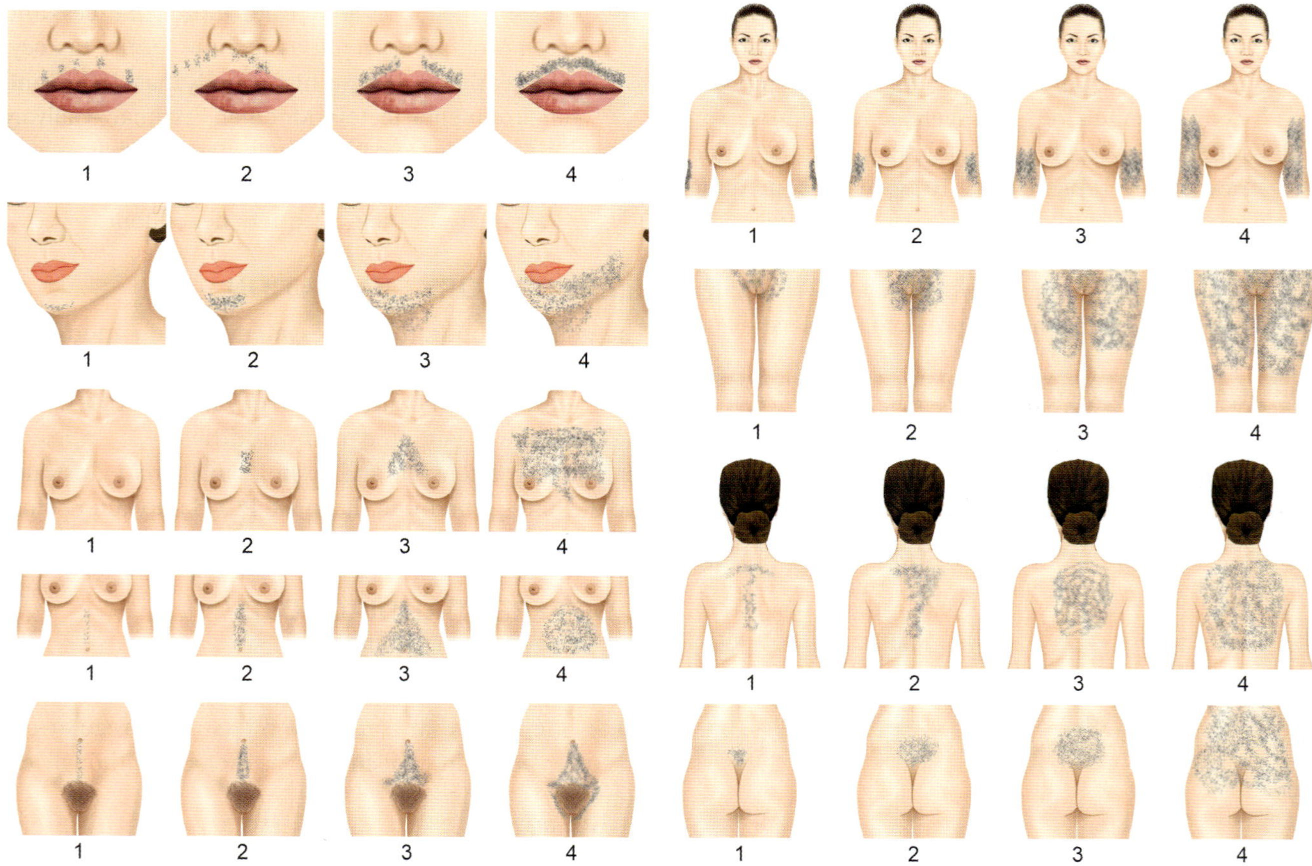

**Fig. 3:** The modified Ferriman–Gallwey (mFG) scoring system to grade hirsutism.
Modified Ferriman-Gallwey scale evaluates terminal hair (pigmented and medullated hair >5 mm in length in 9 androgen-dependent areas), which can be used to assess hirsutism, with a score ≥4–6 indicating hirsutism (0: no hair and 4: adult male pattern of hair).
*Source:* Adapted from the Revel A. Hirsutism. In: DeCherney AH, Nathan L, Laufer N, Roman AS (Eds). Current Diagnosis and Treatment: Obstetrics & Gynecology, 11th edition. McGraw Hill; 2013.

**BOX 1:** Investigations needed for diagnosing PCOS in an adolescent.

- Total testosterone and free testosterone (high-quality assays, such as liquid chromatography tandem mass spectrometry and extraction or chromatography)
- DHEA and DHEAS (to rule out other causes of androgen excess, e.g., tumors and CAH)
- Androstenedione (to rule out other causes of androgen excess, e.g., tumors and CAH)
- Morning serum 17-hydroxyprogesterone, stimulated 17OH-progesterone (to rule out nonclassical CAH)
- LH, FSH, and LH/FSH ratio
- AMH (not recommended in adolescents but used in diagnosing adult PCOS to assess ovarian function and fertility issues)
- TSH and free T4
- Prolactin
- Metabolic parameters
- Liver functions (transaminases to rule out metabolic liver disease)
- Fasting lipid profile
- Fasting blood glucose and glucose tolerance test, HbA1c
- Fasting insulin
- Rule out Cushing syndrome (24-hour urinary cortisol levels)

(AMH: anti-Müllerian hormone; CAH: congenital adrenal hyperplasia; DHEAS: dehydroepiandrosterone sulfate; FSH: follicle-stimulating hormone; HbA1C: hemoglobin A1C; LH: luteinizing hormone; PCOS: polycystic ovary syndrome; TSH: thyroid stimulating hormone; T4: thyroxine) suspected in the presence of 46XX karyotype with clitoromegaly and/or an early-morning, follicular phase 17-hydroxyprogesterone (17-OHP) level of >6 nmol/L (>200 ng/dL) and confirmed at stimulated 17-OHP levels of >35 nmol/L (1,000–1,500 ng/dL).

- Autoimmune thyroid disease
- Hyperprolactinemia
- Cushing's disease/syndrome
- Androgen-secreting tumors.

## ADOLESCENTS "AT RISK" OF POLYCYSTIC OVARY SYNDROME (FIG. 4)

Adolescents who have some features of PCOS but do not meet the diagnostic criteria as per the guidelines, the term "at risk PCOS'" is used. Such adolescents should be kept under close follow-up and reassessment done at or before full reproductive maturity.

*Goals of treatment:* These goals include decreasing the risk of endometrial cancer (unopposed estrogen stimulation leading to endometrial hyperplasia), managing irregular menses (oligomenorrhea and abnormal uterine bleeding), reducing hirsutism and acne, decreasing the risk for development of type 2 diabetes, reducing cardiovascular risks, improving quality of life, and preserving fertility.

### Education, Lifestyle Interventions, and Emotional Wellbeing

Education and counseling should be done in a culturally sensitive manner. Pediatricians should use an empathetic approach, promote self-care, and highlight peer support groups. Lifestyle changes (preferably multicomponent, including diet, exercise, and behavioral strategies) should be recommended in all those with PCOS to achieve reductions in weight, central adiposity, and insulin resistance.

### Pharmacological Intervention

- *Combined oral contraceptive pill (COCP) (combined estrogen and progestin preparations):* The COCP along with lifestyle intervention should be considered in adolescents with PCOS/"at risk" for the management of clinical hyperandrogenism and/or irregular menstrual cycles. The combined preparations suppress the hypothalamic–pituitary–ovarian axis and decrease ovarian and adrenal androgen production. Although the COCP is relatively safe, there are absolute medical contraindications to consider such as migraine, deep vein thrombosis, pulmonary embolism, breast cancer, neuropathy, severe cirrhosis, and liver tumors. COCP containing 30 µg of ethinylestradiol with levonorgestrel, norethisterone (norethindrone), or norgestimate is preferred due to lesser incidence of deep vein thrombosis compared to the preparations with higher estrogenic component.
- *Metformin:* It is a biguanide that acts to decrease hepatic glucose production by increasing peripheral insulin sensitivity. Metformin alongside lifestyle interventions could be considered in adolescents with PCOS/at risk of PCOS. Metformin doses used are 1,500–2,000 mg/day. Mild-to-moderate gastrointestinal side effects can occur, which are self-limiting. *COCP and metformin combination* considered in adolescents with PCOS and a body mass index (BMI) >25 kg/m$^2$ where the above

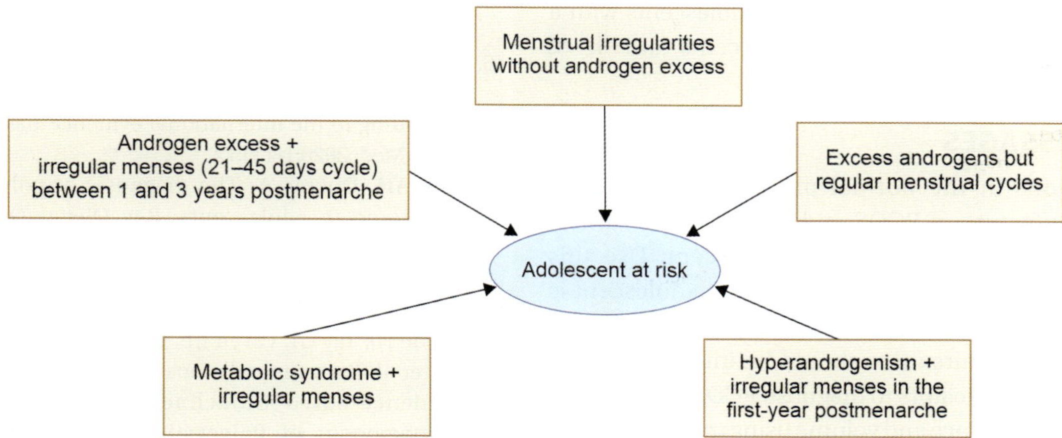


**Fig. 4:** Criteria defining an "Adolescent at risk" of polycystic ovary syndrome (PCOS).

treatment strategies singularly do not achieve desired goals.

- *Antiandrogens:* This can be tried only after usage of COCP along with cosmetic therapy for at least 6 months. Situations where COCPs are contraindicated/poorly tolerated, antiandrogens could be considered to treat hirsutism or androgen-related alopecia. The use of effective contraception is important due to the teratogenic potential of antiandrogens. Spironolactone is commonly prescribed as an androgen receptor blocker along with oral contraceptives. The recommended dose of spironolactone is 50–200 mg/day. Other options include cyproterone acetate, flutamide, and finasteride, but hepatotoxicity is a concern and availability is an issue.

## Topical Treatment

Systemic therapy can work synergistically by topical therapy for hirsutism and acne (e.g., electrolysis, laser therapy, plucking, waxing, shaving, and bleaching). Eflornithine hydrochloride (13.9%) cream (enzyme ornithine decarboxylase blocker) is an option to lessen facial hirsutism and accentuate the effects of laser therapy. Benefits of this cream and other topical strategies are outweighed by their side effects (e.g., burning, folliculitis, etc.) occasionally. For acne, topical retinoic acids are useful adjuncts to oral antibiotics, hormonal therapy, or antiandrogens.

*Models of care and transition:* Primary care is to diagnose, screen, and coordinate multidisciplinary care considering that adolescents with PCOS face multiple health problems and see multiple health professionals. The multidisciplinary care allows the screening and management of comorbidities associated with PCOS and transition to adult care is required for adolescents with a clear diagnosis of PCOS and for adolescents "at risk" of PCOS to ensure their reevaluation.

## ■ KEY MESSAGES

- Aberrations in the normal menstrual cycle are a common feature of PCOS and are often the earliest clinical manifestation in the adolescent. Use this criterion with caution, especially if the adolescent is within 3 years of menarche.
- Severe acne or hirsutism should be interpreted with biochemical indicators to diagnose PCOS.
- Ovarian appearance and volume using transabdominal technique is a less reliable indicator of PCOS due to normal physiological changes in puberty and should not be used. Anti-Müllerian hormone (AMH) is not recommended for a diagnosis of PCOS due to a lack of evidence and specificity.

- Childhood obesity may increase the severity of symptoms of PCOS and undermine the importance of its early diagnosis; hence in patients with hyperandrogenemia, a metabolic workup should be performed. Avoid using obesity with insulin resistance as the lone parameter while diagnosing PCOS.
- Exclusion of the other diagnoses with a similar presentation is crucial.
- Identify the adolescents satisfying the "Adolescent at risk" criteria for PCOS for longitudinal follow-up and thus avoiding unnecessary panic by labeling them as PCOS.
- Special considerations need to be given when assessing, and treating adolescents for PCOS as family's preferences and cultural norms should be considered.

## ■ RECOMMENDED READING

1. Bharali MD, Rajendran R, Goswami J, Singal K, Rajendran V. Prevalence of Polycystic Ovarian Syndrome in India: A Systematic Review and Meta-Analysis. Cureus. 2022;14(12):e32351.
2. Kamboj MK, Bonny AE. Polycystic ovary syndrome in adolescence: diagnostic and therapeutic strategies. Transl Pediatr. 2017;6(4):248-55.
3. Meczekalski B, Niwczyk O, Kostrzak A, Maciejewska-Jeske M, Bala G, Szeliga A. PCOS in Adolescents—Ongoing Riddles in Diagnosis and Treatment. J Clin Med. 2023;12(3):1221.
4. Mousa A, Tay CT, Teede H. Technical Report for the International Evidence-based Guideline for the Assessment and Management of Polycystic Ovary Syndrome. Melbourne, Australia: Monash University; 2023.
5. Peña AS, Codner E, Witchel S. Criteria for Diagnosis of Polycystic Ovary Syndrome during Adolescence: Literature Review. Diagnostics. 2022;12(8):1931.
6. Peña AS, Witchel SF, Hoeger KM, Oberfield SE, Vogiatzi MG, Misso M, et al. Adolescent polycystic ovary syndrome according to the international evidence-based guideline. BMC Med. 2020;18(1):72.
7. Roe AH, Dokras A. The diagnosis of polycystic ovary syndrome in adolescents. Rev Obstet Gynecol. 2011 Summer;4(2):45-51.
8. Rosenfield RL. The Diagnosis of Polycystic Ovary Syndrome in Adolescents. Pediatrics. 2015;136(6):1154-65.
9. Teede HJ, Tay CT, Laven JJE, Dokras A, Moran LJ, Piltonen TT, et al. Recommendations from the 2023 International Evidence-based Guideline for the Assessment and Management of Polycystic Ovary Syndrome. Eur J Endocrinol. 2023;189(2):G43-64.

# 4A.4   Diabetes in Youth

*Dhanya Soodhana, Vijayakumar M*

## ■ INTRODUCTION

India is known as the global epicenter of the diabetes epidemic. The International Diabetes Federation (IDF) estimated that 1.1 million children and adolescents aged 14–19 years were living with diabetes in 2017. With a high genetic predisposition and high susceptibility to environmental insults, the Indian population faces a high risk of diabetes and its complications. Type 1 diabetes mellitus (T1DM) is also showing an increasing trend of 3–5% increase per year. Available Indian data reveals a prevalence of T1DM of over 10/100,000 population with certain urban pockets having cases of over 30/100,000 population. A gradual increase in type 2 diabetes mellitus (T2DM) cases among adolescents is being reported across the country. At referral centers in Lucknow and Chennai, the proportion of children with T2DM is reported as 12% and 26.7%, respectively.

## ■ DEFINITION

The term "diabetes mellitus" describes a complex metabolic disorder that results from defects in insulin secretion, insulin action, or both and is characterized by chronic hyperglycemia. Abnormalities of carbohydrate, fat, and protein metabolism can arise due to inadequate insulin secretion and/or diminished tissue response to insulin. It should be noted that impaired insulin secretion and action can coexist in the same individual. Adolescence is a transitional phase in the development between childhood and emerging adulthood. Healthcare and emotional needs are significantly different from younger children and adults.

The etiology of diabetes is heterogenous; most cases of diabetes can be classified into two broad etiopathogenetic categories:

1. *T1DM:* This occurs due to an autoimmune process characterized by the destruction of β cells, which results in the loss of endogenous insulin production.
2. *T2DM:* This is characterized by the lack of adequate insulin response in the presence of increasing insulin resistance (IR).

It is now recognized that monogenic diabetes, with autosomal dominant inheritance [initially termed maturity-onset diabetes of the young (MODY)], can constitute 1–6% of the children with autoantibody-negative diabetes, who might have been initially classified as T1DM or T2DM.

## ■ DIAGNOSTIC CRITERIA

Diagnostic criteria for diabetes are based on blood glucose level (BGL) measurements and the presence or absence of symptoms. Different strategies can be used to measure BGL, including using a fasting plasma glucose (FPG) value, the 2-hour plasma glucose (2-h PG) value during an oral glucose tolerance test (OGTT), or glycated hemoglobin (HbA1c) criteria **(Box 1)**, and in the absence of unequivocal hyperglycemia, the diagnosis must be confirmed by testing again.

Associated syndromic features, deafness, or optic atrophy should make us think of a mitochondrial disease. A history of exposure to drugs such as glucocorticoids, nicotinic acid, atypical antipsychotics, statins, diazoxide, phenytoin, L-asparaginase (insulin deficiency), β-adrenergic agonists, and growth hormone (GH) should be noted. Infections such as congenital rubella, enterovirus, and cytomegalovirus can predispose to diabetes.

Achieving optimal glycemic control is difficult during adolescence despite recent technological advances. Importance needs to be given to the peer support that adolescents with diabetes can gain through social media. Motivational interviewing by trained psychologists is effective in optimizing outcomes in these individuals.

---

**BOX 1:** Criteria for diagnosis of diabetes.

- Classic symptoms of diabetes or hyperglycemic crisis with plasma glucose concentration ≥200 mg/dL, or
- Fasting (no caloric intake for at least 8 hours) plasma glucose ≥126 mg/dL, or
- 2-hour post-load glucose ≥200 mg/dL during an oral glucose tolerance test (OGTT), or
- Glycated hemoglobin (HbA1c) ≥6.5%

Less consistent use of insulin and other self-care measures can lead to poor glycemic control during this period. During adolescence, prioritizing mental health over other healthcare needs, involving other specialties, and ensuring good interprofessional communication are important. Screening for social health determinants is also very important at this age.

## ■ TYPE 1 DIABETES MELLITUS

### Pathogenesis

Type 1 diabetes mellitus is characterized by chronic immune-mediated destruction of pancreatic β-cells, leading to partial or, in most cases, absolute insulin deficiency. In the majority of cases, autoimmune-mediated pancreatic β-cell destruction occurs at a variable rate and is influenced by different factors, including genes, age, and ethnicity **(Box 2)**.

Youth progress through three stages at variable rates:
- *Stage 1:* It can last for months to many years and is characterized by the presence of β-cell autoimmunity with normoglycemia and a lack of clinical symptoms.
- *Stage 2:* It progresses to dysglycemia but remains asymptomatic.

---

**BOX 2:** Factors contributing to the pathogenesis of type 1 diabetes mellitus.

- *Genetic factors:*
  - HLA DR, HLA DQ, HLA DP
  - Insulin VNTR
  - CTLA 4
  - Other genetic associations (PTPN 22, CTLA 4, TCF7L2, AIRE, FoxP3, STAT3, IFIH1)
- *Epigenetic factors*
- *Environmental factors:*
  - *Infections:* Enterovirus and rubella
  - *Nutrition:* Cow's milk, cereals, and omega 3 fatty acids
  - Obesity
  - Changes in the microbiome
  - Chemical
- *Immunologic factors:*
  - Immune tolerance
  - Cellular and humoral immunity

(AIRE: autoimmune regulator; CTLA: cytotoxic T-lymphocyte antigen; FoxP3: Forkhead Box P3; HLA: human leukocyte antigen; IFIH1: interferon induced with helicase C domain 1; PTPN22: protein tyrosine phosphatase nonreceptor type 22; STAT3: signal transducer and activator of transcription; TCF7L2: transcription factor 7-like 2; VNTR: variable number tandem repeat)

---

- *Stage 3:* It is defined as the onset of symptomatic disease.

Individuals with a first-degree relative with T1DM have a 15-fold increased relative risk of developing T1DM. However, 85% of the individuals with newly diagnosed T1DM do not have a family history of diabetes.

Above the age of 15 years, a male preponderance can be noted in the incidence of T1DM. Children with two or more islet autoantibodies and normoglycemia should be considered to have stage 1 T1DM. Targeted screening and monitoring could help us identify stage 1, stage 2, and presymptomatic stage 3 diabetes and help reduce the incidence of diabetic ketoacidosis (DKA) and rates of hospitalization.

Transient pubertal IR is known to occur in those with or without diabetes and has implications on glycemic control. This decrease in insulin sensitivity is exaggerated in adolescents with diabetes. The increased IR is believed to be mediated by the peak in GH and insulin-like growth factor-1 (IGF-1). GH affects the insulin signaling pathway at the postreceptor level and leads to increased IR. Pattern of increased GH and IR results in exaggerated ketogenesis in adolescents with T1DM, and this could predispose to poor glycemic control and DKA.

### Clinical Features

Type 1 diabetes mellitus in adolescents presents with characteristic symptoms like polyuria, polydipsia, nocturia, enuresis, and weight loss. In some, these symptoms may be accompanied by increased appetite, fatigue, behavioral disturbance, reduced school performance, and blurred vision. Growth impairment and candidiasis can also be the presentation in chronic hyperglycemia. Presentation could be altered sensorium, stupor, or coma if the adolescent is presenting with acute complications such as DKA or hyperosmolar hyperglycemic syndrome (HHS).

### Management

The four main pillars in the management of T1DM include medication (insulin), monitoring, mobility, and medical nutrition therapy. Insulin replacement therapy is essential for the survival of individuals with T1DM and is at present the only treatment available. Daily management of T1DM includes multiple insulin injections and can be administered using a syringe, reusable pen, disposable pen (4–5 times a day), or a continuous subcutaneous pump.

A combination of a short-acting regular insulin or insulin analog such a lispro, aspart, or glulisine (as "bolus" to cover post-meal hyperglycemia) is given three to four times a day and a long-acting insulin glargine, detemir, or degludec (for "basal" insulin coverage) is given once or twice a day. Insulin pumps use only a rapid-acting analog for both the basal and the bolus phases. Basal bolus regimen involves taking three or more injections a day but definitely ensures better glycemic control. The choice of the regimen should be based on the adolescent's motivation, schedule, and financial situation. Adolescents might require a higher daily dose of insulin of 1.2–1.5 units/kg/day owing to their pubertal changes, which lead to physiological IR. The use of Mixtard or other combination insulins should be discouraged in adolescents for their lack of flexibility. Diabetes distress during adolescence could lead to inconsistent use of insulin and poor self-care measures leading to poor glycemic control.

## Complications of Diabetes

Adolescents with T1DM should be cared for routinely by a multidisciplinary team, consisting of a pediatric endocrinologist or a pediatrician with a special interest in diabetes, a diabetes nurse educator, a dietician, and a psychologist/ social worker. They should be monitored every 2–3 months for their general well-being, reviewing the self-monitoring of blood glucose results (SMBG), insulin therapy, growth and pubertal assessment, long-term complications, and their psychosocial state.

*Screening for associated autoimmune disorders* such as autoimmune thyroid disease, celiac disease, primary adrenal insufficiency, and vitiligo is recommended at diagnosis and every year or depending on clinical assessment.

### Acute Complications

- *Diabetic ketoacidosis:* (see in endocrine emergencies)
- *Hyperglycemic hyperosmolar syndrome:* HHS is characterized by extremely elevated serum glucose concentrations and hyperosmolality without significant ketosis. The rates of treatment complications and mortality are significantly higher than in DKA. HHS presents as increasing polyuria and polydipsia accompanied by lethargy, confusion, and dizziness. Despite severe volume and electrolyte losses, hypertonicity preserves intravascular volume, and signs of dehydration are less evident. Intravascular volume may decrease rapidly in children with HHS during treatment, and hence aggressive replacement of intravascular volume is needed to avoid vascular collapse.

*Hypoglycemia:* It is the most common, life-threatening acute complication of diabetes treatment. Blood sugar level of <70 mg/dL is considered to be hypoglycemia in children with T1DM. The brain depends on a continuous supply of glucose for energy although it can use ketone bodies. Adolescents are at a high risk for hypoglycemia and the spectrum might range from mild cognitive impairment to seizure, coma, and even death. The moderate and severe forms of hypoglycemia require the assistance of another person. All adolescents must carry a plastic pouch with three to four teaspoons of powdered sugar or glucose for prompt ingestion in case of symptoms of hypoglycemia such as sweating, anxiety, anger, headache, or blurring of vision. It is important to note that chocolates and ice creams should not be offered during an episode of hypoglycemia, as the fat present in these could delay glucose absorption. Instructions need to be given that in case an adolescent is found unconscious, then it would be better to administer glucagon [weight <25 kg, 0.5 mg subcutaneous (SC) or intramuscular (IM); weight >25 kg 1 mg SC or IM] if available or to form a glucose paste and administer it on the dependent cheek and arrange for the immediate transfer to the nearest medical center. In adolescents with T1DM, recurrent hypoglycemia is known to reduce the BGL that precipitates the counter-regulatory response that is needed to restore euglycemia during a subsequent episode of hypoglycemia. This could lead to hypoglycemia unawareness.

### Chronic Complications

Diabetes can adversely impact growth and pubertal development.
- *Growth:* There is a blunting of pubertal growth spurt with a reduced height velocity. Adult height is at par with normal in a well-managed child and impairment in growth is related to poor glycemic control, which leads to changes in the IGF-1/GH axis.
- *Puberty:* Normal gonadotropin-releasing hormone (GnRH) neuronal function needs the action of both insulin and leptin, and therefore a deficiency can lead to hypogonadism. With newer insulins, pubertal development is usually normal or minimally delayed. Other common problems in adolescent girls with T1DM include ovarian hyperandrogenism and menstrual irregularities. During puberty, body

evidence of autoimmunity (TPO positivity). Treatment should be started only if TSH levels are above 10 mU/L or in the presence of goiter, TPO positivity, and severe growth failure. Obesity is a common cause of subclinical hypothyroidism due to increased hypothalamic TRH production. The thyroid functions usually normalize with a reduction in body weight.

### Nonthyroidal Illness

The physiological response to illness is to reduce metabolism. This is achieved by increased MDI3 expression and decreasing T3 levels. Simultaneously, MDI2 expression is increased, causing increased T4 availability to the pituitary and reduced TSH levels. This constellation of low T3, normal/low T4, and low TSH is characteristic of nonthyroidal illness and should not be considered a marker of central hypothyroidism. Recovery from illness is characterized by elevated TSH, causing a diagnostic dilemma of primary hypothyroidism. Thyroid functions should not be assessed in hospitalized subjects unless it is mandatory to avoid diagnostic confusion. Thyroid hormone treatment should be started only in the presence of persistent and significant elevation of TSH.

### Central Hypothyroidism

Central hypothyroidism is due to pituitary (secondary) or hypothalamic (tertiary) abnormality. The condition is characterized by low FT4 with low or inappropriately normal TSH levels. Isolated acquired TSH deficiency is rare and usually occurs in the setting of hypopituitarism due to central nervous system (CNS) insult, tumor, radiation, and trauma. Cortisol deficiency should be corrected before thyroid hormone replacement in central hypothyroidism.

## Assessment

Hypothyroidism should be suspected with growth failure and normal weight, obesity with short stature, developmental delay, constipation, poor scholastic performance, apathy, myopathy with pseudohypertrophy, precocious puberty with short stature, macroorchidism, menstrual disorders, hyperandrogenism, hyper-prolactinemia, ovarian cysts, pericardial effusion, gastroparesis, euvolemic hyponatremia, and pituitary hyperplasia. Screening for acquired hypothyroidism should be done in children with type 1 diabetes, Turner syndrome, celiac disease, Down syndrome, and autoimmune polyendocrinopathy.

## Diagnosis

Diagnosis and classification of hypothyroidism require estimation of FT4 and TSH levels.
- Low FT4 levels suggest hypothyroidism.
- Normal FT4 levels suggest euthyroid state but indicate subclinical hypothyroidism, if TSH levels are above 10 mU/L.
- Higher TSH in the setting indicates primary hypothyroidism.
- Low FT4 with TSH below 20 mU/L points to central hypothyroidism and the need for a magnetic resonance imaging (MRI) of the hypothalamic–pituitary region and anterior–pituitary functions.

## Evaluation

- Family history of hypothyroidism, autoimmune disorder, and residence in areas endemic for iodine deficiency should be inquired.
- Features of Turner syndrome, celiac disease, type 1 diabetes, and autoimmune polyendocrinopathy should be assessed.
- A thyroid examination should be done to look for thyroid swelling, retrosternal extension, and nodularity. Autoimmunity workup (TPO antibody) should be done to identify autoimmune thyroiditis, while a thyroid scan is performed for dyshormonogenesis (early onset features and developmental delay).
- Ultrasound is indicated for asymmetrical goiter to confirm nodularity. Pituitary function tests and MRI for the hypothalamic–pituitary region are indicated for central hypothyroidism **(Flowchart 2)**.

Key management aspects include timely treatment initiation, follow-up of thyroid functions, and monitoring for growth, development, and puberty.

## Preparation

Oral LT4 is the preferred form of treatment. It is available as a tablet and should be given once a day. Thyroid medication is affected by exposure to light and moisture and should be kept in a closed, dark bottle.

### Dose

Levothyroxine is given at a dose of 100 $\mu g/m^2$/day as younger children require higher doses on a weight basis **(Table 1)**. The treatment should start at 25% of the target dose with gradual increments over 4–6 weeks.

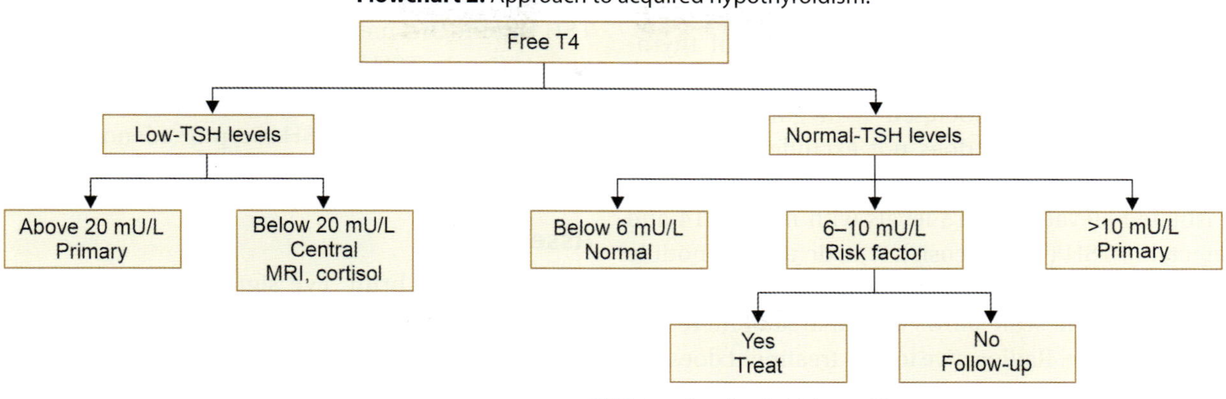

**Flowchart 2:** Approach to acquired hypothyroidism.



(MRI: magnetic resonance imaging; TPO: thyroid peroxidase; TSH: thyroid-stimulating hormone; T4: thyroxine)

| **TABLE 1:** Thyroxine dose in acquired hypothyroidism. | |
| --- | --- |
| **Age** | **Dose (µg/kg/day)** |
| 1–3 years | 4–6 |
| 3–10 years | 3–5 |
| Above 10 years | 2–4 |
| Adults | 1.6 |

## Timing

The drug should be taken at least 4 hours after and 30 minutes before the meal. Intake of calcium, iron, and antacids impairs absorption, emphasizing the need for a gap of at least 6 hours between thyroid medication and these drugs.

## Follow-up

Thyroid functions should be assessed 6 weeks after initiation and dose modification and 3–6 months subsequently. TSH levels can be measured at any time of the day, irrespective of intake, while FT4 levels should be measured before the drug intake. FT4 levels should be kept in a high normal range in children with central hypothyroidism, while TSH levels between 0.4 and 2 mU/L are ideal in primary hypothyroidism.

## Effect of Treatment

Initiation of treatment may cause irritability, headache, and worsening school performance. Persistent headache and vomiting should prompt evaluation for benign intracranial hypertension (fundus examination). Sudden worsening with mildly elevated TSH levels after T4

**Flowchart 3:** Etiology of thyrotoxicosis.

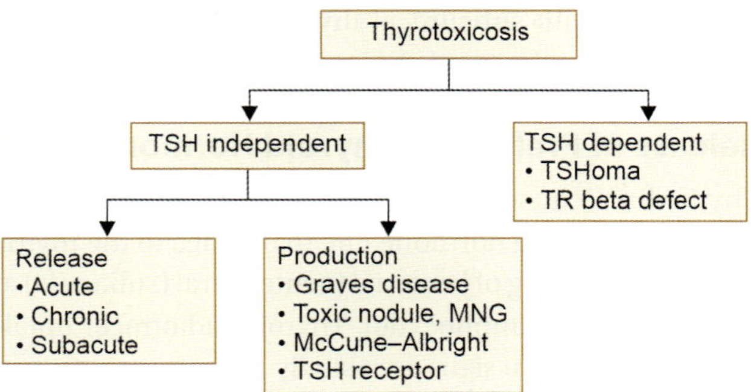



(MNG: multinodular goiter; TR: thyroid receptor; TSH: thyroid-stimulating hormone)

initiation should prompt evaluation for cortisol deficiency. Growth response may take time to manifest due to epiphyseal dysgenesis. Pubertal development may be triggered after initiating thyroid hormones compromising final height. Gonadotropin hormone-releasing hormone (GnRH) analog treatment may be considered in girls with rapid pubertal progress and bone age advancement. Substantially higher thyroid requirements should prompt evaluation for drug administration (timing and adherence), absorption (celiac disease, intake of iron, calcium, sucralfate, orlistat, and antacid), and increased metabolism (rifampicin, phenytoin, and phenobarbitone).

## ■ THYROTOXICOSIS

Thyrotoxicosis is less common compared to hypothyroidism in adolescents but is associated with significant impact. It represents increased production (TSH dependent or independent) or release of thyroid hormones **(Flowchart 3)**.

## Increased Production

Graves disease is the most common cause of thyrotoxicosis due to TSH receptor activating antibody. The condition is usually associated with goiter and eye signs, but their absence does not exclude it. Subjects with iodine deficiency and thyrotoxicosis may present with isolated elevation of T3 levels with normal T4 and undetectable TSH (T3 toxicosis). A toxic thyroid nodule is caused by somatic TSH receptor activating mutation and a radionuclide scan shows a focal area of increased radiotracer uptake. Radioactive iodine treatment does not ablate the remaining thyroid tissue, exposing it to low-dose radiation (due to reduced uptake) and subsequent risk of malignancy. Surgical excision of the lesion is therefore recommended.

Toxic multinodular goiter usually presents in older individuals with subclinical thyrotoxicosis, and surgery remains the treatment of choice.

## Release of Preformed Thyroid Hormone

Thyroiditis causes thyrotoxicosis by the release of preformed thyroid hormone due to damage to the thyroid gland in the setting of bacterial (acute), viral (subacute), or immune insult (lymphocytic). Thyroid radiotracer uptake is reduced, and eye signs are usually absent.

Chronic lymphocytic thyroiditis is associated with immune-mediated damage to the thyroid gland and self-limiting thyroiditis. The condition presents with painless thyroid swelling and has an increased risk of hypothyroidism in the presence of extensive thyroid damage.

Subacute thyroiditis (granulomatous and viral thyroiditis) is associated with neck pain, tenderness, and elevated inflammatory markers [erythrocyte sedimentation rate (ESR) and C-reactive protein (CRP)].

Acute thyroiditis is caused by pyogenic infection and is characterized by severe neck tenderness and elevated inflammatory markers. Antibiotic treatment and drainage are indicated.

## Pointers

Thyrotoxicosis should be considered with weight loss, tremors, anxiety, increased irritability, eye signs, polyuria, and worsening of school performance. It should be excluded in the setting of myasthenia gravis and periodic paralysis. While FT4 levels are usually elevated in most children with thyrotoxicosis, total T3 is a better marker of thyroid status in iodine-deficient areas. T3, FT4, and TSH should be measured in a child with suspected thyrotoxicosis. TSH levels should be undetectable in the presence of elevated thyroid hormones. Detectable TSH in this setting suggests TSH receptor adenoma or thyroid hormone resistance.

## Assessment

- Goiter with bruit, eye signs, increased vascularity on ultrasound, and significant elevation of thyroid hormone levels indicates increased production **(Table 2)**. In contrast, the absence of thyroid swelling and eye signs suggests the release of preformed hormones.
- A thyroid scan helps to distinguish increased production (increased uptake) from the release of preformed hormones (reduced uptake).
- No further evaluation is required in the presence of soft, smooth goiter with bruit and eye signs.
- A thyroid scan should be done in children without these features. TSH receptor antibodies help differentiate Graves disease from thyroiditis. Reduced thyroid scan uptake suggests thyroiditis. A thyroid scan identifies toxic nodules and toxic multinodular goiter.
- Detectable TSH with thyrotoxicosis should prompt evaluation for TSH-secreting adenoma (alpha subunit and MRI of the hypothalamic–pituitary region).

## Management

A thyroid storm is a medical emergency requiring immediate treatment. Antithyroid drugs have a lag response phase and have a limited role in acute

**TABLE 2:** Comparison of features of Graves disease and thyroiditis.

| Feature | Graves disease | Thyroiditis |
| --- | --- | --- |
| Onset | Acute | Chronic |
| Eye signs | Common | Absent |
| Goiter | Common | Absent |
| FT4 | High | High, normal |
| Bruit | May be present | Absent |
| Radionuclide scan | Increased uptake | Reduced uptake |
| Course | Progressive | Self-limiting |
| Treatment | Antithyroid drugs | Symptomatic |

(FT4: free thyroxine 4)

management. Acute management aims to ameliorate symptoms, inhibit thyroid production, and release and activate T4. This involves the correction of hyperthermia and cardiac functions. Digitalis/digoxin is indicated in cardiac failure.

## GRAVES DISEASE

- *Antithyroid drugs:* These are the mainstay of treatment. Propylthiouracil is contraindicated because of the risk of idiosyncratic hepatotoxicity. The initial dose of methimazole or carbimazole is 0.6–1 mg/kg/day followed by a maintenance dose of 0.2–0.5 mg/kg/day. Baseline liver function tests and complete blood count are indicated before starting methimazole. Agranulocytosis is a major cause of concern; throat pain and fever in any patient on methimazole should be considered an emergency. Hepatotoxicity with methimazole is usually dose-dependent and reversible. Cutaneous manifestations like rashes and urticaria are common with methimazole but usually respond to antihistamines.
- *Follow-up:* Thyroid profile should be measured after 6 weeks and then 3 monthly. FT4 levels normalize earlier than TSH and is the initial treatment target. The methimazole dose should be halved once thyroid functions become normal. Antithyroid drugs should be continued for 1–2 years as maximum remission is expected. The remission rate of Graves disease in children is only 15–20%. The likelihood of remission is higher with small goiter, low levels of TSH receptor antibody, and normalization of thyroid functions in the first 3 months of treatment.
- *Radioactive iodine:* It is emerging as a first-line therapy for adolescent Graves disease. High doses are used to ablate thyroid tissue to induce hypothyroidism. Radioactive iodine worsens ophthalmopathy and should be avoided in the presence of active eye disease. *Surgery:* Sub/near-total thyroidectomy should be considered in children with large goiter (above 80 g). Surgery in a child with uncontrolled thyrotoxicosis is associated with a high risk of thyroid storm. Patients should be stabilized using antithyroid drugs or iodine.
- *Thyroiditis:* Symptomatic treatment with beta-blockers is usually sufficient.
    - Lymphocytic thyroiditis improves in over 6–8 weeks with a long-term risk of hypothyroidism.

    - Subacute thyroiditis is treated with beta-blockers, steroids, and nonsteroidal anti-inflammatory drugs (NSAIDs).
    - Acute thyroiditis is an emergency and should be treated with antibiotics and surgery.
- *Toxic nodule:* Surgical resection is the modality of choice for toxic nodules.
- *Thyroid nodule:* These are uncommon in children (2% population prevalence) but have a high risk of malignancy (10–15%) making timely identification and careful management essential. Thyroid nodules may originate from thyroidal or extrathyroidal tissue (cystic nodule or teratoma).
- *Adenoma:* Thyroid adenoma is slow growing, usually smaller than 1 cm, not fixed to the underlying structure, and not associated with change in voice.
- *Ectopic thyroid:* It represents abnormal descent of the thyroid gland located anywhere in the descent path from the foramen cecum to the thyroid cartilage. Ectopic thyroid is visualized as a midline nodule that moves with deglutition but not with tongue protrusion. The thyroid scan is diagnostic of ectopic thyroid.
- *Thyroglossal cyst:* It is a cystic swelling in the path of thyroid descent. It moves with deglutition due to an intact tract for the descent of the thyroid gland. Surgery is advised as it carries a high risk of infection and malignancy in the future.
- *Thyroid carcinoma:* It presents a rapidly enlarging, fixed mass associated with cervical lymph node enlargement. Malignant thyroid nodules may be of papillary (83%), follicular (10%), medullary (5%), or lymphoma (2%) origin.

### Assessment

Careful assessment of thyroid nodules is essential, given the likelihood of malignancy **(Flowchart 4)**.

- *Clinical:* History should focus on the duration and course of swelling. A family history of thyroid malignancy or thyroidectomy should be enquired. Predisposing factors like radiation exposure and cancer syndromes should be inquired. Hard and fixed swelling, >1 cm, and euthyroid status with enlarged lymph nodes suggest malignancy.
- *TSH levels:* The functional lesions have the lowest risk of malignancy (TSH below 0.1 mU/L, <1%). The risk increases with increasing TSH levels. A nuclear scan is recommended where TSH is below 0.1 mU/L, while

**Flowchart 4:** Approach to thyroid nodule.

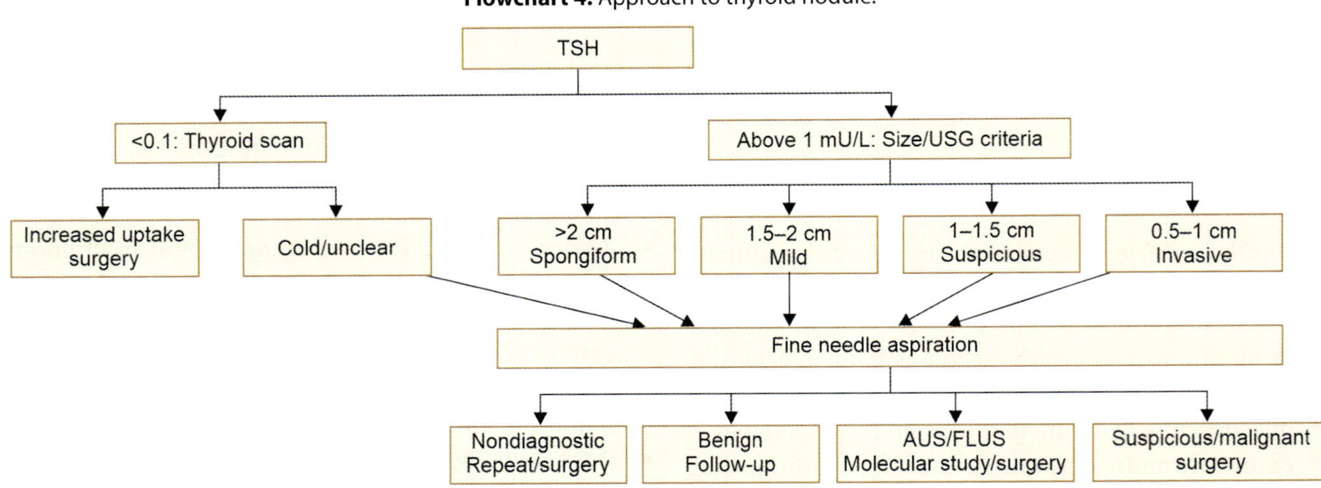

(AUS: atypia of undetermined significance; FLUS: follicular lesion of undetermined significance; TSH: thyroid-stimulating hormone)

in TSH levels between 0.1 and 1 mU/L, the scan is followed by fine needle aspiration cytology (FNAC) in warm or cold nodules. Ultrasound is recommended with levels above 1 mU/L.

- *Ultrasound thyroid:* Features of malignancy on ultrasound include a size of >1 cm, irregular margin, broken calcification, necrosis, and increased vascularity. Malignancy should be considered in children with characteristic features even when the size is <1 cm.
- *Fine needle aspiration (FNA):* Ultrasound-guided FNA should be performed in children with nodules above 1 cm in size and those above 0.5 cm with characteristic features. FNA should be repeated in nondiagnostic cases and where neoplasm is possible (category III). Diagnostic hemithyroidectomy is indicated in the presence of follicular neoplasm (category IV) and suspicion of malignancy (category V). Curative surgery is conducted if FNA is diagnostic of malignancy (category VI).

## Management

Surgical resection is indicated in toxic adenoma after stabilization of thyrotoxicosis. Differentiated thyroid carcinoma should be treated with total thyroidectomy followed by radioactive iodine ablation. Medullary carcinoma should be treated with total thyroidectomy after excluding pheochromocytoma. Genetic study for the *RET* gene should be done in children with a family history of multiple endocrine neoplasia type 2 (MEN2). Prophylactic thyroidectomy is indicated in these cases to prevent the development of thyroid malignancy.

## ■ GOITER

Goiter is a diffuse enlargement of the thyroid gland and needs to be differentiated from the nodule, an isolated swelling of a part of the thyroid gland.

## Etiology

Thyroid enlargement may result from activation of the TSH receptor or infiltration **(Flowchart 5)**.

- *Iodine deficiency:* It is an important cause in endemic areas and presents with mild hypothyroidism and soft goiter.
- *Goitrogens:* These substances inhibit thyroid hormone synthesis, causing enlargement in the thyroid gland. These include iodine-containing agents like amiodarone, thionamide, and lithium. Certain food substances like maize, cauliflower, turnip, and cassava contain goitrin and thiocyanates.
- *Colloid goiter:* Colloid goiter is common during puberty, particularly in girls. It manifests as a euthyroid soft goiter which is self-limiting. There is no role of LT4 treatment.
- *Graves disease:* It is caused by increased production of TSH receptor-stimulating antibodies, which act on the TSH receptor leading to thyroid gland enlargement.
- *Thyroiditis:* It represents inflammation of the thyroid and may rarely present with thyroid enlargement.

**Flowchart 5:** Etiology of goiter.

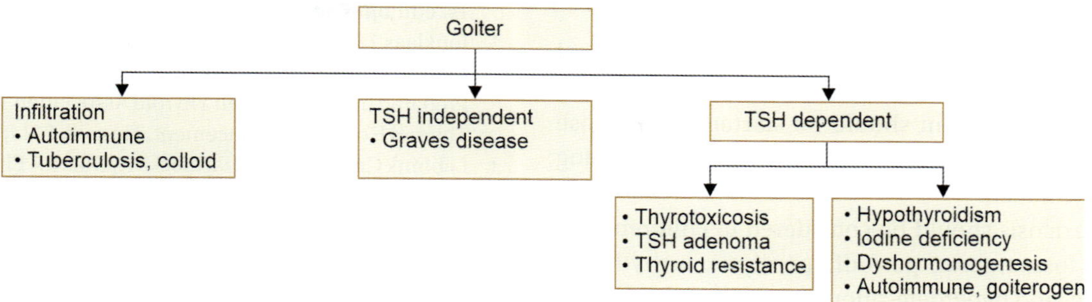


(TSH: thyroid-stimulating hormone)
*Source:* Adapted with permission from Bajpai A, Dave C. (2023). Goiter. MedEClasses Online Course in Pediatric Endocrinology. [online] Available from learning.growsociety.in (Last accessed March, 2024).

**Flowchart 6:** Approach to goiter.

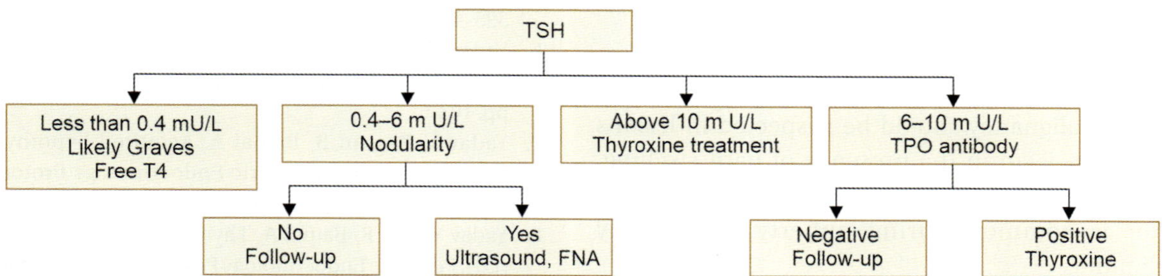


(FNA: fine needle aspiration; TPO: thyroid peroxidase; TSH: thyroid-stimulating hormone; T4: thyroxine)

- *Multinodular goiter:* It is important to identify due to the high risk of malignancy.

## Assessment

- Clinical assessment should include details of a family history of goiter, hypothyroidism, and iodine deficiency.
- Features of hypo- or hyperthyroidism should be assessed.
- Deafness suggests Pendred syndrome.
- Palpation should include the size, surface, and consistency of the swelling.
- Retrosternal extension is assessed by a dull note on percussion. Pemberton sign (discomfort after raising the arms) is another pointer of retrosternal extension. Bruit is indicative of hypervascularity, as in Graves disease.

## Investigations

Diagnostic workup includes thyroid functions (FT4 and TSH) and TPO antibodies. Ultrasonography (USG) helps to identify multinodular goiter **(Flowchart 6)**. A thyroid scan is indicated in children with thyrotoxicosis. FNA is indicated in multinodular goiter with nodules >1 cm or suspicious findings like irregular margins, hypoechoic lesions, calcification, or increased vascularity.

## Management

Management of goiter depends upon the etiology and thyroid functions. T4 supplementation is indicated in children with TSH above 10 mU/L. Suppressive T4 therapy has no role in euthyroid goiter. Surgery is indicated if there are compressive symptoms or mediastinal extension. It involves performing a thyroidectomy. There is a higher risk of complications like hypocalcemia and hoarseness of voice in children than adults.

## ■ KEY MESSAGES

- Initial work-up in a child with suspected thyroid disorders should include TSH and FT4.
- Acquired hypothyroidism should be considered in adolescents with growth failure, obesity, worsening school performance, myopathy, pericardial effusion, and pubertal disorders.

- Mildly elevated TSH levels in obesity do not require treatment.
- Consider central hypothyroidism with low FT4 and inappropriately low (up to 15 mU/L) TSH.
- Thyroid replacement should be started at 25% dose and gradually build up in children with long standing hypothyroidism.
- Thyrotoxicosis should be considered in children with weight loss, tremor, periodic paralysis, arrhythmia, polyuria, and hyperdefecation.
- Thyroiditis should be considered in thyrotoxicosis and no eye sign or goiter.
- Methimazole is the mainstay of treatment in children with Graves disease, radioactive iodine may be considered after the age of 10 years with low chance of remission.
- Thyroid nodules are uncommon in children but have a high risk of malignancy.
- Thyroid malignancy should be suspected in lesions bigger than 1 cm in the presence of hard swelling, associated lymph node and normal thyroid functions.
- Goiter is common during puberty but usually self-limiting.
- There is no role of suppressive thyroxine treatment in euthyroid goiter.

## ◼ RECOMMENDED READING

1. Bajpai A, Dave C. Thyroid physiology and assessment. In: Bajpai A, Dave C, Agarwal N, Patel R (Eds). MedEClasses Pediatric Endocrinology: Basic Endocrinology, volume 1, 1st edition. Kanpur; 2019. pp. 134-43.
2. Jonklaas J, Bianco AC, Bauer AJ, Burman KD, Cappola AR, Celi FS, et al. Guidelines for the Treatment Hypothyroidism: Prepared by the American Thyroid Association Task Force on Thyroid Hormone Replacement. Thyroid. 2014;24:1670-751.
3. Lebbink CA, Links TP, Czarniecka A, Dias RP, Elisei R, Izatt L, et al. 2022 European Thyroid Association Guidelines for the management of pediatric thyroid nodules and differentiated thyroid carcinoma. Eur Thyroid J. 2022;11(6):e220146.
4. Mooij CF, Cheetham TD, Verburg FA, Eckstein A, Pearce SH, Léger J, et al. 2022 European Thyroid Association Guideline for the management of pediatric Graves' disease. Eur Thyroid J. 2022;11(1):e210073.
5. Rivkees S, Baeur A. Thyroid disorders in children and adolescents In: Pediatric Endocrinology Sperling MA (Ed), 5th edition. Philadelphia: Saunders Elsevier; 2020. pp. 395-424.
6. Yadav V, Bansal S, Bajpai A. Goiter. In: Bajpai A (Ed). Pediatric Endocrinology Protocols, 2nd edition. Kanpur; 2023. pp. 103-6.
7. Yadav V, Begum B, Bajpai A. Acquired hypothyroidism. In: Bajpai A (Ed). Pediatric Endocrinology Protocols, 2nd edition. Kanpur; 2023. pp 76-82.
8. Yadav V, Das R, Bajpai A. Thyroid Assessment. In: Bajpai A (Ed). Pediatric Endocrinology Protocols, 2nd edition. Kanpur; 2023. pp. 57-67.
9. Yadav V, Kumar S, Bajpai A. Thyroid Nodule. In: Bajpai A (Ed). Pediatric Endocrinology Protocols, 2nd edition. Kanpur; 2023. pp. 97-102.
10. Yadav V, Udupi G, Bajpai A. Thyrotoxicosis. In: Bajpai A (Ed). Pediatric Endocrinology Protocols, 2nd edition. Kanpur; 2023. pp. 86-96.

# 4A.6 Low Bone Mass

*Anurag Bajpai, Vibha Yadav*

## ◼ INTRODUCTION

Low bone mass is being increasingly identified in adolescents. Prevention, timely identification, and treatment of low bone mass are essential to achieve a good outcome.

## ◼ PATHOPHYSIOLOGY

Low bone mass represents a reduced matrix, or mineral component of the bone, due to an imbalance between bone formation and resorption. Maximum bone mineralization occurs during puberty (40% from 10–18 years). The peak bone mass is achieved around 20 years in girls and 25 years in boys, followed by a gradual decline that increases rapidly after menopause. The most important determinant of bone mineralization is genetics (80%), followed by physical activity (10–15%) and nutrition (5–10%).

## ◼ POINTERS

The key indicators are fragility fractures, underlying conditions, and drugs affecting bone strength. Isolated bone pain is not an indication of bone strength assessment.

**Flowchart 1:** Etiology of low bone mass.

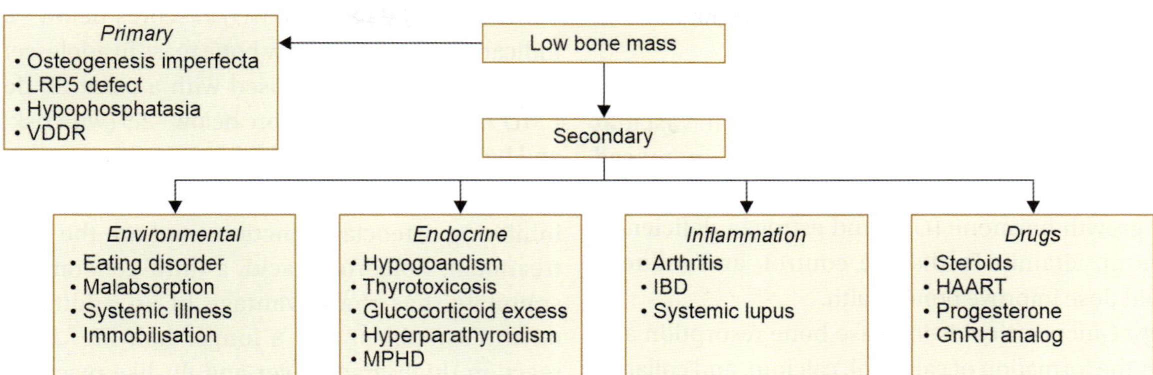


(GnRH: gonadotropin hormone-releasing hormone; HAART: highly aggressive antiretroviral treatment; IBD: inflammatory bowel disease; MPHD: multiple pituitary hormone deficiency; VDDR: Vitamin D dependent rickets)

Fractures are observed in 50% of boys and 40% of girls before adolescence. Significant low bone mass:

- More than two long bone fractures before the age of 10 years and three before the age of 18 years.
- Vertebral fractures are significant at any age.

## ■ CRITERIA

The assessment of bone strength aims to quantify its ability to sustain strain without fracturing. Dual-energy X-ray absorptiometry (DXA) is the most used modality, with site selection guided by age, indication, and physical conditions. The lumbar spine and femur are unreliable before the age of 5 and 18 years, respectively. The results are compared to age and gender-matched population norms and expressed as a Z score.

*Etiology:* Low bone mass represents reduced bone formation (collagen, alkaline phosphatase, and osteoblast regulation) or increased resorption (hypogonadism and enhanced bone turnover). Immobilization, musculoskeletal disorders, osteogenesis imperfecta (OI), and glucocorticoid-induced osteoporosis are the most common causes in adolescents **(Flowchart 1)**.

*Idiopathic juvenile osteoporosis:* It is a reversible low bone mass condition observed and presents around 8–12 years of age, with bone pain and vertebral compression fractures. It tends to improve after puberty. Calcitriol and bisphosphonates may be considered in severe cases. Mild forms of OI (type 1) should be excluded by assessment for blue sclera and hearing defect before establishing the diagnosis.

*Secondary osteoporosis:*

- *Under nutrition:* Undernutrition (malnutrition, anorexia nervosa, celiac disease, and inflammatory bowel disease) compromises bone health by reducing calcium and phosphorus levels and creating an unfavorable hormonal milieu [low insulin-like growth factor 1 (IGF-1), calcitriol, and estrogen levels with high cortisol]. Estrogen deficiency further compromises bone health in anorexia nervosa, causing a high fracture risk (around 32%).
- *Immobilization:* Restricted mobility due to neuromuscular disorders [cerebral palsy and Duchenne muscular dystrophy (DMD)] impairs osteoblast activity, reducing bone formation. Prolonged immobilization causes osteocyte apoptosis while triggering osteoclast activity, further reducing bone mass.
- *Systemic illness:* Systemic illness affects bone health by compromising nutrition, inflammation, and adverse effects of treatment.
- *Cancer treatment:* Acute lymphoblastic leukemia (ALL) compromises bone health due to inflammatory cytokines, infiltration, and the effects of steroids. Spinal fractures are present in 16% at diagnosis. Prolonged steroid exposure and chemotherapy predispose to low bone mass in other cancers.
- *Endocrine causes:* Sex steroid deficiency increases bone resorption while reducing the osteoblast effect. Estrogen deficiency and skeletal defect impair bone strength in Turner syndrome. Hypercortisolism increases bone resorption while lowering bone formation, calcitriol, calcium, and collagen levels. Bone mass improves with treatment of Cushing syndrome.

Bone health is also compromised in thyrotoxicosis, type 1 diabetes mellitus, hyperparathyroidism, and obesity.

- *Inflammatory disorders:* Inflammatory disorders (juvenile chronic arthritis and collagen vascular disorders) reduce bone mass due to increased osteoclast activity and glucocorticoid excess, along with growth hormone (GH) and estrogen deficiency. Calcium, vitamin D, disease control, and reduced steroid dose improve bone health.
- *Drugs:* Glucocorticoids increase bone resorption and lower the formation of calcitriol, calcium, and collagen production. Maximum bone loss occurs within the first 6 months with a predilection for the trabecular bone. Vertebral fractures are common and may manifest as back pain and reduced sitting height. Gonadotropin-releasing hormone (GnRH) analogs or aromatase inhibitors reduce estrogen levels, increasing bone resorption. Highly aggressive antiretroviral treatment compromises bone health.

## ■ ASSESSMENT

The critical aspects of evaluating low bone mass include its confirmation, differentiation of primary from a secondary cause, and delineation of etiology.

*Is it low bone mass?* A DXA Z score below –2 without fracture is classified as low bone mass. Levels above –2 are normal. DXA-derived bone mineral density is the area land underestimates bone strength in short children.

*What is the cause?* Evaluation for systemic illness, treatment (steroids, GnRH analog, and cancer treatment), physical activity, nutritional status, pointers to diagnosis (hearing, sclera color, skin, and joints), and endocrine features is required. The investigations include blood glucose, alanine aminotransferase (ALT), creatinine, calcium, phosphorus, alkaline phosphatase, tissue transglutaminase antibody (TTG), and parathyroid hormone (PTH). Genetic tests are reserved in the presence of clinical features.

## ■ MANAGEMENT

The management aims to prevent fragility fractures, reduce pain, and increase bone mineral density. General measures include nutritional modifications (calcium, phosphorus, and protein) and physical activity (45 minutes five times a week).

*Indication:* Fragility fracture, spinal fractures, and bone mineral density (BMD) Z scores below -2 are the indications for treating low bone mass in adolescents. DXA criteria have been proposed with a pubertal decline in BMD Z score, a BMD Z score below –2.5 (with risk factors), and below –3 (without risk factors).

*Options:* Bisphosphonates reduce bone resorption by inhibiting osteoclast functions and are the mainstay of treatment. Zoledronic acid, a third-generation bisphosphonate, has the advantage of an additional effect on the osteoblast and a longer half-life. Acute phase reaction (high-grade fever and flu-like reaction) occurs with intravenous preparations. Lower dose, prophylactic paracetamol, and slow infusion rate reduce the extent of flare response.

*Glucocorticoid-induced osteoporosis:* Calcium and vitamin D should be given to all on steroids for over 3 months and continued until 3 months after discontinuation. Regular weight-bearing exercise is essential. DXA scan and lateral spine X-ray should be done at baseline to identify low bone mass and vertebral fracture. After 6 months, fracture risk and bone density are reassessed with an annual assessment if a repeat workup is normal. Bisphosphonates are recommended for documented fracture, low bone density, and prednisolone equivalent dose above 0.3 mg/kg/day.

## ■ KEY MESSAGES

- Assesses bone density with vertebral fractures, two or more long bone fractures before the age of 10, and three or more before 18.
- Interpret BMD in the context of puberty, growth, population, and bone age.
- Exclude vitamin D deficiency, metabolic disease of prematurity, and hypophosphatasia before diagnosing osteogenesis imperfecta.
- Consider type III osteogenesis imperfecta with early onset fractures and blue sclera.
- Bisphosphonates are the treatment of choice for osteogenesis imperfecta.

## ■ RECOMMENDED READING

1. Bajpai A, Sen P. Low bone mass. In: Bajpai A (Ed). Pediatric Endocrinology Protocols, 2nd edition. Kanpur; 2023. pp. 42-52.
2. Root WA, Levine MA. Abnormalities of mineral homeostasis in newborn, infant, child and adolescent. In: Sperling MA (Ed). Sperling Pediatric Endocrinology, 5th edition. Philadelphia: Elsevier; 2021. pp. 367-95.

# 4A.7    Menstruation and Related Concerns

*Neema Sitapara*

## ■ NORMAL MENSTRUATION

### Introduction

Menstruation is the monthly physiologic shedding of the endometrium. Menarche, the first occurrence of menstruation, is hallmark of the last stage of female puberty. It usually occurs around 2.5 years of onset of breast budding (thelarche). Age of menarche is determined by genetics, nutrition, racial, and socioeconomic status and is in between 9 and 14 years. Menstrual cycle may last for 2–8 days and recur every 21–45 days. Total blood loss in a cycle varies from 20 to 90 mL. Mean product use is 3–6 pads/tampons per day. Any deviation from normal ranges or recent abnormalities is the indication for seeking medical advice and evaluation. During the first 2 years after menarche, abnormal or irregular menstrual patterns are common due to hypothalamic–pituitary–ovarian (HPO) axis immaturity and anovulatory cycles. First day of menstruation period to the first day of next menstruation consists of a menstrual cycle.

### Pathophysiology

Menstrual cycle is the result of a complex interaction between various glands, organs, and hormones; primarily hypothalamus [gonadotropin-releasing hormone (GnRH)], anterior pituitary [follicle-stimulating hormone/luteinizing hormone (FSH/LH)], and ovaries (estrogen/progesterone). It is divided into proliferative (follicular) and secretory (luteal) phase **(Table 1)**.

### *Follicular or Proliferative Phase*

It lasts from day one of menstruation to ovulation. Levels of estradiol and progesterone fall at the end of the menstrual cycle, which signals secretion of GnRH, LH, and FSH to initiate the next menstrual cycle. FSH stimulates maturation of ovarian follicle. Granulose cells of follicle secrete estradiol. A dominant follicle (Graafian follicle) induces LH surge and ovulation. This phase consists of proliferation and thickening of uterine endometrium.

### *Luteal or Secretory Phase*

In absence of pregnancy, the corpus luteum regresses in next 10–14 days. This is the most consistent phase (14+/–2 days) of menstrual cycle. The endometrium sloughs in the absence of estradiol and progesterone and is shed of vaginally as menstrual discharge. In anovulatory cycles, the follicular growth continues with the stimulation from FSH, but ovulation fails to occur. Corpus luteum is not formed and progesterone is not secreted. When the follicle involutes, estrogen levels drop and withdrawal bleeding occurs, which may be prolonged and heavy. Menstrual discharge remains liquid as it is devoid of thrombin, prothrombin, and fibrinogen.

### Menstrual Myths

Menstruation is a normal biological phenomenon giving the power of procreation to women. It has been socially, culturally, and religiously surrounded by secrecy taboos

**TABLE 1:** Normal menstrual changes (considering 28 days cycle).

| Day | Ovaries | Endometrium | Hormones |
|---|---|---|---|
| 1–5 | Early follicular development | Shedding off as menstruation | Low estrogen and progesterone |
| 5–14 | Follicles enlarge. Primordial follicle mature to Graafian follicle | Endometrial proliferation. Increased stroma, glands, and depth of spiral arteries | GnRH, FSH, estradiol, and LH increase |
| 14th | Ovulation | Changes favoring fertilization and implantation | LH surge |
| 15–28 | Regression of corpus luteum (in absence of pregnancy) | Luteal or secretory phase and sloughing of endometrium at the end | Progesterone and estradiol predominant which reduce at the end |

(FSH: follicle-stimulating hormone; GnRH: gonadotropin-releasing hormone; LH: luteinizing hormone)

**TABLE 2:** Common menstrual myths and strategies for menstrual health.

| Common menstrual myths | Strategies to improve menstrual health |
|---|---|
| • Not entering the "puja" room or kitchen, offering prayers and cooking during menstruation<br>• Menstruating woman or girl can be harmed by using black magic<br>• Food restrictions during menstruation (avoiding sour foods, "hot" and "cold" foods affecting periods)<br>• Exercise/physical activity during menses aggravate dysmenorrhea<br>• Cows become infertile if touched by menstruating women<br>• Avoid bath during menstruation<br>• Avoid vaccination during menstruation | • Raising the awareness for menstrual health and hygiene in adolescent girls and all women<br>• Local education programs at school and community levels<br>• Raising overall female literacy and women participation in decision making<br>• Provision of sanitary napkins at schools and public places<br>• Adequate facilities for sanitation and washing at schools<br>• Awareness in boys to stop stigmatizing periods and empathize with girls during periods |

**BOX 1:** Menstrual hygiene tips.

- Trim pubic hair before periods
- Proper use, frequent changing (6–8 hourly), and environment friendly disposal of menstrual products
- Frequent washing and 3 monthly replacement of reusable cloth
- Use of light fitting, breathable cotton garments
- Adequate hydration (6–8 glasses water) during periods
- Minimum two daily baths and hand wash before and after the use of menstrual product
- Post toilet front to back wash
- Use of nonscented, chemical-free hygiene products

**BOX 2:** Approach to adolescent girls with menstrual complains.

- *Ask for:* Age of menarche, pubertal development, headache, vision, appetite, exercise, diet, galactorrhea, drugs, menstruation in other females and genetic disease in family, menstrual cycle length, frequency, amount, flow, variations, recent changes, pain, and PID symptoms
- *Look for:* Height, weight, BMI, BP, abnormal features, pallor, bleeding tendencies, acne, hirsutism, acanthosis nigricans, and secondary sexual characteristics
- *Keep in mind:* Sexual abuse or relationships and use of contraceptive devices or drugs
- *Assess with:* Rapport, consent, confidentiality and HEADSSS

(BP: blood pressure; BMI: body mass index; HEADSSS assessment tool; PID: pelvic inflammatory disease)

and myths. The core underlying belief being menstruation is impure and a curse, further compounded by ignorance about puberty, menstruation, and reproductive health in women of all age group. Many girls drop out of school with menarche. Poor knowledge, inadequate protection, and washing facilities increases susceptibility to infections and generate huge health and economic burden. **Table 2** shows the common myths associated with menstruation and also the strategies to improve menstrual health.

## Menstrual Hygiene

Each year on May 28, Menstrual Hygiene Day is observed to raise awareness about the importance of access to menstrual products, period education, and sanitation facilities. This can prevent infections, reduce odors, and help women stay comfortable during periods **(Box 1)**.

## ■ DISORDERS OF MENSTRUATION

Common menstrual problems in adolescent girls are premenstrual syndrome (PMS), amenorrhea, dysmenorrhea, abnormal uterine bleeding (AUB), and polycystic ovarian syndrome. Menstruation is a sensitive issue and adolescents should be approached with care and gentleness when they visit primary physicians **(Box 2)**.

## Premenstrual Syndrome

Physical and mental symptoms occurring and recurring before menstruation and affecting a woman's normal life are known as *premenstrual syndrome*. These are most common in age group from 20 to 40 years. It is due to fluctuations in estrogen and progesterone and transitory fluid retention. It includes:

- *Emotional symptoms:* Depression, anger outbursts, irritability, crying spells, anxiety, confusion, social withdrawal, poor concentration, insomnia, increased nap taking, and changes in sexual desire
- *Physical symptoms:* Thirst and appetite changes (food cravings), breast tenderness, bloating and weight gain, headache, swelling of the hands or feet, aches and pains, fatigue, skin problems, gastrointestinal symptoms, and abdominal pain.

Symptoms must be present 5 days before a period, for at least three menstrual cycles in a row, end within 4 days after a period starts and interfere with some normal activities. *Premenstrual dysphoric disorder (PMDD)* is a severe type of PMS that affects 2–6% of women. The diagnostic criteria are given in Diagnostic and Statistical Manual of Mental Disorders 5 (DSM-5).

## Prevention and Treatment

- Psychoeducation about symptoms
- Aerobic exercise of at least 30 minutes, deep breathing and yoga, most days of the week
- Diet rich in complex carbohydrates, calcium, and fibers with reduced intake of fat, salt, sugar, caffeine, and alcohol. Calcium, magnesium, vitamin B-6, and vitamin E supplements
- Nonsteroidal anti-inflammatory drugs (NSAIDs), combined new generation pills in some cases
- Cognitive behavior therapy (CBT) and selective serotonin reuptake inhibitors (SSRIs) in severe cases.

## Amenorrhea

It is lack of spontaneous menstrual periods in a woman of reproductive age. Absence of secondary sexual characters and menarche by 14 years age or absence of menarche by 16 years of age with presence of secondary sexual characters is called *Primary amenorrhea. Secondary amenorrhea* is defined as absence of menstruation for 3 months in a female with previous regular cycles. Common causes of amenorrhea are shown in **Table 3**.

*Approach to a case of amenorrhea:* This is directed at detailed history taking and complete clinical examination followed by hormonal and radiological evaluation **(Flowcharts 1 to 3)**.

**TABLE 3:** Common causes of amenorrhea (pregnancy ruled out).

| *Hypergonadotropic* | *Hypogonadotropic* | *Eugonadotropic* | *Others* |
| --- | --- | --- | --- |
| • Chromosomal (Turner's) <br> • Androgen insensitivity <br> • Ovarian failure (autoimmune disease, chemotherapy and pelvic radiation, congenital thymic aplasia) <br> • Galactosemia, gonadal dysgenesis | • Constitutional, hypothalamic dysfunction (stress, excessive sports and weight loss) <br> • Chronic anovulation Kallmann syndrome, prolactinoma, benign pituitary adenoma hypopituitarism (Sheehan's syndrome, head trauma/ neoplasm), and gonadotropin deficiency | • Outflow obstruction, Müllerian agenesis <br> • Asherman syndrome <br> • Transverse vaginal septum <br> • Cervical stenosis <br> • Imperforate hymen <br> • Male pseudo-hermaphrodite <br> • Vaginal and uterine aplasia | • Other endocrine dysfunctions (CAH, Cushing's syndrome, and thyroid disorders) <br> • Drugs (antipsychotics and antidepressants) <br> • Neoplasms producing androgens, estrogens, or human chorionic gonadotropin <br> • Obesity, PCOS, and substance abuse |

(CAH: congenital adrenal hyperplasia; PCOS: polycystic ovarian syndrome)

**Flowchart 1:** Approach to case of primary amenorrhea (hormonal evaluation).

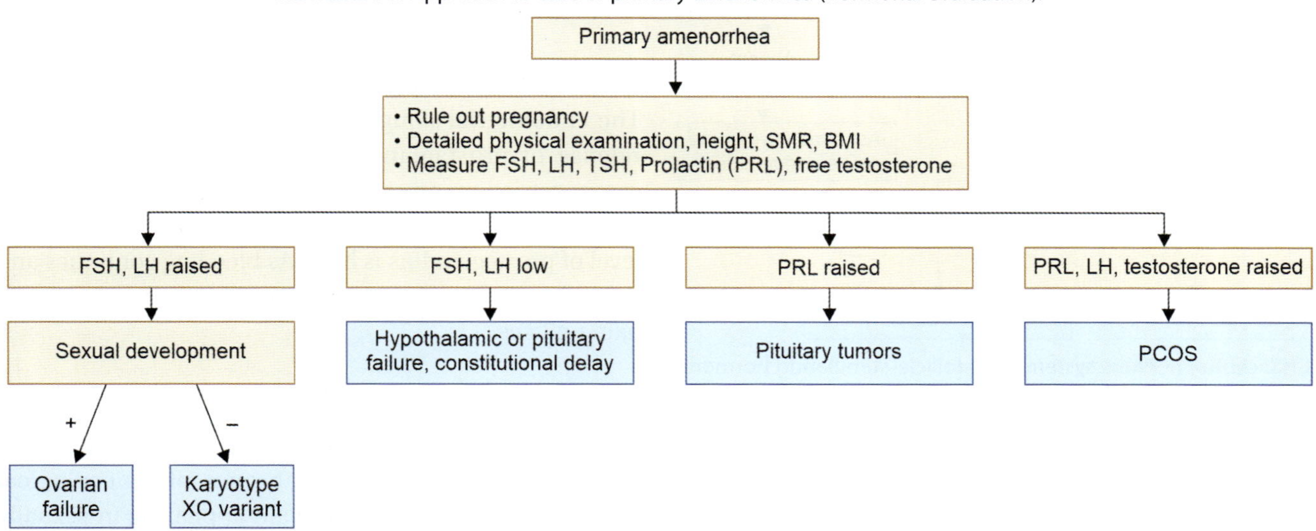


(BMI: body mass index; FSH: follicle-stimulating hormone; LH: luteinizing hormone; PCOS: polycystic ovarian syndrome; TSH: thyroid-stimulating hormone; SMR: sexual maturity rating)

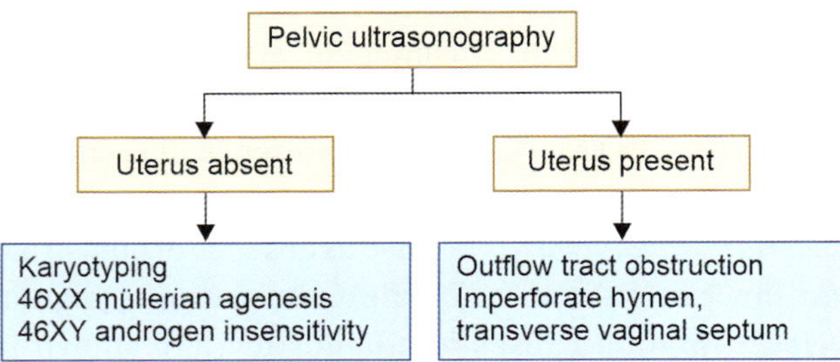

**Flowchart 2:** Approach to case of primary amenorrhea (Radiological evaluation).

**Flowchart 3:** Approach to case of secondary amenorrhea.

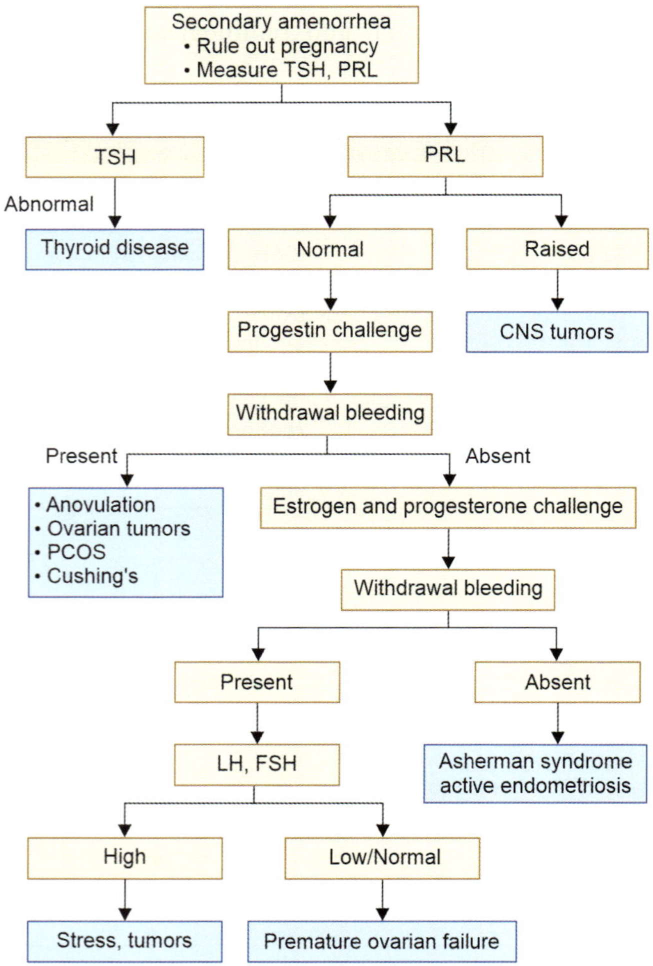

(CNS: central nervous system; FSH: follicle-stimulating hormone; LH: luteinizing hormone; PCOS: polycystic ovarian syndrome; PRL: prolactin; TSH: thyroid-stimulating hormone)

## Management of Amenorrhea

This consists of identification of cause and its treatment **(Box 3).**



(CAH: congenital adrenal hyperplasia; GnRH: gonadotropin-releasing hormone; HRT: hormone replacement therapy; OC: oral contraceptive)

## Dysmenorrhea

Most menstruating females have mild pain for 1–2 days each month, which usually starts during adolescence and tends to decrease with age and after pregnancy. When the pain is severe, long lasting, and impairing normal activities it is termed dysmenorrhea. *Primary dysmenorrhea* occurs without any pelvic pathology, whereas *secondary dysmenorrhea* is associated with organic diseases like endometriosis (most common cause), ovarian cysts, benign uterine tumors, pelvic inflammatory diseases, cervical stenosis, and adhesions. Mild to moderate lower abdominal pain during mid-cycle (13th to 15th day) sometime associated with blood spotting is due to release of the ovum into peritoneal cavity (Mittelschmerz syndrome).

### Pathophysiology of Dysmenorrhea

The endometrial sloughing during menstruation causes release of prostaglandins (PGs). PGF2 alpha causes vasoconstriction, myometrial contractions, and ischemia. PGE2 causes vasodilation. On the first day of a period, the level of prostaglandins is high. As bleeding continues and the lining of the uterus is shed, the level goes down and pain reduces.

### Differential Diagnosis of Dysmenorrhea

Primary dysmenorrhea is usual in adolescents after 6–12 months of menarche in the absence of gynecological symptoms and examination. Pain appearing in sexually active adolescents, after several years of menstruation, presents throughout cycle and with other gynecological symptoms and signs should raise suspicion of secondary causes. The pain of secondary dysmenorrhea often begins 1–2 weeks prior to menses and persists until a few days after the cessation of the bleeding. History suggestive of endometriosis in family and chronic persistent pain is the indications of undergoing ultrasonography (USG) or diagnostic laparoscopy.

## Management

- Exercise, heat application, adequate sleep and hydration, relaxation, and meditation practices help reduce pain.
- *Drug management:* Prostaglandin synthetase inhibitors (naproxen 550 mg load then 275 mg qid, mefenamic acid 500 mg loading then 250 mg qid, and ibuprofen 400–600 mg qid) are effective in approximately 80% of cases.
- NSAIDs unless contraindicated work best if taken early. Acetaminophen is first line of treatment if NSAIDs cannot be used.
- Combined oral contraceptive pills for 3–6 months in persistent and severe cases.
- *Treatment of secondary cause*: Dilation of a narrow cervical os, myomectomy, polypectomy, dilation and curettage, and laparoscopy.

## Abnormal Uterine Bleeding

It is the term used for uterine bleeding that is abnormal in regularity, volume, frequency, or duration [previously described as dysfunctional uterine bleeding (DUB)]. It affects up to 14% of reproductive-age women. The American College of Obstetricians and Gynecologists (ACOG) has endorsed a new PALM-COEIN classification **(Table 4)** developed in 2011 by the International Federation of Gynecology and Obstetrics (FIGO). This also describes a systematic strategy for its evaluation. Excessive blood loss is usually based on the patient's perception of what appears to be heavy bleeding (more than 25 pads or 30 tampons). A severe bleeding episode requiring immediate treatment is defined as acute AUB and that present for 6 months or longer is defined as chronic AUB. Age-wise common causes are given in **Box 4** and routine evaluation for AUB in **Box 5**.

## Complications

It affects quality of life, sex life, mood changes, causes iron deficiency anemia, and increase in overall healthcare burden.

**TABLE 4:** PALM-COIEN classification for AUB.

*AUB (previously called dysfunctional uterine bleeding DUB)*
- Heavy menstrual bleeding (AUB-HMB) *(previously termed menorrhagia)*
- Intermenstrual bleeding (AUB-IMB) *(previously termed metrorrhagia)*

| *PALM structural causes:* | *COEIN nonstructural causes:* |
|---|---|
| • *Polyp* (AUB-P) | • Coagulopathy(AUB-C) |
| • *Adenomyosis* (AUB-A) | • *Ovulatory dysfunctions* (AUB-O) |
| • *Leiomyoma* (submucosal or other) (AUB-L) | • *Endometrial* (AUB-E) |
| • *Malignancy and hyperplasia* (AUB-M) | • *Iatrogenic* (AUB-I) |
|  | • *Not yet classified* (AUB-N) |

(AUB: abnormal uterine bleeding)

**BOX 4:** Age-wise common causes of abnormal uterine bleeding (AUB).

- *13–18 years*—ovarian dysfunction and anovulation
- *19–39 years*—anovulation [e.g., polycystic ovarian syndrome (PCOS)], pregnancy, medication use, endometrial hyperplasia, and structural abnormalities
- *40 years to menopause*—declining ovarian function. (However, it is important to rule out endometrial hyperplasia, carcinoma, and other structural changes.)

**BOX 5:** Evaluation for abnormal uterine bleeding in adolescent.

- *Common laboratory studies:* CBC, PT, aPTT, BT, pregnancy test, and cervical cultures for chlamydia and gonorrhoea
- *Secondary laboratory studies:* In cases of suspected systemic disorder—T3, T4, TSH, RBS, FBS, PRL, FSH, LH, DHEAS, free testosterone, cortisol, and 17-OHP
- *Imaging studies:* Pelvic ultrasound to identify abnormalities of the uterus, endometrial thickness, adnexal abnormalities, and PCOS MRI/CT rare

(aPTT: activated partial thromboplastin time; BT: bleeding time; CBC: complete blood count; CT: computed tomography; DHEAS: dehydroepiandrosterone sulfate; FBS: fasting blood sugar; FSH: follicle-stimulating hormone; LH: luteinizing hormone; MRI: magnetic resonance imaging; PCOS: polycystic ovarian syndrome; PRL: prolactin; PT: prothrombin time; RBS: random blood sugar; TSH: thyroid stimulating hormone; T3: triiodothyronine; T4: thyroxine; 17-OHP: 17-hydroxyprogesterone)

## Treatment

Pharmacotherapy options are the first line with a focus on combined hormonal contraceptives and levonorgestrel-releasing intrauterine systems. Surgical options, such as dilation and curettage, endometrial ablation,

**TABLE 5:** Treatment of AUB.

| Acute AUB | Chronic AUB |
|---|---|
| • In emergency, IV conjugated equine estrogen 25 mg q4–6 hours for 24 hours then switch to oral pills<br>• Ethinylestradiol 35 µg tid for 1 week then once daily for 3 weeks<br>• Oral progestin—medroxyprogesterone acetate (MPA) 20 mg tid for 7 days<br>• Tranexamic acid 1.3 g q8 hourly for 5 days<br>• Oral iron supplementation | • Combined hormonal pills with ethinylestradiol 25–50 µg with progestin 1 tablet daily, weekly patches or rings with 1 week free after 3 weeks<br>• *Others:* Any of following:<br>  – MPA 2.5–10 mg<br>  – Megestrol acetate 40–100 mg<br>  – Norethindrone 2.5–5 mg<br>  – Micronized progesterone 200–400 mg, OD from 5–21 days of cycle if no ovulatory dysfunctions and OD for 2 weeks (q4w if ovulatory dysfunctions)<br>• LNG-IUS (levonorgestrel-releasing intrauterine system) every 5 yearly<br>• Depot MPA 150 mg IM q3mo<br>• Leuprolide acetate 11.25 mg IM q3mo or 3.75 mg IM/month<br>• Danazol 100–400 mg daily in two divided doses<br>• NSAIDs, tranexamic acid during acute on chronic bleeding<br>• Oral iron supplements |

(AUB: abnormal uterine bleeding; IM: intramuscular; NSAIDs: nonsteroidal anti-inflammatory drugs; IV: intravenous)

and hysterectomy should be reserved for patients in whom pharmacotherapy was ineffective or is contra-indicated. For acute AUB, therapy goals include controlling the current bleeding episode, reducing the potential for future episodes, and decreasing blood loss during subsequent menstrual cycles. Detailed treatment is given in **Table 5**.

## Polycystic Ovarian Syndrome

This has been discussed in respective *Chapter 4A.3*.

## KEY MESSAGES

- Menstruation-related problems are common in adolescent girls.
- Information related to menstruation, hygiene, common home remedies, menstrual myths, and abnormalities helps adolescent girls and women to enhance their reproductive health.
- The common menstrual disorders in adolescents are amenorrhea, abnormal/excessive bleeding, dysmenorrhea, and PMS.
- An accurate diagnosis can be obtained by thorough history, complete physical examination, and focused investigations in menstrual disorders.

## RECOMMENDED READING


1. ACOG. (2023). Premenstual Syndrome (PMS). [online] Available from https://www.acog.org/womens-health/faqs/premenstrual-syndrome [Last accessed March, 2024].
2. Bhave SY, Nair MKC, Parthsarathy A, Menon PSN, Greydanus DE (Eds). Bhave's Textbook of Adolescent Medicine. Peepee Publishers; 2006. pp. 95-9.
3. CDC. (2023). Menstrual Hygiene. [online] Available from https://www.cdc.gov/hygiene/personal-hygiene/menstrual.html [Last accessed March, 2024].
4. Garg S, Anand T (Eds). Menstruation related myths in India: Strategies for combating it. J Fam Med Primary Care. 2015;4:184-6.
5. Hale K. (2018). Abnormal Uterine Bleeding: A Review [online] Available from https://www.uspharmacist.com/article/abnormal-uterine-bleeding-a-review [Last accessed March, 2024].
6. Hoffman B, Schorge J, Bradshaw K, Halvorson L, Schaffer J, Corton M (Eds). Williams Gynaecology, 3rd edition. McGraw-Hill Education; 2016. pp. 348-55.
7. Kliegman, Stanton, St Geme, Schor (Eds). Nelson Textbook of Paediatrics, First South Asia Edition, Volume 1. Elsevier; 2015. pp.963-68.
8. Nair MKC, Parthsarathy A (Eds). Sexual Reproductive Health of Young People. New Delhi: Jaypee Brothers Medical Publishers; 2006. pp. 17-22.
9. Pundir J, Coomarasamy A. Gynaecology: Evidence-Based Algorithms. Cambridge University Press. 2016. pp. 28-35.

# 4A.8 — Endocrine Emergencies in Adolescents

*Saurabh Uppal*

## ■ INTRODUCTION

The common endocrine emergencies encountered in the adolescent age group are:

- Diabetic ketoacidosis (DKA)
- Hypoglycemia
- Hypocalcemia
- Adrenal crisis
- Thyroid storm
- Gonadal torsion.

## ■ DIABETIC KETOACIDOSIS

Diabetic ketoacidosis stands as a formidable endocrine emergency demanding expeditious recognition and intervention in adolescents afflicted by diabetes mellitus.

### Pathophysiology

Diabetic ketoacidosis evolves from an intricate interplay of severe insulin deficiency and counter-regulatory hormonal elevation. In adolescents with diabetes, the pathophysiological cascade typically initiates with insufficient insulin, triggering a surge in glucagon, cortisol, and catecholamines. The resultant hepatic gluconeogenesis and glycogenolysis lead to hyperglycemia. Concurrently, lipolysis is accentuated, leading to the release of free fatty acids (FFAs). These FFAs undergo hepatic oxidation, resulting in the production of ketone bodies—acetoacetate, beta-hydroxybutyrate, and acetone. The ensuing ketonemia, along with metabolic acidosis, results from the accumulation of ketoacids. The absence of adequate insulin action fosters unrestrained lipolysis, ketogenesis, and resultant acidosis—a triad characteristic of DKA.

### Diagnostic Criteria

- Hyperglycemia (blood glucose typically exceeding 200 mg/dL)
- Ketonemia
- Metabolic acidosis (arterial/venous pH <7.3 or bicarbonate <15 mEq/L) Clinical presentation often includes polyuria, polydipsia, vomiting, and altered mental status. Ancillary findings such as electrolyte imbalances (hyperkalemia initially due to intracellular–extracellular shift, later transitioning to hypokalemia as treatment ensues) further support the diagnosis.

### Management

#### Fluid Resuscitation

Initiate isotonic saline promptly to address dehydration and restore intravascular volume. Calculate fluid requirements judiciously, factoring in deficits and ongoing losses.

- *Fluid type:* 0.9% NaCl or 0.45% NaCl
- *Bolus dose (0.9% NaCl):* 10–20 mL/kg over 1–2 hours if there are signs of a hypovolemic shock. If moderate dehydration is present, a bolus of 10 mL/kg can be administered.
- Continuous infusion beyond the first hour of therapy should consist of replacement losses (5–10% of current body weight) plus maintenance fluid spread evenly over 48 hours. 5% dextrose is to be added as blood glucose falls below 250 mg/dL and 10% dextrose below 150 mg/dL.

#### Insulin Administration

Administer intravenous regular insulin cautiously to correct hyperglycemia and suppress ketogenesis. It is best achieved by a continuous infusion titrated to achieve a controlled decline in blood glucose, ideally not >90–100 mg/dL/hr.

- *Insulin type*: Regular insulin via continuous infusion started at 0.1 units/kg/hr and hourly monitoring of blood glucose
- *Transition to subcutaneous insulin*: Once ketoacidosis resolves (arterial/venous pH >7.3 and bicarbonate >18 mEq/L), subcutaneous insulin should be started. Temptation to reduce insulin infusion rate as blood glucose reduces should be avoided. Addition of dextrose in maintenance fluid should be titrated below a blood glucose of 250 mg/dL until these insulin transition endpoints are achieved.

#### Electrolyte Correction

Monitor potassium closely, initiating supplementation as required. Start at 40–60 mEq/L if serum levels <3.5 mEq/L;

delay insulin infusion till low potassium is corrected. Add 30–40 mEq/L if serum potassium 3.5–5.3 mEq/L. Routine use of bicarbonate administration is not advisable (unless symptomatic hyperkalemia is present or pH <6.9 with hemodynamic compromise despite aggressive fluid resuscitation).

## Monitoring and Adjustments

Implement vigilant monitoring of blood glucose, ketones, electrolytes, and acid–base status. Adjust insulin infusion rates and fluid replacement in response to evolving clinical and laboratory parameters.

*Monitoring parameters:*
- *Blood glucose:* Hourly
- *Ketones:* Regularly
- *Electrolytes:* Potassium, sodium, chloride
- *Arterial blood gas (ABG):* As needed for acid–base status
- *Neurological status:* Every 2 hours.

*Identification and treatment of precipitating factors:* Identify and address underlying triggers, such as infections or medication noncompliance, to preclude DKA recurrence.

*Transition to subcutaneous insulin:* As clinical and biochemical parameters stabilize, transition to subcutaneous insulin therapy, ensuring seamless continuity of glycemic control. Immediately after resolution of DKA, insulin requirement may be high and children may need insulin doses at 1–3 IU/kg/day for this phase of transition.

## ■ HYPOGLYCEMIA

Hypoglycemia, otherwise uncommon in adolescents but a common concern in adolescents with diabetes, results from excessive insulin or inadequate carbohydrate intake. Clinical manifestations range from autonomic to neuroglycopenic symptoms.

Emergency intervention involves prompt administration of glucose 2 mL/kg of 25% dextrose or 5 mL/kg of 10% dextrose if the patient is unable to take oral glucose in the form of powdered glucose (Glucon D) 7.5 g dissolved in 100–150 mL water. Repeat blood glucose estimation should be done after 20 minutes with a repeat dose administered if necessary. Refractory hypoglycemia may necessitate administration of parenteral glucagon. Preventive strategies encompass personalized insulin regimens, vigilant blood glucose monitoring, and reinforcement of diabetes education.

## ■ HYPOCALCEMIA

Hypocalcemia in adolescents arises from diverse etiologies, such as impaired calcium absorption, increased losses, and diminished parathyroid hormone (PTH) secretion or activity. Notably, nutritional deficiencies, malabsorption syndromes, and chronic renal insufficiency feature prominently in the etiological spectrum. Critical illness, sepsis, or extensive blood transfusions may precipitate hypocalcemia through citrate-mediated chelation or altered calcium homeostasis. Anxiety-induced hyperventilation, poor compliance with medication for a preexisting calcium disorder, and vitamin D deficiency during pubertal growth spurt are other common etiologies encountered in this age group.

The parathyroid glands play a pivotal role in calcium regulation. Hypocalcemia may result from hypoparathyroidism or impaired PTH function, compromising the stimulation of renal calcium reabsorption and bone resorption. Furthermore, vitamin D deficiency, whether nutritional or due to malabsorption, impedes intestinal calcium absorption, exacerbating the hypocalcemic state.

### Diagnosis

Hypocalcemia often manifests with neuromuscular irritability, including perioral numbness, tetany, seizures, and, in severe cases, laryngospasm. ECG findings may reveal QT prolongation, indicative of impaired myocardial repolarization.

Serum calcium concentration is below the age-specific reference range. Importantly, assessment of ionized calcium provides a more accurate reflection of the physiologically active form, especially in situations where hypoalbuminemia may be present. Concurrent evaluation of serum phosphate, magnesium, and alkaline phosphatase aids in elucidating potential underlying causes. Documentation of a Vitamin D replete status is important before committing to another diagnosis as the etiology of hypocalcemia.

### Management

The therapeutic approach to adolescent hypocalcemia necessitates a multifaceted strategy addressing both acute manifestations and underlying etiologies.

### *Acute Symptomatic Hypocalcemia*

Administer intravenous 10% calcium gluconate solution (0.5 mL/kg) over 10 minutes diluted in 100 mL normal saline preferably in a large vein and under ECG monitoring to detect iatrogenic arrhythmia. After initial stabilization, start maintenance infusion of 10% calcium gluconate at 1–5 mL/kg/day or oral calcium supplements at 50–75 mg/kg/day in four divided doses. For adolescents, the maximum dose of oral calcium supplements is 2 g/day. Concurrent vitamin D supplementation facilitates intestinal calcium absorption.

### Addressing Underlying Etiologies

Identification and correction of underlying causes, such as vitamin D deficiency, hypoparathyroidism, or renal dysfunction, constitute a cornerstone in preventing recurrence.

### Regular Monitoring

Serial monitoring of serum calcium levels, along with adjustments in supplementation, ensures optimal control and mitigates the risk of hypercalcemia. In chronic hypocalcemia secondary to hypoparathyroidism or pseudohypoparathyroidism, the aim of treatment is to keep calcium levels in the low normal range to prevent hypercalciuria and nephrocalcinosis. In these situations, calcitriol [15 ng/kg/day (up to 1.5 µg/day)] and alfacalcidol [25 ng/kg (up to 2 µg/day)] needs to be administered. Spot urine calcium creatinine ratio should be repeated every 6 months to document normocalciuria. Oral calcium supplements may be necessary if the adolescent's diet is deficient in calcium. The absorption of calcium from milk and other dairy products is better than that obtained from supplements. Above a dose of 500 mg, the absorption of calcium reaches a plateau so multiple divided doses are preferred if higher doses are needed in adolescents.

## ■ ADRENAL CRISIS

Adrenal crisis, an acute and life-threatening manifestation of adrenal insufficiency, necessitates swift recognition and precise intervention to mitigate morbidity and mortality in the adolescent population. Adrenal crisis ensues from an acute insufficiency of glucocorticoids, mineralocorticoids, or both, typically stemming from primary adrenal disorders or abrupt withdrawal of exogenous glucocorticoid therapy. In adolescents, the most common etiology is underlying autoimmune adrenalitis, contributing to the insidious destruction of the adrenal cortex. This process culminates in compromised cortisol and aldosterone production, leading to systemic consequences.

The lack of cortisol, a crucial stress hormone, results in impaired glucose metabolism, diminished anti-inflammatory responses, and compromised vascular tone regulation. Concurrent aldosterone deficiency contributes to electrolyte imbalances, particularly hyperkalemia and hyponatremia, predisposing the individual to profound hemodynamic instability.

*Precipitating factors:* Adrenal crisis may be precipitated by stressors such as infection, trauma, surgery, or psychological distress. Abrupt cessation of exogenous glucocorticoid therapy, particularly in individuals on chronic steroid regimens or in cases of unwarranted steroid misuse, poses a notable risk. Moreover, adrenal crisis can be the initial presentation in adolescents with undiagnosed adrenal insufficiency.

*Clinical Presentation:* Profound weakness, fatigue, abdominal pain, nausea, vomiting, and altered mental status. Hypotension refractory to fluid resuscitation, hyponatremia, hyperkalemia, and hypoglycemia may be evident.

## Laboratory Findings

Serum cortisol levels markedly below the normal range.

Elevated adrenocorticotropic hormone (ACTH) levels are indicative of a primary adrenal insufficiency.

*Ancillary investigations:* Blood gas analysis may reveal metabolic acidosis. Electrocardiogram (ECG) may demonstrate characteristic changes associated with hyperkalemia.

## Management

### Immediate Resuscitation

Intravenous fluid resuscitation with isotonic saline at 20 mL/kg to address hypovolemia and hypotension is done. Administration of intravenous hydrocortisone as the glucocorticoid of choice in a dose of 100 mg/m$^2$/day in four divided doses over the first 24 hours and tapered over the next 2–3 days after clinical stability is recommended. Hypoglycemia needs prompt correction with 2.5 mL/kg of 10% dextrose; repeat if necessary after 20 minutes. IV DNS (5%) may be required at 1.5–2 times maintenance if recurrent hypoglycemia is present. Mineralocorticoid replacement with fludrocortisone is necessary only when transitioned to oral therapy. Hyperkalemia may require intravenous administration of calcium gluconate and insulin with glucose.

## Monitoring and Ongoing Treatment

- Continuous monitoring of hemodynamic parameters, electrolytes, and blood glucose
- Initiation/dose adjustment of long-term glucocorticoid and mineralocorticoid replacement as appropriate, addressing the underlying adrenal insufficiency

Identification and management of precipitating factors:
- Thorough investigation and treatment of underlying triggers, such as infections or stressors, to prevent recurrence.
- *Patient and family education:* Comprehensive education on steroid replacement therapy, stress dosing, and recognition of adrenal crisis symptoms for both patients and caregivers.

## ■ THYROID STORM

*Triggers and precipitating factors:* Thyroid storm (also known as thyrotoxic crisis) is a rare but an acute life-threatening manifestation of thyrotoxicosis that presents with multisystem involvement. It is more common with Graves' disease but can occur with other hyperthyroid states like multinodular goiter and toxic thyroid adenoma. Precipitating factors are uncontrolled hyperthyroidism, infection, trauma, or nonadherence to antithyroid medications. Stressors, such as surgery or diabetic ketoacidosis, can exacerbate the hypermetabolic state.

The clinical presentation is caused by a sudden increase in thyroid hormones and hyperadrenergic manifestations, including hyperpyrexia, tachycardia, and hypertension. Profound alterations in mental status, ranging from agitation to delirium, are common. Gastrointestinal symptoms, such as vomiting and diarrhea, contribute to the multisystem involvement. Recognition of these features is paramount, given their potential to escalate swiftly and precipitate life-threatening complications.

The diagnosis of a thyrotoxic state is clinical. Serum thyroid function tests confirm the diagnosis. Very high levels of thyroid hormones are not a prerequisite for the diagnosis. Additional laboratory findings may be hypercalcemia, hyperglycemia, raised WBC count, and markers of end-organ dysfunction, such as hepatic transaminases and cardiac biomarkers.

Treatment consists of beta-blockers and glucocorticoids to alleviate acute symptoms, and antithyroid medications, such as methimazole and oral iodine to attenuate thyroid hormone synthesis. Supportive measures include fluid resuscitation, cooling strategies, and meticulous management of associated complications. Patient education on adherence, trigger recognition, stress management, and timely intervention is very important.

## ■ TESTICULAR TORSION

Although a urologic emergency, it is important for the adolescent medicine practitioner to be aware of this important emergency. Torsion is marked by the abnormal twisting of the spermatic cord, leading to compromised blood flow to the testicle and triggering hormonal changes that impact Leydig cell function responsible for testosterone production.

Clinical signs include sudden-onset severe testicular pain, scrotal swelling, and nausea. Physical examination may reveal the "bell-clapper" deformity, and Doppler ultrasound is essential for diagnosis.

Urgent medical attention is imperative due to the potential consequences of ischemia, including hormonal changes affecting testosterone production. Prompt surgical intervention involves detwisting the spermatic cord and may include orchidopexy to prevent future torsion. Postoperatively, monitoring testosterone levels is crucial, with hormonal supplementation considered if deficiency persists. Counseling must be provided to adolescents and their families regarding the risk of recurrence and the importance of prompt medical attention if symptoms reoccur.

## ■ OVARIAN TORSION

Ovarian torsion, akin to testicular torsion, is characterized by the abnormal rotation of the ovary around its vascular pedicle. This rotation leads to compromised blood flow to the ovary, resulting in ischemia and necessitating prompt intervention. Clinical manifestations include sudden-onset pelvic pain, often accompanied by nausea and vomiting. Physical examination may reveal tenderness, an adnexal mass, or asymmetry in pelvic organ position. Ultrasound aids in confirming the diagnosis by detecting reduced or absent blood flow to the affected ovary. Surgical intervention involves untwisting the ovary, addressing any adnexal pathology, and securing the ovary to prevent future torsion.

## ■ KEY MESSAGES

- Management of diabetic ketoacidosis is aimed at correction of acidosis. Insulin infusion is guided by pH and bicarbonate levels rather than blood glucose levels.

- Adequate fluid and insulin replacement contribute to early recovery from DKA.
- In an adolescent with hypocalcemia, an underlying undiagnosed disorder of calcium axis must be considered.
- Vitamin D replete status must be documented before committing to another etiology for hypocalcemia.
- Diagnosis of adrenal crisis requires a high index of suspicion, especially in the setting of acute metabolic stress. Empirical use of parenteral steroid may be considered while awaiting results.
- Hyperadrenergic symptoms in a child on antithyroid medications should be taken as a thyroid storm needing prompt management.
- Acute severe lower abdominal pain in an adolescent should alert the clinician to the possibility of gonadal torsion. A good physical examination can rule out torsion.

## ■ RECOMMENDED READING

1. Abisad DA, Glenn Lecea EM, Ballesteros AM, Alarcon G, Diaz A, Pagan-Banchs P. Thyroid storm in pediatrics: a systematic review. J Pediatr Endocrinol Metab. 2022;36(3): 225-33.
2. Calimag APP, Chlebek S, Lerma EV, Chaiban JT. Diabetic ketoacidosis. Dis Mon. 2023;69(3):101418.
3. Dasgupta R, Renaud E, Goldin AB, Baird R, Cameron DB, Arnold MA, et al. Ovarian torsion in pediatric and adolescent patients: a systematic review. J Pediatr Surg. 2018;53(7):1387-91.
4. Edwards BL, Dorfman D. High-risk Pediatric Emergencies. Emerg Med Clin North Am. 2020;38(2):383-400.
5. Root AW, Diamond FB Jr. Disorders of calcium and phosphorus metabolism in adolescents. Endocrinol Metab Clin North Am. 1993;22(3):573-92.
6. Rushworth RL, Chrisp GL, Bownes S, Torpy DJ, Falhammar H. Adrenal crises in adolescents and young adults. Endocrine. 2022;77(1):1-10.

# Part B: Systemic Conditions

***Sub-section Editors:*** *Samir Shah, Poonam Bhatia, Shailaja Mane*

## 4B.1 | Common Skin and Hair Problems in Adolescents

*R Prema, Harikishan Kumar Y, Chitra Dinakar, JS Nikhil Ram*

### ■ INTRODUCTION

Skin diseases are a major health problem affecting a high proportion of the population in India. Skin diseases can place a heavy emotional and psychological burden on patients that may be far worse than the physical impact. Increased consciousness, especially among the youth about their body and beauty, further aggravates their anxiety. Adolescent dermatological problems contribute about one-third of all consultations in the setting of both pediatrics and dermatology outpatient services. The prevalence of skin diseases in adolescents varies considerably in different parts of the world. Atopic dermatitis is the most prevalent dermatosis in the Middle East and Western countries. In India, according to the Global Burden of Disease (GBD) study, acne vulgaris affects about 85% of young adults aged 12–15 years. Its prevalence in males was slightly higher when compared to females as sebaceous glands begin to develop at an age of 7–8 years due to adrenarche and sebum production related to testosterone levels. Infections and infestations are also the most common skin problems, seen in nearly half of the adolescent cases followed by dermatitis (25%). Of these, bacterial infections contribute to 27.29% and scabies and pediculosis in 10.16% of the cases. Fungal and viral infections are observed in 4.65% and 3.68% of the cases, respectively. Allergic reactions like urticaria, papular urticaria, and drug reactions are reported in 6.5% of the children. Disorders of hair and nails are seen in 5.2% of the children.

### ■ CLASSIFICATION OF COMMON PEDIATRIC DERMATOSES

Classification of common pediatric dermatoses is given in **Box 1**.

---

**BOX 1:** Classification of common pediatric dermatoses.

- Infestations and infections
- *Dermatitis and eczema:* Seborrheic dermatitis, atopic dermatitis
- Urticaria
- *Pigmentary disorders:* Vitiligo, café-au-lait macules
- *Diseases of hair:* Alopecia areata
- *Disorders of appendages:* Acne vulgaris
- *Miscellaneous conditions:* Papular urticaria, miliaria rubra, miliaria crystallina

---

### ■ MANAGEMENT OF COMMON SKIN PROBLEMS AMONG ADOLESCENTS

Management of common skin problems among adolescents is given in **Table 1**.

### ■ ACNE VULGARIS

#### Definition

Acne vulgaris can be defined as a chronic, self-limiting, inflammatory disease of the pilosebaceous unit, manifesting generally in adolescence with pleomorphic lesions like comedones, papules, pustules, nodules, and cysts, and these may lead to scarring. It is the most prevalent skin disease in the pediatric population and is nearly universal in that most individuals will be affected by it at some point in their lives. Acne vulgaris is multifactorial in origin, and several factors affect the severity of acne like androgens, sebaceous hyperplasia with seborrhea, and altered cornification and differentiation. The organism—a terminology change from *Propionibacterium acnes* to *Cutibacterium acnes*—has been proposed based upon genomic analysis, inflammation, and immune response.

**TABLE 1:** Management of common skin problems among adolescents.

**Infections**

| Bacterial | Etiology | Typical lesions | Management |
|---|---|---|---|
| Impetigo | *Staphylococcus aureus, Streptococcus pyogenes* | Small papulovesicles or pustules rupture to form honey-colored crusted plaques with erythema (**Figs. 1A and B**) | Topical fusidic acid and mupirocin 2–3 times a day |
| Folliculitis and furuncle | Coagulase-positive *Staphylococcus* organisms | Erythematous papules and pustules with perilesional erythema centered on hair follicles (**Figs. 2 and 3**) | Topical mupirocin and fusidic acid 2–3 times a day |

| Fungal | | | |
|---|---|---|---|
| Tinea versicolor | *Malassezia furfur* | Patchy and scaly discoloration of skin on upper chest and back and upper extremities (**Fig. 4**) | • Potassium hydroxide test from skin scraping<br>• Topical selenium sulfide or oral fluconazole |
| Tinea corporis | Trichophyton, Microsporum, Epidermophyton | Annular lesion with erythematous border and scaly with clear center | • KOH mount of the scale<br>• Terbinafine and Itraconazole |

| Viral | | | |
|---|---|---|---|
| Viral warts | Human papilloma virus 1, 2, 4, and 7 | Hyperkeratotic verrucous papules which occur as multiple lesions | Cryodestruction |
| Molluscum contagiosum | Molluscum contagiosum virus | Multiple asymptomatic pearly white papules with central umbilication (**Figs. 5A and B**) | Curette, cryotherapy, and topical tretinoin |

| Infestations | | | |
|---|---|---|---|
| Scabies | Mite sarcoptes scabiei var hominis | Transmitted by skin-to-skin contact. Manifests as nocturnal pruritus on face, palms, and soles in infants (**Figs. 6 and 7**). Waist, wrists, and ankles in older children | • Identification of mites, eggs in skin scrapings by light microscopy<br>• Permethrin cream, oral ivermectin |

| Dermatitis | | | |
|---|---|---|---|
| Seborrheic dermatitis | *Malassezia ovalis* yeast | Yellow greasy scales on an erythematous base seen on scalp, eyebrows, eyelids, nasolabial folds, ears, sternal area, axilla, and groin (**Figs. 8 and 9**) | Selenium sulfide, ketoconazole, topical corticosteroids |

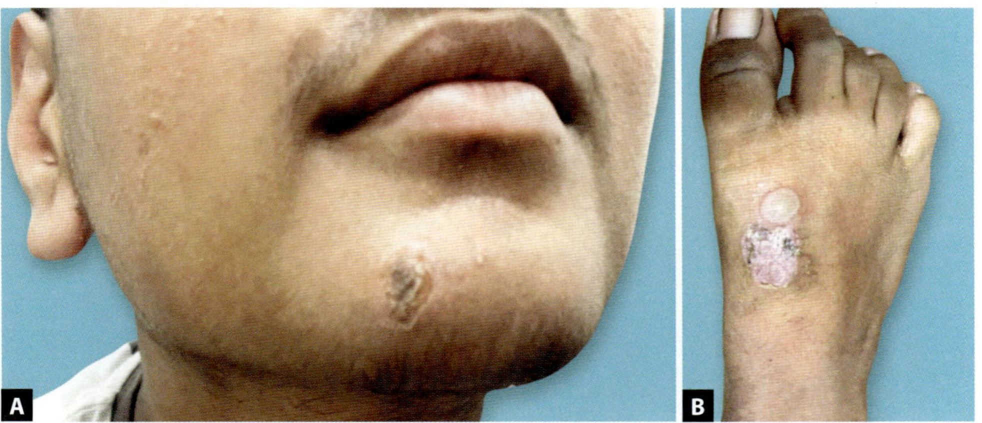


**Figs. 1A and B:** Multiple crusted plaques seen on the (A) face and (B) foot in impetigo.

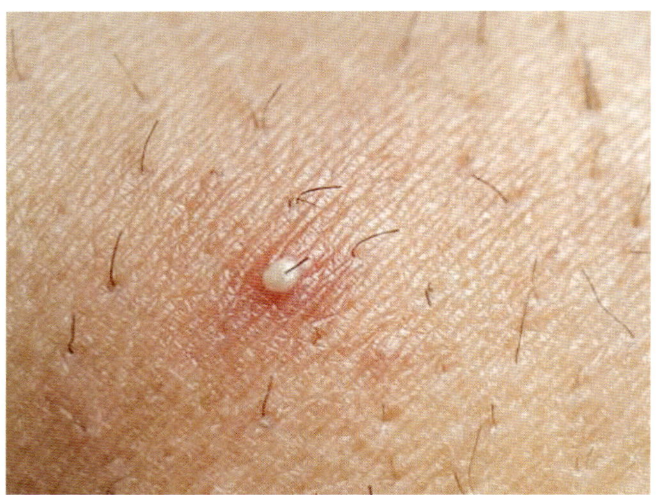

**Fig. 2:** Follicular pustule with rim of erythema.

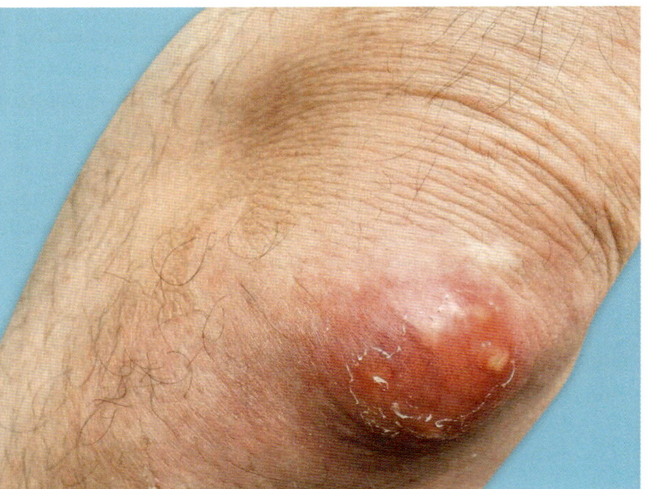

**Fig. 3:** Furuncle on the elbow.

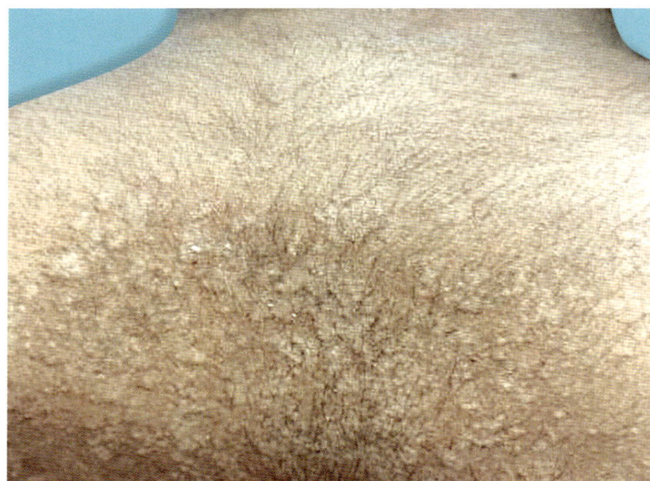

**Fig. 4:** Typical furfuraceous scales in pityriasis versicolor.

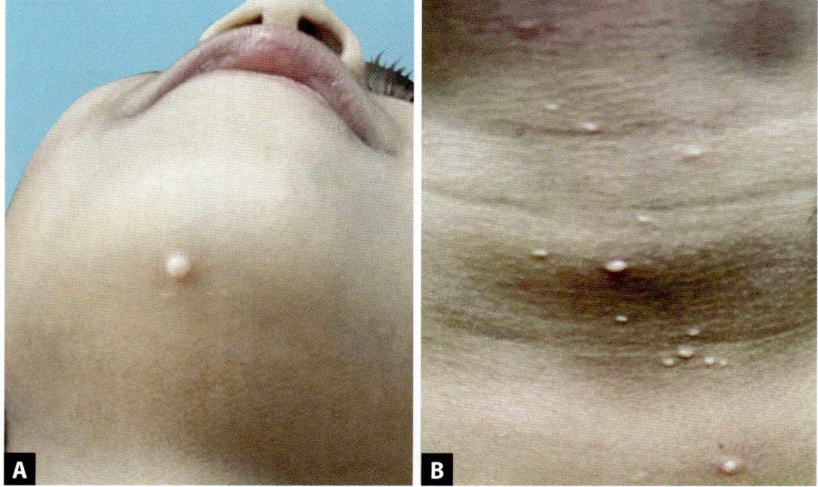

**Figs. 5A and B:** Multiple umbilicated papules seen in molluscum contagiosum.

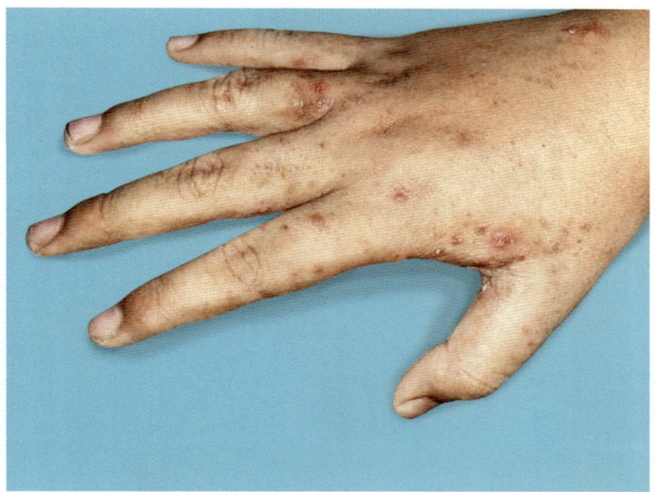

**Fig. 6:** Web space and fingers involvement in scabies.

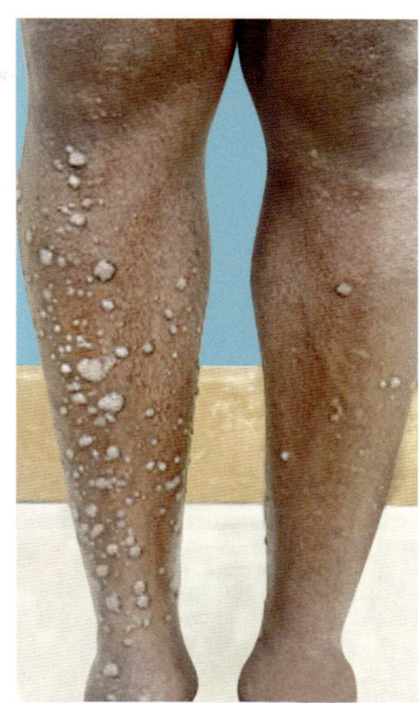

**Fig. 8:** Multiple warts on the lower limbs.

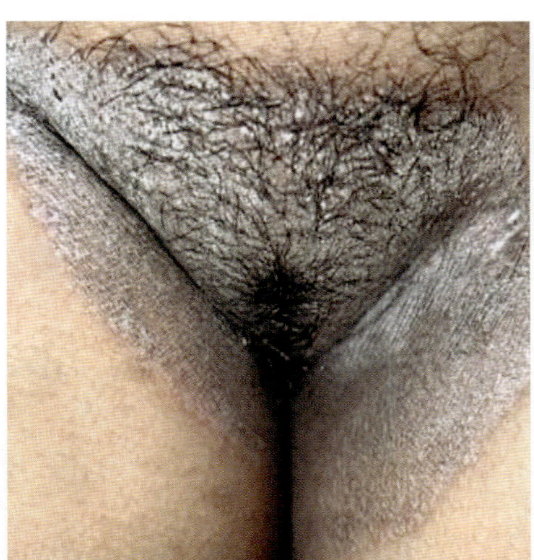

**Fig. 7:** Hyperpigmented erythematous plaques with scaling in tinea corporis.

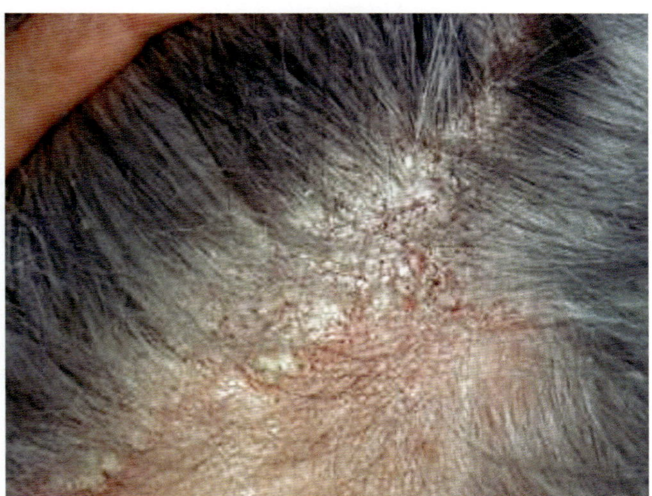

**Fig. 9:** Seborrheic dermatitis involving the scalp.

## Clinical Features

Acne vulgaris was graded by Indian authors, using a simple grading system **(Figs. 10A to D)**, which classifies acne vulgaris into four grades as follows:

- *Grade I (Mild):* Comedones, occasional papules
- *Grade II (Moderate):* Comedones, many papules, few pustules
- *Grade III (Severe):* Predominantly pustules, nodules, and abscesses also called acne conglobata (AC)
- *Grade IV (Cystic):* Mainly cysts or abscesses, widespread scarring

## General Measures in Management of Acne (Flowchart 1)

- Education and counseling on making the patient understand about the disease
- Avoid the use of oils, pomades, and heavy cosmetics.
- Avoid the excess consumption of fats, oils, and dairy products.
- Regular face wash and maintenance of personal hygiene
- Elimination of emotional stress by reassurance
- Awareness regarding premenstrual flare and seasonal variation.

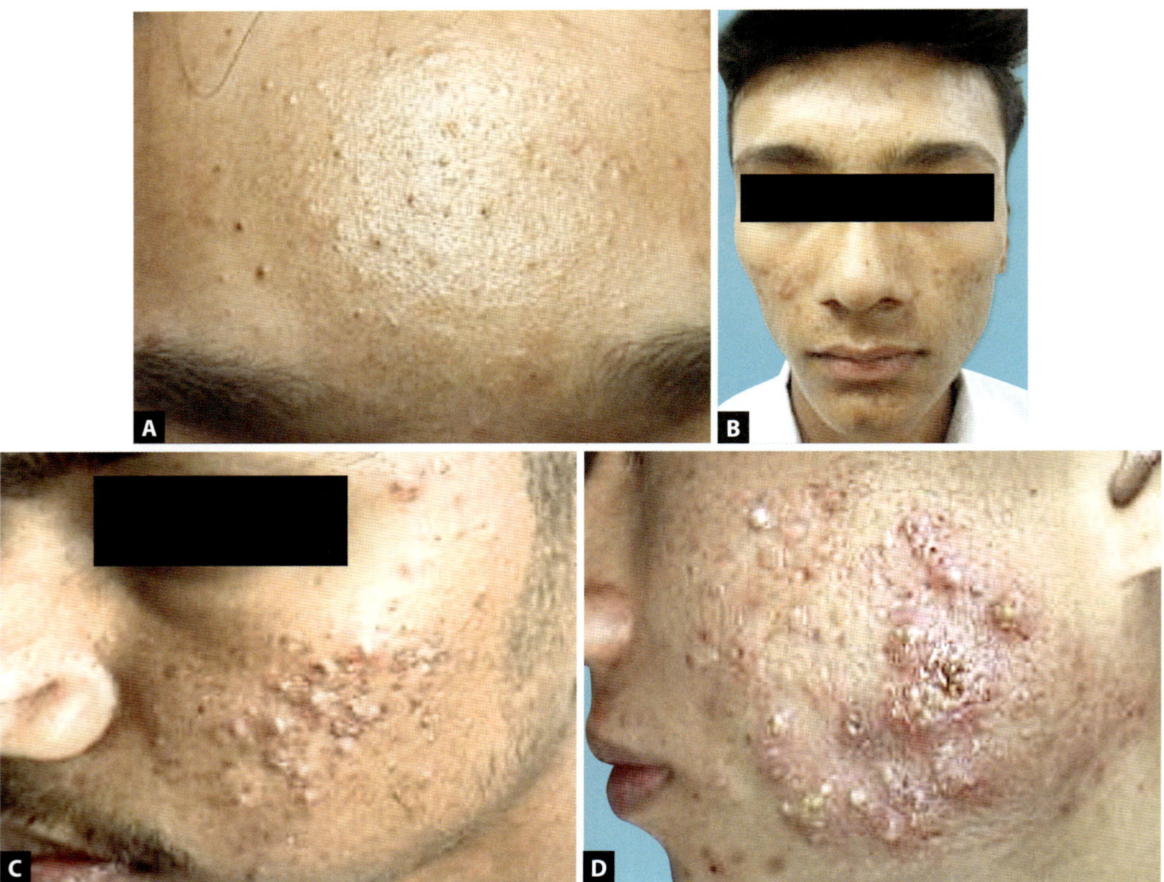

**Figs. 10A to D:** (A) Grade 1 acne; (B) Grade 2 acne; (C) Grade 3 acne; (D) Grade 4 acne.

Mainstay of Treatment:

**Flowchart 1:** Management of acne.

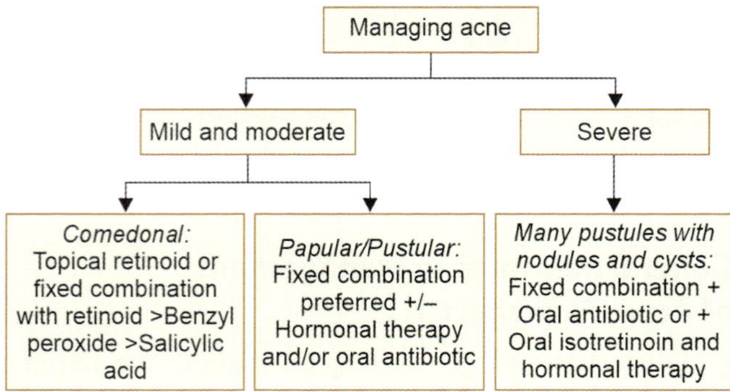

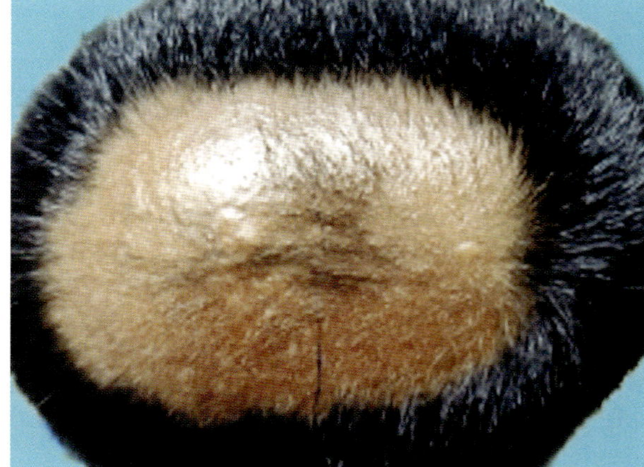

**Fig. 11:** Alopecia areata on the scalp.

## ■ HAIR LOSS: ALOPECIA AREATA

### Definition

Alopecia areata (AA) is a common, chronic inflammatory disease directed against the anagen hair follicle, causing nonscarring alopecia of the scalp, beard, and/or body hair **(Fig. 11)**. AA has been hypothetically attributed to various etiological factors including infectious, metabolic, vascular, endocrine, nutritional, neuropathic, and trophoneurotic.

## Clinical Features

Alopecia areata is characterized by sudden onset of (nonscarring) hair loss in one or several circumscribed areas in the scalp. Although it usually involves the scalp, AA can also affect the beard, eyebrows, eyelashes, and other body areas.

## Diagnosis and Treatment

Diagnosis of AA is easy and straightforward just based on clinical evaluation. Microscopy of completely plucked hair shows a "mixed telogen–dystrophic anagen pattern" in AA. Although spontaneous regrowth occurs in AA, treatment is advised in order to hasten the resolution process. Topical mid (betamethasone dipropionate 0.05% lotion) to potent steroid (clobetasol propionate 0.05% lotion) for a period of 4 weeks is the treatment of choice. Intradermal injection of triamcinolone acetonide at a concentration of 2.5 mg/mL for the eyebrows and 10 mg/mL for the scalp ($0.1 \ mL/cm^2$) is an alternative option. Three doses are given at 3 weekly intervals.

## ■ KEY MESSAGES

- Skin diseases can adversely affect the quality of life of an individual. Adolescence is a critical time in biophysical development, and adverse skin conditions during this period can alter the growth in self-confidence and self-esteem and social engagement.
- Adolescent self-esteem is easily threatened when a highly visible skin disorder becomes a focus for unwelcome peer attention.
- Skin diseases in children may lead to considerable discomfort and embarrassment and unnecessary absence from school and workplace which delivers notable impact on psychosocial behavior and quality of life.

- Infections and infestations are very common in residential schools due to their poor hygienic practices.
- The role of cosmetology also plays a very important role in adolescent skin health; many topical agents available as over-the-counter drugs maybe overused by the adolescents for reasons like skin brightening or as skin fairness agents. Parents and doctors must have a strict vigil over this as it may lead to conditions like irritant contact dermatitis, topical steroid damaged facies, etc.
- Mental and psychological support is always a must for adolescents with body dysmorphic disorder (BDD), a mental health condition where an individual spends a lot of time worrying about flaws in their appearance, and mostly these flaws are unnoticeable to others.

## ■ RECOMMENDED READING


1. Joseph N, Kumar GS, Nelliyanil M. Skin diseases and conditions among students of a medical college in southern India. Indian Dermatol Online J. 2014;5:19-24.
2. Krowchuk D, Mancini A. Acne. In: Pediatric Dermatology, 2nd edition. New Delhi: Jaypee Brothers Medical Publishers; 2015. pp. 21-131.
3. Poojary S, Jaiswal S. Skin at different ages. In: Sacchidanand S, Oberoi C, Inamdar A (Eds). IADVL Textbook of Dermatology, 4th edition. Mumbai: Bhalani Medical House Book; 2018. pp. 202-3.
4. Sanfilippo AM, Barrio V, Kulp-Shorten C, Callen JP. Common Pediatric and Adolescent Skin Conditions, J Pediatr Adolesc Gynecol. 2003;16(5):269-83.
5. Sethuraman G, Bhari N. Common Skin Problems in Children. Indian J Pediatr. 2014;81:381-90.
6. Thappa, D.M. Common skin problems. Indian J Pediatr. 2002;69:701-6.
7. Xu L, Liu KX, Senna MM. A Practical Approach to the Diagnosis and Management of Hair Loss in Children and Adolescents. Front Med. 2017;4:112.

# 4B.2 Common Gastrointestinal Problems in Adolescents

*Prashant Kariya*

## ■ INTRODUCTION

Adolescence is a pivotal stage of life marked by rapid growth and development, making it particularly susceptible to gastrointestinal (GI) disorders. GI disorders can significantly impact the well-being of adolescents, often manifesting as a range of uncomfortable and disruptive symptoms. Common GI disorders in this age group include recurrent vomiting and chronic abdominal pain (CAP).

*Recurrent vomiting can be due to:*
- Gastroesophageal reflux disease (GERD)
- Cyclical vomiting syndrome (CVS)
- Corrosive GI injury

*Chronic abdominal pain can be due to:*
- Organic causes (10–15%) like irritable bowel syndrome (IBS), inflammatory bowel disease (IBD), and celiac disease
- Functional abdominal pain (FAP) (70–85%)
- Psychogenic (5%).

## ■ GASTROESOPHAGEAL REFLUX DISEASE

Gastroesophageal reflux disease is a condition where stomach contents flow back into the esophagus, causing symptoms and potential complications. A study by Akinola et al., found a high GERD prevalence in adolescents at 32.8%.

Treatment for GERD involves various strategies, including lifestyle modifications and the use of specific drugs. These methods include the following:

- *Lifestyle modifications:*
  - Weight reduction is recommended for individuals who are obese or overweight.
  - Elevating the head end of the bed during sleep
  - Consuming small, frequent meals
  - Avoiding the intake of caffeinated drinks, alcohol, smoking, chocolates, as well as deep-fried, oily, and smoked foods
- *Drug therapies:*
  - H2-receptor antagonists (H2RA) drugs
    - Ranitidine at 3–5 mg/kg/day
  - Proton-pump inhibitors (PPI)
    - Omeprazole at 0.5–1 mg/kg/day
    - Lansoprazole at 1–4 mg/kg/day

These are generally taken 30 minutes before breakfast for 6–8 weeks.

### Cyclical Vomiting Syndrome

Cyclic vomiting syndrome is a disorder characterized by the occurrence of recurrent, discrete, and self-limited episodes of vomiting. Diagnosis is primarily established using symptom-based criteria, and it is important to note that patients typically present with negative findings in laboratory tests, radiographic imaging, and endoscopic examinations.

In a recent consensus statement on the diagnosis of CVS in children, *NASPGHAN* (North American Society for Pediatric Gastroenterology, Hepatology, And Nutrition) introduced criteria that consist of the following elements:

**TABLE 1:** Gastroesophageal reflux disease (GERD).

| Clinical features | • *Esophageal manifestations:* Vomiting, retrosternal heartburn, dysphagia, odynophagia<br>• Extraesophageal manifestations involve ear, nose, throat (ENT) and oral cavity<br>  – Chronic laryngitis, chronic sinusitis, otitis media, hoarseness of voice, night cough, sore throat, postnasal drip, nasal congestion, halitosis, dental erosions, paroxysmal laryngospasm and recurrent wheeze, aspiration pneumonia, laryngeal and subglottic stenosis, laryngeal and pharyngeal carcinoma |
|---|---|
| Complications | Peptic strictures, Barrett's esophagus, adenocarcinoma |
| Investigations | Upper GI endoscopy is commonly employed to assess mucosal changes, the presence of hiatus hernia, and the development of strictures. Meanwhile, the gold standard tests for GERD diagnosis include the 24-hour pH monitoring test and impedance manometry |

- A minimum of 5 episodes overall or at least 3 episodes occurring within a 6-month time frame.
- Recurrent attacks are characterized by vomiting and nausea, lasting for a duration of 1–10 days, and separated by at least 1 week.
- Consistency in the presentation of symptoms and episodes (stereotypy).
- During episodes, vomiting should take place at least 4 times per hour for a minimum of 1 hour.
- The child should return to their baseline health status between these episodes.
- The condition should not be attributed to another underlying disorder.

## ▪ TREATMENT APPROACH

For 1–2 months or cycles, implement lifestyle changes:
- Offer reassurance, emphasizing that episodes are not self-induced.
- Encourage keeping a "vomiting diary" to identify triggers.
- Discourage fasting.
- Promote good sleep hygiene to avoid sleep deprivation.
- Suggest avoiding trigger foods like chocolate, cheese, monosodium glutamate (MSG), and antigenic foods.
- Discourage excessive energy expenditure; recommend extra carbohydrates during fasting-induced episodes.
- Provide fruit juices, sugary drinks, and snacks between meals, before exertion, or at bedtime.
- For migraine management, encourage regular aerobic exercise while avoiding overexertion.
- Promote regular meal schedules, emphasizing no skipped meals.
- Recommend moderation or avoidance of caffeine.

### Pharmacotherapy

*Acute Attack*
- *Fluid, electrolyte, and nutritional management:* 0.45% NS with KCL—1.5 times the maintenance dose to be started. If required for a prolonged time, then add peripheral parental nutrition with amino acids. If required, symptomatic treatment can be added like:
  - *Antiemetics*: Ondansetron: 0.3–0.4 mg/kg/dose intravenously every 4–6 hours (up to 20 mg)
  - *Sedatives:* Diphenhydramine 1.0–1.25 mg/kg/dose intravenously every 6 hours or Lorazepam 0.05–0.1 mg/kg/dose intravenously every 6 hours
  - *Analgesics (nonsteroidal and narcotic) agents:* Ketorolac 0.4–1.0 mg/kg intravenously every 6 hours

### Prophylactic Treatment

- The first choice is tricyclic antidepressants. *Amitriptyline:* Start with 0.25–0.5 mg/kg bedtime, which can be increased to 5–10 mg weekly with a maximum dose of 1.0–1.5 mg/kg. Monitor ECG changes, mainly QT interval, before starting and 10 days after starting. Side effects may include constipation, sedation, arrhythmia, and behavioral changes, particularly in young children.
- The second choice is beta-blockers, specifically propranolol.
- *Dose:* 0.25–1.0 mg/kg/day, often given as 10 mg BD or TDS
- Monitor the resting heart rate and ensure that it remains at or above 60 beats per minute. Side effects include lethargy and decreased exercise tolerance.
- Contraindicated for individuals with asthma, diabetes, heart disease, or depression. When discontinuing, a tapering regimen should be followed for 1–2 weeks.

## ▪ CHRONIC ABDOMINAL PAIN

Chronic abdominal pain is a persistent challenge in pediatrics, especially when it lasts over 2 months. Adolescents are significantly affected, with 15–17% experiencing CAP. It can be categorized into three groups: (1) Functional (70–85%), (2) organic (10–15%), and (3) psychogenic (5%). IBS is a common cause of CAP in adolescents, while organic causes include conditions like peptic ulcer disease (PUD), chronic pancreatitis, and intestinal tuberculosis.

### Functional Abdominal Pain

Functional abdominal pain characterizes pain that lacks an identifiable anatomical, biochemical, metabolic, inflammatory, immunologic, or neoplastic basis.

Red flag signs indicating organic abdominal pain in adolescents include:
- Severe, unrelenting pain
- Sudden onset of pain
- Abdominal tenderness or guarding or rigidity
- Weight loss
- Anemia, jaundice
- Blood in the stool
- Abnormal physical examination findings like mass in the abdomen or organomegaly
- Family history of GI disorders
- Previous abdominal surgery
- Prolonged fever without an apparent cause

Common investigations for organic abdominal pain vary according to the suspected cause and include:
- Complete blood count (CBC)
- Serum amylase and lipase levels
- Abdominal ultrasound
- Stool studies (e.g., stool occult blood, culture, or microscopy)
- Upper GI series
- Endoscopy [esophagogastroduodenoscopy (EGD)]
- Colonoscopy
- Computed tomography (CT) scan
- Magnetic resonance imaging (MRI)
- Biopsy of affected tissue, when necessary.

## Organic Causes of Chronic Abdominal Pain

### Peptic Ulcer Disease

Peptic ulcer disease in adolescents is a relatively rare but serious condition characterized by open sores in the lining of the stomach or the upper part of the small intestine.

*Types*
*Gastric ulcers:* Develop in the lining of the stomach

*Duodenal ulcers:* Occur in the upper part of the small intestine (duodenum)

*Erosive esophagitis:* Severe inflammation and ulcers in the esophagus.

*Clinical features:*
- Abdominal pain, typically in the upper abdomen
- Nausea and vomiting
- Loss of appetite
- Weight loss
- GI bleeding, leading to dark or bloody stools
- Anemia from chronic bleeding
- Heartburn and acid reflux in cases of erosive esophagitis.

## Investigations

- *Endoscopy:* Direct visualization of ulcers
- *Upper GI series:* X-ray examination with contrast to identify ulcers
- *Stool tests:* To detect blood in the stool
- *Helicobacter pylori testing:* Blood, stool, or breath tests to determine if the bacterium *H. pylori* is present

*Management:*
- *Medications:* Proton-pump inhibitors (PPIs) to reduce stomach acid, antibiotics for *H. pylori* eradication, and antacids

- *Lifestyle changes:* Avoiding spicy and acidic foods, smoking, and alcohol. Eating smaller, more frequent meals
- *Endoscopic therapy:* For severe bleeding ulcers, endoscopy may be used for hemostasis.

### Irritable Bowel Syndrome

Irritable bowel syndrome is relatively common among adolescents, with an estimated prevalence of around 10–15%.

*Clinical features:*
- Abdominal pain and discomfort
- Altered bowel habits, including diarrhea, constipation, or both
- Bloating and distension
- Mucus in the stool
- Urgency to have a bowel movement
- Relief of symptoms after a bowel movement
- Symptoms often worsen with stress

> **Rome III Diagnostic Criteria**
>
> To diagnose IBS, the Rome III criteria are commonly used, which include the presence of recurrent abdominal pain or discomfort at least 3 days per month for the past 3 months, associated with two or more of the following:
> - Improvement with defecation
> - Onset associated with a change in frequency of stool
> - Onset associated with a change in form (appearance) of stool
> - No evidence of IBD or neoplasia

*Investigations:*
- *Stool studies:* To rule out infections and malabsorption
- *Blood tests*: To check for inflammation or celiac disease
- *Colonoscopy or sigmoidoscopy:* For individuals with alarm symptoms (e.g., bleeding, unexplained weight loss) or those not responding to treatment

*Management:*
- *Dietary modifications:* Adjusting the diet to alleviate symptoms [e.g., low-FODMAP (Fermentable Oligosaccharides, Disaccharides, Monosaccharides, and Polyols) diet]
- *Medications:* Antispasmodics, fiber supplements, or medications to manage diarrhea or constipation
- *Stress management:* Behavioral therapies and relaxation techniques
- *Lifestyle changes:* Regular exercise, adequate sleep, and maintaining a routine.

## TABLE 2: Comparison of organic abdominal pain versus functional abdominal pain in adolescents.

| Aspect | Organic Abdominal pain | Functional abdominal pain |
|---|---|---|
| Etiology | Underlying anatomical or physiological cause | No identifiable anatomical or physiological cause |
| Onset | Sudden or acute onset | Gradual or chronic onset |
| Duration | Prolonged | Shorter |
| Night pain | Present | Absent |
| Severity | Moderate to severe | Mild to moderate |
| Location | Usually localized | Diffuse |
| Physical examination | Tenderness, guarding, or palpable masses | Nonsignificant |
| Diagnostic tests | Conclusive | Nonconclusive |
| Response to treatment | Good | Variable |

## ◼ KEY MESSAGES

- *Be vigilance for GI symptoms:* Be attentive to recurrent vomiting or CAP in your adolescent, as these may be indicative of underlying GI disorders.
- *GERD awareness:* Understand the symptoms of GERD, such as heartburn and chronic cough, and seek medical advice if persistent. Lifestyle modifications for GERD like encouraging weight management, elevate the head during sleep, and avoid triggers like caffeine, alcohol, and certain foods are recommended.
- *CVS recognition:* Be aware of CVS symptoms, including recurrent vomiting episodes, and maintain vomiting diary and avoid triggers.
- *CAP evaluation:* Recognize that CAP can have organic, functional, or psychogenic causes, necessitating thorough evaluation.
- *Red flag signs for organic pain:* Be alert to red flag signs indicating organic abdominal pain, such as severe pain, weight loss, or abnormal physical examination findings.

- *IBS awareness:* Understand IBS symptoms, including abdominal discomfort and altered bowel habits, and seek medical attention for appropriate diagnosis.
- *Overall well-being:* Prioritize your adolescent's overall well-being by promoting a healthy lifestyle, including regular exercise, adequate sleep, and stress reduction. Regular medical checkups are crucial for early detection and management of gastrointestinal issues.

## ◼ RECOMMENDED READING


1. Akinola MA, Oyedele TA, Akande KO, Oluyemi OY, Salami OF, Adesina AM, et al. Gastroesophageal reflux disease: prevalence and Extraesophageal manifestations among undergraduate students in South West Nigeria. BMC Gastroenterol. 2020;20(1):160.
2. American Academy of Pediatrics Subcommittee on Chronic Abdominal Pain; North American Society for Pediatric Gastroenterology Hepatology, and Nutrition. Chronic abdominal pain in children. Pediatrics. 2005;115(3): e370-81.
3. Chey WD, Leontiadis GI, Howden CW, Moss SF. ACG Clinical Guideline: Treatment of *Helicobacter pylori* Infection. Am J Gastroenterol. 2017;112(2):212-39.
4. Drossman DA. Rome III: the new criteria. Chin J Dig Dis. 2006;7(4):181-5.
5. Fleisher DR, Matar M. The cyclic vomiting syndrome: a report of 71 cases and literature review. J Pediatr Gastroenterol Nutr. 1993;17(4):361-9.
6. Hungin APS, Raghunath AS, Wiklund I. Beyond heartburn: a systematic review of the extra-oesophageal spectrum of reflux-induced disease, Family Pract. 2005;22(6):591-603.
7. Kim JS. Acute abdominal pain in children. Pediatr Gastroenterol Hepatol Nutr. 2013;16(4):219-24.
8. Li BU, Lefevre F, Chelimsky GG, Boles RG, Nelson SP, Lewis DW, et al. North American Society for Pediatric Gastroenterology, Hepatology, and Nutrition. North American Society for Pediatric Gastroenterology, Hepatology, and Nutrition consensus statement on the diagnosis and management of cyclic vomiting syndrome. J Pediatr Gastroenterol Nutr. 2008;47(3):379-93.
9. Malmborg P, Grahnquist L. Crohn's disease in children and adolescents: a long-term follow-up. J Pediatr Gastroenterol Nutr. 014;58(2):152-8.

# 4B.3   Bronchial Asthma

*Harmesh Singh Bains*

## ■ INTRODUCTION

Bronchial asthma is one of the common respiratory problems in adolescents. The characteristic features of bronchial asthma include recurrent attacks of cough, wheeze, tightness in the chest, and shortness of breath. There is chronic inflammation of airways, with its reversible and variable hyperresponsiveness.

## ■ DEFINITION

The definition of bronchial asthma includes the following characteristics:

- Hyperresponsiveness of airway to triggers
- Inflammation of airway
- Diffuse and reversible airway obstruction.

## ■ PATHOPHYSIOLOGY

The diffuse obstruction in the airway is due to the following factors:

- There is inflammatory edema of airway mucosal lining.
- There is smooth muscle spasm of airway.
- Mucus secretion and different types of cellular collection in the airway.

## ■ TRIGGERS OF BRONCHIAL ASTHMA

Various triggers for bronchial asthma include the following:
- Viral infections
- *Environmental factors:* Indoor and outdoor: cigarette smoke, mosquito repellents, *agarbatti*, automobile exhaust, smoke from firewood. Insects, dust mite, dampness, pollens grains, and domestic animals like dog and cat
- Exercise
- Endocrinal factors.

## ■ ASSESSMENT

### History

A brief and relevant history and quick physical examination should be carried out so as to initiate treatment.

*History should include:*
- Duration and precipitating cause (if known) of the current exacerbation/triggers

- *Severity of asthma symptoms:* Breathlessness, waking during sleep, whistling sound
- *Type of cough:* Dry/wet/exercise induced/recurrent or chronic persistent
- Diurnal variation (nocturnal/daytime/early morning)/ seasonal variations
- *History of atopy/eczema/allergic rhinitis:* Personal or in family members
- Previous hospital admissions and response to treatment
- Previous emergency room visits or hospitalizations.

### Clinical Examination

- *General appearance:* Consciousness, work of breathing, and color CBC)
- *Vital signs:* Pulse, respiration rate, temperature, blood pressure, oxygen saturation, use of accessary muscles, and ability to complete sentences
- *Rule out:* Foreign body, pneumonia, atelectasis, pneumothorax, pneumomediastinum
- Auscultate for bilateral wheeze/rhonchi; unilateral or localized signs

*Asthma is unlikely if the following features are observed:*
- Unilateral rhonchi or wheeze—foreign body, congenital anomaly
- Failure to thrive, poor weight gain, chronic diarrhea, clubbing
- Chronic productive cough
- *Involvement of multiple systems:* Gastrointestinal tract (GIT), hematological, cardiovascular system (CVS), central nervous system (CNS)
- *Onset in early infancy:* Congenital anomalies
- Fever

## ■ CLINICAL DIAGNOSIS

History of more than three wheezing attacks in a year; response to bronchodilators and no other cause of wheezing.

*Oxygen saturation:* Oxygen saturation by pulse oximetry should be regularly monitored. A saturation <92% is an indication for hospitalization.

*Lung function tests; peak expiratory flow (PEF) or forced expiratory volume in 1 second (FEV1):* It is important to record PEF or FEV1 before starting the treatment; spirometry may not be immediately possible. There will be reduced FEV1. FEV1/FVC will be <80% in asthma. Repeat the FEV1 after 10–15 minutes of giving 200–400 µg salbutamol; there should be more than 12% increase.

*Arterial blood gas (ABG):* ABG is indicated in the following situations:

- PEF or FEV1 <50% of the predicted value
- No response to initial treatment; deterioration during initial treatment.

*Chest X-ray:* It is not routinely indicated in bronchial asthma. It may be normal or may show hyperinflation. It may be required to rule out cases of pneumothorax, pneumonia, or an inhaled foreign body.

*Blood tests:* CBC may be normal. There may be eosinophilia in atopy.

*Serum total IgE:* It is not helpful in diagnosing asthma.

*Allergy tests:* Allergy testing is not routinely recommended in asthma. It may be helpful in cases with a history of allergic rhinitis, food allergy, and difficult-to-control asthma. Allergen should be chosen on the basis of history; fixed panels are not useful.

The recommended tests include in vivo skin prick test (gold standard) and in vitro blood test for allergen-specific IgE estimation.

*Comorbid conditions:* A careful evaluation for comorbid conditions should be done.

- Allergic rhinitis, sinusitis, adenoidal hypertrophy
- Obstructive sleep apnea syndrome
- Obesity
- GERD
- Anxiety, depression.
  Approach to an adolescent with acute exacerbation of asthma (IAP guidelines) is given in the **Flowchart 1**.

*Treatment:* It is important to assess the level of control before starting treatment **(Table 1)**:
- Control of symptom
- Risk of future adverse outcomes

## ■ HIGH-RISK FACTORS FOR EXACERBATIONS

There are modifiable and nonmodifiable risk factors.

### Modifiable Risk Factors

- Uncontrolled asthma symptoms, psychological problems, and poor adherence

- Seasonal "flare-up", comorbidities
- Exposure to irritants and triggers.

### Nonmodifiable Risk Factors

- Ever intubated or intensive care unit admissions
- More than one severe exacerbation requiring hospitalization in the last 1 year.

## ■ MANAGEMENT FOR ADOLESCENTS TO CONTROL SYMPTOMS AND MINIMIZE FUTURE RISK (TABLE 2)

*Track 1:* Inhaled corticosteroids (controller) and formoterol (reliever)

*Track 2:* Inhaled corticosteroids and other relievers short acting beta agonists (SABA).

Intravenous salbutamol can be used in severe asthma cases with no response to other treatments. The inhaled drugs may not have adequate effect because of severe or complete airway obstruction due to bronchoconstriction. These patients need an intensive care setting.

In the management of bronchial asthma, the severity is graded as given in **Table 3**.

The features in life-threatening asthma are as follows:
- Cyanosis
- Silent chest
- Fatigue
- Alteration in sensorium
- Poor respiratory efforts
- Oxygen saturation—90%; peak expiratory flow rate (PEFR)—30%
- Immediate care of life-threatening asthma **(Flowchart 2)**
- Continue SABA nebulization every 1 hour or continuously.
- Start Ipratropium nebulization every 30 minutes, three times, and then every 6 hours for 24 hours.
- Monitor vitals and observe for 1–2 hours.
- If need be, give magnesium sulfate IV infusion over 30 minutes.
- There may be need of continuous IV infusion of terbutaline.
- IV aminophylline should be reserved solely for adolescents with a severe asthma exacerbation, who have failed to respond to the maximal therapy with continuous inhaled beta 2-agonists, IV corticosteroids, and IV magnesium sulfate.

**Flowchart 1:** Approach to an adolescent with acute exacerbation of asthma (IAP guidelines).

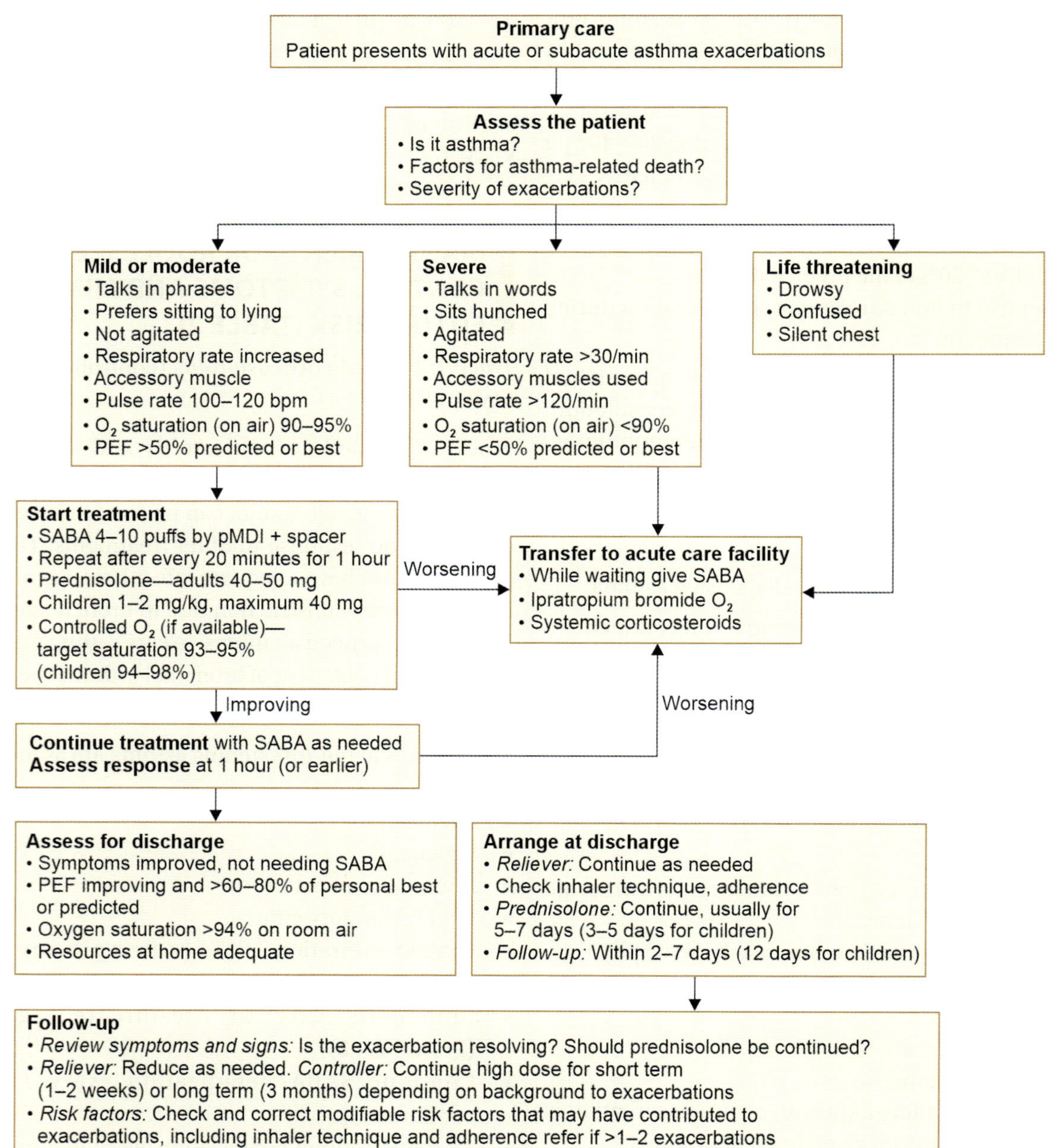



(PEF: peak expiratory flow; pMDI: pressurized metered-dose inhaler; SABA: short-acting beta-agonist)

| **TABLE 1:** GINA guidelines for assessment of asthma control. | | | |
|---|---|---|---|
| **Asthma symptoms control** | **Level of asthma symptoms control** | | |
| Symptoms in the past 4 weeks | Well controlled | Partly controlled | Uncontrolled |
| More than twice/week symptoms during day? | Yes/No | Yes/No | |
| Any night waking due to asthma? | None of those | 1–2 of those | 3–4 of those |
| SABA reliever for symptoms more than twice/week? | Yes/No | Yes/No | Yes/No |
| Limitation of activities? | Yes/No | Yes/No | Yes/No |

(GINA: global initiative for asthma; SABA: short-acting beta-agonists)

**TABLE 2:** Management for adolescents to control symptoms and minimize future risk of asthma.

| Duration of symptoms and severity | Treatment option | | |
| --- | --- | --- | --- |
| | Controller | Reliever | Alternative reliever |
| Less than 4–5 days/wk | Low-dose ICS | Formoterol | SABA |
| On most days of week or waking with asthma once a week or more | Low-dose maintenance ICS | Formoterol | LABA |
| On all days/waking with asthma once or more in a week and low lung function | Medium-dose maintenance ICS | Formoterol | LABA |
| Severely uncontrolled asthma | SC oral steroids/high-dose ICS | Formoterol | LAMA |

(ICS: inhaled cortcosteroids; LABA: long acting beta-agonist; LAMA: long-acting muscarinic antagonist; SABA: short-acting beta-agonist; SC: short course)

**TABLE 3:** Grading of severity in the management of bronchial asthma.

| Clinical parameter | Mild | Moderate | Severe |
| --- | --- | --- | --- |
| Initial impression (CBC):<br>• Consciousness<br>• Work of breathing<br>• Color | Normal<br>Normal/minimal chest indrawing<br>Normal | Anxious<br>Chest indrawing<br>Normal | Agitated<br>Chest indrawing, nasal flare<br>Pale |
| Vitals:<br>• Respiration rate<br>• Pulsus paradoxus<br>• Oxygen saturation (%) | Increased<br><10 mm<br>>95 | Increased<br>10–20 mm<br>90–95 | Increased<br>>20 mm<br><90 |
| Dyspnea | Nil | Moderate | Severe |
| Speech | Can speak sentence | Can speak phrase | Difficulty in speech |
| Peak expiratory flow rate (PEFR) (%) | >80 | 60–80 | <60 |

- Monitor serum potassium, CBC, X-ray chest, and blood gases.
- *Sustained 4–6 hours:* Stop Aminophylline infusion in 24 hours. Taper and discontinue terbutaline drip. Omit ipratropium nebulizer in 24 hours. Reduce SABA.
- *Discharge criteria:* Comfortable, normal sleep, and eating well.

## ■ KEY MESSAGES

- Asthma is one of the common problems of adolescence.
- Asthma triggers should be identified.
- A careful evaluation for comorbid conditions should be done: Allergic rhinitis, sinusitis, adenoidal hypertrophy, obstructive sleep apnea syndrome, obesity, GERD, anxiety, and depression.
- X-ray chest is not routinely indicated in bronchial asthma. It may be required to rule out cases of pneumothorax, pneumonia, or an inhaled foreign body.
- Allergy testing is not routinely recommended in asthma.
- The four essential components of asthma management are patient education, minimizing exposure to asthma triggers, monitoring for changes in symptoms or lung functions and, pharmacologic therapy.
- Management in adolescents includes control symptoms and minimize future risk.
- Track 1 includes ICS and formoterol used as controller and reliever.
- Track 2 includes ICS and alternative reliever, i.e., SABA.

**Flowchart 2:** Management of asthma exacerbation in an acute care facility (IAP).

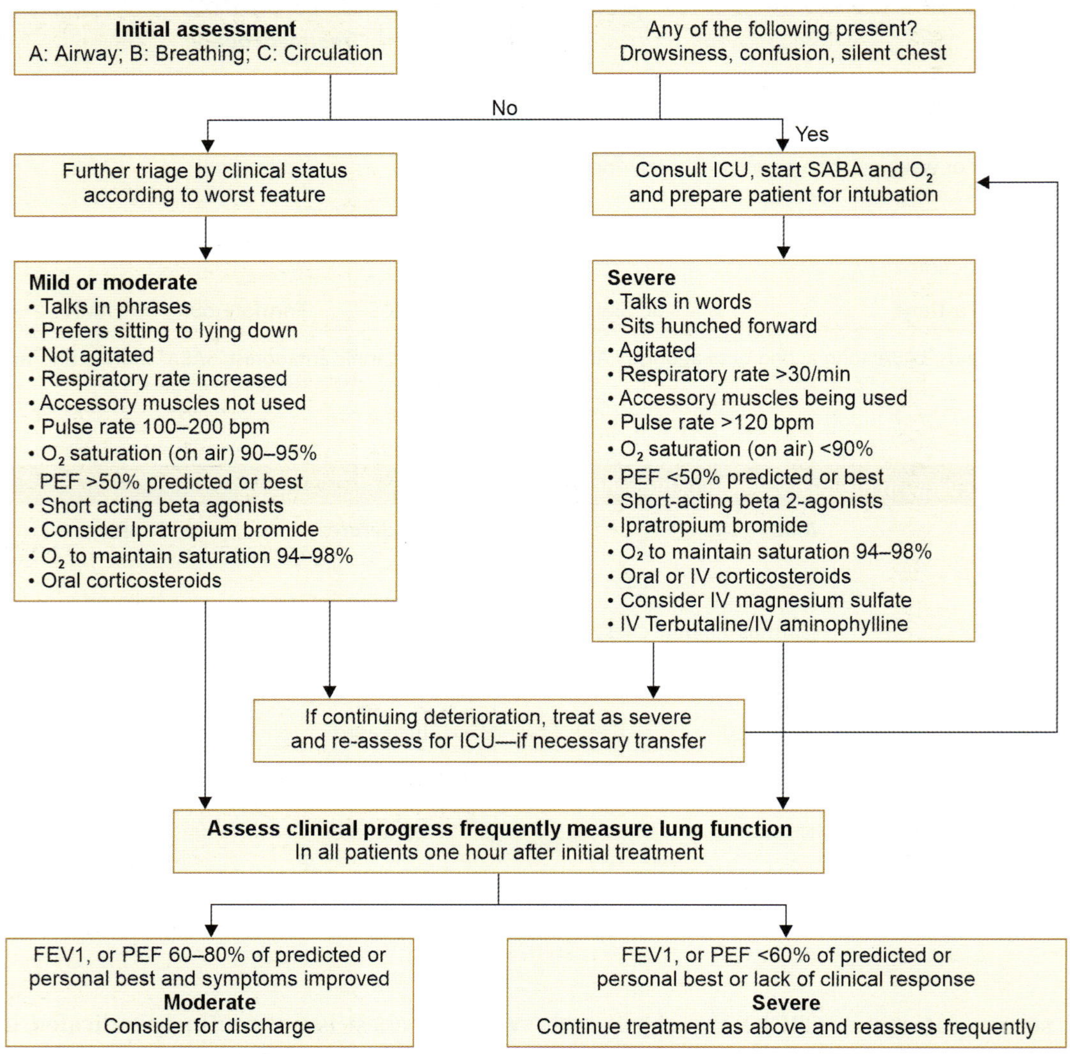


(ICU: intensive care unit; PEF: peak expiratory flow; SABA: short-acting beta-agonist)

## ■ RECOMMENDED READING


1. Bitsko MJ, Everhart RS, Rubin BK. The Adolescent with Asthma. Pediatric Respir Rev. 2014;15:146-53.
2. Cheng ZR, Tan YH, Teoh OH, Lee JH. Keeping pace with adolescent asthma: a practical approach to optimizing care. Pulm Ther. 2022;8:123-37.
3. Global Initiative for Asthma (GINA). (2023). [online] Available from www.ginasthma.org [Last accessed March, 2024].
4. Mehta PN. Asthma and the school going child. Indian Pediatr. 2002;39:731-8.
5. Sethi GR, Bajaj M, Sehgal V. Management of Acute Asthma. Indian Pediatr. 1998;35:745-62.

# 4B.4　Common ENT Problems in Adolescent

*Shreeya Kulkarni*

## ■ DEAFNESS

### Introduction

Deafness and hearing loss are widespread and found in every country. Currently 1.5 billion people, i.e., 20% of global population are deaf. Hearing loss or deafness varies from very minimal loss to complete deafness. Patients initially may not notice it. They will notice when their day-to-day activities are hampered. That also depends on age, gender, education, profession, and associated symptoms.

### Etiology

#### Classification of Hearing Loss

- *Organic:*
  - Conductive hearing loss (CHL)
  - Sensorineural hearing loss (SNHL)
  - Mixed hearing loss
- *Nonorganic:* Malingering—psychogenic

#### Causes of Conductive Hearing Loss

- *External auditory canal:* Wax, foreign bodies, otitis externa, congenital and acquired stenosis, exostoses, osteomas, tumors, and cyst
- *Tympanic membrane (TM):* Perforations [traumatic, acute suppurative otitis media (ASOM), chronic suppurative otitis media (CSOM)], *tympanosclerosis, and retraction*
- *Ossicles:* Fixation (otosclerosis, tympanosclerosis, and congenital) and discontinuity (traumatic, inflammatory, and cholesteatoma)
- *Middle ear:* Eustachian tube dysfunction, otitis media with effusion, adhesive otitis media, hemotympanum, cholesteatoma, and tumors (benign and malignant)

#### Causes of Sensorineural Hearing Loss

- *Congenital:* Genetic and nongenetic
- *Infections (viral, bacterial, or spirochetal):* Labyrinthitis and meningitis
- *Trauma:* To labyrinth and cranial nerve (CN) VIII in fractures of temporal bone and ear surgery
- *Ototoxic drugs:* Streptomycin and gentamicin
- *Endolymphatic hydrops:* Primary or idiopathic (Ménière's disease) and secondary
- *Tumors:* Acoustic neuroma
- *Systemic diseases:* Diabetes, multiple sclerosis, syphilis, hypothyroidism, kidney disease, autoimmune disorders, and blood dyscrasias
- *Miscellaneous:* Sudden idiopathic SNHL, familial progressive SNHL, noise-induced hearing loss (NIHL), and presbycusis.

### Clinical Features, Investigations, and Diagnosis

**Table 1** shows clinical features of conductive and sensorineural hearing loss.

### Management

#### Conductive Hearing Loss

Most cases are managed by medical or surgical means.
- Removal of canal obstruction, e.g., impacted wax, foreign body, osteoma, exostosis, benign or malignant tumors, or meatal atresia
- Removal of fluid—myringotomy with or without grommet insertion
- *Removal of pathology in middle ear:* Mastoidectomy, tympanoplasty, cholesteatoma removal, repair of perforation (myringoplasty), ossicular reconstruction (ossiculoplasty) removal of small middle ear tumors, and stapedectomy for otosclerotic fixation.
- *Hearing aid:* In cases where surgery is not possible, failed, or refused.

#### Sensorineural Deafness

Depending upon the cause medical treatment is done. In few cases operative procedure like cochlear implants and sac decompression is done.

## ■ OTITIS MEDIA

It is the inflammation of middle ear cleft.

### Classification

Otitis media can be classified as shown in **Flowchart 1**.

**TABLE 1:** Clinical features of conductive hearing loss and sensorineural hearing loss.

| Features | Conductive hearing loss | Sensorineural hearing loss |
|---|---|---|
| Site of lesion | External and middle ear | Internal ear, CN VIII, and central auditory connections |
| Speech understanding | Good | Poor |
| Intolerance to loud sounds | Absent | Present in cochlear lesions |
| Speech of the patient | Low voice | Loud voice |
| Common associated symptom | Otorrhea/earache | Tinnitus |
| Profound hearing loss | Never | Common |
| Rinne test | Negative (BC >AC) | Positive (AC >BC) |
| Weber test | Lateralized toward worst ear | Lateralized toward better ear |
| Absolute bone conduction | Normal | Reduced |
| Pure-tone audiometry (PTA) | Air-bone gap present | Absent |
| PTA: Recruitment | Absent | Present in cochlear lesions |
| PTA: Tone decay | Absent | Present in CN VIII lesion |
| PTA: Thresholds | Never >60–70 dB | Can be >60–70 dB |
| Speech discrimination | Not affected | Poor |

(AC: air conduction; BC: bone conduction; CN: cranial nerve)

**Flowchart 1:** Classification of otitis media.

```
                            Otitis media
                   ┌─────────────┴──────────────┐
                 Acute                        Chronic
            ┌──────┴──────┐              ┌──────┴──────┐
       Suppurative  Nonsuppurative  Suppurative  Nonsuppurative
            │            │              │              │
       • ASOM       • OME        • Tubotympanic—     • OME/glue ear
       • Viral OM   • Otic         safe/perforation  • Adhesive OM
       • ANOM         barotrauma • Attico-antral—    • Tympanosclerosis
                                    unsafe/cholesteatoma
```

(ANOM: acute necrotizing otitis media; ASOM: acute suppurative otitis media; OM: otitis media; OME: otitis media with effusion).

### Acute Suppurative Otitis Media

*Definition:* Acute inflammation of middle ear cleft with pyogenic organisms

*Etiology:* Routes of infection—via Eustachian tube. It is the most common route, via external ear. Infection occurs due to traumatic perforation of TM or blood-borne. Causative organisms include *Streptococcus pneumoniae, Streptococcus pyogenes, Staphylococcus aureus,* and sometimes *Pseudomonas aeruginosa.*

*Clinical features:* Patient complains of otorrhea, earache, deafness, high-grade fever, and malaise. In early stage, TM appears congested, red and bulging, and then about to rupture. Later on there is blood-tinged discharge with small perforation.

*Treatment:*
- Antibacterial therapy—co-amoxiclav augmentin, 40 mg/kg, cefixime (III generation), taxim-O, and biotax-O 8 mg/kg
- Decongestant nasal drops—oxymetazoline (Nasivion) or xylometazoline (Otrivin); oral nasal decongestants or combination of decongestant and antihistaminic
- Analgesics and antipyretics—paracetamol
- Ear toilet. If there is discharge in the ear, it is dry-mopped with sterile cotton buds.

## Otitis Media with Effusion

*Introduction:* This is an insidious condition characterized by accumulation of nonpurulent effusion in the middle ear cleft **(Fig. 1)**.

*Etiology:* Malfunctioning of Eustachian tube due to adenoid hyperplasia, chronic rhinitis and sinusitis, chronic tonsillitis, benign and malignant tumors of nasopharynx, and palatal defects; allergy; seasonal or perennial allergy; unresolved otitis media; and viral infections.

*Clinical features:* Symptoms—hearing loss, mild earaches, and delayed and defective speech. Signs—TM is often dull and opaque with loss of light reflex.

*Investigations:* Audiometry—CHL; impedance audiometry—presence of fluid.

*Treatment:*
- *Medical:*
  - Decongestants in the form of nasal drops, sprays, or systemic decongestants help to relieve edema of Eustachian tube.
  - *Antiallergic measures:* Antihistaminics or sometimes steroids may be used in cases of allergy.
  - Antibiotics for upper respiratory tract infections or unresolved ASOM
- *Surgical:*
  - Myringotomy and aspiration of fluid
  - Grommet insertion to provide continued aeration
  - *Surgical treatment of causative factor:* Adenoidectomy and tonsillectomy

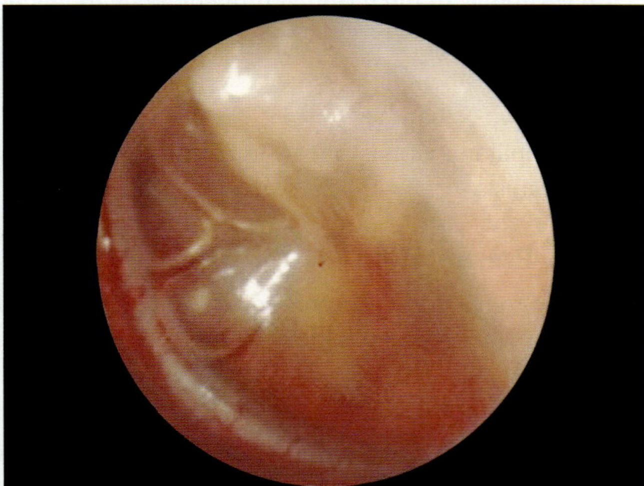
**Fig. 1:** Otitis media with effusion.

## Chronic Suppurative Otitis Media

Chronic suppurative otitis media is a long-standing infection of a part or whole of the middle ear cleft characterized by ear discharge. Incidence of CSOM is higher in developing countries, because of poor socioeconomic standards, poor nutrition, and lack of health education.

*Types of CSOM:*
- Tubo-tympanic/safe or benign type is associated with a central perforation. There is no risk of serious complications.
- Attico-antral/unsafe or dangerous type is associated with an attic or a marginal perforation. The disease is often associated with a bone eroding process, such as cholesteatoma, granulations, or osteitis. Risk of complications is high.

## ■ DISORDERS OF VOICE

- *Puberphonia (mutational falsetto voice):* It is seen in adolescence.
- *Rhinolalia aperta (hypernasality):* It is due to open nasopharynx, e.g., cleft palate.
- *Rhinolalia clausa (hyponasality):* It is due to obstructed nasopharynx, e.g., adenoids.
- *Hoarseness:* Any change in voice quality from harsh, rough or weak voice, is usually referred to hoarseness. It is caused by laryngeal dysfunction.

### Treatment

Treatment of the cause is important. Voice therapy helps in functional causes.

## JUVENILE NASOPHARYNGEAL ANGIOFIBROMA

### Introduction

Juvenile nasopharyngeal angiofibroma (JNA) is a highly vascular histologically benign, yet locally aggressive, head and neck tumor.

### Origin

It originates from posterior nasal and nasopharyngeal region in adolescent males.

### Clinical Features

*Unilateral nasal obstruction and epistaxis in a young adolescent male patient:* Hallmark of JNA, epistaxis—profuse, recurrent, and usually from one nostril, snoring, mouth breathing, adenoid facies, and rhinolalia clausa.

## Investigations and Diagnosis

*Nasal endoscopy and CT scan of paranasal sinuses with contrast:* Both are the gold standard for diagnosis of JNA. Biopsy is avoided for risk of hemorrhage.

## Treatment

Surgery remains the mainstay and treatment of choice for JNA.

## ■ SLEEP APNEA

Sleep apnea is the absence of movement of air at the level of nose and mouth during sleep.

*Consequences of sleep apnea:*
- Congestive heart failure/cor pulmonale
- Polycythemia and hypertension

## Clinical Features

Clinical features include adolescent body mass index—overweight, 25–29%; and obesity, 30–34.9.

## Investigations

Polysomnography is the "gold standard" for diagnosis of sleep apnea.

## Management

Management includes nonsurgical—weight reduction, and surgical intervention is applied according to pathology.

## ■ TONSILLITIS

Inflammation of tonsil is called tonsillitis, which can be acute or chronic **(Fig. 2)**.

## Etiology

The causes of tonsillitis include primary infection of tonsil or secondary to upper respiratory tract infection (URTI).

## Clinical Features

- *Symptoms*: Pyrexia, sore throat, difficulty in swallowing, malaise, and body ache
- *Signs:* Breath is fetid, tonsils are swollen, congested and exudates are seen in the crypts, and jugulodigastric lymph nodes are enlarged and tender.

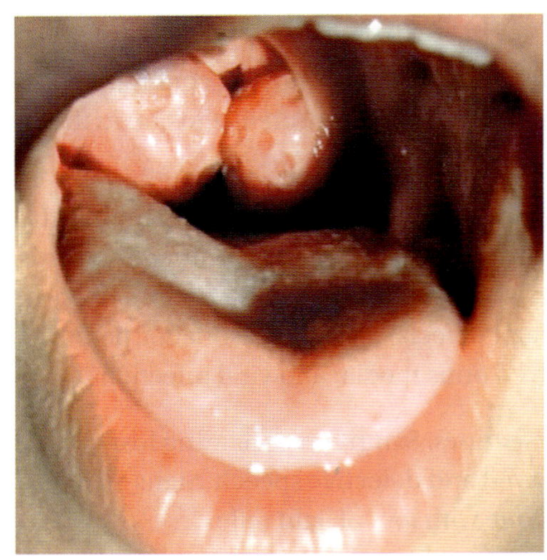

**Fig. 2:** Tonsillitis.

## Investigations

Investigations include total count, differential count—leukocytosis with neutrophilia.

## Treatment

Bed rest, drink plenty of fluids, antibiotics, analgesic, anti-inflammatory drugs, throat gargles, and *tonsillectomy* are the definitive treatments in chronic tonsillitis.

## ■ RECURRENT RESPIRATORY PAPILLOMATOSIS

### Introduction

Recurrent respiratory papillomatosis (RRP) is a potentially life-threatening disease characterized by the development of papillomata anywhere in the respiratory tract from the nasal vestibules to the terminal bronchi. Male to female ratio is 3:2.

### Etiology

Human papilloma virus is the cause of recurrent respiratory papillomatosis.

### Clinical Presentation

Hoarseness and stridor, chronic cough, and paroxysms of choking are the clinical symptoms.

### Treatment

Treatment of recurrent respiratory papillomatosis includes surgical treatment, coblation, and tracheostomy a last resort.

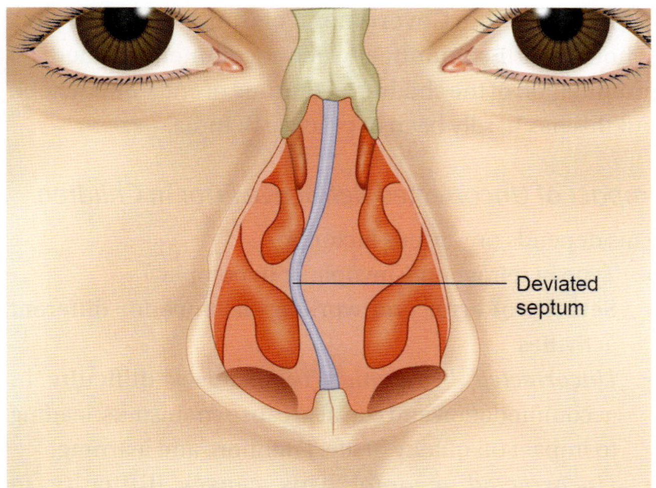

**Fig. 3:** Deviated nasal septum.

## DEVIATED NASAL SEPTUM DEVIATED NASAL SEPTUM

About 50% of the population has some deviated nasal septum (DNS), but most of them are asymptomatic. Nasal obstruction, which may be unilateral or bilateral, is the most common symptom of headache; epistaxis can occur. External deformity can be associated with DNS and can be disturbing to the young adolescent males.

The treatment is surgical. Septoplasty may be done with endoscopic surgery under general or local anesthesia. It is combined with rhinoplasty if there is significant external deformity **(Fig. 3)**.

### ■ KEY MESSAGES

- Conductive deafness is mostly curable.

- Otitis media is completely curable if diagnosed in time. Unsafe otitis media needs surgical intervention at the earliest.
- Juvenile angiofibroma can present as severe epistaxis in adolescent age.
- Sleep disorders can be very disturbing problem in obese or over weight adolescents.
- Tonsillar infection and adenoid enlargements need to be treated surgically if causing troublesome symptoms.
- RRP is notorious for cure.
- Many ENT-related problems in adolescent age group require early detection and timely intervention.
- Deviated nasal septum with external deformity can be very disturbing in adolescence.

### ■ RECOMMENDED READING


1. Bansal M (Ed). Diseases of Ear, Nose and Throat with Head and Neck Surgery, 3rd edition. New Delhi: Jaypee Brothers Medical Publishers; 2021.
2. Dhingra PL, Dhingra S (Eds). Diseases of Ear, Nose and Throat, 7th edition. Elsevier Health Science; 2017.
3. Kirtane MV (Ed). Endoscopic Endonasal Surgery: Sinuses and Beyond, 1st edition. New Delhi: Jaypee Brothers Medical Publishers; 2015.
4. Watkinson JC, Clarke RW (Eds). Scott-Brown's Otorhinolaryngology and Head and Neck Surgery. Volume 2: Paediatrics, The Ear, and Skull Base Surgery, 8th edition. CRC Press; 2018.
5. Watkinson JC, Clarke RW (Eds). Scott-Brown's Otorhinolaryngology and Head and Neck Surgery. Volume 1: Basic Sciences, Endocrine Surgery, Rhinology, 8th edition. CRC Press; 2018.
6. Watkinson JC, Clarke RW (Eds). Scott-Brown's Otorhinolaryngology and Head and Neck Surgery: Volume 3: Head and Neck Surgery, Plastic Surgery, 8th edition. CRC Press; 2018.


# 4B.5 Common Ophthalmic Problems

*Santosh S Bhide*

### ■ INTRODUCTION

Many changes take place in our body during the period of adolescence, i.e., from 13 to 18 years of our life. This process starts as early as 6 years and continues up to 20 years of life.

Physical changes occurring during this period are obviously seen, but there is significant development of eye during this period.

At birth, the eye is normally mildly hyperopic, and this error reduces over the next several years.

The risk of myopia in childhood is associated with a range of socioenvironmental factors, with indoor lifestyle and with more time on schooling and other near-work tasks. Myopia is more associated with urban location.

Near tasks related to mobile phones, tablets, and other technologies are common and influence refractive error in both rural and urban locations.

## CHANGES IN EYE DURING ADOLESCENCE (TEENAGERS AND YOUNG ADULTS)

Axial length of eyeball is 16.8 mm at birth and 23.6 mm at the age of 20 years.

Growth of eyeball occurs mainly immediately after birth and continues even during puberty.

Visual skills continue to mature during adolescence.

*Visual skills are:*
- Visual acuity—for distance and near
- Accommodation—for far and for near
- Eye tracking—for tracking moving objects and while reading sentences
- Visual perception—cortical perception and cognitive sense
- Binocular vision—for depth perception.

## COMMON OCULAR PROBLEMS IN TEENAGERS AND YOUNG ADULTS

- Refractive errors
- Eye strain—asthenopia
- Computer vision syndrome
- Inflammatory conditions—infections and allergic
- Seborrheic blepharitis
- Trauma—sports and occupational
- Contact lens-related issues.

### Refractive Errors in Teenagers

Good visual acuity plays an important role in the development of child for learning and communication.

Uncorrected refractive error has become a major public health challenge for all of us.

Uncorrected refractive error is the second largest cause of blindness globally.

An estimated 19 million children are visually impaired worldwide of which 12 million are due to refractive errors, which could be easily corrected.

Many screening programs are being carried out in schools, but there is still a lack of accurate data in the prevalence of visual impairment.

Active screening and timely intervention at the right time will not only help in vision restoration but will also influence a child's growth and development.

In 1960, the Government of India constituted a school health committee which recommended medical examination of the children at the time of entry into school, but this has hardly been in practice in India.

### *Impact of Uncorrected Refractive Error in Children*

This depends on various factors:
- Type of refraction—myopia or hyperopia
- Severity of error and working distance for different activities
- *Uncorrected hyperopia:* This causes difficulty in accommodation and can also cause strabismus, leading to impact on quality of life, attention, and learning.
- *Uncorrected myopia:* This causes difficulty in visualizing distant objects, leading to negative impact on distance tasks, such as viewing a blackboard, impacting not only educational outcomes but also self-esteem and well-being.
- Uncorrected anisometropia in early childhood may result in amblyopia with associated loss of depth perception, impacting activities of daily living.

Early detection and correction of childhood refractive error is therefore important to prevent these adverse effects. Pediatrician can play very crucial role in screening and early detection of refractive errors in children. Use of spectacle is the main option for children with refractive error. Contact lenses is another safer option for correction.

Laser vision correction, LASIK (laser-assisted in-situ keratomileusis), PRK (photorefractive keratectomy), SMILE (small incision lenticule extraction), and ICL (implantable contact lens) are various modalities for correction on refractive errors in young adults. Patient should be at least 21 years of age, and his refractive error should be stable before considering him for surgery. Thorough eye checkup is mandatory before these procedures.

### Ocular Allergy in Children and Young Adolescent

Allergic conjunctivitis is a spectrum of clinical conditions. It can be acute or chronic. It can also vary in severity. It is often associated with asthma, rhinoconjunctivitis, and is often considered as comorbidity. Ocular symptoms in asthma and allergic rhinitis are often underestimated and undertreated.

Family history of atopy, gender, early sensitization, food allergy, and atopic dermatitis are the risk factors for allergic rhinoconjunctivitis. It is more common in girls.

Most common symptoms of ocular allergy are itching, tearing, and ocular hyperemia.

### Treatment of Ocular Allergy

In mild to moderate cases, cold compresses can relieve symptoms by decreasing stimulation of nerves and by reducing vasodilatation. Preservative-free artificial tears are highly recommended due to its lubricating action and safety in long-term usage.

Topical antihistaminics like olopatadine, alcaftadine, and epinastine relieve itching and have dual action and safe to use.

Mast cell stabilizers like cromolyn are effective in mild to moderate symptoms.

Nonsteroidal anti-inflammatory drugs (NSAIDs) like ketorolac, though reduce symptoms, are often not tolerated and have side effects.

Topical steroids like loteprednol, fluorometholone, dexamethasone, and prednisolone have excellent anti-inflammatory action and reduce symptoms, but should not be used for long duration due to potent side effects like steroid-induced cataract and glaucoma.

Topical immunomodulators like cyclosporin and tacrolimus can be used judiciously under supervision. Use of preservative-free artificial tears along with other topical drops help in reducing irritation caused by other medicines and thus improves tolerability and compliance of the patient.

Excessive and continuous rubbing of eyes by child in ocular allergic conditions is thought to be one of the causes of keratoconus in children and young adults. One should be vigilant if there are frequent changes in refractive error of patient and if patient does not get clear vision in spite of full correction of error.

## Ocular Trauma

Ocular traumas are the leading cause of acquired unilateral blindness in the pediatric age group.

It is devastating trauma in the pediatric age group and is an important cause of morbidity in children. Worldwide, ocular trauma admissions in children account for 8–14% of total emergency trauma admissions, and the incidence of severe visual impairment or blindness ranges from 2–14%.

Eye injuries are both a significant socioeconomic burden and an important cause of morbidity that causes parents to worry about their children.

Most eye injuries can be prevented with simple protective measures.

Ocular injuries are usually caused by sharp objects, toys, wooden sticks, pencils, various sports activities, and stones in children.

Traumas are generally classified into two types as globe and adnexal. The most common emergency admission is with open globe injuries and requires urgent intervention.

Incidence of ocular trauma varies from region to region; there is also variation with demographic data like age and gender.

Pediatric acute eye trauma remains an important source of preventable monocular blindness. Children are vulnerable to ocular trauma and need more supervision. Toys, playgrounds, and entertainment places must be under parental supervision. The great majority of ocular traumas could be prevented, especially by wearing protective goggles during at-risk activities. Sharp objects such as pens, scissors, needles, knives, and household chemicals such as acidic or alkaline cleaning materials should be out of the reach of children. Awareness and education are needed to implement preventive measures and prevent sequelae. Parents must repeat educational warnings to their children handling sharp objects.

## Computer Vision Syndrome

Use of computers in school going children is on the rise following coronavirus disease 2019 (COVID-19) pandemic. Work from home has also led to excessive use of computers in young adults.

Computer vision syndrome (CVS) is also referred to as digital eye strain. It is a group of eye and vision-related problems that result from prolonged use of computer, tablet, e-reader, and cell phone **(Fig. 1)**.

The most common symptoms associated with CVS or digital eye strain are:

- Eyestrain
- Headaches
- Blurred vision
- Dry eyes
- Neck and shoulder pain

*These symptoms may be caused by:*
- Poor lighting
- Glare on a digital screen
- Improper viewing distances
- Poor sitting posture
- Uncorrected vision problems

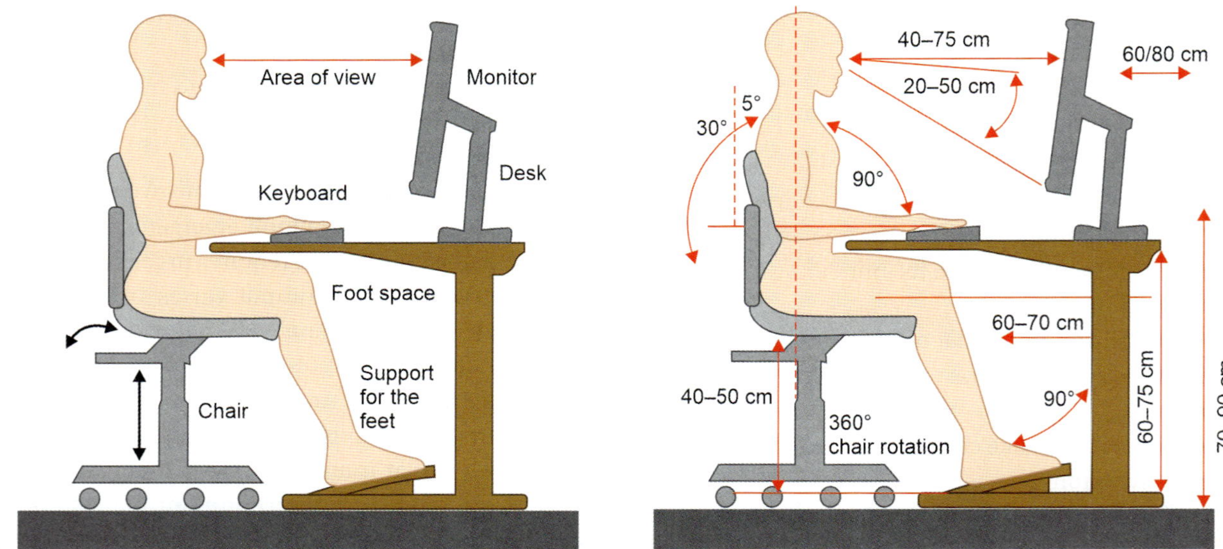



**Fig. 1:** Proper sitting posture.

- A combination of these factors
- Frequent blinking of eyes during use of computers causes dryness of eyes leading to CVS.
- Improper sitting posture aggravates symptoms of CVS.

## KEY MESSAGES

Tips for maintaining good eye sight:
- Regular eye checkup from ophthalmologist
- Protection of eyes from ultraviolet (UV) rays by wearing sunglasses
- Use of safety goggles to prevent occupational eye injuries
- Avoid self-medications and over the counter use of steroid drops in allergy
- Proper diet—green leafy vegetables, carrot, papaya, milk, and fish
- Do not smoke—quit smoking

## RECOMMENDED READING


1. Abbott J, Shah P. The epidemiology and etiology of pediatric ocular trauma. Surv Ophthalmol. 2013;58:476-85.
2. Al-Mahdi HS, Bener A, Hashim SP. Clinical pattern of pediatric ocular trauma in fast developing country. Int Emerg Nurs. 2011;19:186-91.
3. American Optometry Association.
4. Bourne RR, Dineen BP, Huq DM, Ali SM, Johnson GJ. Correction of refractive error in the adult population of Bangladesh: Meeting the unmet need. Invest Ophthalmol Vis Sci. 2004;45:410-7.
5. Brophy M, Sinclair SA, Hostetler SG, Xiang H. Pediatric eye injury–related hospitalizations in the United States. Pediatrics. 2006;117:e1263-71.
6. Desai T, Vyas C, Desai S, Malli S. Pattern of ocular injuries in paediatric population in western India. NHL J Med Sci. 2013;2:37-40.
7. GBD 2019 Blindness and Vision Impairment Collaborators Vision Loss Expert Group of the Global Burden of Disease Study. Causes of blindness and vision impairment in 2020 and trends over 30 years, and prevalence of avoidable blindness in relation to vision 2020: the right to sight: an analysis for the global burden of disease study. Lancet Glob Health. 2021;9:e144-60.
8. Gilbert C, Jugnoo SR, Graham EQ. Visual impairment and blindness in children. In: Gordon JJ, Darwin CM, Robert AW, Sheila KW (Eds). The Epidemiology of Eye Diseases, 2nd edition. London: Arnold Publication; 2003. pp. 260-83.
9. Ipe A, Shibu P, Skariah R. Prevalence of refractive errors and the extent of correction possible with conservative methods, among patients visiting a tertiary care hospital in South Kerala Age. 2016;6:16-45.
10. Mela EK, Mantzouranis GA, Giakoumis AP, Blatsios G, Andrikopoulos GK, Gartaganis SP. Ocular trauma in a Greek population: review of 899 cases resulting in hospitalization. Ophthalmic Epidemiol. 2005;12:185-90.
11. Pascolini D, Mariotti SP. Global estimates of visual impairment: 2010. Br J Ophthalmol. 2012;96:614-8.
12. Reichman NE, Corman H, Noonan K. Impact of child disability on the family. Matern Child Health J. 2008;12:679-83.
13. Resnikoff S, Pascolini D, Mariotti SP, Pokharel GP. Global magnitude of visual impairment caused by uncorrected refractive errors in 2004. Bull World Health Organ. 2008;86:63.
14. Rizal SOJ. Epidemiology and visual outcomes of pediatric ocular trauma cases in a tertiary hospital. Philipp J Ophthalmol. 2014;39:27-32.
15. Thompson C, Kumar N, Billson F, Martin F. The aetiology of perforating ocular injuries in children. Br J Ophthalmol. 2002;86:920-2.

# 4B.6 Common Dental Problems in Adolescents

*Aishwarya Kulkarni*

## ■ INTRODUCTION

Adolescence is a crucial period in an individual's life marked by significant physical, emotional, and social changes. Amidst these transformations, one often overlooked aspect of adolescent health is dental well-being. Dental problems in adolescents are a common concern that can have lasting impacts on their overall health and quality of life. This stage of life is characterized by a unique set of challenges and risk factors that can predispose adolescents to a range of oral health issues. In this context, it is essential to explore the various dental problems that affect adolescents, their causes, consequences, and the importance of early intervention to ensure that these young individuals can maintain healthy smiles well into adulthood. This chapter delves into the intricate world of dental health during adolescence, shedding light on the issues that can arise, the factors that contribute to them, and the strategies to mitigate them.

## ■ VARIOUS DENTAL CONCERNS

### Developmental Issues

#### Etiology

Developmental in origin, i.e., could be due to mutations in genes, inheriting pattern, or systemic disturbances like intoxications, perinatal and postnatal problems, malnutrition, infectious diseases, and a range of other medical conditions.

#### Explanation

Developmental tooth defects are irregularities in tooth morphology that occur during tooth formation. Various defects can occur, but the primary three include those that affect the mineralization of tooth enamel—dental fluorosis, enamel hypoplasia, and amelogenesis imperfecta. Hypomineralized teeth often wear more poorly or fracture more easily than normally formed teeth, and they may be aesthetically compromised and/or more susceptible to tooth decay.

The impact of a congenitally missing permanent tooth on the developing dentition can be significant. When treating adolescent patients who are congenitally missing teeth, many factors (e.g., aesthetics; patient age; growth potential; and orthodontic, periodontal, and oral surgical needs) must be taken into consideration.

The atypical eruption of permanent teeth during adolescence may lead to various issues such as root resorption, bone loss, gingival problems, space constraints, and aesthetic considerations. Detecting and addressing incorrectly positioned teeth early can result in a healthier and more aesthetically pleasing smile. Prevention and treatment options may encompass removing baby teeth, surgical procedures, or a combination of endodontic, orthodontic, periodontal, and restorative treatments.

### Tooth Decay

#### Etiology

Tooth decay also known as dental caries can be caused due to one or combination of multiple factors, such as dietary sugar, biofilm formation, role of host, and eventual effect of time due to lack of overall oral hygiene.

#### Explanation

A significant history of cavities in early childhood stands as the most potent indicator for experiencing cavities in adolescence and beyond into adulthood. In cases where the risk factors for dental caries persist from childhood, the likelihood of developing cavities in permanent teeth will continue to rise throughout adolescence. Immature permanent tooth enamel, a total increase in susceptible tooth surfaces, and environmental factors such as diet, independence to seek care or avoid it, moreover, neglecting oral hygiene, and other social factors can further contribute to the increasing prevalence of cavities during adolescence.

### Dental Emergency

#### Etiology

Physical injury or trauma, especially due to sports and other outdoor/indoor activities, is the cause of dental emergency.

*Explanation*

Increased physical growth and coordination during adolescence and the desire of some to participate in sports, along with an increased capacity and freedom for risk-taking behavior, raise the likelihood of traumatic orofacial injury. These accidents may lead to dental injuries like tooth chipping, fractures, or, in some cases, complete tooth loss.

## Periodontal Problems

### Etiology

Biofilms are commonly linked to the development of periodontal diseases. To thrive in a specific environment, microbes must adhere to tooth surfaces and proliferate in sheltered areas such as tooth crevices and periodontal pockets. The buildup of microbes on tooth surfaces is referred to as dental plaque.

*Explanation*

Adolescence is a pivotal time for periodontal health. Evidence shows that irreversible periodontal tissue damage often starts in late teens to early adulthood. Gingival disease is common during this phase. Factors like dental caries, mouth breathing, tooth crowding, and eruption can lead to gingivitis in adolescents. Hormonal shifts during puberty might also play a role. Increased sex hormones are believed to modify gingival response, leading to heightened inflammation, even with minimal plaque presence.

Gingivitis refers to gum inflammation triggered by the buildup of biofilm (plaque) along the gumline. On the other hand, periodontal disease, characterized by chronic inflammatory infection, results in gum inflammation, bleeding, and in its advanced stages, potential loss of alveolar bone, tooth mobility, and eventual tooth loss.

Adolescents can face a range of dental conditions, including dental plaque biofilm gingivitis, nondental plaque-induced gingival disease, various forms of periodontitis (chronic, aggressive, and necrotizing), periodontal issues linked to systemic diseases, periodontal abscess, endodontic-periodontal lesions, gingival recession, occlusal trauma, and peri-implant diseases. The severity of these conditions is assessed through clinical and radiographic examinations, often classified by staging and grading the clinical presentation. Early diagnosis becomes crucial, particularly when systemic risk factors such as poorly controlled diabetes, leukemia, smoking, or malnutrition are present.

## Orthodontic Problems

### Etiology

The majority of malocclusions are of genetic origin, but some can be acquired. Inherited issues encompass problems like crowded teeth, excessive gaps between teeth, additional or missing teeth, and an array of irregularities affecting the jaws, teeth, and facial structure. Acquired malocclusions may result from factors such as accidents causing trauma, habits like thumb-sucking or pacifier use, airway obstruction due to enlarged tonsils and adenoids, dental conditions, or the premature loss of primary or permanent teeth. Regardless of their origin, many of these issues not only impact tooth alignment but also influence facial development and appearance.

*Explanation*

Common orthodontic problems seen in children include overbites, open bites, underbites, and spacing issues. For many adolescents, the presence and impact of malocclusion become significant. Malocclusion involves the misalignment of teeth and jaws, which can have far-reaching consequences. It can affect oral functionality, alter facial aesthetics, increase the risk of dental injuries, and diminish overall quality of life. While some malocclusions are primarily cosmetic, more severe cases can significantly impact periodontal health, chewing ability, speech, and psychosocial development. Notably, the appearance becomes a pivotal concern just as this age group often begins orthodontic treatment with appliances or braces.

## High-risk Behavior and Habits

### Etiology

The use of alcohol and illicit drugs is the risk factor for poor oral health outcomes in adolescents that can extend into adulthood and lead to substance misuse or abuse and behaviors in adulthood that may have negative oral health outcomes as well. Smoking has systemic as well as dental effects like staining on teeth and change in the natural microbes in oral cavity and alteration in salivary flow making teeth more susceptible to caries and plaque and other gum diseases.

## Explanation

Increased alcohol consumption is correlated with a heightened risk of oral human papillomavirus (HPV) infection in older adolescents and young adults. Moreover, alcohol intake elevates vulnerability to oral and dental ailments. Engaging in heavy episodic drinking has been connected to a greater occurrence of cavities among adolescents, possibly stemming from increased consumption of sugar-sweetened beverages (SSBs) and suboptimal dental hygiene practices.

The influence of various risk factors on alcohol and drug use, such as temperament, family, peers, and environment, varies throughout different stages of development. Younger adolescents tend to have higher rates of inhalant use and misuse of prescription medication, whereas older adolescents are more exposed to and likely to use alcohol and illicit drugs. This transition corresponds with a phase of exploration, identity development, and reduced parental monitoring, which often coincides with increased availability of alcohol and drugs.

Evaluating the influence of tobacco consumption on the oral health of adolescents can present challenges. Nevertheless, it is important to recognize that both regular and occasional teenage users may experience various issues, including teeth discoloration, receding gums, periodontitis, halitosis, dental cavities, tooth fractures, and the development of leukoplakia.

## Orofacial Pain and Temporomandibular Disorders

### Etiology

The most common causes of orofacial pain in adolescents are tooth decay and gingival-related problems caused by abscess (infection) of the tooth or the gums. Injuries due to sports or other trauma to face can also cause this type of pain. Stress and parafunctional habits like bruxism and clenching or nail biting can also serve as a cause.

### Explanation

Discomfort can also arise from the eruption of the third molar, commonly referred to as the wisdom tooth. Pain may occur when the tooth's path of eruption is obstructed, or when it only partially emerges, leading to inflammation in the surrounding gum tissue, a condition known as pericoronitis. Another form of orofacial pain that tends to manifest during adolescence is the recurring aphthous ulcer, commonly called a canker sore. These are typically roundish, ulcer-like sores that develop inside the mouth, often on the inner surfaces of the lips, cheeks, or tongue. Additionally, recurrent herpetic infections, commonly known as cold sores, can also be problematic. These oral infections may be related to changes in diet, emotional stress, and hormonal changes as well as sun exposure and can be transmitted through intimate behavior. They usually disappear on their own in 10–14 days.

Temporomandibular joint (TMJ) disorders can manifest at any stage of life, but they seem to be more common during adolescence. While the symptoms of temporomandibular disorder (TMD) may emerge at an earlier age in adolescents than in adults, the underlying causes of the disorder are likely to be consistent across different age groups. Similar to adults, factors associated with TMD in adolescents show more occurrence in females compared to males such as experiencing negative somatic and psychological symptoms. Habits like night bruxism can also lead to temporomandibular stress and subsequent pain.

## ■ MANAGEMENT

### Caries or Tooth Decay

#### Primary Prevention

- *Fluoride:* Fluoridation has proven to be safe and highly effective in prevention and control of caries. Fluoride can be advantageous for adolescents not only during their teenage years but also into early adulthood. While it is generally considered unnecessary to introduce fluoride into developing enamel beyond the age of 16 years for systemic benefits, topical advantages can still be achieved through the use of optimally fluoridated water, professionally administered or prescribed fluoride compounds, as well as fluoride-containing toothpaste.
- *Oral hygiene:* Adolescents become more independent and toothbrushing may become less of a priority. Encouragement and motivation are essential to promote regular brushing with fluoride toothpaste and consistent flossing among adolescent patients. It is important to discuss oral hygiene in order to highlight the benefit of the topical effect of fluoride, removal of plaque from tooth surfaces, and also decrease halitosis and improve aesthetics.
- *Diet management:* Many adolescents are exposed to and consume high quantities of refined carbohydrates and acid-containing beverages in the form of soda,

high-energy sports drinks, and junk food and with introduction of coffee. Diet analysis and adjustment can prove beneficial for the adolescent. Reduction in sugar intake and avoiding snacking in-between meals are important.

■ *Sealants:* Sealant placement is an effective caries-preventive technique that should be considered on an individual basis. Sealants have been recommended for any tooth, primary or permanent, that is judged to be at risk for pit and fissure caries. The risk of developing cavities can rise as a result of alterations in patient habits, shifts in oral microflora, or changes in physical health. In such cases, unsealed teeth may benefit from the application of dental sealants.

### Secondary Prevention

■ *Professional preventive care:* Professional preventive dental care, on a routine basis, may prevent oral disease or disclose existing disease in its early stages. Adolescents who do not receive regular dental check-ups may require immediate professional evaluation and comprehensive treatment due to advanced issues, such as severe cavities, gum disease, or other oral problems.

■ *Restorative options:* Five strategies are available:
  1. Complete caries removal, and restoration
  2. Partial caries removal, and restoration
  3. No caries removal, seal with restoration
  4. No caries removal, leave cavity, or make lesion self-cleansing, provide prevention
  5. Extraction, or a reevaluation with possible extraction in the event of pain or sepsis development.

In permanent molars, noncavitated occlusal dentin lesions and radiographically in the outer one-third of the dentine can be sealed and monitored. To examine permanent teeth with proximal lesions located in the outer one-third of the dentine for enamel damage or cavities penetrating into the dentin, orthodontic separators can be employed for separation. Subsequently, follow-up X-rays should be captured to reassess the lesions within a year. When making a decision about whether to use a stainless steel crown, replace a flawed restoration, or simply observe and reevaluate, it is crucial to take into account the expected lifespan of a primary tooth with existing restoration issues.

## Malocclusion and Orthodontic Issues

■ Any tooth/jaw positional problems that present significant esthetic, functional, physiologic, or emotional dysfunction are potential difficulties for the adolescent, e.g., single or multiple tooth malpositions, tooth size and jaw size discrepancies, and craniofacial disfigurements. Malocclusion can affect the oral health quality of life for adolescents. Adolescents with Class II and III malocclusions or anterior overjet greater than 6 mm reported a significant impact on their oral health-related quality of life.

■ Evaluation of third molars, including radiographic diagnostic aids, should be an integral part of the dental examination of the adolescent.

## Orofacial Pain and TMD

Majority of the time patients visit the physician when they have discomfort or dysfunction. Examples of symptoms include headaches, joint locking episodes (open lock/TMJ subluxation), pain associated with mandibular function (chewing), and limitations in opening. Reducing pain, regaining normal range of motion, and regaining normal jaw and masticatory function are the objectives of TMD treatment. Numerous TMDs have the potential to be self-limiting and cyclical, with intervals of total symptom remission. Evaluating the cause of the symptom is crucial for the further treatment planning for instance night guards can be given for adolescents with bruxism.

## High-risk Behavior and Habits

Managing high-risk behavior in children involves education, open communication, positive role modeling, setting boundaries, supervision, emotional support, peer influence awareness, and involvement in constructive activities. If necessary, seek professional help, especially if risky behavior persists. Encourage responsible decision-making, teach coping mechanisms, and be prepared for crises. Each child is unique, so tailored approach to their specific needs and circumstances. It is important to remember that managing high-risk behavior in adolescents is an ongoing process that requires patience, understanding, and consistent effort. The approach may need to be adapted to their specific needs and parents should seek medical and other professional counseling help if needed.

## Periodontal Disease (Gingivitis/Periodontitis)

It's important for individuals with periodontal disease to work closely with their dental professionals to develop a personalized treatment plan tailored to their specific needs and the severity of their condition. Early detection and intervention can help prevent the progression of periodontal disease and preserve oral health.

1. *Nonsurgical Treatments:*
   - *Professional dental cleanings:* Regular cleanings by a dental hygienist or dentist can remove plaque and tartar buildup, preventing the progression of gum disease.
   - *Scaling and root planing:* This deep cleaning procedure involves removing plaque and tartar from below the gumline (scaling) and smoothing the root surfaces (root planing) to remove bacteria and promote gum healing.
   - *Antimicrobial therapy:* Antibacterial mouth rinses or gels may be prescribed to reduce bacterial load in the mouth and promote healing.

2. *Surgical Treatments:*
   - *Flap Surgery:* In cases where deep pockets have formed between the gums and teeth, flap surgery may be performed to lift the gums, remove tartar, and reposition the gums for better hygiene access.
   - *Bone grafts:* If periodontal disease has caused bone loss around the teeth, bone grafting procedures may be necessary to regenerate lost bone tissue and support the teeth.
   - *Soft Tissue Grafts:* Gum grafts may be used to replace or augment gum tissue that has been lost due to periodontal disease, helping to cover exposed tooth roots and reduce sensitivity.
   - *Guided tissue regeneration:* This surgical procedure involves placing special membranes or materials between the gum tissue and bone to encourage the regeneration of lost bone and periodontal ligament.

3. *Maintenance Therapy:*
   - *Ongoing monitoring:* Regular dental check-ups and periodontal evaluations are essential for monitoring the progress of treatment and preventing recurrence of periodontal disease.
   - *Periodontal maintenance cleanings:* After initial treatment, patients may require more frequent cleanings (often every three to four months) to maintain gum health and prevent further progression of the disease.
   - *Home care education:* Patients should receive guidance on proper oral hygiene techniques, including brushing, flossing, and interdental cleaning devices, to effectively control plaque buildup and prevent future gum disease.

## ■ CONCLUSION

Adolescence is a critical phase marked by unique dental challenges and risk factors, including gingival disease, periodontitis, hormonal influences, and various other oral health issues. Early intervention and effective oral hygiene practices are essential to mitigate these problems and maintain healthy smiles into adulthood. Adolescents must be educated about the importance of oral health, and healthcare providers should emphasize the significance of regular dental check-ups. Recognizing and addressing periodontal conditions, especially in cases with systemic risk factors, is of paramount importance. As adolescents navigate the complexities of this developmental stage, addressing their dental health needs can contribute to their overall well-being and quality of life in the long run.

## ■ KEY MESSAGES

- It is advisable to brush teeth twice a day with tooth-paste containing fluoride to ensure ongoing topical advantages.
- Professional fluoride treatments should be tailored to the individual patient's caries risk, as assessed by their dental provider.
- Home-applied prescription strength topical fluoride products [e.g., 0.4% stannous fluoride gel, 0.5% fluoride gel or paste, 0.2% sodium fluoride (NaF) rinse] can be employed as necessary based on an individual's caries history or risk level.
- Systemic fluoride intake via optimal fluoridation of drinking water or professionally prescribed supplements is recommended to 16 years of age. Supplements should only be considered once a comprehensive assessment of all other potential sources of fluoride has been conducted.
- Adolescents should be educated and motivated to maintain personal oral hygiene through daily plaque removal, including flossing, with the frequency and technique based on the individual's oral hygiene needs.
- Professional removal of plaque and calculus is recommended highly for the adolescent, with the frequency of such intervention based on the individual's assessed risk for caries/periodontal disease as determined by the patient's dental provider.

- Diet analysis, along with professionally determined recommendations for maximal general and dental health, should be part of an adolescent's dental health management.
- Adolescents at risk for caries should have sealants placed. An individual's susceptibility to cavities can vary with time, making it important to periodically reevaluate the need for dental sealants during adolescence.
- Supplemental medical history topics regarding questions on pregnancy, alcohol and drug use, oral piercings, tobacco use, sexual activity, and eating disorders should be included in the adolescent dental record.
- Periodic visits to the dentist are required for preventive care as well as early identification of an issue. Adolescents and parents should be aware about maintenance of oral hygiene.

## ■ RECOMMENDED READING


1. American Academy of Pediatric Dentistry. Adolescent oral health care. The Reference Manual of Pediatric Dentistry. Chicago, Ill.: American Academy of Pediatric Dentistry; 2023. pp. 317-26.
2. Dean JA. Mcdonald and Avery's Dentistry for the Child and Adolescence, 4th edition.
3. Kini V, Patil RU, Pathak T, Prakash A, Gupta B. Diagnosis and management of periodontal disease in children and adolescents: a brief review. J Dent Allied Sci 2016;5:78-83.
4. Marwah N (Ed). Textbook of Paediatric Dentistry, 3rd edition. New Delhi: Jaypee Brothers Medical Publishers (P) Ltd.; 2016.
5. Oral Health Clinical Advisory Network. (2019). Clinical guidelines for child and adolescent oral health. [online] Available from chrome-extension:// efaidnbmnnnibpcajpcglclefindmkaj/https://www. nzohcan.org.nz/wp-content/uploads/2019/09/OHCAN_ Clinical-Guidelines-for-Child-and-Adolescent-Oral-Health_2019-July_online-2-3-2.pdf [Last accessed March, 2024].
6. Oral Health in America: Advances and Challenges. Bethesda (MD): National Institute of Dental and Craniofacial Research (US); 2021. Section 2B, Oral Health Across the Lifespan: Adolescents.
7. Romero-Reyes M, Uyanik JM. Orofacial pain management: current perspectives. J Pain Res. 2014;7:99-115.

# Part C: Seemingly Trivial Health Issues

***Sub-section Editors:*** *Poonam Bhatia, Samir Shah, Shailaja Mane*

## 4C.1 — Sleep Disorders

*Bharath Reddy, Newton Luiz*

## ■ INTRODUCTION

As per the American Academy of Sleep Medicine recommendations, an adolescent is required to sleep 8–10 hours every night to ensure general well-being, cardiovascular health, and metabolic and mental health. Chronic sleep deprivation is associated with an increased prevalence of obesity, diabetes mellitus, immune dysfunction, and a higher risk of cardiac disease, stroke, and Alzheimer's disease. 20% of serious and fatal road traffic accidents in the USA are caused by drowsy drivers.

## ■ ADOLESCENT SLEEP PHYSIOLOGY

The onset of puberty corresponds with a biologically mediated change in circadian physiology: There is a shift in the release of melatonin (the sleep hormone) to a later hour, leading adolescents to delay sleep. Physiologically, adolescents can stay awake at night and typically take longer to fall asleep compared to prepubertal teenagers. The homeostatic drive for sleep, which intensifies with prolonged wakefulness, tends to accumulate at a slower rate in adolescents.

## ■ SLEEP DEPRIVATION

The most common sleep-related issue in adolescents is sleep deprivation. 62–72% adolescents sleep <8 hours each night. Various factors of sleep deprivation include studies, meeting with friends of the same and other gender, TV, social media, working for pocket money, and time spent on sports, games, and online gaming compete for their time, and they often go to bed 1–2 hours later than adults.

*Any adolescent who needs to be routinely woken up for school, frequently falls asleep in school, or sleeps 2 hours more in the weekends and holidays than on school days should be considered as sleep deficient.* Parents are frequently unaware that adolescents and youth have a higher sleep requirement than adults and attribute their sleepiness to laziness. Parents may serve as poor models by going to bed at irregular times, falling asleep while watching TV, and sleeping excessively on weekends.

### Consequences of Sleep Deprivation

Excessive daytime sleepiness results in drowsiness, yawning, lethargy, and a tendency to doze off in the classroom. While this is easily recognizable as sleep deficit, most of the other manifestations go unrecognized:

- *Cognitive:* Impaired attention, concentration, and memory consolidation. This affects studies.
- *Emotional:* Mood swings and irritability, impacting interpersonal relationships, and increased risk of developing depression and anxiety.
- *Impaired motor skills:* Decreased co-ordination and slower reaction time, increasing the risk of road traffic accidents.
- *Increased risky behaviors:* Due to impulsivity and poor decision-making. Drives recklessly, tries out drugs, and indulges in unprotected sex.
- *Increased stress levels:* Causes anxiety, and elevates levels of hormones like cortisol and epinephrine, which reduce immune function, increase glucose levels, increase hunger and obesity, and increase blood pressure.
- Migraine

As sleep problems are great mimics, they should be ruled out in every child suspected to have attention-deficit/hyperactivity disorder (ADHD), migraine, and behavioral or academic problems.

## ■ POOR SLEEP HYGIENE

The most common cause of sleep deprivation in adolescents is poor sleep hygiene. This refers to habits

## INVESTIGATIONS

- A smartwatch provides useful data on sleep duration and quality and sleep-wake patterns.
- Polysomnography (PSG) is the gold standard for assessing sleep stages, and sleep disruptors such as OSA and periodic limb movement disorder (PLMD).

## RESTLESS LEGS SYNDROME

The characteristic feature is a powerful urge to move the legs, usually associated with strange sensations in the lower limbs, which interferes with the ability to fall asleep. Walking, stretching, or even rubbing the limbs will result in immediate but temporary relief of these symptoms, which tend to be worse at rest, especially at bedtime. The incidence is 2% in adolescence, and increases with age. It is worsened by alcohol or caffeine intake, sleep deprivation, antidepressants, low iron stores even without anemia, and pregnancy. There is a sixfold increase in prevalence among first-degree relatives. The pathogenesis is uncertain and is probably multifactorial. One suggested mechanism is that iron is a cofactor for tyrosine hydroxylation, which is needed for dopamine synthesis, and these persons seem to have some dopaminergic dysfunction. Restless legs syndrome (RLS) is more common in certain systemic illnesses, especially renal disorders. Management is by avoiding aggravating factors and by iron supplementation for 3 months if serum ferritin is <50 µg/L. If this proves inadequate pramipexole, which increases dopamine levels in the CNS, is highly effective.

## PERIODIC LIMB MOVEMENT DISORDER

The adolescent may be totally unaware of this common disorder that causes excessive daytime sleepiness. During sleep there are repeated jerking movements affecting mainly the lower limbs, each movement lasting only a few seconds, usually occurring every 20–40 seconds, but this can go on for minutes or even hours. Usually, the movement is minimal: the big toe extends and the ankle dorsiflexes repeatedly. However, he may kick around a lot, move all over the bed, and even fall off it. The next morning, he complains of muscle pains or daytime sleepiness.

Polysomnography reveals PLMD in >10% of adolescents who complain of insomnia or daytime drowsiness. These movements occur infrequently in healthy individuals, and it is considered a disorder only when they are severe enough to disturb sleep.

> **BOX 4:** BEARS sleep screening tool.
>
> - **Bedtime:** Do you have any problems falling asleep at bedtime?
> - **Excessive daytime sleepiness:** Do you feel sleepy a lot in the day? In school? While driving?
> - **Awakenings:** Do you awaken a lot at night? Do you have trouble getting back to sleep?
> - **Regularity and duration:** At what time do you usually go to bed on school days? During weekends? How much sleep do you usually get?
> - **Snoring:** (Ask the parent) Does your teenager snore loudly or nightly?

Periodic limb movement disorder and RLS have the same etiological factors, may act by a similar mechanism, and are managed in the same manner. PLMD is very common in adolescents diagnosed as ADHD, and the management of PLMD often dramatically relieves their ADHD symptoms.

## SCREENING

BEARS is a simple and free-to-use sleep screening tool **(Box 4)**.

## PRIMARY NOCTURNAL ENURESIS

This parasomnia occurs in deep sleep. The prevalence is 2–5% in early adolescence, and comes down to <1% in adults. It is more common in males, and if one or more parents had primary nocturnal enuresis (PNE) in childhood. It is a matter of great shame to the adolescent, who cannot participate in a school excursion, or stay overnight at a cousin's or friend's house, for fear that the secret would become public knowledge.

One must first rule out secondary causes: Ask about daytime urinary problems, snoring, and constipation; examine for spinal problems or a distended bladder; and do routine urine tests.

Behavioral therapy works most of the time. Ask when is dinnertime and bedtime. Enquire into fluid intake in the evening.

- Is there plentiful fluid intake close to bedtime (with dinner, or even afterward)? The bladder capacity of a 10-year-old is only 360 mL ("age + 2" ounces).
- Does bedtime occur soon after dinner? More than 50% of the "solid" food we consume is fluid (rice is one-third grain and two-thirds water). It takes around 2 hours for the food to be digested and urine to be produced.

*Advise behavioral therapy:*

- Drink as much water as you want in the daytime. But no fluids for 3 hours before bedtime.
- Have dinner 2–3 hours before bedtime.
- Take only one-third glass of water (2 ounces) along with dinner. Avoid spicy food, watery foods, and milk at dinnertime.
- Visit the washroom 30 minutes before bedtime, and again immediately before going to bed.

Most adolescents with PNE lack motivation and feel helpless, yet success depends on their cooperation. Ask them to write down the days 1–31 on a piece of paper. Every morning they (or a parent) should tick √ if the bed is dry, and × if it is wet. There will usually be notable improvement in a week if they cooperate.

If behavioral therapy is inadequate, prescribe imipramine 25–50 mg HS, which can be given for 3–6 months. A minority will require oral desmopressin acetate 0.2–0.6 mg 2 hours before bedtime. Also effective is an auditory/vibratory alarm that goes off when the adolescent wets, setting off a moisture sensor in the underwear.

## ■ FUTURE GOALS

The incidence of sleep deprivation is increasing in adolescents, which requires strategies from all stakeholders, healthcare professionals, parents, schools, and the community. An American Academy of Pediatrics policy statement states that delayed school start times for middle and high schools will increase overall sleep time, decrease levels of daytime sleepiness, improve mood, increase school attendance, and reduce car crashes.

## ■ KEY MESSAGES

- Sufficient sleep is a biological necessity, not a luxury.
- Insufficient sleep is the most common sleep-related issue faced by adolescents.
- Parents are unaware that adolescents need 8–10 hours of sleep daily.
- Adolescents deliberately sacrifice sleep to find time for study, sports, work, TV, social media, and friends of the same and other gender.
- Insufficient sleep often manifests as headache, mood disorders, difficulty studying, hyperactivity and impulsivity, or cognitive defects.
- Adolescents should be taught good sleep hygiene.
- In primary insomnia, the adolescent is so anxious about his inability to asleep that his agitation further interferes with his ability to fall asleep.

- RLS and progressive limb movement disorder can often be treated with iron supplements.
- BEARS is a simple and effective screening tool for sleep disorders.
- PNE is a common, distressing, yet eminently treatable parasomnia.

## ■ RECOMMENDED READING


1. de Bruin EJ, Bögels SM, Oort FJ, Meijer AM. Improvements of adolescent psychopathology after insomnia treatment: results from a randomized controlled trial over 1 year. J Child Psychol Psychiatry. 2018;59(5):509-22.
2. Dewald-Kaufmann JF, Oort FJ, Meijer AM. The effects of sleep extension and sleep hygiene advice on sleep and depressive symptoms in adolescents: a randomized controlled trial. J Child Psychol Psychiatry. 2014;55(3):273-83.
3. Gradisar M, Dohnt H, Gardner G, Paine S, Starkey K, Menne A, et al. A randomized controlled trial of cognitive-behavior therapy plus bright light therapy for adolescent delayed sleep phase disorder. Sleep (Basel). 2011;34(12):1671-80.
4. Kansagra S. (2020). Sleep Disorders in Adolescents. [online] Available from https://publications.aap.org/pediatrics/article/145/Supplement_2/S204/34446/Sleep-Disorders-in-Adolescents?autologincheck=redirected [Last accessed March, 2024].
5. Levenson JC, Shensa A, Sidani JE, Colditz JB, Primack BA. Social media use before bed and sleep disturbance among young adults in the United States: a nationally representative study. Sleep. 2017;40(9):zsx113.
6. Marx R, Tanner-Smith EE, Davison CM, Ufholz LA, Freeman J, Shankar R, et al. Later school start times for supporting the education, health, and well-being of high school students. Cochrane Database Syst Rev. 2017;7(7):CD009467.
7. Owens JA. Sleep Medicine. In: Kliegman RM, St Geme JW, Blum NJ, Shah SS, Tasker RC, Wilson KM (Eds). Nelson Textbook of Pediatrics, 21st edition. Philadelphia: Elsevier; 2020. pp. 172-84.
8. Paruthi S, Brooks LJ, D'Ambrosio C, Hall WA, Kotagal S, Lloyd RM, et al. Consensus statement of the American Academy of sleep medicine on the recommended amount of sleep for healthy children: methodology and discussion. J Clin Sleep Med. 2016;12(11):1549-61.
9. Sadock BJ, Sadock VA, Ruiz P. Kaplan and Sadock's Synopsis of Psychiatry, 11th edition. Philadelphia: Wolters Kluwer; 2015. pp. 533-63.
10. Scammell TE, Saper CB, Czeisler CA. Sleep Disorders. In: Jameson JL, Fauci AS, Kasper DL, Hauser SL, Longo DL, Loscalzo J (Eds). Harrison's Principles of Internal Medicine, 20th edition. Philadelphia: McGraw-Hill Education; 2018. pp. 166-76.

# 4C.2    Headache in Adolescents

*JC Garg*

## ■ INTRODUCTION

Headaches are common and greatly influence the quality of life in adolescence. On one hand it could be pointer toward serious intracranial pathology or mental disorders, which might result in school absence, decreased extracurricular activities, or poor academic achievement.

Prevalence of adolescent headache ranges from 57–82%. Before puberty boys are affected more than girls; later it occurs more frequently in girls. 20% of adults suffering from headaches have the onset before the age of 10 years.

Based on cause headaches are divided into primary and secondary headaches.

- *Primary headaches:* This type of headache does not have any underlying disease.
  - Migraine
  - Tension-type headache
  - Cluster headache
- *Secondary headaches:* This type of headache is secondary to some underlying pathology.
  - Infections—sinusitis, otitis media (OM), meningitis, and encephalitis
  - Trauma—head/neck
  - Vascular—cranial/cervical
  - Nonvascular intracranial
  - Intracranial space-occupying lesion (ICSOL)—raised/low intracranial pressure (ICP), postepileptic, tumor, meningitis, and subarachnoid hemorrhage
  - Substance abuse—withdrawal/overdose
  - Facial pain from cranium, neck, eyes, ears, nose, sinuses teeth, and mouth
  - Disorders of homeostasis
  - Psychiatric disorders.

## ■ EVALUATION

When an adolescent presents with complaints of headaches, it is important to ask a series of questions to understand the context and potential causes. So, history taking is the key to successful diagnosis.

### History

- *Frequency and duration:* How often do you experience these headaches? How long do they usually last?

- *Location and intensity:* Can you describe where you feel the pain in your head? On a scale of 1 to 10, how intense is the pain?
- *Triggers:* Are there any specific activities, foods, stressors, or environments that seem to bring on these headaches?
- *Associated symptoms:* Do you experience any other symptoms alongside the headache, like nausea, sensitivity to light or sound, dizziness, or vision changes?
- *Sleep and hydration:* How is your sleep pattern? Do you drink enough water throughout the day?
- *Stress and emotional well-being:* Have you been feeling stressed, anxious, or overwhelmed lately? Any recent major changes or emotional challenges?
- *Medical history:* Do you have any history of head injuries, previous headaches, or any chronic medical conditions?
- *Medications and supplements:* Are you taking any medications or supplements regularly?
- *Lifestyle habits:* How much time do you spend on screens (computer, phone, and TV)? Do you maintain a regular meal schedule and balanced diet? Eye strains due to excessive mobile use and excessive study?

How and when headache started, sudden, first headache? Have you had like before this? Do you get a headache every day?

Do you have the same kind of headaches all the time? How long does your headaches last? How the headache pain feels—pounding, squeezing, stabbing, or something else?

What do you do when you get a headache? When you get a headache what makes your headache feel better or worse?

### HEEADSSS Screening

HEEADSSS screening is an essential tool to screen psychosocial issues of adolescents, especially those who suffer from recurrent headaches. HEEADSSS screening questionnaire gives a wealth of information regarding teens behavior, peers, contributor of stress, etc.

Discussing about confidentiality is essential before proceeding with the questions.

*Home:*
- Tell me something about family dynamics.
- Do you want to share something related to your home environment?

*Education:*
- Has there been any change in your educational performance?
- Does your headache affect your school attendance?
- Has there been any change in school?

*Eating:*
- Does headache affects your appetite?
- What do you feel about your body?

*Activity:*
- How do you spend your leisure time?
- How often do you play outdoor sports?
- How much time do you spend on screen?

*Drugs:*
- What is your opinion regarding use of drugs?
- Do any of your friends smoke or uses drugs?

*Sexuality:*
- Are you in romantic relationship?
- How comfortable are you with your gender?

*Suicide:*
- For any reason do you feel stressed out?
- At any point of time do you feel harming yourself?

*Safety:*
- Are you a member of any gang?
- Do you possess any arm?

Few other questions are essential to find out etiology of headache, such as:
- Are there any prodromal symptoms, like irritability, carving, and tiredness?
- Is headache acute, chronic, recurrent, chronic progressive, and chronic nonprogressive?

These questions provide valuable insights into potential triggers or underlying causes of the headaches. Depending on the responses, it may be necessary to seek further medical evaluation or advice from a healthcare professional.

## Physical Examination

Thorough physical examination is done to assess etiology of headache.
- Examination of eye for tension, undiagnosed refractive errors

**BOX 1:** Red flags.

| | |
|---|---|
| • Fever | • Seizures |
| • Altered sensorium | • Trauma—physical/ emotional |
| • Hypertension | |
| • Abnormal neurological examination | • Neck rigidity |
| | • Abnormal fundus |
| • Acute, severe, headache | • Chronic progressive occipital headache |
| • Recent change in character/ frequency of headache | |
| • Early morning headache | |

- Examining neck—stiffness, or restricted moments of neck
- Look for pallor—to rule out anemia as chronic anemia can cause frequent headache.
- Palpate for tenderness over sinuses—sinusitis
- Look for tenderness over jaw—temporomandibular joint pain
- Facial puffiness and generalized anasarca could be because of some renal pathology
- Blood pressure monitoring is done and primary or secondary causes of hypertension

*Approach:*
- Screen for red flags **(Box 1)**
- *Headache:* Onset, site, duration, frequency, aura, triggers, and relievers
- Family history, chronic disease, and medication
- *HEEADSSS:* Rule out psychopathological factors, look for stressors and strengths
- Body mass index (BMI), blood pressure (BP), Eye, ENT (Ear, Nose, and Throat), and dental examination
- Mental status examination

| PedMIDAS | |
|---|---|
| It was developed to assess migraine disability in pediatric and adolescent patients validated for ages 4–18 years | |
| *Disability grade* | *PedMIDAS score* |
| Little/none | 0–10 |
| Mild | 11–30 |
| Moderate | 31–50 |
| Severe | >50 |

## ■ MANAGEMENT OF PRIMARY HEADACHE

Treatment for acute headache includes:
- Ibuprofen (7.5–10 mg/kg), paracetamol (20–15 mg/kg), naproxen (2.5-5mg/kg), triptans (rizatriptan 10 mg, almotriptan 12.5 mg, sumatriptan 10 mg nasal, zolmitriptan 2.5 mg, and 5 mg nasal)

- Metoclopramide (10 mg BID) may be used as an adjunct. Treatment of underlying cause or disease.

## PREVENTION

To improve quality of life of these children, several non-pharmacological measures can be applied, such as:

- Maintaining headache diary helps to identify triggers and methods, which help in relieving symptoms.
- *Healthy lifestyle:* Regular diet and sleep, minimum 60 minutes physical activity
- Managing chronic diseases
- *Stress management:* Meditation, progressive muscle relaxation, and abdominal breathing. All these techniques help to decrease activity of overactive sympathetic system, which is tuned to generate flight and fight response.
- Cognitive behavior therapy (CBT) helps in managing mental health diseases.
- *Biofeedback:* In this, through sensors, therapist teaches how to reduce tension in particular muscle, thereby reducing number of episodes of headache associated with any stress.

*Chronic daily headache (CDH):* When adolescent suffers from headache on daily basis for at least 4 h/day or more than 15 days a month or daily for 3 months then they are said to suffer from CDH. Following could be the cause of such headaches:

- Obesity
- Sleep disorders
- *Mental disorders:* Depression, anxiety, drug use, etc.
- Sexual abuse
- Medication overuse like acetylsalicylic acid (ASA), nonsteroidal anti-inflammatory drugs (NSAIDs), and acetaminophen/paracetamol for >15 days/month for over 3 months

*Prophylactic treatment:*

- The patient has more than two migraine attacks per month
- *Indication:* >3/month, PedMIDAS score >30, and frequent school absences
- The patient has single attacks that last longer than 24 hours.
- The headaches cause major disruptions in the patient's lifestyle.
- The patient has complicated migraine.

Following medications are recommended:

- *Flunarizine:* 5–10 mg/day HS (adverse effects body-weight gain and drowsiness)
- *Antiepileptics*: Topiramate <2 mg/kg/dose; valproate 15–20 mg/kg
- *Propranolol:* 2–3 mg/kg/day TDS (contraindicated in asthma, heart failure, and diabetes)
- *Cyproheptadine:* 0.2–0.4 mg/kg/day HS
- *Amitriptyline:* 0.1–2 mg/kg
- *Nutraceuticals:* Riboflavin and magnesium
- Melatonin for regulating sleep.

## KEY MESSAGES

- Headaches are common in children and adolescents.
- A detailed history including HEEADSSS screening is essential for headache in adolescents.
- Screening for red flags is essential for timely treatment of acute headache.
- Intracranial imaging is indicated only when neurological signs or focal deficits are clinically evident.
- Management of primary headache includes lifestyle changes, biobehavioral therapy, and pharmacotherapy.

## RECOMMENDED READING

1. American Migraine Foundation. (2023). Breathing exercises for migraine. [online] Available from https://americanmigrainefoundation.org/resource-library/breathing-exercises-for-migraine/ [Last accessed March, 2024].
2. Assarzadegan F, Asgarzadeh S, Hatamabadi HR, Shahrami A, Tabatabaey A, Asgarzadeh M. Effect of slow-paced respiration on migraine characteristics: a randomized controlled trial. Iran J Neurol. 2021;20(1):19-25.
3. Garza I, Schwedt TJ. Diagnosis and management of chronic daily headache. Semin Neurol. 2020;40(3):287-93.
4. Goadsby PJ, Holland PR, Martins-Oliveira M, Hoffmann J, Schankin C, Akerman S. Pathophysiology of migraine: a disorder of sensory processing. Physiol Rev. 2017;97(2):553-622.
5. Headache Classification Committee of the International Headache Society (IHS). Classification and diagnostic criteria for headache disorders, cranial neuralgias, and facial pain. Cephalalgia. 1988;8(Suppl 7):1-96.
6. Yu S, Liu R, Zhao G, Yang X, Qiao X, Feng J, et al. The prevalence and burden of primary headaches in China: a population-based door-to-door survey. Headache. 2012;52(4):582-91.

# 4C.3 Fainting

*Kalpana Datta*

## ■ INTRODUCTION

*Fainting*, or the medical term syncope, is defined as an abrupt, transient, complete loss of consciousness, associated with an inability to maintain postural tone, with rapid and spontaneous recovery. It is most often benign but may sometimes herald a more serious and potentially life-threatening cause.

The loss of consciousness is because of a lack of cerebral blood flow or cerebral hypoperfusion most commonly due to a transient disturbance of normal reflexive mechanisms of the autonomic nervous system in regulating heart rate, blood pressure, and peripheral vascular resistance (neurocardiogenic syncope or vasovagal syncope). It is estimated that 20% of all children will experience at least one episode of fainting or syncope before the end of adolescence, so it is not an uncommon problem. Before the age of 6 years, however, syncope is unusual except in patients with seizure disorders, breath-holding episodes, or primary cardiac dysrhythmias.

A typical presentation in an adolescent is loss of consciousness triggered by a specific event such as pain, medical procedure, emotional distress, sitting or standing upright, and often accompanied by an early prodrome of dizziness, nausea, diaphoresis, and pallor.

## ■ CAUSES OF SYNCOPE

Syncope can be classified into three major categories: Neurally mediated syncope (NMS), cardiovascular syncope, and noncardiovascular syncope **(Box 1)**. The most common cause of syncope in young patients is vasovagal syncope (NMS). The second category or cardiovascular syncope though having a small representation is a major cause of anxiety due to its potentially life-threatening causes.

Neurally mediated syncope typically begins with a prodrome that lasts several seconds to minutes, progressing to a brief period of unconsciousness. Prodromal symptoms include light headedness, dizziness, nausea, shortness of breath, pallor, diaphoresis, and visual changes. These episodes are often triggered by one of many provocative events, such as emotional stress, fear, anxiety, or a

---

**BOX 1:** Causes of syncope.

*Neurally mediated syncope*
*Cardiovascular syncope:*
- *Primary:*
  - Left ventricular outflow obstruction
  - Right ventricular outflow obstruction
  - Pulmonary hypertension
  - Eisenmenger
  - Cardiomyopathy
- *Arrhythmias:*
  - Tachyarrhythmias:
    - Long QT syndrome
    - Brugada syndrome (familial ventricular fibrillation)
    - Wolff–Parkinson–White syndrome
    - Supraventricular tachycardia
    - Ventricular tachycardia:
      - Postoperative
      - Idiopathic
      - Right ventricular dysplasia
- *Bradyarrhythmias:*
  - Sick sinus syndrome
  - Heart block
- *Noncardiovascular syncope:*
  - Basilar migraine
  - Seizures
  - Vertigo
  - Hyperventilation
  - Situational (cough, micturition, stretch, hair grooming, and defecation)
  - Breath-holding spells

---

sudden change in posture. Anemia, dehydration, hunger, physical exhaustion, and a crowded or poorly ventilated environment can all act as a precipitant.

Vasodepressor syncope that is associated with exercise has been well described in adolescent patients and most commonly occurs immediately after the termination of an activity.

Cardiac syncope is less common than NMS, but a thorough evaluation of any syncopal event is mandated to ensure the detection of potentially life-threatening cardiac causes. Cardiac causes can be divided in two broad categories: *Primary cardiac anomalies* (right or left heart obstruction, hypertrophic or congestive

> **BOX 2:** Risk factors that suggest cardiac syncope.
>
> - Little or no prodrome
> - Loss of consciousness lasting longer than 5 minutes
> - Exercise-induced syncope
> - Chest pain or palpitations
> - History of cardiac disease

cardiomyopathies, pulmonary hypertension, cyanotic spells in cyanotic heart defects) and *arrhythmias* that can lead to syncope [long QT syndrome, Brugada syndrome, postoperative atrial flutter or ventricular tachycardia (VT), Wolff–Parkinson–White (WPW) syndrome, and idiopathic VT or VT associated with arrhythmogenic right ventricular dysplasia].

Clinical features that suggest an underlying cardiac problem or the *Red flags of syncope* are listed in **Box 2**.

## CLINICAL EVALUATION AND INVESTIGATION

History taking and physical examination are crucial in the evaluation for syncope. The history will indicate whether the diagnosis is related to cardiac causes **(Box 2)**, NMS (prodrome, associated symptoms, triggering event), or noncardiac syncope (migraine, history of seizures, etc.). A positive family history of syncope, cardiomyopathy, or sudden death will indicate potentially serious cardiac causes like long QT syndrome and familial hypertrophic cardiomyopathy. NMS associated with exercise does exist, but a more serious cardiac cause should always be excluded in exercise-related syncopal event.

The physical examination should emphasize on a complete cardiac evaluation. An electrocardiogram (ECG) should always be included in all initial evaluations of syncope in children to exclude long QT syndrome, ventricular hypertrophy, obstructive cardiac lesions or cardiomyopathies; manifest preexcitation of WPW or any other arrhythmias.

In cases in which an arrhythmia is suspected, a 24-hour ambulatory monitor should be used to eliminate frequent ectopy, VT, supraventricular tachycardia, bradycardia, intermittent WPW, heart block, or pauses.

When the history, physical examination, and ECG suggest NMS, no further diagnostic tests are needed. However, if the diagnosis is not clear or any of the following red flags like exercise-induced syncope that occurs during exertion, chest pain that precedes an episode of fainting, seizure activity, recurrent syncope (more than two or three episodes), abnormal cardiac examination is there, further work up is necessary.

An echocardiogram should be done to rule out cardiomyopathies or malformations. In NMS diagnosed based on history, physical examination, and ECG, a tilt table test can be used to confirm the diagnosis; however, its use is controversial in pediatrics.

For exercise-induced syncope, an exercise stress test is recommended.

## ■ MANAGEMENT

Treatment and therapy for syncope are dependent on the cause. As in adolescents it is mostly benign, reassuring and educating the patient and family, focusing on preventing, or limiting the severity of future episodes is the key.

*Behavioral modification* is the primary treatment for NMS. Understanding the settings that lead to individual syncopal events aids in tailoring specific recommendations. The patient is advised to avoid dehydration, long periods of standing, irregular mealtimes, also to recognize prodrome, and assume supine position at onset. When syncope persists despite behavioral changes, medical therapy can be used and usually includes a beta-blocker or fludrocortisone; however, this is reserved for patients with frequent attacks and severe symptoms who fail conservative management. Avoidance of potentially toxic drugs is the rule; however, disopyramide has been used with success in some cases.

For cardiac syncope, the treatment is directed to the underlying cause. Pacemaker therapy is rarely used.

## ■ CONCLUSION

Syncope in adolescents in most cases is neurally mediated with a natural history of spontaneous resolution with age. Conservative measures like patient reassurance and education should be tried before introducing pharmacotherapy. Cardiac syncope is potentially life-threatening and should always be excluded by use of simple evaluative measures including history, physical examination, and ECG.

## ■ KEY MESSAGES

- *Fainting*/syncope is an abrupt, transient, and complete loss of consciousness.
- It is most often benign, but can have a more serious and potentially life-threatening cause.

- A typical presentation is loss of consciousness triggered by specific events, such as pain, medical procedure, emotional distress, sitting, or standing upright.
- Syncope can be classified into three major categories: NMS, cardiovascular syncope, and noncardiovascular syncope.
- Cardiac syncope though less common than NMS is potentially life-threatening and should always be excluded.
- A thorough history-taking and physical examination are crucial in the evaluation for syncope. An ECG should always be included in all initial evaluations of syncope.
- Treatment for syncope is dependent on the cause: Reassurance, education, and behavioral modification in NMS. Treatment of underlying cause in cardiac syncope.

## ■ RECOMMENDED READING

1. Calkins H, Seifert M, Morady F. Clinical presentation and long-term follow-up of athletes with exercise-induced vasodepressor syncope. Am Heart J. 1995;129:1159-64.
2. Côté JM. Syncope in children and adolescents: Evaluation and treatment. Paediatr Child Health. 2001;6(8): 549-51.
3. Lewis AL, Zlotocha J, Henke L, Dhala A. Specificity of head-up tilt testing in adolescents: Effects of various degrees of tilt challenge in normal control subjects. J Am Coll Cardiol. 1997;30:1057-60.
4. Luckstead EF. Cardiovascular evaluation of the young athlete. Adolesc Med. 1998;9:441-55.
5. Manolis AS. Evaluation of patients with syncope: Focus on age-related differences. J Am Coll Cardiol. 1994;3:13-8.
6. Morillo CA, Leitch JW, Yee R, Klein GJ. A placebo-controlled trial of intravenous and oral disopyramide for prevention of neurally-mediated syncope induced by head-up tilt. J Am Coll Cardiol. 1993;22:1843-8.
7. Wolff GS. Unexplained syncope: Clinical management. Pacing Clin Electrophysiol. 1997;20:2043-7.
8. Writing Committee Members, Shen WK, Sheldon RS, Benditt DG, Cohen MI, Forman DE, Goldberger ZD, et al. 2017 ACC/AHA/HRS guideline for the evaluation and management of patients with syncope: a report of the American College of Cardiology/American Heart Association task force on clinical practice guidelines and the heart rhythm society. Heart Rhythm. 2017;14: e155-217.

# 4C.4     Chest Pain

*DB Kadam*

## ■ INTRODUCTION

Chest pain is a common frightening symptom dealt by physician in day-to-day practice. Adolescent chest pain creates panic in patients and parents but carries different significance than that of adult patient. In this age group, chest pain is rarely due to serious life-threatening condition.

## ■ INCIDENCE AND PREVALENCE

In literature, there are very few studies mentioned about this symptom.

A study on 3,700 patients showed 76% musculoskeletal etiology, 12% exercise-induced asthma, 8% gastrointestinal (GI), 4% had psychogenic cause, and only 1% had cardiovascular disorder indicating lower incidence of cardiac disorder.

Another study from Korean Journal of Pediatrics consisting of 517 patients showed respiratory cause in 9.3%, musculoskeletal in 8.8%, GI cause in 2.9%, psychogenic in 1.4%, pneumonia in 1.2%, cardiovascular was 3.8%, and biggest chunk of idiopathic in 73.6%. Cardiac cause included 13 patients with arrhythmia and one patient with Kawasaki disease.

In tropical country like India, etiological factors are varied and things like worm infestation, pulmonary eosinophilia, costochondritis, and pubertal gynecomastia accounts for more patients.

Incidence of various disorders will vary with age group, socioeconomical status, and genetic background.

## ■ ETIOPATHOGENESIS AND CLINICAL FEATURES

### Cardiac Conditions

- *Mitral valve prolapse (MVP) syndrome:* Palpitations with premature ventricular contractions and chest pain which is recurrent and atypical anginal pain. This can occur at rest and with activity.

- *Hypertrophic cardiomyopathy:* Chest pain on exertion, breathlessness, pedal edema, syncope, and arrhythmia with possible history of sudden cardiac deaths in family.
- *Aortic stenosis:* Triad of syncope, angina, and dyspnea. Chest pain is typical anginal and at rest also.
- *Coarctation of the aorta:* Labored breathing, hypertension (predominant), cold feet/legs, leg cramps, and nose bleeds
- *Classic angina due to early atherosclerotic disease from hyperlipidemias or diabetes mellitus:* Substernal, crushing, or choking-type radiating down the left arm or up into the jaw, may be associated with vomiting, diaphoresis, altered mental status, or dyspnea.
- *Coronary artery abnormalities:* Kawasaki disease, anomalous coronary arteries, and myocardial bridge. Kawasaki disease is associated with rashes, swollen glands, strawberry tongue, red eyes, and swollen and red hands and feet. These conditions will have typical anginal pain with electrocardiography (ECG) changes.
- *Variant angina:* After recreational drug use—cocaine, amphetamines, marijuana, and synthetic cannabinoids. Glue sniffing and inhalational intoxicants can also produce atypical anginal pain.
- *Pericarditis and myocarditis:* Sharp, precordial, or retrosternal pain exacerbated by lying down and local pressure, sometimes radiating to the left shoulder, and often associated with fever.
- *Dilated cardiomyopathy:* Presents with sign and symptoms of heart failure with anginal chest pain.
- *Tachyarrhythmias:* Pounding heartbeats, dyspnea, and syncopal attacks. Persistent tachycardia for >20 minutes is associated with hypotension and anginal pain.
- *Aortic aneurysm or dissection:* Severe, tearing type of pain often radiating to the back. Features of Marfan syndrome should be looked for.
- *Multisystem inflammatory syndrome in adults (MIS-A) (COVID-related):* MIS presents with fever, anginal pain, features of cardiac failure, and/or renal insufficiency.

## Other Noncardiac Causes

### Respiratory

- *Airway foreign body:* Definite history available with hyperacute onset, dyspnea, and cough.
- *Spontaneous pneumothorax:* Sudden onset hemi-thoracic pain with dyspnea
- *Pleuritis:* Local sharp cutting pain with deep inspiration and cough. It can be primary pleuritis or secondary to pneumonia, and pulmonary embolism.
- *Pulmonary embolism:* Sudden onset anginal pain with dyspnea and cough
- *Pulmonary hypertension:* Palpitation and right-sided failure associated
- *Eosinophilic tracheitis:* Substernal burning or choking pain with bronchospasm
- *Glue sniffing:* Dry cough with constricting chest pain
- *Mediastinitis:* Substernal pain, fever, tachycardia, and cardiac failure
- *Sickle cell disease with acute chest syndrome:* Acute onset severe Bowring type of pain and dyspnea
- *Tumor (chest wall, pulmonary, or mediastinum):* Pain depends upon site and nature of tumor.

### Musculoskeletal

- *Costochondritis:* This is the most common cause; history of viral infection 2 weeks prior followed by pain and tenderness at costochondral junction, the most common at third and fourth costochondral junction on left side, is also a cause of costochondritis.
- *Precordial catch syndrome:* Sudden onset catch like pain during inspiration in intercostal space due to impeachment of intercostal nerve.
- *Intercostal myalgia:* It is associated with prolonged bouts of cough. It has associated intercostal tenderness.
- *Muscle strain:* It occurs with sudden jerky movement in odd position. Site depends upon involved muscle like trapezius and serratus anterior.
- *Slipping rib syndrome:* It is associated with rib dislocation at costochondral junction.
- *Fibromyalgia:* This rheumatic condition is associated with prolonged fever and enthesopathy.
- *Pectus excavatum or carinatum:* Unusual to produce any chest pain.

### Gastrointestinal

- *Gastroesophageal reflux disease:* This is the second most common cause seen in practice. Gastroesophageal reflux disease causes substernal burning or choking pain after food or lying down. Waterbrash can be present. This is mostly associated with consumption of fast food and in obese patient.

- *Medication-induced ("pill") esophagitis:* This is classically seen in patients on doxycycline. Esophagitis leading to stricture is of serious consequence.
- *Esophageal foreign body:* Either history is present in mentally challenged persons or in patients who takes nonvegetarian diet.
- *Esophageal spasm and achalasia:* Reflux symptoms are more common with chest pain. Early morning vomitus containing day prior night food is classical finding.
- *Gastritis:* Typically will have pain and tenderness in epigastric region with anorexia.
- *Peptic ulcer:* Epigastric pain with pain-food-relief cycle.
- *Cholecystitis and pancreatitis:* Both are unusual causes for chest pain but will have epigastric pain with occasional radiation to lower sternal region.
- *Nontraumatic esophageal rupture—Boerhaave syndrome:* This follows intractable vomiting episodes and presents as sudden onset left-sided hemithoracic pleural pain.

## Psychiatric

In psychiatric disorders, restlessness, agitation, and dramatization are more common. This is associated with poor schooling, lack of attention, and interpersonal conflicts. This can be confused with organic conditions as will have tachycardia, sweating, and hyperventilation.

- Anxiety
- Hypochondriasis
- Depression
- Somatization
- Panic disorder with or without hyperventilation syndrome.

## Issues Related to Breast

- *Male adolescents:* Gynecomastia—pubertal gynecomastia with breast pain and occasional galactorrhea can be present.
- *Female adolescents:* Pregnancy, thelarche, mastitis, and fibrocystic disease are the uncommon conditions for chest pain. Adolescent pregnancy can come as a surprise with breast pathologies.

## Skin Conditions

- *Herpes zoster:* This is the third common condition for severe chest pain. Easily identifiable after dermatomal blister eruptions. Difficult prior to that only clue is dermatomal hyperesthesia. This is common in juvenile diabetes.
- *Hair root infections:* Single or multiple boils in phase of inflammation can present as chest pain. Easily distinguishable by erythema, induration, and local tenderness.

## Neurological Conditions

- Radicular pain due to spinal tumor/fracture
- Syringomyelia
- Craniovertebral anomaly

These are uncommon causes of chest pain and are associated with other neurodeficits and signs.

## ■ EVALUATION

- Evaluation primarily depends on suspected etiology on history and examination.
- With first encounter we should look for red flag findings as described below, suggestive of serious etiology.

*Electrocardiography changes:*
- Primary investigation like ECG has to be interpreted differently.
- *Persistent juvenile T-wave pattern (PJTWP):* It should not be confused with ischemic heart disease. Right-sided dominance can be seen till 16–20 years of age.
- Shallow T-wave inversions limited to V1-V3/V4, asymmetric morphology of the inverted "T" wave, and no significant ST segment deviation
- Diagnosis of PJTWP should be achieved only after excluding other dangerous causes, such as anterior ischemia, posterior myocardial infarction (MI), severe chronic obstructive pulmonary disease (COPD), pulmonary embolism, and pulmonary hypertension.

*X-ray will be diagnostic in:*
- Pneumonia
- Pleural effusion
- Pneumothorax
- Aortic aneurysm
- Boerhaave syndrome

*2D echo:* It is essential for MVP, rheumatic fever, pericarditis, pulmonary embolism, and myocardial infarction.

*Ultrasonography (USG) thorax and abdomen:* USG is done to rule out pulmonary and GI causes.

*Red flag symptoms:* Severe acute chest pain, breathlessness, giddiness, altered mental status, fatigue, vomiting, diaphoresis, and fever
*Red flag signs:*
- Tachycardia >120 beats/min

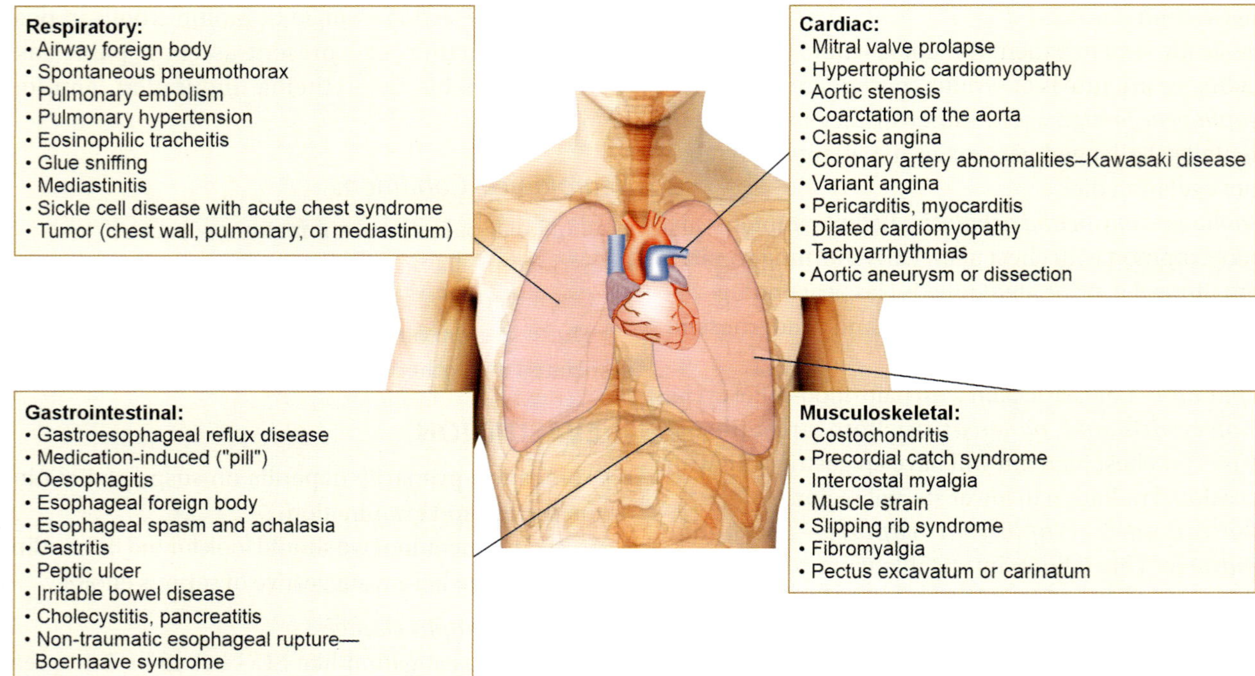


**Fig. 1:** Causes of chest pain.

**Flowchart 1:** Approach to a patient with chest pain.

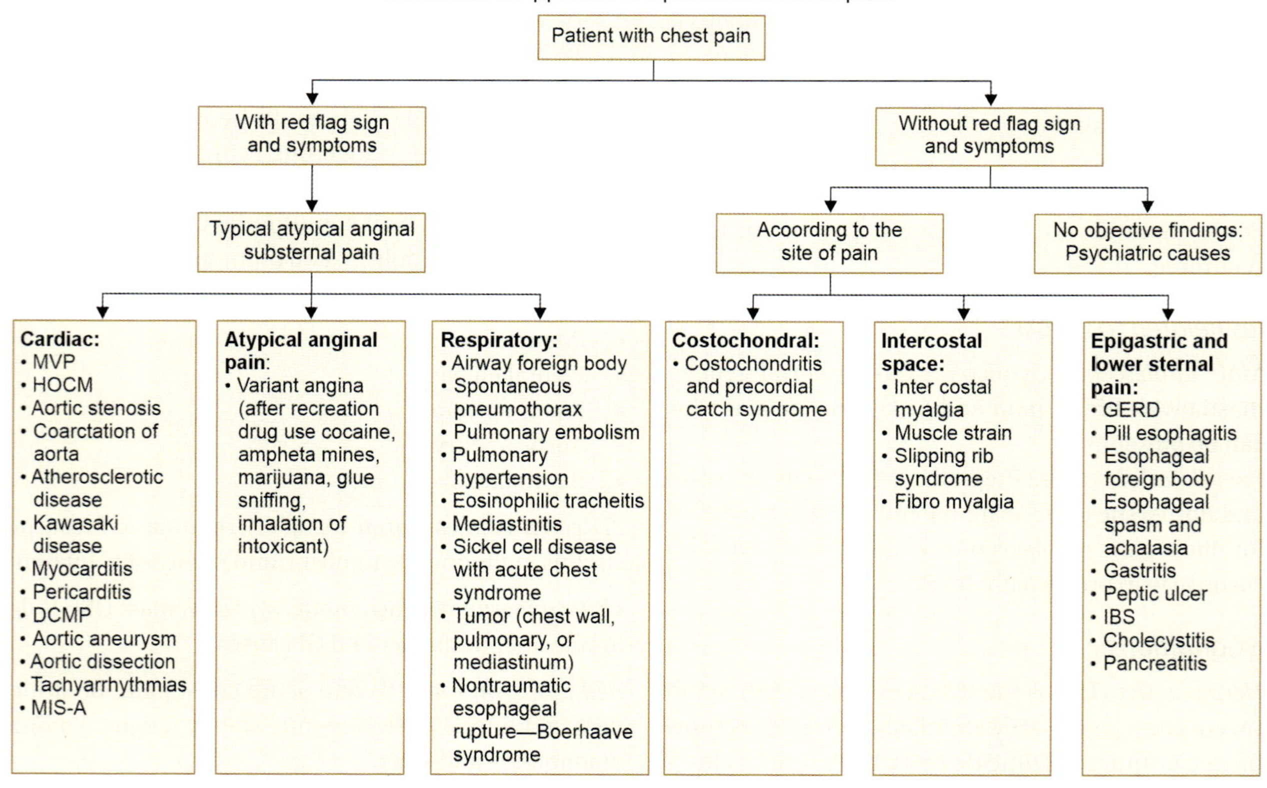


(DCMP: dilated cardiomyopathy; HOCM: hypertrophic obstructive cardiomyopathy; GERD: gastroesophageal reflux disease; IBS: inflammatory bowel syndrome; MIS-A: multisystem inflammatory syndrome in adults; MVP: mitral valve prolapse)

- Tachypnea >24 beats/min
- Blood pressure (BP) <20 mm Hg for the age group or systolic BP <90 mm Hg
- Oxygen saturation (SPO$_2$) <94%
- Presence of sweating, cyanosis, and anxious look
- Fever >100°F

## ■ TREATMENT

- It depends essentially on the primary condition. Cardiac, respiratory, and GI conditions have typical protocol management.
- Musculoskeletal conditions should be treated with muscle relaxants, analgesics, and anti-inflammatory drugs.
- Psychiatric conditions and drug addictions will need counseling and antidepressants or mood elevators.
- Amitriptyline is found to be more useful.

## ■ KEY MESSAGES

- Chest pain is a common symptom in adolescent practice.
- Serious etiology for this is unusual.
- Red flag signs and symptoms should be looked for.

- Costochondritis, reflux esophagitis, and underlying psychiatric disorder are the common causes.
- ECG, X-ray chest, and 2D echo are for basic evaluation.
- Treatment depends upon cause.

## ■ RECOMMENDED READING


1. Chun JH, Kim TH, Han MY, Kim NY, Yoon KL. Analysis of clinical characteristics and causes of chest pain in children and adolescents. Korean J Pediatr. 2015;58(11):440-5.
2. Foussas SG, Adamopoulou EN, Kafaltis NA, Fakiolas C, Olympios C, Pisimissis E, et al. Clinical characteristics and follow-up of patients with chest pain and normal coronary arteries. Angiology. 1998;49(5):349-54.
3. Geggel R, Endom E, Redding G, Drutz JE, Fleisher GR. Nontraumatic chest pain in children and adolescents: Approach and initial management. [online] Available from https://www.uptodate.com/contents/nontraumatic-chest-pain-in-children-and-adolescents-approach-and-initial-management [Last accessed March, 2024].
4. ScientificPhotoLibrary. Ribcage and heart. [online] Available from https://sciencephotogallery.com/featured/rib-cage-and-heart-samantha-elmhurstscience-photo-library.html [Last accessed March, 2024].
5. Veeram Reddy SR, Singh HR. Chest pain in children and adolescents. Pediatr Rev. 2010;31(1):e1-9.


<table>
<tr><td>4C.5</td><td><h1>Speech and Language Disorders</h1></td></tr>
</table>

# 4C.5 Speech and Language Disorders

*Sneha Jay Bhalerao*

## ■ INTRODUCTION

### Communication

"Communication" is the exchange of information using a socially accepted system of symbols and behaviors. It can be verbal as well as nonverbal. Humans communicate with gestures, posture, and facial expression, which is nonverbal communication, and spoken language can be defined as verbal mode of communication.

### Language

Language can be referred as a code for transforming the mental events such as thoughts and memories into events that can be perceived by other people. Language can be divided into two parts: Expressive language and receptive language.

### Speech

Speech is the oral expression of language. These sound patterns are produced as a result of respiration, phonation, resonation, and articulation. An important point is that language is the code, whereas speech is the sensorimotor production of that code.

## ■ COMPONENTS OF COMMUNICATION

**Flowchart 1** shows the components of communication.

## ■ DISORDERS OF SPEECH PRODUCTION

Disorders of speech can be defined by any change to the structures or physiologic function of the speech mechanism. Most speech disorders in children are due to functional mislearning or are caused by organic anomalies,

**Flowchart 1:** Components of communication.

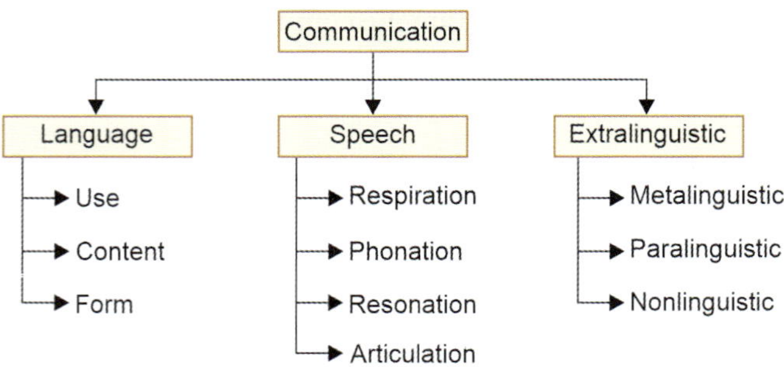

which can affect oral, pharyngeal, or laryngeal structures or neuromuscular functions. Oropharyngeal anomalies include macroglossia, asymmetries related to hemifacial microsomia, or cleft palate, and laryngeal changes include alterations to the vocal folds, such as laryngeal papilloma or intubation trauma.

Speech disorders occur when there is disruption in the neuromotor coordination of respiration, laryngeal, and articulatory functions, e.g., muscular dystrophy and cerebral palsy.

## Cleft Lip and Palate

Intact palatal structures are very important for the development of normal speech. The velopharynx closes to direct airflow orally for most speech sounds and opens to permit nasal resonance on nasal speech sounds (in English: "m," "n," and "ng"). When dynamic function of the velopharynx is disrupted, speech is hypernasal in quality. Also, feeding disorders, misarticulations, and hypernasality are very common in children with cleft lip and palate.

## Dysarthria

Dysarthria is a speech sound disorder caused by medical conditions that impair the muscles or nerves that activate the oral mechanism (Caruso and Strand, 1999). Dysarthric speech may be difficult to understand due to weak, imprecise, and abnormally slow or rapid speech movements. Neuromuscular conditions, including stroke, infections (e.g., polio and meningitis), cerebral palsy, and trauma, can cause dysarthria.

## Speech Disfluency or Stuttering

Fluency is an aspect of speech production that refers to continuity, smoothness, rate, and effort in speech. Stuttering, the most common fluency disorder that is, it is an interruption in the flow of speaking characterized by repetitions (sounds, syllables, words, and phrases), sound prolongations, blocks, interjections, and revisions, which may affect the rate and rhythm of speech. These disfluencies may be accompanied by physical tension, negative reactions, secondary behaviors, and avoidance of sounds, words, or speaking situations. Cluttering is another fluency disorder; it is characterized by a perceived rapid and/or irregular speech rate, which results in breakdowns in speech clarity and/or fluency. These are not readily controllable and may be accompanied by other movements and by emotions of negative nature such as fear, embarrassment, or irritation.

## Childhood Apraxia of Speech

Childhood apraxia of speech (CAS) is a complex neurodevelopmental disorder in which the ability to plan and sequence speech movements is impaired in the absence of paralysis or weakness of the oral musculature, thereby decreasing the precision, consistency, and intelligibility of speech. The child's connected speech is likely to be limited to vowel sounds and also speech appears to be effortful. Children who have CAS are often described as "groping" for accurate placement of the articulators when they try to produce consonant speech sounds with intact auditory comprehension skills. Hence, when a child demonstrates inconsistent production of consonants and vowels on repeated productions of syllables or words, lack of smooth transitions between sounds and syllables, or inappropriate inflection patterns (prosody), hence should be referred for a full speech and language evaluation.

## ■ SPEECH DELAY OR DISORDER

### Articulation Disorders

It is very common for a child who is learning to speak to simplify adult productions of words and speech sounds. For example, a child might say "icem" instead of "icecream. The speech of the child should be 50% intelligible by age 36 months and about 75% intelligible by the age of 48 months. Persistent speech production issues may reflect difficulty with learning or coordinating articulatory placement for individual sounds (e.g., "th" for "s"), which is called an articulation disorder.

### Phonological Disorders

Phonological processes can be final consonant deletion (ca for cat), cluster reduction (pot for spot), reduplication (wawa for water), weak syllable deletion (nana for banana), etc. Formal assessment and detailed analysis of speech sounds are very necessary to differentiate articulation problems from phonologic disorders of speech production or from CAS.

## DISORDERS OF LANGUAGE

### Speech and Language Delay

Speech delay is defined as when the child's conversational speech sample is either more incoherent than would be expected for age or is marked by speech sound error patterns not appropriate for age. Often a "wait-and-watch" policy leads to late diagnosis and intervention for children with speech delay. It is really necessary to go for early intervention.

### Autism

According to Diagnostic and Statistical Manual of Mental Disorders 5 (DSM-5) diagnostic criteria for autism spectrum disorder (ASD), the prototypical features of ASD are: Social communication and social interaction deficits that are persistent in multiple contexts for all three criteria, which included deficits in social reciprocity, deficits in nonverbal communication, deficits in developing and maintaining relationships appropriate to developmental level and restricted, and repetitive patterns of behaviors and interests. ASDs included the wide range and severity of symptoms, which included "classic autism," Asperger's syndrome, Rett syndrome, childhood disintegrative disorder, and pervasive developmental disorders. Autism is a complex condition characterized by a wide range of symptoms that can include communication problems such as lack of eye contact, reduced interest in vocal exchange, lack of recognition of and response to voices, onset of babbling after age 9 months, decreased or absent prespeech behaviors such as social waving, alterations in speech rate and rhythm, and failure to develop the speech. The most common characteristic across the children who have autism is difficulty in the social use of communication and language (pragmatics). They may also demonstrate problems with reading and writing.

### Hearing Impairment

Congenital hearing loss can affect child's speech as well as language. Hearing impairment is a factor that directly compromises the individual's language, which can affect emotional and academic defects by delayed development of communicative ability. This can vary according to the type and degree of hearing loss.

## DISORDERS OF VOICE

*Dysphonia:* It occurs when the laryngeal structures, including the vocal cords, do not function correctly. For example, a voice that sounds hoarse or breathy may be due to growths on the vocal cords, allergies, paralysis, infection, or excessive vocal abuse when speaking.

*Aphonia:* A complete inability to produce any sound which may be caused by inflammation, infection, or injury to the vocal cords.

*Puberphonia:* Puberphonia is a psychogenic voice disorder. One of the treatments for this is a speech therapy. The persistence of adolescent voice even after puberty in the absence of organic cause is known as puberphonia. This condition is commonly seen in males. The patient has an unusually high-pitched voice persisting beyond puberty. This disorder is grouped under psychogenic voice disorders. The most common symptoms include pitch breaks, hoarseness, breathiness, difficulty in vocal projection, and visible laryngeal muscle tension. One of the reasons of puberphonia is increased laryngeal muscle tension causing laryngeal elevation, embarrassment of the newly achieved vocal pitch, failure to accept the new voice, social immaturity, etc.

## SPEECH–LANGUAGE EVALUATION

The child's medical, developmental, and psychosocial histories are obtained before the evaluation by chart review, parent interview, or both. The goal of the evaluation is to assess the child's speech and language function relative to age and developmental expectations. The evaluation begins with understanding the child's eye contact, use of social greetings, shyness, or willingness to engage in play. Assessments may include observing the parent–child interaction, involving the child in play activities to elicit a spontaneous speech and language sample, and administering a standardized test of articulation, comprehension, and expressive language use. Standardized tests for speech and language (REELS, COM-DEALL, 3D-LAT etc.) allow speech therapist to understand the receptive language age and expressive language age of the child. Articulation tests allow the speech–language pathologist (SLP) to elicit all the speech sounds in the language in each word position, within a few minutes.

Also standardized test like PAT used for evaluation of errors made at each sound position (initial, medial, and final) in a word. Stuttering Severity Index (SSI) is used for evaluation fluency disorders for understanding and evaluating the repetitions, prolongations, and blocks. In patients with voice disorders (puberphonia/dysphonia), the perceptual [grade, roughness, breathiness, asthenia, and strain (GRABAS)] and acoustic analyses [multidimensional voice program (MDVP)] were performed once prior to onset of therapy and repeated prior to planning discharge from therapy for understanding the changes acoustically as well as instrumentally and accordingly intervention is planned. The SLP evaluates all the data obtained and should review the findings with the parents at the time of the evaluation or at follow-up. Recommendations may include no further assessment or treatment, waiting and reevaluating, giving parents some tips for facilitating communication at home, or direct service intervention.

## ▌SCREENING ASSESSMENT TOOLS FOR AUTISM SPECTRUM DISORDER

**Table 1** depicts the screening assessment tools for autism spectrum disorder.

Individuals suspected of having ASD based on screening results are referred to an SLP, and other professionals as needed, for a comprehensive assessment.

## ▌TESTS USED FOR EVALUATION IN ADOLESCENTS

Tests used for evaluation in adolescents are mentioned in **Table 2**.

## ▌TREATMENT

When therapy is recommended, the primary goal is to give the child a reliable way to exchange ideas and information in his daily social and educational environment. Treatment is planned according to the disorder type and severity, the child's age, and the etiology of the problem and also according to the specific communication needs of each child. Any speech or language intervention requires involvement of that child's family and educators also.

*Therapy for speech disorders:* Treatment for articulation impairments targets the correct production of specific consonant or vowel sounds and then generalize them into bisyllables, words, sentences, and passages (natural speech), whereas treatment for systematic mislearning of the phonologic system in the language addresses the patterns of error, rather than teaching each sound individually. In treatment for CAS, oral-motor strengthening exercises have often been recommended to strengthen and increase range of movement in the oral mechanism. Because few speech production disorders relate to muscular weakness or reduced range of motion, the finding of limited efficacy of oral exercises is not surprising. For a child with age less than 3 years with speech and language developmental delay, child is reinforced for usage of new behaviors to communicate using language stimulation activities which parents also can use at home. Older preschoolers and school-aged children can benefit

**TABLE 1:** Screening assessment tools for autism spectrum disorder.

| Test | Age range | Authors | Year |
|---|---|---|---|
| Modified checklist for autism in toddlers (M-CHAT) | 16–30 months | Robins, Fein, and Barton, 2009 | 2009 |
| Quantitative CHAT (Q-CHAT) | 18–24 months | Allison C, Baron-Cohen S, Wheelwright S, Charman T, Richler J, Pasco G, and Brayne C | 2008 |

**TABLE 2:** Tests for evaluation in adolescents.

| Test name | Author(s) | Year |
|---|---|---|
| Clinical evaluation of language fundamentals—5*B | H Wiig, Semel, and Secord | 2013 |
| Clinical evaluation of language fundamentals—5 metalinguistics | Wiig and Secord | 2014 |
| Comprehensive receptive and expressive vocabulary test—3 | Wallace and Hammill | 2013 |
| Comprehensive test of phonological processing—2 | Wagner, Torgesen, Rashotte, and Pearson | 2013 |
| Peabody picture vocabulary test—4*B | H Dunn and Dunn | 2007 |
| *SCAN—3:* A tests for auditory processing disorders in adolescents and adults | Keith | 2009a |
| *SCAN—3:* C tests for auditory processing disorders for children | Keith | 2009b |
| Test of auditory processing skills—3 | Martin and Brownell | 2005 |

*Most common tests are mentioned here.

from individual or group therapy that focuses on their specific language needs (i.e., vocabulary, longer word combinations, or the use of more grammatically complex utterances).

*Therapy for the child who is nonverbal:* When a child is not able to use speech to communicate, the primary goal of speech language therapy is to establish a reliable means of communication using the child's capacity for communication skills, which may include the use of gestures, idiosyncratic signs, more formal "baby signs," or an established manual sign language. Children who have severe impairments in speech production may benefit from the use of communication technology, ranging from the use of a picture communication board to a speech generating device to a computer-based system that features access to word processing and voice output.

*Therapy of a child with voice disorder:* The voice therapy treatment protocol for puberphonia included therapy techniques commonly applied for achieving lowering of pitch such as humming while gliding down the pitch scale, phonation of vowel sounds with a glottal attack, use of vegetative sounds, and digital manipulation of thyroid cartilage during vowel production. The therapy techniques were practiced according to patient's comfort, ease of production, and improvement in pitch and simultaneously all the patients practiced relaxation exercises to reduce the compensatory laryngeal tension. During the course of therapy, the patients were asked to note the difference in their habitual pitch and lowered pitch and counseling were done regarding the use of this "new voice."

## AUDIO-RELATED DISORDERS

These include hearing loss which can be due to congenital defect, ear infection, autoimmune diseases, head trauma, and exposure to loud noises.

Early identification hearing problems in children are very important, because it can have potential effect on developing language and communication skills. Newborn hearing screening program is developed for the early identification of the congenital hearing impairment. The primary justification for early identification of hearing impairment in infants relates to the impact of hearing impairment on speech and language acquisition, academic achievement, and social and emotional development. The first 3 years of life are most critical for speech and language acquisition. Early auditory deprivation interferes with the development of neural structures necessary for hearing and the goal of early identification and intervention is to minimize the adverse effects. Neonatal and infant screening programs use test procedure like otoacoustic emission (OAE) and auditory brain stem response (ABR), which have been established worldwide for this purpose.

Identification of type and severity of hearing loss can be done using test named pure-tone audiometry. If the child has sensorineural hearing loss then child can go for hearing aid after the hearing aid trial.

## RECENT ADVANCES

- Telehealth services experienced exponential growth during the coronavirus disease 2019 (COVID-19) pandemic. Telehealth technology included not only computers with external hardware and specialized software to commercially available equipment but also handheld portable devices with built-in audiovisual components and publicly available videoconferencing platforms. Clinicians anticipate that new developments have the potential to continue improving telehealth service delivery, bolstering the viability of telehealth long after the COVID-19 pandemic is gone.
- The novel COVID-19 pandemic has led to sudden, widespread use of telepractice, which included providing services to children who use aided augmentative and alternative communication (AAC). Most SLPs were using telepractice to provide both direct and consultation services to children who used aided AAC. They realized the improved AAC technologies, young children with complex communication needs will have better tools to maximize their development of communication, language, and literacy skills, and attain their full potential.

## PARENTAL GUIDELINE

- Early identification is important.
- Early intervention is necessary.
- Parental involvement is very necessary. With therapy parents will have to work on child at home also.
- Taking treatment from correct resources is important.
- Patient should go to pediatricians first and accordingly go to speech therapist if have speech, language, and swallowing difficulty and should go to occupational therapist if have hyperactivity and hypersensitivity.
- Treatment from a team according to the disorder of a child is very necessary.

## ■ KEY MESSAGES

- Early identification and early intervention of disorder are very important. The goal of early identification is to initiate early intervention, which has been shown to improve outcomes in child.
- Newborn hearing screening program is developed for the early identification and early intervention of children with congenital hearing impairment.
- Team approach is important.
- Formal assessment and detailed analysis of disorders are very necessary. (For example, to differentiate articulation problems from phonologic disorders of speech production or from CAS.)
- Younger the age at cochlear implantation, better the auditory performance. Therefore, regular aural–verbal rehabilitation and speech and language therapy are essential for younger children with hearing impairment to achieve the highest level of hearing function.
- Alternative and augmentative communication (aided or unaided) can be used for children with communication difficulty. Evidences found that AAC is useful in autism (regardless of severity) also.
- Telerehabilitation can be used for those who cannot reach therapist physically and it has found very useful.
- Children with voice disorder, articulation disorders, and fluency disorders do not follow any age limit for the speech therapy.
- Parents' role in communication disorders is very important as they are considered as a main factor in the team.
- Inclusion of special children in society allows them to participate fully with acknowledging their inherent value and worth as contributing members. Inclusive environments provide them opportunities to learn, grow, and develop essential life skills. Also, interacting with peers from diverse backgrounds enhances social, emotional, and cognitive development, contributing positively to their overall well-being.

## ■ RECOMMENDED READING


1. Arnold GE, Winckel F, Wyke BD (Eds). Disorders of Human Communication. Springer.
2. Campbell DR, Goldstein H. Evolution of Telehealth Technology, Evaluations, and Therapy: Effects of the COVID-19 Pandemic on Pediatric Speech-Language Pathology Services. Am J Speech Lang Pathol. 2022;31(1): 271-86.
3. Chenausky KV, Brignell A, Morgan A, Gagné D, Norton A, Tager-Flusberg H, et al. Factor analysis of signs of childhood apraxia of speech. J Commun Disord. 2020;87: 106033.
4. Light J, Drager K. AAC technologies for young children with complex communication needs: State of the science and future research directions. Augment Altern Commun. 2007;23(3):204-16.
5. Reed V (Ed). An Introduction to Children with Language Disorders, 5th edition. Pearson; 2017.
6. Sharp HM, Hillenbrand K. Speech and language development and disorders in children. Pediatr Clin North Am. 2008;55(5):1159-73, viii.
7. Sunderajan T, Kanhere S. Speech and language delay in children: Prevalence and risk factors. J Fam Med Prim Care. 2019;8(5):1642.

# Part D: Infections

***Sub-section Editors:*** *Shailaja Mane, Poonam Bhatia, Samir Shah*

## 4D.1 | Tuberculosis in Adolescents

*Shivananda S, Geeta Patil*

### ■ INTRODUCTION

Eleven percent of cases of tuberculosis (TB) occur in the pediatric age group 0–19 years. Among them, the highest proportion occur in children <5 years and in older adolescents (15–19 years. It was recently estimated that 1.5 million children and adolescents get TB infection every year. The National Strategic Plan 2017–2025 hopes to eliminate TB by 2025.

Adolescents are an important risk group for transmission due to their high social mobility and the infectiousness of the disease **(Box 1)**. TB disease and its treatment can interrupt education and employment, and disrupt relationships with family and peers. Adolescents are hypersensitive to the stigma of the disease label, yet contact tracing is very important in this group. They are less compliant to therapy as it lasts many months. Though one-fourth of the global population consists of adolescents and the majority live in low- and middle-income countries (LMIC) where TB incidence is high, TB eradication policies and guidelines have not studied the importance of TB transmission in adolescents and young adults (AYA, ages 10–24 years), always grouping them with either children or adults.

### ■ PRESENTATION

Adolescents may approach a clinician or the health services with clinical features suggestive of TB, or as a part of contact tracing, or because of a suggestive incidental finding on X-ray or other investigations. 50–90% of TB cases in adolescence and adulthood result from reactivation of a previously dormant primary infection **(Box 2)**.

> **BOX 1:** Factors associated with an increased incidence of TB.
>
> - Coinfection with HIV
> - Poor socioeconomic status
> - Overcrowding
> - Smoking
> - Indoor air pollution

(HIV: human immunodeficiency virus; TB: tuberculosis)

Intrathoracic TB is most common. There is a predilection for the apical or posterior segment of upper lobes or the superior segment of the lower lobes. Focal or patchy heterogeneous consolidation, consolidation with cavitation, and pleural effusion are common X-ray findings; tuberculomas are seen occasionally. Cervical lymphadenopathy is the next most common site of disease, as in adults. Miliary and meningeal disease are uncommon **(Box 3)**.

> **BOX 2:** Clinical symptoms.
>
> - *Cough:* Persistent cough for 2 weeks or more
> - *Fever:* Persistent fever for 2 weeks or more
> - *Lethargy:* Persistent unexplained lethargy or decrease in activity
> - *Weight loss:* More than 5%, within 3 months
> - Hemoptysis
> - *Night sweats:* Excessive nighttime sweating that soaks the bed or clothes
> - *Swollen lymph node:* Painless, enlarged cervical, submandibular or axillary lymph node
> - *Others:* Pain in abdomen, joint pain, swelling, breathlessness, chest pain, and back pain

> **BOX 3:** Physical signs suggestive of extrapulmonary tuberculosis (TB).
>
> - *TB lymphadenopathy:* Nontender enlarged cervical lymph node mass (>2 × 2 cm) with or without sinus formation
> - *Spinal TB*: Presence of kyphosis or gibbus
> - *Tuberculous meningitis:* Meningitis with onset over more than 5 days
> - *Pleural effusion:* Unilateral dullness with pleuritic pain in a child who is not acutely sick
> - *Pericardial TB:* Pericardial effusion, distant or muffled heart sounds, or signs of new-onset heart failure
> - *Abdominal TB:* Nonacute distended abdomen with or without ascites
> - *Osteoarticular TB:* Nontender swollen joints with painful or abnormal gait

## ■ INVESTIGATIONS

*Chest X-ray* is still the first line of investigation. The World Health Organization (WHO) recommends computer-assisted detection (CAD) software for the automated interpretation of chest X-ray in adults and adolescents above 15 years. While younger children often present with hilar lymphadenopathy or miliary disease, adolescent presentation is similar to that of adults, such as apical consolidation, cavitation, and pleural effusion **(Figs. 1A to D)**.

High-resolution computed tomography (HRCT) is occasionally useful for a CT-guided biopsy and may suggest TB, but mostly it is used to rule out the other differentials. *Chest ultrasonography (USG)* may help to decide on the best spot for fine-needle aspiration cytology (FNAC) or aspiration of a pleural fluid.

*Mantoux test* using 2TU PPD RT23 is considered positive if the induration is 10 mm or more. In HIV coinfected cases, 5 mm may be taken as the cut-off. Mantoux test is no longer recommended as the test solutions available today are different from the original standard solutions and are not reliable.

*Interferon-gamma release assay (IGRA)*, like the Mantoux test, elicits delayed-type hypersensitivity when it is positive. It does not require a repeat visit for test reading, and does not cross-react with BCG (Bacillus Calmette–Guérin) vaccination, but it is expensive. A positive test indicates the presence of TB infection in an individual but cannot confirm the presence of disease.

*Serology* [immunoglobulin M (IgM), IgG, and IgA antibodies], commercial polymerase chain reaction (PCR) tests, and BCG tests are not recommended as TB diagnostic tools as they are often inaccurate. Erythrocyte sedimentation rate (ESR) is nonspecific.

*Microbiological studies:* Adolescents can expectorate sputum for smear and microbiological studies. Induced

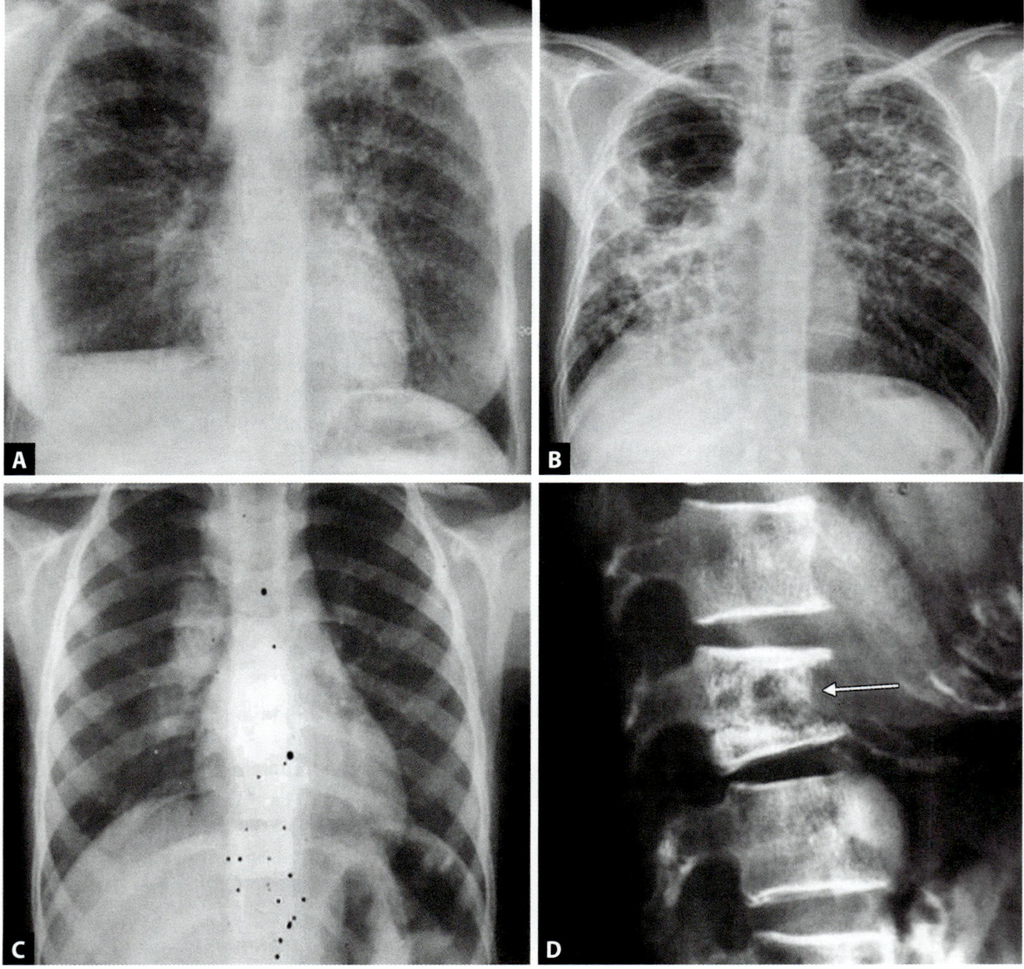

**Figs. 1A to D:** (A) Pleural effusion; (B) Fibrocaseous tuberculosis (TB); (C) Lymphadenopathy; and (D) Spinal TB.

sputum (saline-induced coughing) gives higher culture yields than spontaneously produced samples. Adolescents with pulmonary TB often have "microbiologically confirmed" disease (i.e., smear, culture, or PCR positive), but negative test results do not rule out TB. It is better to send multiple samples on the same day, which is as effective as samples collected on separate days, and makes sample collection easier.

The Xpert MTB/RIF (Mycobacterium tuberculosis/resistance to rifampin) [cartridge-based nucleic acid amplification test (CBNAAT)] should be used as an initial diagnostic test for TB and rifampicin-resistance detection in sputum rather than smear microscopy/culture. CBNAAT is highly specific but sensitivity is less than the culture. Culture detects 35–45% of cases.

Pleural fluid aspirate should be sent for biochemical, cytological, and smear examination by Ziehl–Neelsen (ZN) stain. A tuberculous effusion fluid is a straw-colored exudate, with hundreds of mononuclear cells, with high proteins (>3 g/dL), and forms a cobweb on standing. Culture and NAAT are positive only in 5%. However, a pleural biopsy is 80% positive if subjected to histopathology, ZN staining, and cultures.

In adolescents with peripheral lymphadenopathy, FNAC is safe and feasible, and has good sensitivity and specificity. Invasive sampling is necessary for meningeal, abdominal, renal, genitourinary, and musculoskeletal TB.

## ■ MANAGEMENT

Management of TB is mentioned in **Boxes 4 to 6**.

---

**BOX 4:** Components and skills.

- Management of TB drugs
- Look for clinical signs that indicate the need for urgent care
- Identify comorbidities, including undernutrition and HIV status
- Manage adverse events like hepatotoxicity due to drugs, and IRIS
- Implement infection control measures
- Educate patients and their families and caregivers
- Provide psychological and socioeconomical support
- Involve family members in decisions regarding treatment
- Support treatment adherence
- Contact investigation
- TB prophylaxis to eligible family members
- Report to monitor and notifications and treatment

(HIV: human immunodeficiency virus; IRIS: immune reconstitution inflammatory syndrome; TB: tuberculosis)

## Pediatric Tuberculosis Management Essentials, Based on Childhood Tuberculosis Guidelines (Updated 2021) National Tuberculosis Elimination Program and Indian Academy of Pediatrics (IAP)

As the weight gain happens during treatment dose should be adjusted accordingly **(Table 1)**. Care giver to be identified. Adherence to the full course of treatment should be emphasized and reinforced.

The WHO in its consolidated TB guidelines 2022 has given a recommendation to shorten the therapy from 6 months to 4 months for nonsevere TB.

Pyridoxine supplementation 10 mg/day is recommended to all patients receiving INH (isoniazid). When

---

**BOX 5:** The principles of TB treatment are the same in all age groups.

- 2HRZE + 4HRE. E is added in continuation phase due to high resistance to H (13%)
- All drugs are given together. Fixed drug combinations replace combi packs
- Daily treatment is superior to intermittent regimes
- If poor response after 2 months, investigate for drug resistance
- Category II (retreatment regime) is removed
- Retreatment cases with no drug resistance treated with same standard regime
- *Rifampicin resistance:* Managed as MDR-TB

(HRE: isoniazid and rifampicin with ethambutol; HRZE: isoniazid, rifampicin, pyrazinamide, ethambutol; MDR-TB: multidrug-resistant tuberculosis)

---

**BOX 6:** Regimen for TB (RS-TB) NTEP guidelines 2020.

- *2HRZE + 4HRE:* For all new microbiologically confirmed RS pulmonary or extrapulmonary TB. (2HRZE + 10HRE in neuro and spinal TB)
- *2HRZE + 4HRE:* For all new clinically diagnosed pulmonary or extrapulmonary TB. (2HRZE + 10HRE in neuro and spinal TB). Do molecular testing in all such cases for TB diagnosis and RS
- Previously treated TB (recurrent, treatment after loss to follow up, treatment after failure) should be evaluated for drug resistance. If found to be rifampicin (and INH) sensitive, they should be restarted on the regimen as for a new case
- *Lymph node TB:* 2HRZE + 4HRE
- *TBM:* 2HRZE + 10HRE
- *Osteoarticular:* 2HRZE + 10HRE

(HRE: isoniazid and rifampicin with ethambutol; HRZE: isoniazid, rifampicin, pyrazinamide, ethambutol; NTEP: National Tuberculosis Elimination Program; RS-TB: rifampicin-sensitive tuberculosis; TBM: tuberculous meningitis)

**TABLE 1:** Drug doses, first line.

| Drug | Range (mg/kg/day) | Average (mg/kg/day) | Maximum (mg) |
|---|---|---|---|
| Rifampicin—R | 10–20 | 15 | 600 |
| Isoniazid—H | 7–15 | 10 | 300 |
| Pyrazinamide—Z | 30–40 | 35 | 2,000 |
| Ethambutol—E | 15–25 | 20 | 1,500 |
| Streptomycin—S | 15–20 | 20 | 1,000 |

**BOX 7:** When to suspect drug resistance.

- There is contact with a person with confirmed DR-TB or with presumed DR-TB (source case did not respond to treatment/failed treatment or is currently retreated for TB or recently died from TB)
- Adolescent with TB is not responding to first-line treatment after 2–3 months despite adherence (and is not considered living with HIV on ART)
- Adolescent previously treated for TB (especially within the past 12 months) presents with recurrence of disease (either a true relapse or reinfection)
- Extensively drug-resistant TB (XDR; MDR with additional resistance to at least one fluoroquinolone and at least one second-line injectable agent)
- Drug susceptibility tests (DSTs) confirm diagnosis of RR (rifampicin resistance) TB from clinical samples or cultured isolates

(ART: antiretroviral therapy; DR-TB: drug-resistant tuberculosis; HIV: human immunodeficiency virus; MDR: multidrug-resistant; XDR: extensively drug resistant TB XDR)

resistance to first-line medication develops, second-line agents such as kanamycin, capreomycin, and amikacin are administered as an injection, and fluoroquinolones such as moxifloxacin, gatifloxacin, and levofloxacin are administered orally **(Box 7)**. In 2019, the WHO recommended use of novel drugs in rifampicin-resistant TB treatment, which includes delamanid and bedaquiline.

*Monitoring:* Clinical follow-up should be done every month during treatment, and every 6 months for 2 years after completion of treatment to pick up relapses early. Monitor dosage of drugs, adherence, adverse events, HIV status, nutrition, comorbidities, and response to treatment.

*Adverse events:* Generally well tolerated. The most important side-effect is hepatotoxicity. Ethambutol can be used safely in children. Routinely patients are monitored clinically and not by laboratory investigations.

*Adherence:* Poor adherence is the most common cause of treatment failure. Adolescents desire autonomy, and they

**BOX 8:** Adolescents who should receive tuberculosis preventive therapy (TPT).

- In contact with active case of pulmonary TB patients (DSTB as well as DRTB), who are found not to have TB disease by an appropriate clinical evaluation
- Living with HIV (+ART)
- Living with HIV who had successfully completed treatment for TB disease earlier should receive a course of TPT after completing treatment of TB to prevent recurrence

(ART: antiretroviral therapy; DRTB: drug-resistant tuberculosis; DSTB: drug-sensitive tuberculosis; HIV: human immunodeficiency virus)

give importance to short-term social benefits than long-term health gains. Adherence counseling before initiation of treatment therapy is of paramount important.

Treatment failure also suggests the possibility of rifampicin resistance/multidrug-resistant TB (RR/MDR-TB) and needs additional diagnostic evaluations. This is more common in adolescents living with HIV. Young adolescents with culture-negative, nonsevere RR TB disease have been shown to have excellent outcomes with total treatment duration of 12 months.

*Adolescents living with HIV* should be treated for both TB and HIV. TB is the main cause of mortality among adolescents living with HIV. Extrapulmonary and disseminated disease patterns are more common; TB is typically paucibacillary, and chest radiographic appearances are not typical. The WHO recommends that adolescents with TB living with HIV should be treated irrespective of the degree of immunosuppression, ART, history of previous TB treatment, and pregnancy. It is common to wait for 4 weeks to get accustomed to TB treatment before starting ART. An unusual side-effect is IRIS (immune reconstitution inflammatory syndrome).

## Tuberculosis Preventive Therapy

This consists of 6 months daily INH (5 mg/kg/day, maximum 300 mg/day) + 3 months weekly INH and rifapentine **(Box 8)**.

Tuberculosis preventive therapy is also required for household contacts of drug-resistant pulmonary TB.

## ■ KEY MESSAGES

- Adolescents and young adults (ages 10–24 years) are an important but understudied population in global efforts to end TB.
- TB is curable and preventable.

- Reactivation or post primary TB is common in adolescence.
- The principles of TB treatment are the same in adolescents and adults.
- 2HRZE (isoniazid, rifampicin, pyrazinamide, ethambutol) + 4HRE (isoniazid and rifampicin with ethambutol) are the regime followed.
- Monitoring is mainly by clinical follow up every month during treatment, and every 6 months for 2 years after completion of treatment.
- Poor medication adherence and loss to follow-up are serious concerns, and adherence counseling before initiation of treatment therapy is very important.
- Adolescents living with HIV should be treated for both TB and HIV.

## ■ RECOMMENDED READING


1. Kalpana S. Management of Childhood Tuberculosis. Indian J Pract Pediatr (Pulmonol). 2023;25(2):123.
2. Ministry of Health and Family Welfare, New Delhi. Paediatric TB Management Guideline 2022. NTEP Central TB Division. [online] https://tbcindia.gov.in/showfile.php?lid=3668 [Last accessed March, 2024].
3. Pediatric TB Management Essentials, Based on Childhood TB Guidelines (updated 2021) National TB Elimination program and IAP.
4. WHO operational handbook on tuberculosis: Module 5: Management of tuberculosis in children and adolescents. (2022). [online] Available from chrome-extension://efaidnbmnnnibpcajpcglclefindmkaj/https://iris.who.int/bitstream/handle/10665/352523/9789240046832-eng.pdf?sequence=1 [Last accessed March, 2024].
5. World Health Organization. Global Tuberculosis Report 2020. World Health Organization: Geneva, Switzerland; 2020.


# 4D.2   Infections in Adolescents

*G V Basavaraja, Ravishankara Marpalli*

## ■ INTRODUCTION

An estimated 1.7 million adolescents (age 10–19 years) were living with human immunodeficiency virus (HIV) in 2021 with around 90% in the World Health Organization (WHO) African Region. While there have been substantial declines in new infections amongst adolescents from a peak in 1994, adolescents still account for about 10% of new HIV infections, with three-quarters amongst adolescent girls.

Children and young adolescents aged under 15 years represent about 11% of all people with tuberculosis (TB) globally. This means 1.1 million children and young adolescents aged under 15 years fall ill with TB every year, and more than 225,000 of them lose their lives.

Adolescents and young adults usually present with bacteriologically infectious TB characterized by cavities seen on chest X-rays. The notification rates in adolescents aged 15–19 years are relatively high compared with younger adolescents.

Diarrhea and lower respiratory tract infections (pneumonia) are estimated to be among the top five causes of death for adolescents 10–14 years, with mortality rates being particularly high in African low- and middle-income countries.

## ■ UPPER RESPIRATORY TRACT INFECTIONS

### Common Cold

It refers to a mild upper respiratory viral illness. The common cold is a separate and distinctly different entity than influenza, pharyngitis, acute bronchitis, acute bacterial rhinosinusitis, allergic rhinitis, and pertussis. The common cold is associated with an enormous economic burden as assessed by lost productivity and expenditures for treatment and loss of school days. The average incidence of the common cold is two to three per year in adolescents. Common viruses are metapneumovirus, bocavirus, rhinovirus, adenovirus, enterovirus, and coronavirus 2 and its variants.

Other infections like infectious mononucleosis, influenza, pertussis, pharyngitis, and sinusitis are other common problems apart from common cold during adolescent age group. As obesity is on rise, which is proinflammatory condition, the pathology of any disease is aggravated then normal weight adolescents.

Recent study has shown dengue fever has got stormy course in obese adolescents.

*Risk factors* for increased severity of upper respiratory tract infection (URTI) other than obesity are underlying chronic diseases, congenital immunodeficiency disorders,, malnutrition, and cigarette smoking.

## Sexually Transmitted Infections

Sexually transmitted infections (STIs) are common in adolescents. Approximately two-thirds of incident chlamydia infections and one-half of incident gonococcal infections occur in adolescents. Repeated acquisition of STIs is common. Almost 40% of the annual incidence of chlamydial or gonococcal disease occurs in adolescents previously infected with the causative organisms. Repeated acquisition of STIs is a risk factor for subsequent development of HIV infection.

*Risk factors for acquisition of STIs in adolescents include:*
- Behavioral
- *Biologic:* Cervical ectopy or cervical immaturity, which refers to the area of ectocervix that is covered by columnar epithelium after puberty. Columnar epithelium is thought to be more susceptible than squamous epithelium (that replaces columnar epithelium upon maturation) to sexually transmitted organisms such as *Neisseria gonorrhoeae, Chlamydia trachomatis,* and human papillomavirus (HPV). Young females with immature cervical epithelium have higher levels of several cervicovaginal and regulatory cytokines and chemokines than females with mature cervical epithelium. Vaginal microbiota plays an important role in vaginal immune and inflammatory responses. This microbiota, especially in terms of populations of various species of *Lactobacillus,* may be particularly variable after puberty and first sexual experiences.
  - Residing in a detention facility
  - Mood disorders (which may increase the risk of substance use)
  - Food insecurity (associated with increased risk behaviors and with STI positivity)
  - Adverse childhood experiences, including maltreatment, sexual abuse, and sexual trafficking.

## ▪ SPECIAL CONCERNS

- *Consent and confidentiality:* Concerns about privacy and confidentiality
- *Pregnancy:* Pregnancy or fear of pregnancy sometimes motivates care-seeking with a chief complaint of genital symptoms.

## ▪ EVALUATION FOR SEXUALLY TRANSMITTED INFECTIONS

Adolescents with symptoms of STI should be evaluated for STI with examination and/or diagnostic tests. The type of the examination depends upon the suspected infection. Remember speculum and bimanual pelvic examinations may cause anxiety and/or discomfort and are not always necessary.

An external genital examination is done for evaluation of genital lesions that may be caused by genital herpes, primary syphilis, or HPV. Oral and anal/rectal examinations for signs of STI also are indicated based upon exposure risk.
- *Discharge syndromes:* Urethral or vaginal discharge and dysuria could be there in gonorrhea, trichomonas, chlamydia, candidiasis, and bacterial vaginosis.
- *Genital ulcer syndrome*—genital herpes, primary syphilis, and chancroid. Nonsexually acquired vulvar ulcers may occur in association with viral illness, Crohn disease, vasculitis, and Behçet syndrome. Patients with an ulcerative STI are at increased risk for coinfection with other STIs.
- *Pelvic inflammatory disease (PID):* PID encompasses a wide spectrum of clinical presentations and may be challenging to diagnose. It should be suspected in sexually active adolescents who present with pelvic discomfort.
- *Dermatologic syndromes:* The most common is genital warts (condylomata acuminata) caused by HPV. HPV types 6 and 11 are the most common causes of genital warts.

Other STI and infections that can be transmitted by sexual activity that may present with skin rash include:
- Secondary syphilis
- Disseminated gonococcal infection
- Pediculosis pubis caused by the crab louse
- Scabies

*Oral lesions:* STIs with oral manifestations include:
- *Syphilis:* Chancres are the initial manifestations of primary syphilis. They usually occur on the genitalia but may occur on the lips, tongue, and tonsils.
- *N. gonorrhoeae:* Gonococcal pharyngitis is usually acquired by oral sexual exposure. Clinical

manifestations include sore throat, pharyngeal exudates, and/or cervical lymphadenitis.

- HPV
- Herpes simplex virus

*Diagnostic testing for STI:* Adolescents who are tested for STI should also receive testing and counseling for HIV infection.

*Counseling:* Adolescents who undergo diagnostic testing for STI should be counseled about STI prevention. They should be instructed to practice abstinence while waiting for definitive test results. Those who are being treated for a STI (other than HIV) should be instructed to avoid sexual intercourse until they and their partner(s) have completed antimicrobial therapy.

## Challenges to Treatment

*Self-treatment:* Self-treatment with topical medications, antibiotics, or vaginal or rectal douching may delay treatment.

*Incomplete adherence:* Single-dose observed therapy is preferable when available, particularly for adolescents treated in the emergency department. Approximately 30–40% of adolescents treated for STI in the emergency department failed to take their prescriptions.

*Partner notification:* Many adolescents prefer to notify partners themselves. It is better the clinician does it to inform all the partners

*Expedited partner therapy (EPT):* EPT refers to the provision of appropriate antibiotics to patients with STIs for delivery to partners.

*Reinfection:* A high prevalence of *C. trachomatis* and *N. gonorrhoeae* (reinfection rather than treatment failure) is observed in patients. To avoid reinfection, patients and sexual partners who are being treated for an STI other than HIV should abstain from sexual activity until they have been adequately treated.

Individuals recently treated for chlamydia or gonorrhea should be retested approximately 3 months after treatment is completed and whenever they next seek medical care within the following 3–12 months.

## Prevention

The comprehensive approach to STI prevention is based on some major strategies, such as:

- Accurate sexual health assessment (including sexual orientation and gender identification), with education and counseling on ways to avoid STIs
- Pre-exposure vaccination for vaccine preventable STIs
- Identification of both asymptomatic and symptomatic individuals with STIs
- Effective diagnosis, treatment, counseling, and follow-up of infected individuals
- Evaluation, treatment, and counseling of sex partners of infected individuals
- Antimicrobial pre- or postexposure prophylaxis (PrEP/ PEP) against certain STIs.

## HUMAN IMMUNODEFICIENCY VIRUS INFECTION

Exposure to HIV can be a consequence of many of the risk-taking behaviors that occur among adolescents **(Box 1)**.

## Counseling and Testing

Human immunodeficiency virus testing should be incorporated into routine adolescent healthcare maintenance. Advantages of routine testing for HIV are:

- Routine testing allows the identification of acute HIV infections and early initiation of antiretroviral therapy (ART).
- Acute infection is associated with higher viral loads and higher infectivity compared with chronic infection. Initiating ART in the acute or early stage of infection will decrease onward infection.
- Early initiation of treatment is associated with improved clinical outcomes.

**BOX 1:** Risk factors.

- Multiple sexual partners
- Injection drug use by patient or a sexual partner
- Male-to-male sexual contact
- History of sexually transmitted diseases or patients seeking care for sexually transmitted infection
- More than one sexual partner in the last 6 months or since last HIV test
- Sex partner with known or suspected HIV
- Exchange of sex for drugs or money by patient or a sexual partner
- Admittance to jail or other detention facility
- Residence in areas with high prevalence of HIV
- Inadequate sex education
- Socioeconomic challenges, including poverty
- Housing and food insecurity
- Lack of medical insurance or limited access to confidential sexual health services
- Stigma and misperceptions about HIV
- Feelings of isolation, especially among gay, bisexual, or transgender adolescents

(HIV: human immunodeficiency virus)

- It is important to subsequently notify partners and provide them with screening.
- An estimated 10–60% of individuals with early HIV infection will not experience symptoms. Routine testing helps to identify those asymptomatic persons.

## Clinical Features

Incubation period is 2–4 weeks, but sometimes can go up to 10 months.

The constellation of symptoms is also known as the acute retroviral syndrome. The most common findings are fever, lymphadenopathy, sore throat, rash, myalgia/arthralgia, diarrhea, weight loss, and headache. None of these findings is specific for acute HIV infection, but certain features, especially prolonged duration of symptoms and the presence of mucocutaneous ulcers, are suggestive of the diagnosis. The presence and increased severity and duration of symptoms appear to be poor prognostic factors.

Nontender lymphadenopathy primarily involves the axillary, cervical, and occipital nodes. Adenopathy often develops during the second week of the illness, showing a specific immune response to HIV.

Sore throat is a frequent manifestation of acute HIV infection. The physical examination reveals pharyngeal edema and hyperemia, usually without tonsillar enlargement or exudate.

Painful mucocutaneous ulceration is one of the most distinctive manifestations of acute HIV infection. Shallow, sharply demarcated ulcers with white bases surrounded by a thin area of erythema may be found on the oral mucosa, anus, penis, or esophagus.

Opportunistic infections such as oral and esophageal candidiasis, cytomegalovirus (CMV) infection (proctitis, colitis, and hepatitis), *Pneumocystis jirovecii* pneumonia, and prolonged, severe cryptosporidiosis can occur.

## Laboratory Features

In early HIV infection, which is a period of rapid viral replication and infection of CD4 T cells, the viral RNA level is typically very high (e.g., >100,000 copies/mL) and the CD4 cell count can drop transiently. The leukocyte count and lymphocyte subset counts vary during the acute illness.

Please send a combination antigen/antibody test in addition to an HIV virologic (viral load) test. Also send for drug resistance testing and screening for STIs, and other coinfections.

## Diagnosis

Human immunodeficiency virus diagnosis is mentioned in **Flowchart 1**.

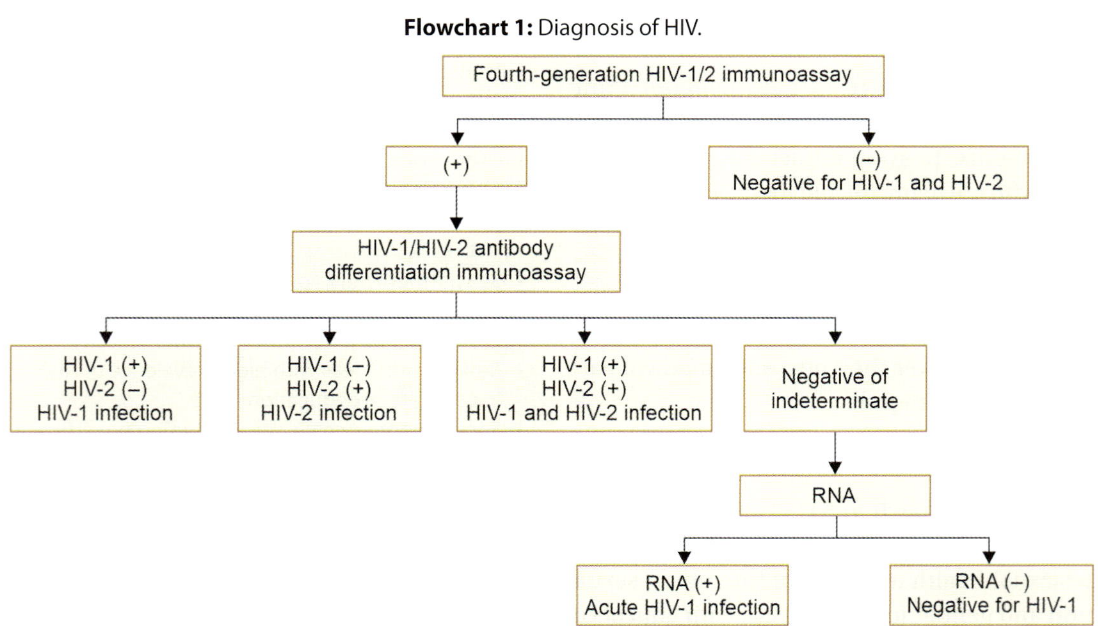

**Flowchart 1:** Diagnosis of HIV.



(HIV: human immunodeficiency virus; RNA: ribonucleic acid)

## Goals of Therapy

The goal is to achieve and maintain viral suppression, which will decrease HIV-associated complications and prevent transmission to others.

There are four classes of antiretroviral drugs typically used in initial regimens. These include:

1. Nucleoside (and nucleotide) reverse transcriptase inhibitors (NRTIs)
2. Non-nucleoside reverse transcriptase inhibitors (NNRTIs)
3. Protease inhibitors (PIs)
4. Integrase strand transfer inhibitors (INSTIs)

*Preferred regimen:*

- Bictegravir–emtricitabine–tenofovir alafenamide
- Dolutegravir plus tenofovir alafenamide–emtricitabine

*Alternative regimen:*

- *Integrase strand transfer inhibitor-based regimens:*
  - Dolutegravir–abacavir–lamivudine
  - Elvitegravir–cobicistat–emtricitabine–tenofovir alafenamide
  - Raltegravir plus tenofovir alafenamide–emtricitabine
- *Protease inhibitor-based regimens:*
  - Atazanavir (boosted with ritonavir or cobicistat) plus tenofovir alafenamide–emtricitabine
  - Darunavir (boosted with ritonavir or cobicistat) plus tenofovir alafenamide–emtricitabine
- *Non-nucleoside reverse transcriptase inhibitors-based regimens:*
  - Doravirine plus tenofovir alafenamide-emtricitabine
  - Efavirenz plus tenofovir alafenamide-emtricitabine
  - Efavirenz–emtricitabine–tenofovir disoproxil fumarate
  - Rilpivirine–emtricitabine–tenofovir alafenamide

*Two-drug regimens:* Dolutegravir–lamivudine.

The management of ART can be complex and should be delivered by or in consultation with providers with specific training. Special considerations are given for regimen selection in those who are planning to conceive, are pregnant, and/or are from resource-limited settings.

*Other management considerations:* Important components of the management of adolescents with HIV include:

- Immunizations
- Consistent use of condoms and frequent STI screening
- Prevention of pregnancy; preconceptual counseling and access to expert obstetric care to avoid vertical or partner transmission and ensure healthy outcomes
- Monitoring response to therapy, immune status and comorbidities, and appropriate use of prophylactic measures for prevention of opportunistic infections
- Monitoring for noninfectious complications and promotion of healthy lifestyle
- Transition planning and support and anticipatory guidance around life transitions that may impact engagement in care.

## ACUTE INFECTIOUS CYSTITIS IN ADOLESCENTS

Cystitis is the inflammation of the urinary bladder, usually caused by infection, which can occur alone or in conjunction with pyelonephritis.

Acute bacterial cystitis is defined as significant bacteriuria [i.e., ≥100,000 colony-forming units (CFU)/mL of a uropathogen from a clean catch urine sample or ≥50,000 CFU/mL of a uropathogen from a catheterized urine sample] in a patient with an inflammatory response and lower urinary tract symptoms (e.g., dysuria and frequency).

*Uncomplicated cystitis:* Uncomplicated cystitis is limited to the lower urinary tract.

*Complicated cystitis:* Complicated cystitis is defined by coexisting upper urinary tract infections (UTIs), multiple drug-resistant uropathogens, or hosts with special considerations (e.g., anatomic or physiologic abnormality of the urinary tract, indwelling bladder catheter, malignancy, and diabetes).

Most uropathogens originate in the gastrointestinal tract, migrate to the periurethral area and the urethra, and ascend to the bladder, where they stimulate a host response. However, cystitis may be caused by any pathogen that colonizes the periurethral area and urinary tract, including nonenteric bacteria, fungi, viruses, and parasites.

### Risk Factors

Risk factors include female sex, sexual activity, abnormalities of the urinary system, bladder stones, and diabetes.

### Clinical Features

Patients with acute infectious cystitis usually present with lower urinary tract symptoms (e.g., dysuria, frequency, urgency, and abdominal or suprapubic pain), and/or hematuria.

The history of the acute illness should include:

- *Recent illness:* It may suggest adenovirus infection or acute poststreptococcal glomerulonephritis, both of which may be associated with hematuria.
- *Recent antibiotics:* It may be associated with pathogens other than *Escherichia coli* and resistant pathogens.
- *Urethral discharge:* It may be associated with urethritis and in males, possibly epididymitis.
- *Vaginal discharge:* It may be associated with vaginitis or cervicitis.
- *Sexual activity:* It increases the risk of acute infectious cystitis and expands the list of pathogens to be considered (e.g., *Staphylococcus saprophyticus and Trichomonas vaginalis*)
  - Use of barrier contraception with spermicidal agents in sexually active females—predisposes to UTI by altering the normal vaginal flora and may contribute to chemical cystitis.

## Laboratory Evaluation

The laboratory evaluation of an adolescent with possible cystitis typically includes a urinalysis (dipstick and microscopic examination) and urine culture.

*Choice of agent:* The choice of empiric antibiotic therapy is guided by clinical features, age, local resistance patterns, and urine Gram stain, if performed. When urine culture results are available, antibiotic therapy can be tailored according to susceptibilities of the identified uropathogen.

## ■ RECURRENT SIMPLE CYSTITIS

Recurrent simple cystitis is common among young, healthy women who have anatomically and physiologically normal urinary tracts. Recurrent UTI refers to ≥2 infections in 6 months or ≥3 infections in 1 year.

## Risk Factors

### Behavioral Risk Factors

Sexual intercourse and diaphragm-spermicide use are strong and independent risk factors for acute simple cystitis.

- Spermicide use during the past year
- Having a new sex partner during the past year
- Having a first UTI at or before 15 years of age
- Having a mother with a history of UTIs

### Biologic or Genetic Factors

This results in greater propensity for uropathogenic coliforms to adhere to the uroepithelial cells of such girls.

## ■ BALANITIS AND BALANOPOSTHITIS

Balanoposthitis describes inflammation of the glans penis and the foreskin (prepuce) in uncircumcised males. Balanitis refers to the inflammation of the glans penis alone. Posthitis is the inflammation of the prepuce alone.

Acute balanitis and balanoposthitis may be classified into infectious, irritant, and traumatic causes. Sexual activity, coexisting chronic diseases (especially diabetes mellitus), and immunodeficiency [especially HIV/acquired immunodeficiency syndrome (AIDS)] increase the risk of infectious balanoposthitis.

In adolescents, 14–18% of men are *Candida albicans* carriers.

*Bacterial:* The most common causes of balanitis and balanoposthitis in postpubertal patients include *Gardnerella vaginalis* and anaerobic bacteria. Anaerobic infections are most the common, caused by *Bacteroides* spp. and may be accompanied by nonspecific urethritis.

Group B streptococci also cause balanoposthitis, presenting in 13% of adult males with penile inflammation. Males can be asymptomatic carriers and present with nonspecific erythema with or without exudates.

Sexually transmitted infections by *N. gonorrhoeae*, *C. trachomatis*, or rarely, *Treponema pallidum* have also been described. Group A *Streptococcus* is rarely isolated in the postpubertal male but has been documented to be sexually transmitted after fellatio.

*Viral:* HPV and herpes simplex virus types 1 and 2.

*Protozoan: T. vaginalis* causes an erosive balanoposthitis following sexual contact. Anogenital contact has been associated with *Entamoeba histolytica* balanoposthitis.

## Clinical Features

Common symptoms in patients with balanitis and balanoposthitis include pain, genital itching and irritation, groin rash, and dysuria. Balanoposthitis is also characterized by penile, but not urethral discharge, foul odor exudate, preputial swelling, tenderness, erythema lymphadenopathy, or lymphadenitis. Scarring between the glans and prepuce causes meatal stenosis and phimosis. Balanitis is characterized by swelling, tenderness, and erythema of the glans penis, meatus, and/or penile shaft, and/or lymphadenopathy or lymphadenitis.

## Diagnosis

The presence of inflammation of the glans penis and/or foreskin on direct inspection establishes the diagnosis. Gram stain and bacterial culture of preputial secretions to be done, including KOH microscopy and fungal culture. Group A *Streptococcus* culture should be obtained in those with pharyngitis, a history of oral-genital contact, or persistent disease. Patients with balanitis or balanoposthitis, who are sexually active, have genital ulcers, or urethral drainage should have appropriate specimens to evaluate for the STIs.

## Management

### General Measures

General measures include sitz bath to the penis [soaking of the penis in warm water containing a weak salt solution two to three times per day is advised while inflammation persists], avoidance of irritants, and reinforcement of proper foreskin hygiene.

### Treatment by Etiology

Therapy guided by appropriate laboratory studies can be opted. Nonspecific balanitis and balanoposthitis can be treated by empirical application of topical antibiotic ointment (e.g., polysporin or bacitracin) four times daily or mupirocin cream twice daily helps reduce dysuria and may prevent secondary bacterial infection.

Most patients respond to general care augmented by appropriate topical therapy within 7 days. Up to 10% of patients have recurrence of balanoposthitis.

Proper hygiene and avoidance of forceful retraction are the most important interventions to prevent balanoposthitis.

## ■ RECOMMENDED READING


1. Centers for Disease Control and Prevention (CDC). HIV prevention practices of primary care physicians—United States, 1992. MMWR Morb Mortal Wkly Rep. 1994;43(47):869-73.
2. District of Columbia Department of Health. CDC Fact Sheet: Information for Teens and Young Adults: Staying Healthy and Preventing STDs. Washington, DC: District of Columbia Department of Health. [online] Available from https://www.cdc.gov/std/life-stages-populations/stdfact-teens.htm [Last accessed March, 2024].
3. Fisher JD, Fisher WA, Cornman DH, Amico RK, Bryan A, Friedland GH. Clinician-delivered intervention during routine clinical care reduces unprotected sexual behavior among HIV-infected patients. J Acquir Immune Defic Syndr Hum Retrovirol. 1994;7(8):777-83.
4. Stanford Children's Health. Sexually transmitted diseases in adolescents. Palo Alto, CA: Stanford Children's Health. [online] Available from https://www.stanfordchildrens.org/en/topic/default?id=sexually-transmitted-diseases-in-adolescents-90-P01654 [Last accessed March, 2024].
5. World Health Organization. (2021). Sexually transmitted infections among adolescents: the need for adequate health services. Geneva, Switzerland: World Health Organization. [online] Available from https://www.who.int/publications/i/item/9789240071476 [Last accessed March, 2024].
6. World Health Organization. Treatment and care in children and adolescents. Geneva, Switzerland. [online] Available from https://www.who.int/teams/global-hiv-hepatitis-and-stis-programmes/hiv/treatment/treatment-and-care-in-children-and-adolescents [Last accessed March, 2024].


# 4D.3 | Adolescent Immunization

*Kripasindhu Chatterjee, SG Kasi, Vipin Vashistha*

## ■ INTRODUCTION

India has a "young population" profile, with 22% of the population (about 253 million) consisting of adolescents (10–19 years). India has the largest adolescent population in the world. Of these, 12% belong to the 10–14 years age group and nearly 10% are in the 15–19 years age group. Thus, every fifth person in India is an adolescent. Adolescents accounted for 230 million or 15.5% of total disability adjusted life years (DALYs) worldwide, much of this due to vaccine-preventable diseases (VPDs). Health issues that arise in adolescence may impact their health status in adulthood.

## BURDEN OF COMMUNICABLE DISEASES IN ADOLESCENTS

### Global

In 2019, globally among people aged 0–24 years, there were 3.0 million deaths and 30.0 million years of healthy life lost to disability [as measured by years lived with disabilities (YLDs)] from communicable diseases (CDs) corresponding to a total disease burden of 288.4 million DALYs. This burden represents 57.3% of the total CD burden across all ages.

For children and adolescents, specifically, CD accounted for 44.1% of the total 6.9 million deaths in this age group, 16.6% of the total disability, and 37.9% of the total 760.0 million all-cause DALYs **(Table 1)**.

Communicable disease burden among children and adolescents in countries of low sociodemographic development accounted for 58.2% of all CD deaths and 56.0% of all CD DALYs among children and adolescents. More than half of the mortality among children and adolescents in settings of low sociodemographic development was caused by CDs compared with just 5.6% of deaths and 7.1% of DALYs in settings of high sociodemographic development.

In children and adolescents, three disease groups: (1) Enteric infections, (2) lower respiratory tract infections, and (3) malaria accounted for 60% of CD burden.

In 2013, in younger adolescents (age 10–14 years), CDs accounted for 54% of deaths in girls and 47% in boys. Intestinal infections, diarrheal diseases, and lower respiratory infections were the major causes for death in this age group.

Communicable diseases accounted for 43% of disabilities in girls and 41% in boys.

In 2013, in the older age group (15–19 years), 42% of deaths among older adolescent girls and 31% of deaths in older boys resulted from CDs.

In this age group, CDs accounted for 34% of DALYs in girls and 27% in boys.

As compared to 1990, deaths and DALYs due to CDs decreased in both girls and boys in the 10–19 years age group.

## VACCINE-PREVENTABLE DISEASES IN ADOLESCENTS

The burden of VPDs in adolescents in India is not well defined. Available studies indicate a lack of protective antibodies in a significant proportion of adolescents.

### Diphtheria

India account for ~92% of reported diphtheria cases in the world. In a recent review done in 2016, 41% of cases occurred in those >10 years of age. In a study done in 2,400 school children aged 6–17 years studying the various government schools in Hyderabad, only 56% had protective levels of immunoglobulin G (IgG) antidiphtheria titers of >0.1 IU/mL.

### Pertussis

The incidence of pertussis in adolescents in India is unknown. In a recently published article titled "prospective multinational serosurveillance study of B. pertussis infection among 10–18 years subjects from 8 Asian countries", with 200 subjects from India, high titers of anti-PT IgG >62.5 IU/mL, indicative of B. pertussis infection within the past 12 months, was found in 18% of subjects. In a study done in Vellore on 281 subjects, of whom all had received three primary vaccines and one booster, 42.7% had received the second booster and 5.3% had received the adolescent booster of pertussis-containing vaccines, around 7% of adolescents had evidence of recent infection, and 54% of the adolescents tested had no detectable antibodies, suggesting waning

| **TABLE 1:** Estimates of deaths, YLDs, and DALYs (communicable-disease specific), in 2019. | | | |
|---|---|---|---|
| | *Mortality (% due to communicable diseases)* | *YLDs (% due to communicable diseases)* | *DALYs (% due to communicable diseases)* |
| *10–14 years* | | | |
| Male | 47.2 | 15.5 | 26.8 |
| Female | 41.2 | 17.6 | 27.8 |
| *15–19 years* | | | |
| Male | 33.9 | 11.5 | 20.0 |
| Female | 25.8 | 13.2 | 20.0 |

(DALYs: disability adjusted life years; YLDs: years lived with disabilities)

immunity and susceptibility to pertussis, which can lead to periodic epidemics.

## Tetanus

In 2016, India accounted for 3,781 of the 10,300 cases of tetanus reported worldwide. In a serosurvey of schoolchildren 7–17 years in Hyderabad, only 64% were immune to tetanus.

## Measles, Mumps, and Rubella

In a serosurvey of students from Manipal university, the prevalence of serological susceptibility to measles was 9.5%, mumps 32%, rubella 16.6%, and varicella 25.8%.

Involvement of adolescents has been reported in mumps outbreaks in Rajasthan and Orissa. Susceptibility to rubella has been reported in 7–66% of adolescent females. In a multicenter serosurvey, about 20–30% of adolescents and young adults were found susceptible to varicella at the age of 11–20 years.

## Hepatitis A

The shifting epidemiology of hepatitis A infections has increased the incidence of this infection in adolescents with greater morbidity.

## Human Papilloma Virus

India has a female >15 years population of 483.5 million; all are potentially at risk for cervical cancer. In 2012, India had 123,907 cases of cervical cancer and 77,348 deaths due to cervical cancer. The prevalence of human papilloma virus (HPV) 16/18 in women with normal cytology is 5%, in women with cervical intraepithelial neoplasia (CIN) 1–28.2%, in women with CIN 2/3 62.8%, and in cervical cancer 83.2%.

The prevalence of HPV was found to be 12.3% in Indian tribal girls and young women. The overall HPV prevalence varied with age—it was 19.2% in young adults (18–25 years), 11.4% in adolescents (13–17 years), and 6.6% in preadolescent girls (9–12 years). In a study done in 12 schools around Delhi and NOIDA in children 8–17 years of age, the prevalence of HPV was 3.2% in girls and 2.1% in boys; 33.4% were <13 years of age.

## Dengue

In a nationally representative community-based survey done from June 19, 2017, to April 12, 2018, the overall seroprevalence of dengue virus (DENV) infection in India was 48.7% [95% confidence interval (CI) 43.5–54.0],

increasing from 28.3% (21.5–36.2) among children aged 5–8 years to 41.0% (32.4–50.1) among children aged 9–17 years, and 56.2% (49.0–63.1) among individuals aged between 18 and 45 years. The seroprevalence was high in the southern [76.9% (69·1–83·2)], western [62.3% (55.3–68.8)], and northern [60.3% (49.3–70.5)] regions.

Evidence of recent dengue infection (positive capture IgG capture ELISA among individuals with past exposure to dengue) was highest in the 9–17 years age group compared to lower and higher age groups.

## IMMUNIZATION COVERAGE IN ADOLESCENTS

Vaccine coverage in adolescents lags far behind the uptake rates in the population aged under 5 years. Even in a developed country like USA, in 2022, up to date coverage with HPV vaccine was only 62.6%. Coverage rates in low- or middle-income countries (LMICs) are much lower, and there is a lack of data from many of these countries. In India, tetanus and diphtheria (Td) is the only vaccine recommended for adolescents in the National Immunization Program (NIP), while the Japanese encephalitis (JE) vaccine is offered in hyperendemic areas. In campaign mode, measles and rubella (MR) vaccine is offered till 15 years of age. Even in the private sector, coverage with the "exclusive adolescent vaccines" is poor.

## ADOLESCENT IMMUNIZATION SCHEDULES

Vaccines for adolescents are considered under four groups:
1. Exclusive adolescent vaccines
2. Catch-up vaccines
3. Vaccines for adolescents in special situations
4. Vaccines for the adolescent traveler.

### Exclusive Adolescent Vaccines

Tetanus, diphtheria, and pertussis (Tdap) and HPV vaccines are the *"exclusive"* adolescents' vaccines.

### Catch-up Vaccines

Catch-up vaccines include measles, mumps, and rubella (MMR), hepatitis B, hepatitis A, varicella, and typhoid-TCV (typhoid conjugate vaccine).

### Vaccines for Adolescents in Special Situations

These vaccines include influenza, pneumococcal, JE vaccines, rabies, and meningococcal.

**TABLE 2:** Composition per dose.

| | Diphtheria | Tetanus | PT | Pertactin | FHA | FIM 2 and 3 |
|---|---|---|---|---|---|---|
| Boostrix | 2 IU | 20 IU | 8 µg | 2.5 µg | 8 µg | |
| Adacel | 2 IU | 20 IU | 2.5 µg | 3 µg | 5 µg | 5 µg |

(FHA: filamentous hemagglutinin; FIM: fimbriae; PT: pertussis toxin)

## Vaccines for the Adolescent Traveler

These vaccines include meningococcal, yellow fever (YFV), JE vaccines, and rabies.

## Tetanus, Diphtheria, and Pertussis Vaccine

Two Tdap brands are presently marketed in India, Boostrix™ and Adacel™ **(Table 2)**.

Contraindications for Tdap are:

- Anaphylaxis after a previous dose of any Tdap antigen-containing vaccine or to any component of the vaccine
- Encephalopathy of undetermined cause within 7 days of administration of a previous pertussis antigen-containing vaccine.

Tetanus, diphtheria, and pertussis vaccines have shown moderate efficacy against polymerase chain reaction (PCR) positive pertussis. Postlicensure studies of Tdap have reported vaccine effectiveness ranging from 65.6 to 78.0% among adolescent populations. However, immunity wanes to levels as low as 8.9% (95% CI –30.6 to 36.4%) by ≥4 years after vaccination. Hence, Tdap is moderately effective in the prevention of pertussis in adolescents for a short period of time and does not play a significant role in reducing transmission.

Tdap is now recommended as a single dose between 10 and 12 years of age. This dose is to be administered in the adolescent age group even if Tdap was administered earlier at 4–6 years. While Boostrix is licensed >4 years of age, Adacel is licensed for use between 11 and 54 years.

## Human Papilloma Virus Vaccines

Three vaccines against HPV are marketed in India:

1. Gardasil™, which is a quadrivalent vaccine containing serotypes 6, 11, 16, and 18
2. Gardasil 9™, which contains 6, 11, 16, 18, 31, 33, 45, 52, and 58.
3. Cervavac™, which is a quadrivalent vaccine containing serotypes 6, 11, 16, and 18, and manufactured by Serum Institute of India.

All three vaccines are manufactured by recombinant DNA technology that produces noninfectious viral-like particles (VLPs) comprising the HPV L1 protein.

Clinical trials with Gardasil-4 and Gardasil-9 have used efficacy against CIN 2/3 and adenocarcinoma in situ (AIS) caused by HPV strains contained in the concerned vaccine as primary end-points, which have been accepted by the regulatory authorities. Cervavac has been licensed on basis of immunological noninferiority to Gardasil-4. Neither vaccines have significant cross-protection over a longer period of time. Although the regulatory studies were done in women 16–25 years, the vaccine is licensed from the age of 9 years as bridging studies have shown higher antibody responses in the preadolescents. The immune protective correlates are not known.

Adolescent immunization with the HPV vaccines is important for the following reasons:

- HPV vaccine being a prophylactic vaccine should be administered before exposure to sexual activity and sexual exposure is unlikely in the 9–14 years age group.
- The vaccine can be amalgamated with existing Tdap visit at 10 years.
- Bridging studies have conclusively demonstrated that the immune response is superior in the younger age groups.
- Vaccinating before 15 years of age needs only two doses and hence is cost saving.

## Quadrivalent Vaccine (Gardasil™)

This vaccine contains a mixture of L1 proteins of HPV serotypes 6, 11, 16, and 18, adjuvanted with amorphous aluminum hydroxyphosphate sulfate. Each 0.5 mL dose of this vaccine contains L1 protein of HPV-6: 20 µg, HPV-11: 40 µg, HPV 16: 40 µg, and HPV 18: 20 µg with 225 µg of the adjuvant.

The phase 3 studies showed that three doses at 0, 2, and 6 months resulted in a vaccine efficacy (VE) of 99% against types 16, 18 related CIN-2/3 and AIS, and 99–100% efficacy against vaccine-type related genital warts, vaginal intraepithelial neoplasia (VaIN), and vulvar intraepithelial neoplasia (VIN), in per protocol analysis. Follow-up studies have shown undiminished protection till 14 years.

## Quadrivalent Vaccine (Cervavac™)

Each dose of 0.5 mL contains:

The phase 2/3 study involved a cohort of 2,307 subjects in two age groups of 9–14 years and 15–26 years, including both female and male subjects.

In girls 9–14 years receiving two doses of CERVAVAC versus women 15–26 years receiving three doses of Gardasil, the Geometric Mean Fold Rise (GMFR) for all four serotypes was >1,000-fold. Noninferiority was demonstrated for high risk (oncogenic) HPV types as lower bound of geometric mean titer (GMT) ratio CI was above 0.5. Similar findings were demonstrated in boys 9–14 years receiving two doses of CERVAVAC versus women 15–26 years receiving three doses of Gardasil, in women 15–26 years receiving three doses CERVAVAC versus women 15–26 years receiving three doses of Gardasil and men 15–26 years receiving three doses of SIIPL-qHPV versus women 15–26 years receiving three doses of Gardasil.

Noninferiority was also demonstrated in girls 9–14 years receiving two doses of CERVAVAC versus girls of age 9–14 years receiving two doses of Gardasil and boys 9–14 years receiving two doses of CERVAVAC versus girls of age 9–14 years receiving two doses of Gardasil.

At 7 months the seroconversion rates were 100% in both cohorts.

## Nonavalent Vaccine (Gardasil-9)

This vaccine contains 6, 11, 16, 18, 31, 33, 45, 52, and 58. It provides ~15% additional protection as compared to Gardasil 4. In India, it is expected to cover ~98% of all cervical cancer-causing strains.

The vaccines have very good safety record. The Centers for Disease Control and Prevention (CDC), EMEA, World Health Organization (WHO), and other leading health organizations closely monitor the safety of HPV vaccines and have declared the vaccines to be safe.

## ADVISORY COMMITTEE ON VACCINES AND IMMUNIZATION PRACTICES (ACVIP) RECOMMENDATIONS

*HPV 4 (Gardasil):*
- In India, this vaccine is licensed only for females.
- 9–14 years: Two doses: With 6–12 months interval between doses

- Immunocompromised individuals: Three dose 0-2-6 months
- 15–45 years: Three doses: 0–2–6 months

*Cervavac TM SII:*
- Boys and girls 9–14 years: Two dose: with 6–month interval between doses
- Males and females 15–26 years: Three doses: 0–2–6 months. Not licensed beyond 26 years

*Gardasil 9:*
- Boys and girls 9–14 years: Two doses: with 6–months interval
- 15–26 years (only for females): Three doses: 0–2–6 months
- Immunocompromised individuals: Three doses at 0–2–6 months

*Dengue vaccines:*

Although not an adolescent-specific vaccine, it is expected that when available in India, it will be used in adolescents.

*Dengvaxia* is a live-attenuated tetra-valent chimeric vaccine, constructed by using YFV viral backbone of the strain 17D (YF17D). It is administered in a three doses at 0–6–12 months.

Efficacy varied by region, serotype, baseline serostatus, and age.

In Southeast Asian countries, the overall efficacy was 56.5% (43.8–66.4), type 1: 50.0% (24.6–61.0), type 2: 35% (–9.2–61.0), type 3: 78.2% (52.9–90.8), and type 4: 75.3 (54.5–87.0).

Overall efficacy in seropositive individuals was 74.3% (53.2–86.3) and in seronegative individuals 35.5% (–26.8–66.7). The efficacy was 74.4% (59.2–84.3) in the 12–14 year age groups and much lower in the younger age groups.

The RR of hospitalization increased over time for vaccine recipients who were <9 at the time of vaccination; hence, the vaccines is recommended only for those who are seropositive.

DENGVAXIA is approved for use in individuals 6 through 16 years of age with laboratory-confirmed previous dengue infection and living in endemic areas.

*Qdenga:* It is a live-attenuated dengue vaccine based on the complete DENV-2 genome. It has an attenuated DENV-2 PDK-53 backbone and the PrM and E proteins of types 1, 3, and 4 inserted into this backbone.

The overall VE was 80.2%.

In seropositives, it was 82.2 and 74.9% in the seronegatives.

Vaccine efficacy against type 1 was 73.7%, type 2 97.7%, type 3 62.6%, and type 4 63.2%.

Vaccine efficacy was uniform across age groups: 4–5 years: 72.8%; 6–11 years: 80.7%; and 12–16 years: 83.3%.

The VE against virologically confirmed + hospitalization in the seropositive was 94.4% and 97.2% in the seronegatives.

It is licensed for use for the prevention of dengue disease caused by any serotype in individuals 6–45 years of age. It is to be used in a two-dose schedule of 0–3 months. Neither vaccines are presently marketed in India.

*Coronavirus disease (COVID) vaccine:* Altogether four COVID vaccines have been approved in India in pediatric population and all are under emergency use authorization (EUA) and from the age of 12 years onward. These are:

- *Covaxin$^{TM}$:* It is a whole virus inactivated vaccine, administered in a two-dose schedule at least 28 days apart.
- *Corbevax$^{TM}$:* It is a protein subunit vaccine and schedule is same as Covaxin.
- *Covovax$^{TM}$:* It is a recombinant nanoparticle vaccine, administered intramuscularly (IM) as two doses schedule on days 0–21 days
- *ZyCoV-D$^{TM}$:* It is a DNA plasmid vector vaccine, administered as 0.1 mL ID, in three dose schedule on days 0–28–56.

## Catch-up Vaccines

Catch-up vaccines include MMR, hepatitis B, hepatitis A, varicella, and typhoid-TCV.

- Adolescents without a history of medically documented disease or vaccination record should receive two doses of MMR and varicella at interval of 4–8 weeks. Adolescents who have received a single dose of these vaccines, a second dose is to be recommended. Vaccination with MMR and varicella vaccines is mandatory for admission to universities in Europe and USA.
- Adolescents without a record of previous hepatitis B vaccination should receive three doses in a schedule of 0–1–6 months.
- Adolescents without previous history of medically documented disease or no record of previous immunization should receive two doses of inactivated hepatitis A vaccine at 0–6 months or a single dose of the live-attenuated hepatitis a vaccine. Prevaccination estimation of anti-hepatitis A IgG may be considered.
- A single dose of a TCV is also recommended.

For adolescents in *special situations*, the following vaccines are recommended:

- *Influenza:* Adolescents at higher risk for developing severe influenza include pregnant adolescents, obese patients with body mass index (BMI) >40 kg/m$^2$, younger than 19 years who are on chronic aspirin or salicylate-containing medication, sickle cell disease, other immune compromised conditions, and adolescents with chronic systemic illnesses such as respiratory, cardiac, renal, neurological, hepatic, or metabolic diseases.
- *Pneumococcal:* Immunosuppressed states, anatomical or functional asplenia, sickle cell disease, other hemoglobinopathies, cerebrospinal fluid (CSF) leaks, chronic heart disease (excluding hypertension), chronic lung disease (including asthma), and chronic liver disease. The schedule is single dose of pneumococcal conjugate vaccine 13 (PCV13) followed by the 23-valent polysaccharide vaccine at least 8 weeks later.
- *JE vaccines:* It is approved up to 18 years in districts declared as endemic for JE. The vaccines are administrated in a schedule of two doses of 0.5 mL of either of the two available inactivated JE vaccines (JENVAC and JEEV), 4 weeks apart.
- *Rabies:* Postexposure prophylaxis (PEP) in a schedule of 0-3-7-14 to 28 days for PEP along with RIG/Mab for Class 3 bites.

## ■ BARRIERS TO ADOLESCENT VACCINATIONS

Various barriers exist to adolescent immunization. Adolescents rarely participate in preventive health services. Missed opportunities are common. There is generally a low perceived threat due to the disease, fear of adverse effects, and internet and media sources that give misinformation about vaccines, especially vaccine safety is another important barrier against immunization.

## ■ THE WAY FORWARD

Uptake of adolescent vaccinations can be increased making immunization services available at timings that are suitable for adolescents attending schools, colleges, or employed and utilizing the schools as a base for immunization programs. Moreover, exclusive adolescent specific immunization charts should be utilized. Demand has to be created by providing information about necessary vaccinations, having patient reminder systems through SMS and having vaccination certificates for school requirements. A strong and unambiguous health care provider recommendation is crucial for acceptance of vaccinations. This is particularly important for acceptance of the HPV vaccines.

Rarely do adolescents present for identified routine preventive health care. Their contact with healthcare services is primarily for illnesses, injuries, and sexual or mental health issues. These contacts can be utilized for delivery of appropriate vaccines. Adolescents may not be accompanied by parents or caregivers during these contacts. Thus, the prerequisite for parental consent for vaccination can present a significant barrier to improve adolescent vaccine uptake in these settings.

Granting adolescents the authority to agree to vaccination without parental permission would allow them to catch up on any missed childhood vaccines and participate in school-based and community-based vaccination programs.

The legal age of consent tends to coincide with the age of majority, which is 18 years in most countries. It implies that, for adolescents 12–17 years, consent is normally required from their parent or legal guardian for vaccinations. To circumvent this barrier, some countries have fixed the age of consent at younger ages, specifically to allow HPV vaccination.

## ■ KEY MESSAGES

- In India, adolescent immunization is still in its infancy, although adolescent have a significant burden due to VPDs.
- Tdap and HPV vaccines are the exclusive adolescent vaccines. MMR, hepatitis B, hepatitis A, varicella, and typhoid-TCV are the catch-up vaccines. Adolescents with comorbid conditions need influenza, pneumococcal, JE, and rabies vaccines. The adolescent traveler should be immunized with meningococcal, yellow fever, JE, and rabies vaccines according to standard recommendations.
- Barriers to adolescent immunization include missed opportunities, low public awareness about the need for immunization coverage in this age group, misperceptions about vaccine safety, and lack of knowledge about the importance of immunizations.
- Adolescent immunizations uptake can be enhanced by interventions in the healthcare systems and increasing demand for the vaccines.
- School-based vaccination programs are the most appropriate settings for adolescent vaccination programs.

## ■ RECOMMENDED READING

1. Biswal S, Reynales H, Saez-Llorens X, Lopez P, Borja-Tabora C, Kosalaraksa P, et al. Efficacy of a Tetravalent Dengue Vaccine in Healthy Children and Adolescents. N Engl J Med. 2019;381:2009-19.

2. Bruni L, Albero G, Serrano B, Mena M, Collado JJ, Gómez D, et al. (2023). ICO/IARC Information Centre on HPV and Cancer (HPV Information Centre). Human Papillomavirus and Related Diseases in India. Summary Report 22 October 2021. [online] Available from chrome-extension:// efaidnbmnnnibpcajpcglclefindmkaj/https://hpvcentre. net/statistics/reports/IND.pdf [Last accessed March, 2024].

3. Edwards KM, Decker MD. Pertussis vaccines. In: Plotkin SA, Offit PA, Orenstein WA, Edwards KM (Eds). Plotkin's Vaccines, 7th edition. Philadelphia: Elsevier; 2018. pp. 711-61.

4. GBD 2019 Child and Adolescent Communicable Disease Collaborators. The unfinished agenda of communicable diseases among children and adolescents before the COVID-19 pandemic, 1990–2019: a systematic analysis of the Global Burden of Disease Study 2019. Lancet. 2023;402:313-35.

5. Humiston SG, Rosenthal SL. Challenges to Vaccinating Adolescents: Vaccine Implementation Issues. Pediatr Infect Dis J. 2005;24:S134-40.

6. Jennifer SL, Basker MM, Verghese VP, Anandan S, Sethuvel DPM, Abirami SB, et al. A Seroepidemiological Survey for Pertussis among Adolescents. Indian J Pediatr. 2021;88(5):509.

7. Kasi SG, Shivananda S, Marathe S, Chatterjee K, Agarwalla S, Dhir SK, et al. Indian Academy of Pediatrics (IAP) Advisory Committee on Vaccines and Immunization Practices (ACVIP): Recommended Immunization Schedule (2020-21) and Update on Immunization for Children Aged 0 Through 18 Years. Indian Pediatr. 2021;58:44-53.

8. Kjaer SK, Sigurdsson K, Iversen OE, Hernandez-Avila M, Wheeler CM, Perez G, et al. A pooled analysis of continued prophylactic efficacy of quadrivalent human papillomavirus (Types 6/11/16/18) vaccine against high-grade cervical and external genital lesions. Cancer Prev Res (Phila). 2009;2:868-78.

9. Kumar MS, Kamaraj P, Khan SA, Allam RR, Barde PV, Dwibedi B, et al. Seroprevalence of Dengue Infection Using IgG Capture ELISA in India, 2017–2018. Am J Trop Med Hyg. 2021;105(5):1277-80.

10. Pingali C, Yankey D, Elam-Evans LD, Markowitz LE, Valier MR, Fredua B, et al. Vaccination Coverage Among Adolescents Aged 13–17 Years—National Immunization Survey–Teen, United States, 2022. MMWR Morb Mortal Wkly Rep. 2023;72(34):912-19.

11. World Health Organization. Review of the epidemiology of Diphtheria—2000-2016. [online] Available from https:// www.who.int/immunization/sage/meetings/2017/ap ril/1_Final_report_Clarke_april3.pdf?ua=1. [Last accessed March, 2024].

# Part E: Adolescents with Distinctive Circumstances

***Sub-section Editors:** Samir Shah, Poonam Bhatia, Shailaja Mane*

## 4E.1 Concerns of Adolescents with Chronic Health Conditions

*Madhushree Deshpande*

### ■ INTRODUCTION

Globally, 1.3 million adolescents died from preventable/treatable causes in 2012 [World Health Organization (WHO)]. Moreover, about 35% of the global burden of the disease has its roots in adolescence like half of the mental health problems of adults begin by 14 years of age, and most cases are undetected and untreated.

Since adolescents constitute about one fifth of the total Indian population, India's achievement of most of the United Nation's Sustainable Development Goals and their targets will depend on the development and well-being of these adolescents, directly or indirectly.

Adolescent programs mainly focus on health education for sexual and reproductive health, nutritional education and supplementation, anemia control, immunization, and counseling. There is no comprehensive program to address all the needs of adolescents. The program to cover awareness on congenital and noncommunicable diseases presenting in adolescence age running a chronic course till adulthood, and morbidity due to diseases, along with the life style adopted should be properly taken care of.

### ■ DEFINITION

Chronic illness is defined as a disease that requires a minimum of 3 months of continuous medical care, permanent lifestyle changes, and continuous behavioral adaptation to the unpredictable course of the disease.

### ■ PREVALENCE

Approximately 10–30% of adolescents world over suffer from chronic diseases with a prevalence of 1 in 10 adolescents. The steady increase in the incidence of disease could be due to improved treatment of diseases, which were once thought to be untreatable or fatal (cystic fibrosis).

### Commonly Occurring Chronic Health Disease/Illness in Adolescent Age

- *Lungs and upper respiratory tract:* Bronchial asthma, cystic fibrosis
- *Heart:* Congenital heart disease, rheumatic heart disease, cardiomyopathy, and hypertension
- *Blood and bone marrow:* Thalassemia, sickle cell anemia, leukemia, and lymphoma
- *Kidney:* Chronic kidney failure and postinfectious nephritis sequel
- *Liver:* Chronic hepatitis, cirrhosis, portal hypertension, and chronic liver disease
- *Brain/central nervous system (CNS):* Epilepsy (seizure disorders), malignancies, tumors, postinfection sequel, and poststroke
- *Gastrointestinal:* Celiac disease, Crohn's disease, ulcerative colitis, and irritable bowel syndrome (IBS)
- *Endocrine:* Type 1 diabetes mellitus (T1DM) and type 2 diabetes mellitus (T2DM) and hypothyroidism
- *Skin:* Allergies, winter eczema, and seborrheic dermatitis
- *Orthopedic:* Bone tumors and malignancies, congenital deformity, and developmental dysplasia
- *Chromosomal:* Down syndrome, Turner syndrome, Klinefelter syndrome, and fragile X syndrome
- *Nutritional:* Obesity, undernutrition, anorexia nervosa, and bulimia
- *Psychiatric:* Depression, bipolar disorder, and obsessive–compulsive disorder
- *Hearing, vision disorders, and other disabilities:* Since birth or later due to accident/diseases
- *Inborn errors of metabolism:* Galactosemia and phenylketonuria
- *Storage disorders:* Gaucher disease, Pompe disease, Niemann–Pick disease, and Tay–Sachs disease

- *Immunodeficiencies:* Congenital and acquired
- *Environmental:* Lead poisoning and survivors of nuclear radiation exposure, poisonous gas exposures, and pollution effects
- *Urogenital:* Intersex disorders
- *Autoimmune disorders:* T1DM, rheumatoid arthritis, systemic lupus erythematosus (SLE), lupus, psoriasis, and Hashimoto's thyroiditis.

## ■ FACTORS RELATED TO

- *Age of onset:* It has been noticed that the younger the patient, the more is the adaptability and less is the psychosocial destructivity in the disease. Children adapt easily to chronic illness, which begins early in life or is congenital.
- *Visible effects of the disease:* The chronic disease results in visible physical changes, like typical hemolytic facies in children with thalassemia major, which may result in body image issues in children. It may develop a sense of personal devaluation and low self-esteem.
- *Severity of impairment:* For adolescents to grow normally, physically, and psychologically, it is important for them to involve more actively socially and with friends and peers. The severity of illness has a noticeable impact on normal development.
- *Course of disease:* The diseases running in a chronic, continuous course produce stable condition and cause consistency in adaptation to the disease for better or worse. The disease which fluctuates between remission and exacerbation, such as nephrotic syndrome and asthma, leads to frequent changes in self-perception causing mood swings and change in behavior pattern.

## ■ IMPACT OF CHRONIC DISEASE ON ADOLESCENTS

Chronic disease affects the growth and development. Chronic illness is always associated with psychosocial impact throughout life. Adolescence is a period marked with psychosocial and identity issues, which pose a difficult and unique challenge for adolescents, families, and treating physician. The provision for proper assessment and interventions will surely yield a favorable outcome to improve behavior, improve quality of life, and promote near-normal functions. The effects of chronic disease vary with severity, type of the disease, stage of the disease, and other factors.

## Effect on Physical Health

Chronic disease directly affects growth and developmental potential resulting in small stature, delayed puberty, undernutrition, malnutrition, and micronutrient deficiencies.

Children with genetic diseases grow at a variable rate, and a disease-specific growth chart should be used to assess their growth and height velocity (Down syndrome and Turner disease).

Restricted physical activity further results in obesity due to either disease or treatment. Obesity makes the adolescent more vulnerable to T1DM, hypertension, and metabolic syndrome. Other developmental changes due to pubertal hormones are related to changes in growth, metabolic rate, fat, muscle growth or redistribution, and breast and genital development. T1DM is the most common disease occurring now, with a steady increasing trend being observed in adolescents worldwide. The estimated prevalence for T1DM in adolescents of 19 years or younger is 1 in 1,000 youths.

## Effect on Emotional and Mental Health

It has been noted that in general, adolescents cope with emotional challenges in a better way than the adults. Chronic illness poses a constant challenge to the autonomy and peer involvement causing stress of standing out. Hence, the coping mechanisms, which are in developing stage, make them vulnerable to mental illness as follows:

- Anxiety, adjustment disorders, depression, and suicide in both adolescents and their parents; the effect on cognition can be subtle
- Behavioral problems and school being missed out, leading to low school performance
- Substance abuse
- *Eating disorders:* Anorexia nervosa and bulimia
- Mood disturbances and others.

## Effect on Chronic Mental Health

The most important concern is that the most commonly used screening tools have not been validated with children who are cognitively impaired or have life experiences that are very atypical. Increased psychosocial distress in virtually all domains of life like hyperactivity–inactivity, emotional symptoms, peer problems, conduct problems, adjustment disorder, lower self-esteem, stress, internalizing and externalizing behavior, stigmatization, anxiety, and depression may increase due to increased stressors. Family rejection, physical or sexual abuse and various health problems may further aggravate mental health vulnerabilities in adolescents.

## Sociocultural, Educational, and Vocational Aspects

The effect on cognition and learning can be subtle, causing poor school performance, due to repeated absence from school, poor health, or admission to hospital. Along with educational disadvantage, they find it difficult to get a good job and financial independence as adults. It is the foremost responsibility of healthcare professionals to improve adolescents' transition from education to the workforce. They should encourage development of vocational capacity according to the disease process. Encourage the adolescent to engage in part-time jobs and working for the parents. Finding suitable work experience and placements and identifying strengths and abilities rather than disabilities are crucial. The early-stage interventions and continuous reassessment of adolescents for vocational readiness, educational achievement, communication skills, self-esteem, expectations, and work experience are needed.

## Effect on Activity

Adolescents with juvenile arthritis, IBD, and other conditions with chronic pain limit the outdoor activity, which keeps them in physical deconditioning, increased pain, and reduced functioning in future also. The regular activity should be individualized depending upon the severity of the disease. When they will start listening to the call of their body, it will reduce the chance of exertion and push them when needed.

## Effect on Sleep

Poor sleep reduces immune function and causes poor concentration, increased anxiety, depression, and behavioral symptoms. To address the sleep problems, they may have to resort to psychoeducation and monitor sleep habits, such as consistent sleep/wake cycle, reducing screen time, late-night caffeine use, and bright lights at bedtime, and following regular bedtime routine to prepare the body to sleep. Adolescents with insomnia need cognitive behavioral therapy (CBT) or more targeted sleep interventions such as a sleep diary to track sleep, stimulus-control intervention (bed only for sleep), sleep-restriction therapy, and relaxation techniques.

## ◼ EFFECT ON COPING SKILLS

Adolescents fail to manage typical teen stressors and illness-related stressors. The stressors are balancing school and medical management schedule, adherence to treatment, communicating with treating professionals about illness, and managing chronic pain. They should be trained to follow life skills like self-awareness, self-esteem, problem-solving, coping with stress and emotions, and setting goals in life. The CBT skills includes learning to identify the challenge, restructure distorted or unhelpful thoughts and learn to practice selfhelp strategies to bring out positive health behavior.

## Effect on Families

Normal parenting gets disturbed and becomes more evident by chronic diseases of the adolescent such as dependency on parents, extra time of the parents, financial burden, and parental feelings of guilt, frustration, anxiety, or sometimes depression. The grandparents and other family members should be involved in discussions regarding management plans and sharing responsibilities and finances so that each member will feel connected to the adolescent with chronic disease.

## Effect on Siblings

The siblings usually feel left out and ignored, which makes them jealous and develop hatred toward the child. The siblings are worried that they may suffer from the same disease and compare their lives to other children in fear. They also have a fear of losing a diseased child. If the siblings are involved actively in the care of a diseased adolescent and are given responsibility, they develop empathy and connectedness, and their problems like feeling left out are taken care of.

## Effect on Substance Abuse and Sexuality

A study on substance misuse and sexual function in adolescents with chronic disease was carried out using a modified questionnaire evaluation. A study on substance misuse and sexual function in adolescents with chronic disease was carried out by screening tool such as "CRAFT" screening tool for substance abuse/dependence on high-risk behavior. It has been noted that the frequencies of alcohol/tobacco and illicit drugs abuse were similar in both groups, that is, chronically diseased adolescent (CD) and healthy adolescent (30% vs. 34%), and likewise the frequencies of bullying (42% vs. 41%). The study comparing CD using alcohol, smoking, and illicit drugs and CD who are not using these found that the median current age is (15 vs. 14 years). A trend of low frequency of drug therapy was observed in patients who use substances (70% vs. 82%). A positive correlation was observed between CRAFT score and current age in CD. CD using substance was more likely to have sexual intercourse, thus posing a greater risk for unwanted pregnancy, sexually transmitted infections (STI), human immunodeficiency virus (HIV), vaginitis, and other health-related risky sexual behaviors. The study showed that female CD reflected a higher rate of use of drugs and sexual activity.

## Effect of Screen Time/Social Media

Judicious use of screen time for healthy media use and to follow digital rules and digital hygiene positively for the purpose of information, connectedness, and treatment is a boon for an adolescent with restricted activity. These adolescents can interact with the children with the same disease, attend group counseling, and join disease-specific groups. The various disease-specific groups include thalassemia, cystic fibrosis, celiac disease, leukemia, and many more. Group counseling and child interaction sessions can be attended in hospitals. Encourage the adolescent to participate in activities, camps, and group meetings for similar children to realize that they are not alone. The adolescent can interact with an adult with the same disease as a role model, who successfully led the life and achieved their goals. Excessive/addictive use of digital media causes physical, psychosocial, and neurological adverse impacts on their illness. Use of mobile phones, duration, content, media type, and number of devices are key determinants of screen time safety.

## EFFECT OF "ADOLESCENCE" ON CHRONIC HEALTH DISEASE

The developmental changes of adolescence will reciprocally affect chronic illness and their treatment. Indulgence in risky behaviors will compromise their physical and mental health. For physiological reasons, few diseases run in an unstable course during adolescence (the hormonal changes of pubertal growth spurts decreased insulin sensitivity and make diabetes difficult to manage).

Lung functions deteriorate during adolescence in cystic fibrosis.

## APPROACH TO CARE/TREATMENT OF ADOLESCENTS WITH CHRONIC HEALTH DISEASE

The approach to care/treatment of adolescents with chronic health diseases is as follows:

- *Age limit and office practice:* Pediatrician should be well versed with knowledge about when and where to transfer the adolescent for further care. The age and development should be taken into consideration. The decision to transfer should be made after involving family and adolescent on a one-to-one basis. A summary of medical history, therapies, medications, surgery, and vaccination in writing should be provided for a successful transition, as this is the key to care coordination.
- *Networking:* During transfer for care, the clinician should be aware about the groups and organizations that provide physical and emotional support to the patients and their families. The information includes supporting family through lay groups, home healthcare providers, social service agencies, and educators.
- *Education:* Educate the adolescents to avoid the situations that exacerbate their disease and take measures to minimize the exacerbation. Adolescents should be trained in self-care skills to minimize the effects of the disease.
- *Training regarding solving disparity between developmental needs and healthcare needs:* The different ways to resolve the conflicts between needs and development process are as follows:
  - Ensure the participation of adolescents in decision-making process related to the disease.
  - Find opportunities to train the adolescent in self-care skills.
  - Always give them advice regarding coping skills to solve the upcoming problems in regard to the disease.
  - Inform them of the concerns arising out of their illness.
  - The information about side effects and treatment alternatives should be given.
  - Ensure that adolescents should be consulted in decision-making about the disease.

## CHALLENGES IN EXISTING ADOLESCENT HEALTH SERVICES

In India, many programs are available like adolescent-friendly health services (AFHS) through adolescent clinics addressing all health needs. But the main target point is to give services on reproductive and sexual health while other issues are not focused. In 2014, Rastriya Kishor Swasthya Karyakram (RKSK) was launched under the Ministry of Health and Family Welfare (MoHFW), but similar services are already run by other ministries also. Adolescents with chronic medical disease will benefit from acceptance-based therapeutic approach. It teaches them a strategy to learn to accept and cope with worries, fears, and uncertainty regarding illness. Acceptance and commitment therapy are most useful for the adolescents with chronic health disease.

## KEY MESSAGES

- Adolescents constitute the largest workforce in India and their well-being should be assured to achieve the developmental goals of the country.
- Due to advances in treatment, there is a steady rise in the number of adolescents suffering from chronic illnesses.
- These chronic ailments significantly impact their physical, psychological, and behavioral health issues.
- Adherence to the treatment protocols is the major cause of concern for parents as well as healthcare providers.
- The transfer to the adult physician should carry a summary of medical histories, therapies, medications surgery, and vaccination in writing, which will be helpful for a successful transition, and this is the key to care coordination.
- During transfer for care, the clinician should be aware of the groups and organizations that provide physical and emotional support to the patient and their families.
- The approach to care and treatment of adolescents with chronic illnesses depends on various factors like age of the adolescent, awareness of the adolescent, and involvement of the family members in treating them.
- Along with managing their chronic illnesses, these children should be equipped with various life skills like self-awareness, self-esteem, coping with stress and emotions, problem-solving, and decision-making.
- Child Illness and Resilience Program (CHIRP) aims to increase coping and function in four areas including physical functioning (exercise, activity, sleep, and nutrition), school functioning (attendance and academic performance), social functioning (peer relationship, interpersonal relationship, and family communication), and coping skills (coping, stress management, and lifestyle management).
- The goals of treatment are to reduce barriers to managing illnesses, facilitate coping with illnesses, and improve functioning and not to teach adolescents to manage chronic medical conditions perfectly.

## RECOMMENDED READING


1. Araújo P, Carvalho MG, van Weelden M, Lourenço B, Queiroz LB, Silva CA. Substance misuse and sexual function in adolescents with chronic diseases. Rev Paul Pediatr. 2016;34(3):323-9.
2. Bhave SY, Greydanus DE, Pemde HK, Shivananda, Prajapati NC, Rao MIS. Chronic illness and disability-special problems. In: Bhave SY, Nair MKC, Parthasarathy A, Menon PSN, Greydanus DE (Eds). Bhave's Textbook of Adolescent Medicine. New Delhi: Jaypee Brothers Medical Publishers (P) Ltd; 2006. pp. 734-48. (Chapter 22)
3. Indian Academy of Pediatrics (IAP). (2023). Guidelines for parents. Chronic disease in children. [online] Available from https://iapindia.org/pdf/Ch-100-Care-of-chronic-illness-IAP-Parental-Guideline.pdf [Last accessed March, 2024].
4. Russo K. Assessment and treatment of adolescents with chronic medical conditions. J Health Serv Psychol. 2022;48(2):69-78.
5. Sivagurunathan C, Umadevi R, Rama R, Gopalakrishnan S. Adolescent health: Present status and its related programmes in India. Are we in the right direction? J Clin Diagn Res. 2015;9(3):LE01-6.
6. Stenberg U, Haaland-Øverby M, Koricho AT, Trollvik A, Kristoffersen LR, Dybvig S, et al. How can we support children, adolescents and young adults in managing chronic health challenges? A scoping review on the effects of patient education interventions. Health Expect. 2019;22(5):849-62.
7. Suris JC, Parera N. Sex, drugs and chronic illness: health behaviours among chronically ill youth. Eur J Public Health. 2005;15(5):484-8.
8. UNICEF. (2022). How to support adolescents with chronic conditions in their transition to adult healthcare? [online] Available from https://www.unicef.org/kazakhstan/en/press-releases/how-support-adolescents-chronic-conditions-their-transition-adult-healthcare [Last accessed March, 2024].
9. Yeo M, Sawyer S. Chronic illness and disability. BMJ. 2005;330(7493):721-3.

# 4E.2 — Overview of Malignancies and Hematological Disorders

*Intezar Mehdi, Suma TL*

## INTRODUCTION

Adolescents and young adults (AYAs) belong to a special category of population, 15–39 years of age, in hemato-oncological settings across the globe. The cancer outcomes in this particular age group differ from the younger children and older population, thus making them a challenging category with respect to holistic and age-appropriate care. They have very distinctive psychosocial needs that necessitate their personal involvement in their own cancer care. Leukemias, lymphomas, bone sarcomas, gonadal germ cell tumors (GCTs), brain tumors, and thyroid cancers are some of the common cancers affecting the AYA. They exhibit different pharmacological toxicity profiles, and hence, both gonadal and nongonadal toxicities are of particular concern. Anticipatory vomiting is more common in adolescents. The need for fertility preservation prior to the administration of chemotherapy drugs and radiation is important in the AYA. The risks of mortality and morbidity confound the survival rates, and hence modifications in treatment protocols and improved supportive care take a pivotal role. AYAs present with concerns of autonomy, emotional and economic independence, employment, and disruption of education.

## ACUTE LYMPHOBLASTIC LEUKEMIA

Acute lymphoblastic leukemia (ALL) is the most common type of leukemia in children and adolescents and comprises about 80% of all leukemias and about one third of all childhood cancers. ALL is a heterogeneous disease affecting a wide range of population, and hence behave differently at a biological level. Survival outcomes have improved for the 10–24-year age group significantly over the last 2 decades; even then, these statistics are not as great as one would notice in the 1–10-year age group who have an overall survival of >90%. The most common symptoms are fever, lymphadenopathy, fatigue, and pallor owing to anemia, petechiae, and bleeding. Most symptoms are due to thrombocytopenia and anemia. Painless enlargement of the testes in boys, bone pain, and limp due to excess stress on the bone marrow, and in uncommon cases neurological symptoms due to central nervous system (CNS) involvement may also be seen. National Cancer Institute (NCI) criteria take ages <1 year and >10 years as the unfavorable age group along with white blood cell (WBC) counts >50,000/cu.mm at the time of diagnosis as a high-risk feature. Hypoploidy, *MLL* rearrangements and fusions, $t(17; 19)$, iAMP21, and the Philadelphia chromosome BCR/ABL1 are some of the poor prognostic cytogenetics found in precursor B-cell ALL. In the T-cell immunophenotype, *HOX11L2* generally confers a poor outcome, and *HOX11* and *MLL-ENL* are associated with a favorable outcome. AYAs have a higher incidence of BCR/ABL1 translocations and T-cell immunophenotype. After risk stratification, these children receive protocol-based, combination chemotherapy treatment largely based on a Berlin–Frankfurt–Münster (BFM) backbone pioneered in the 1980s. The first course is called induction that lasts for 28 days and consists of 4 drugs: Dexamethasone/prednisolone, vincristine, anthracyclines (daunomycin), and L-asparaginase (or pegylated asparaginase). Intrathecal therapy is administered with methotrexate for the management of cerebrospinal fluid (CSF) sanctuary sites and the marrow is evaluated at the end of induction for morphological and minimal residual disease (MRD) remission. The poor prognostic genotypes are treated with allogeneic hematopoietic stem cell transplantation (HSCT) at the first clinical remission whereas majority of the others receive chemotherapy alone. Induction is followed by consolidation, interim maintenance with high-dose methotrexate or escalating doses of methotrexate, delayed intensification, and ends with maintenance chemotherapy consisting of oral 6 mercaptopurine (MP) and methotrexate. The entire treatment lasts 2–3 years depending on the protocol. Most standard protocols have now moved away from prophylactic craniospinal irradiation. 5-year survival rates for adolescents aged 15–19 years increased from 36% (1975–1984) to 78% (2011–2017), and with continued understanding and collaborative efforts, will continue to improve in the future.

## ACUTE MYELOGENOUS LEUKEMIA

Acute myelogenous leukemia (AML) represents 15–20% of leukemias in children and approximately 33% in AYAs. AML is sometimes a second malignant neoplasm (SMN) in AYA, especially in those who have received intensive chemotherapy and radiotherapy in the past. The prognosis worsens with advancing age. Children with AML are sicker than those with ALL. The overall survival rates in AYA are between 50 and 60%. The incidence is 0.6% in children with ALL/solid tumors. M3 AML/acute promyelocytic leukemia (APML) accounts for 25–30% of AMLs seen in AYA. The frequency of unfavorable cytogenetics increases with age, karyotypes like [–7/del (7), –5/del (5q) or 5p, inv (3)/t (3; 3), t (6; 9), and complex karyotypes, 12p, 17p, and 11q23/MLL aberrations. The treatment involves intensive induction courses of cytarabine and anthracyclines at dosages adequate to achieve morphological and molecular remission, followed by either high-dose cytarabine or HSCT depending on the risk stratification, cytogenetics, and availability of a human leukocyte antigen (HLA) matched donor. The overall survival (43%) and treatment-related mortality rate for AYA has historically been inferior to that for children and superior to that for older adults. APML is now treated according to risk stratification with all-trans retinoic acid (ATRA) and arsenic trioxide (ATO) reducing the usage of anthracyclines and thus decreasing treatment-related complications.

## LYMPHOMAS

Childhood lymphoma [including Hodgkin lymphoma (HL) and non-Hodgkin lymphoma (NHL)] is the third most common childhood malignancy. Approximately 7–8% childhood cancers are NHL. The incidence of both is higher in the second decade of life. Epstein–Barr virus (EBV) infections, human immunodeficiency virus (HIV), immune deficiency disorders, and deoxyribonucleic acid (DNA) repair syndromes are associated with lymphomas, especially Burkitt lymphomas (BL) and HL. Excision lymph node biopsy and not fine needle aspiration cytology (FNAC) is the preferred diagnostic and confirmatory test for lymphoma. Histopathology coupled with immunohistochemistry (IHC) can help clinch the diagnosis. Rarely, cytogenetics and molecular studies may be required on tissue histopathology examination (HPE) for diagnosis and risk stratification or prognostication of NHL. Staging evaluation includes positron emission tomography-computed tomography (PET-CT) scan, bone marrow biopsy, and CSF study (NHL).

Hodgkin lymphoma is curable in >90% children. It is characterized by painless lymphadenopathy of waxing and waning nature in the neck, axilla, or inguinal area. It can be associated with fever of 38°C or higher, drenching night sweats, and weight loss of 10% or more of baseline weight in the previous 6 months (B symptoms).

Hodgkin lymphoma is further classified into:
- Classical HL (mixed cellularity, lymphocyte predominant, lymphocyte depleted, and nodular sclerosis)
- Nodular lymphocyte predominant HL (NLPHL).

Early favorable risk HL after staging workup is treated with anthracyclines or alkylator-based combination chemotherapy like ABVD, BEACOPP, OEPA/COPDAC. Most protocols are standardized and have excellent results. These children do not need radiation to the involved group of lymph nodes once they achieve metabolic remission on PET. Advanced HL can also be cured by combination chemotherapy regimens and treatment is decided by interim PET response. If there is residual disease in the lymph node regions, they are treated with targeted radiation therapy with advanced techniques like intensity-modulated radiation therapy (IMRT). Relapsed/refractory HL can be treated with high-dose chemotherapy followed by autologous stem cell rescue. Targeted therapies like brentuximab (anti-CD30) and rituximab (anti-CD20) are now being used in the upfront treatment of HL.

Non-Hodgkin lymphoma in childhood and adolescence is predominantly of following types:
1. *Lymphoblastic lymphoma:* T- and B-cell type
2. Mature B-cell lymphoma [diffuse large B-cell lymphoma (DLBCL), BL, and primary mediastinal B cell]
3. Anaplastic large cell lymphoma

More than 80% children survive NHL when treated well according to their stage, risk stratification, and involvement of marrow and CSF sanctuary at diagnosis.

Lymphoblastic lymphoma T-cell type can present with anterior mediastinal mass causing airway compression and superior mediastinal syndrome, presenting as a medical emergency. Coexisting pleural and pericardial effusions can complicate the situation further. Pleural fluid analysis and flow cytometry done on pleural samples can confirm the diagnosis. Children with superior vena cava (SVC) syndrome should not be sedated for any procedure.

Lymphoblastic lymphomas are treated with leukemia-based protocols.

Burkitt lymphoma and DLBCL are very aggressive malignancies and are treated with short and highly intensive chemotherapy regimens. The first course is a cytoreductive chemotherapy regimen followed by four to six courses of pulse high-dose chemotherapy.

Tumor lysis syndrome, either laboratory/clinical or both in the form of hyperuricemia, hyperkalemia, hyperphosphatemia, and hypocalcemia, is often present at diagnosis or after initiation of treatment.

This is managed with aggressive hydration, allopurinol (xanthine oxidase inhibitor—to prevent renal damage), and management of dyselectrolytemia. Since BL and DLBCL are CD20 positive, rituximab can be used for effective clearance of the disease. Relapsed/refractory DLBCL and BL can be treated with high-dose chemotherapy followed by autologous stem cell rescue, chimeric antigen receptor (CAR) T-cell therapy, and allogeneic HSCT. Anaplastic large-cell lymphoma (ALCL) is rare and managed with cytoreductive prophase followed by four to six courses of intense chemotherapy. Brentuximab, *ALK* inhibitors like crizotinib, and HSCT are used in relapse and refractory settings.

## ■ SARCOMAS

Osteosarcoma (OS) is the most common malignant bone tumor in children with incidence peaking in the second decade of life, followed by Ewing sarcoma. Bone tumors tend to present with pain and swelling with or without the restriction of joint movements. Osteosarcoma involves long bones more commonly, whereas Ewing sarcoma affects flat bones. More often than not, trivial sports injuries or incidents of trauma bring them to clinical attention. Night pain and systemic symptoms like fever and weight loss may follow in a few cases. Paraosteal OS, central low-grade OS, and periosteal OS are morphologically and clinically distinct OS subtypes with better prognosis.

The staging evaluation involves magnetic resonance imaging (MRI) of the involved bone covering distal and proximal joints followed by PET-CT scan to look for metastasis. The confirmatory test is a core needle biopsy done preferably by the orthopedic team that would eventually plan the definitive surgery following the rules of surgical planes and excise the biopsy tract in toto with the tumor. Histopathology alone can suffice in the case of osteosarcoma, recognized by the presence of neoplastic cells interspersed around the osteoid matrix.

Osteosarcoma is treated according to three-drug protocol—Methotrexate, cisplatin, and doxorubicin (EURAMOS-1 trial). Alternative chemotherapy regimens comprising ifosfamide, cisplatin, and doxorubicin are also used in some centers. Most patients need preoperative chemotherapy followed by limb-salvage surgery for tumor necrosis evaluation and then postoperative chemotherapy. Nonmetastatic OS has a survival rate of 70%, whereas metastatic cases do poorly. Rotationplasty and vascularized allografts are a few other surgical techniques employed.

Vincristine, doxorubicin, and cyclophosphamide (VDC) alternating with ifosfamide and etoposide (IE) on an every 2-week schedule has become the standard of care for patients with Ewing's sarcoma.

Ewing sarcoma shows small blue round cells with clear to lightly eosinophilic cytoplasm, evenly dispersed chromatin, indistinct nucleoli, and sometimes pseudo-rosettes. Immunohistochemistry strongly expresses CD99 and shows *FLI1* expression in >80% of the cases.

Unlike OS, Ewing sarcoma can be treated with surgery and radiation for local control. Metastatic Ewing sarcoma, especially extrapulmonary metastasis, has a dismal prognosis. There are some reports that say high-dose chemotherapy with busulfan and melphalan followed by autologous stem cell rescue may benefit some patients.

## ■ GERM CELL TUMORS

Germ cell tumors are rare in childhood and adolescence accounting for <4% of all childhood cancers. The incidence is higher among 15–19-years-old and AYAs fare worse than younger children.

In male prepubertal children, teratomas comprise a majority of observed tumors, accounting for up to 40% of testicular tumors. The most common malignant histology is yolk sac tumor. In AYAs, majority are mixed nonseminomas, with tumors consisting of more than one malignant histology and a higher proportion of embryonal carcinoma and choriocarcinoma. Serum tumor markers alpha-fetoprotein (AFP), human chorionic gonadotropin (HCG), and lactate dehydrogenase (LDH) play important diagnostic roles, and their higher levels correlate with an increased burden of disease and they are used for risk assignment as well as for treatment-response assessment.

In girls, immature teratomas and dysgerminomas account for approximately 80% of tumors. Mixed GCTs are the most common nongerminomatous GCT in this age group.

Children's Oncology Group (COG) staging system is most followed for risk stratification. Cisplatin/carboplatin with etoposide and bleomycin (JEB/PEB) chemotherapy regimens are the standard of care. Adolescent patients had the lowest 3-year event-free survival (EFS) at 60% compared to younger children with EFS of 87%.

Aplastic anemia and thalassemia (beta thalassemia major) are the two common hematological problems that deserve to be discussed in this chapter.

## ■ APLASTIC ANEMIA

Aplastic anemia (AA) is characterized by pancytopenia with a hypocellular bone marrow in the absence of abnormal infiltration by leukemia/lymphoma cells/or any malignant cells.

AA can be inherited or acquired; some of the congenital disorders presenting with AA are inherited bone marrow failure syndromes (IBMFS) like Fanconi anemia, dyskeratosis congenita, Shwachman–Diamond syndrome, and Diamond Blackfan anemia.

The disease presents with symptoms like fatigue, pallor, infections due to neutropenia, and easy bruisability secondary to thrombocytopenia. Secondary aplastic anemia (SAA) or acquired AA can be triggered with viral infections like EBV, HIV, parvovirus, cytomegalovirus (CMV), human herpesvirus (HHV6), and hepatitis virus. The etiology in SAA is an autoimmune attack directed at hematopoietic progenitor cells by cytotoxic T cells that target hematopoietic stem cells leading to apoptosis and hematopoietic failure. Detailed history with attention to vaccination, intake of any alternative medications, need for transfusions and clinical examination looking for height, limb abnormalities, and neurocutaneous markers are important. Bone marrow aspiration and trephine biopsy looking for cellularity in the marrow help ascertain the degree of hypocellularity. A close differential diagnosis for SAA is pediatric myelodysplastic syndrome (MDS), which needs a patient and observant hematopathologist eye for diagnosis.

Severe AA has <25% cellularity with absolute neutrophil count <200. Peripheral blood stress cytogenetics, flow cytometry for paroxysmal nocturnal hemoglobinuria (PNH) clone (when indicated), and IBMFS clinical exome sequence studies are necessary for ruling out associated problems. Patients who have an HLA-matched sibling unaffected donor can proceed to allogeneic HSCT directly; the procedure is preferably done before 20 transfusions

to prevent alloimmunization in the recipient. The overall cure rate with early matched sibling/family donor HSCT would be around 80%. Immunosuppressive therapy (IST) with antithymocyte globulin (ATG) and cyclosporin A is quite effective in patients without a matched sibling donor; the response rate to this treatment is about 70%. Relapse is common after discontinuation of therapy, and clonal evolution to hematological malignancies like MDS/AML is a reality.

## ■ THALASSEMIAS

Thalassemia is an inherited benign hematological disorder caused by the absence or dysfunction of globin genes resulting in ineffective erythropoiesis and hemolytic anemias. It is broadly classified into alpha thalassemia and beta thalassemia. Beta thalassemia is further classified into thalassemia major, thalassemia intermedia, and thalassemia minor. The prevalence of thalassemia is more in tropical and subtropical regions.

The clinical spectrum of the disease varies from nontransfusion-dependent thalassemia to transfusion-dependent anemia warranting chronic transfusions and iron chelating to curb iron overload. Without treatment, the disease would be lethal causing morbidity and premature mortality. The traditional curative approach in beta-thalassemia major is an allogeneic HSCT with a matched sibling donor. When this is not feasible, other options for HSCT can be HSCT from a matched related donor, matched unrelated donor, or haploidentical donor with either parent as a donor. However, the risks and complications are worse with alternate donor HSCT. Results of HSCT are best if HSCT is done at an early age, preferably before 7 years of age and before iron overload-related complications develop. Adolescents who have not had HSCT as a curative option will develop iron-overload complications related to the heart and liver responsible for morbidity and mortality. Other most important notable complications in this age group are those related to endocrine problems. Delayed puberty, hormonal dysfunction involving thyroid hormones and sex hormones, and diabetes mellitus are some of the complications in this age group. Bone mineral density issues and bone-related problems are the other major issues. Psychosocial problems and school and college performances are other challenges in the AYA group.

Currently, novel therapeutic strategies are developing to cure thalassemia of which gene therapy is showing promising results. By correcting ineffective erythropoiesis, it obviates the need for regular transfusions. It is especially beneficial for children who do not have a matched donor. However, the current standard of care remains both regular transfusion and chelation. The only curative option at present is allogeneic hematopoietic transplantation depending on the availability of the donor.

## ■ KEY MESSAGES

- AYAs have very distinctive psychosocial needs that necessitate their personal involvement in their own cancer care.
- Leukemias, lymphomas, bone sarcomas, gonadal GCTs, brain tumors, and thyroid cancers are some of the common cancers affecting the AYA.
- AYAs exhibit different pharmacological toxicity profiles, and hence both gonadal and nongonadal toxicities are of particular concern. The need for fertility preservation prior to the administration of chemotherapy drugs and radiation is important in the AYA.
- The risks of mortality and morbidity confound the survival rates, and hence modifications in treatment protocols and improved supportive care take a pivotal role.
- AYAs present with concerns of autonomy, emotional and economic independence, employment, and disruption of education.
- Survival rates in adolescents with ALL are inferior compared to children; however, with a better understanding of the pathophysiology and coordinated team approach, survival rates have improved.
- Incidence of adverse cytogenetics and molecular features is more common in adolescents with AML and their survival is also inferior.
- Children with lymphoblastic lymphoma, especially T cell, present with SVC syndrome, which is an oncological emergency. Children with SVC syndrome should not be sedated for any procedure.
- The most common age group for bone sarcomas like osteogenic and Ewing sarcoma is around adolescence.
- Thalassemia and aplastic anemias are two important hematological issues that are very challenging to handle in AYAs.

## ■ RECOMMENDED READING


1. Bielack SS, Carrle D, Hardes J, Schuck A, Paulussen M. Bone tumors in adolescents and young adults. Curr Treat Options Oncol. 2008;9(1):67-80.
2. Bigenwald C, Galimard JE, Quero L, Cabannes-Hamy A, Thieblemont C, Boissel N, et al. Hodgkin lymphoma in adolescent and young adults: insights from an adult tertiary single-centre cohort of 349 patients. Oncotarget. 2017;8(45):80073-82.
3. Boissel N, Baruchel A. Acute lymphoblastic leukemia in adolescent and young adults: treat as adults or as children? Blood. 2018;132 (4):351-61.
4. Creutzig U, Kutny MA, Barr R, Schlenk RF, Ribeiro RC. Acute myelogenous leukemia in adolescents and young adults. Pediatr Blood Cancer. 2018;65(9):e27089.
5. DeZern AE, Guinan EC. Aplastic Anemia in Adolescents and Young Adults. Acta Haematol. 2014;132(3-4): 331-9.
6. Fonseca A, Frazier AL, Shaikh F. Germ Cell Tumors in Adolescents and Young Adults. J Oncol Pract. 2019;15(8): 433-41.
7. Karponi G, Zogas N. Gene therapy for beta-thalassemia: Updated perspectives. Appl Clin Genet. 2019;12:167-80.
8. Minard-Colin V, Brugières L, Reiter A, Cairo MS, Gross TG, Woessmann W, et al. Non-Hodgkin lymphoma in children and adolescents: progress through effective collaboration, current knowledge, and challenges ahead. J Clin Oncol. 2015;33(27):2963-74.
9. Sanchez-Villalobos M, Blanquer M, Moraleda JM, Salido EJ, Perez-Oliva AB. New insights into pathophysiology of β-thalassemia. Front Med (Lausanne). 2022;9:880752.
10. Stock W. Adolescents and young adults with acute lymphoblastic leukemia. Hematology Am Soc Hematol Educ Program. 2010;2010(1):21-9.

# 4E.3 Health Issues in the Tribal Adolescents: A Cause for Concern and a Call for Action

*Shubhada Khirwadkar*

## ■ UNDERSTANDING THE TRIBAL LANDSCAPE

India, a land of rich cultural diversity, is home to numerous tribal communities that have distinct languages, traditions, and lifestyles. Of the 243 million Indian adolescents (the largest in the world in terms of absolute numbers), 2 million (9%) belong to Scheduled Tribes (STs) and live in underserved, rural/tribal areas. Though adolescents from different regions share common developmental experiences, tribal adolescents represent a significant demographic group facing unique health challenges.

Tribal communities in India often reside in remote, difficult-to-access, hilly, forest regions with limited access to healthcare facilities. Tribal adolescents live in a community which has its own culture and tradition, steeped in deep-rooted myths about medical conditions which are usually treated by traditional faith healers. The remoteness, inadequate transport facilities, meagre economic opportunities, and fear about unfamiliar modern medical techniques lead to their low health-seeking behavior which in turn impacts their overall health and well-being. They rarely utilize the existing health care facilities to their full potential. Tribal-specific cultural, environmental, geographic, and socioeconomic factors present formidable challenges in proposing solutions for adolescent health. Hence, policy changes need to be effectively planned and executed by policy makers and health professionals.

## ■ KEY HEALTH ISSUES

It is important to understand that the health issues in tribal adolescents need to be looked at with a tribal-specific sociodemographic perspective, to comprehensively tackle them.

The diseases prevalent in adolescents living in tribal areas can be broadly classified into categories as shown in **Table 1**.

### Malnutrition

Malnutrition remains a pervasive issue among tribal adolescents due to inadequate dietary diversity and limited access to nutritious food. Undernutrition leads to thinness

**TABLE 1:** Diseases prevalent in adolescents living in tribal areas.

| | |
|---|---|
| Malnutrition | Low birth weight, lower body size, stunting, iron, vitamin A, D, B complex deficiency |
| Reproductive and sexual health | Early marriage, teenage pregnancy, high IMR, MMR, U5MR, ASMR |
| Infections | Respiratory infections, tuberculosis, diarrhea, malaria, filaria, typhoid, hepatitis, skin infections, STD, HIV |
| Accidents and injuries | Burns, falls, wild animal bites, snake bites, RTI, violence due to conflicts, suicides |
| Substance abuse | Alcohol, tobacco in various forms, drugs in northeast |
| Hereditary diseases | Sickle cell disease, G6PD deficiency |
| Speciality problems | Orthopedic, surgical, ophthalmic, ENT, gynecological, orodental |
| Noncommunicable diseases | Hypertension, cardiac issues, diabetes, stroke, cancer |
| Mental health problems | Depression, anxiety, addictions, agrarian suicides (more in conflict-ridden, Naxalite areas) |

(ENT: ear nose throat; G6PD: glucose-6-phosphate dehydrogenase; HIV: human immunodeficiency virus; IMR: infant mortality rate; MMR: maternal mortality rate; RTI: road traffic injury; STD: sexually transmitted disease; U5MR: under-5 mortality rate)

(weight for age) and stunting (height for age), slowing of growth and sexual maturity, and compromised immune systems. Anthropometric studies reveal that the median body mass index (BMI) by age/sex, though comparable with their rural counterparts, is below the median National Health and Nutrition Examination Survey (NHANES) reference values. About 63% of tribal adolescent boys and 42% of girls are undernourished (<5th BMI age percentiles of NHANES). The overall prevalence of stunting (height for age < median −2 SD) is 42% among boys and 46% among girls, which is higher than that reported for their rural counterparts (39% each for boys and girls).

Adolescence is the last chance to rectify growth lag that may have occurred during early childhood. Multiple nutrition surveys in different tribal regions of the country indicate that the average intake of all the nutrients (especially the income elastic foods such as pulses, milk and milk products, oils and fats, and sugar and jaggery) by adolescent boys and girls of the tribes is below the recommended dietary allowances (RDA) in all the age groups. The deficit in the intake of energy is higher among boys than girls in older adolescents (13–17 years) compared to younger adolescents (10–12 years).

Inadequate nutrition in adolescence leads to anemia, which is among the top 15 causes of global morbidity and mortality. In some tribal regions, iron deficiency among tribal adolescent girls is as high as 60%. The prevalence of anemia (higher in households with poorest wealth quintiles) decreases with a higher level of mother's schooling. Ironically, the targets for weekly iron and folic acid supplements (WIFS) for girls under Rashtriya Kishor Swasthya Karyakram (RKSK) are higher for girls who are in school than those out of school. Studies have established that there is a direct link between anemia, diet pattern and food intake, land holding, type of employment, poverty, illiteracy, and village-level facilities. Hence, increasing girls' access to education is important to reduce anemia as they would then be able to receive benefits of both RKSK and Mid-Day Meal programs **(Fig. 1)**.

## Reproductive and Sexual Health

The World Health Organization (WHO) has identified that 15–19-year age-group girls are highly vulnerable for unsafe sex, abortion, and pregnancy-related complications.

Young tribal girls often enter the reproductive age facing greater health risks of early marriage, frequent pregnancies, unsafe deliveries, and sexually transmitted diseases, which pose risks to both the mother and the child's health. With their low social status, they seek treatment only when the ailment is well advanced. Moreover, pregnancy is not considered a condition that requires medical treatment, nourishment, or care, hindering efforts to deliver antenatal services.

When undernourished girls enter adolescent growth spurt with simultaneous pregnancy, there is competition in the body itself for resources, which severely impacts their health negatively.

Adolescent mothers tend to be shorter, underweight, and anemic. The children born to them are shorter for their age, have lower birth weights for height, and are at a higher risk of death and disease throughout infancy than children born to adult mothers. They also have cognitive impairment, developmental problems, and a greater susceptibility to illness which damages their ability to work during adulthood.

Unprotected sexual exploration in adolescence with multiple partners being a culturally accepted norm in many tribal communities causes sexually transmitted diseases which often go undetected and untreated. Accessible reproductive health services are frequently unavailable to both tribal boys and girls. Reproductive health of adolescent girls is more pathetic with their shy nature and precise social barriers in accessing the services.

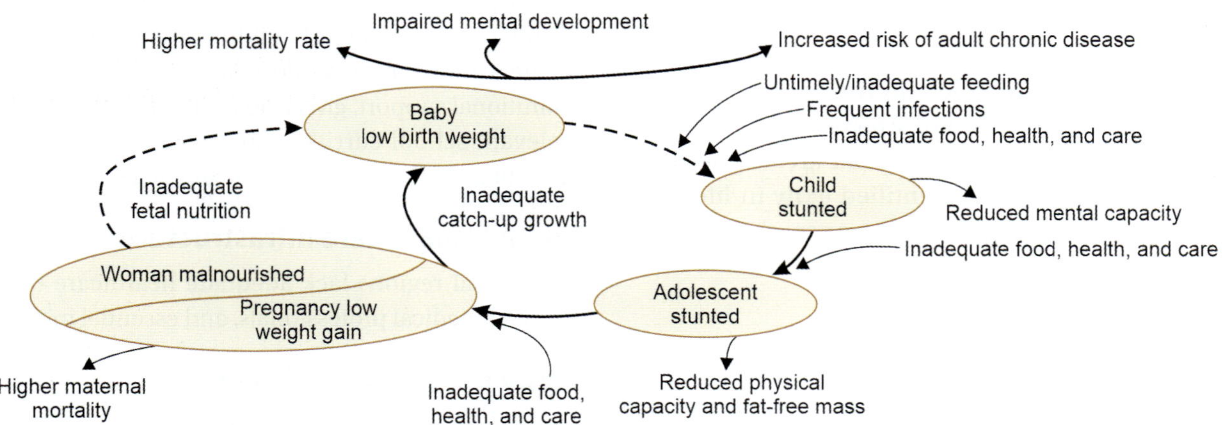


**Fig. 1:** Poor nutrition throughout the life cycle of an adolescent.
*Source:* Adapted from the ACC/SCN-appointed Commission on the Nutrition Challenges of the 21st Century. [online] Available from https://www.ncbi.nlm.nih.gov/pmc/articles/PMC7113978/ [Last accessed March, 2024].

## Infections

The 8.6% tribal population constitutes 30% of all cases of malaria (>60% *Plasmodium falciparum*) and as much as 50% of the mortality associated with malaria. The estimated prevalence of tuberculosis (TB) (per 100,000) is 703 cases against 256 in the nontribal population. Also, only 11% pulmonary TB get treated based on smear-positive reporting. Unsafe drinking water combined with unhygienic sanitary practices still make diarrheal diseases, hepatitis, and typhoid a major cause of morbidity and mortality in poor tribal adolescents.

## Substance Abuse

More than 72% tribal men (15–54 years) use tobacco and more than 50% consume alcohol against 56% and 30% nontribal men, respectively. Smoking in tribal adolescents is attributed to easy availability of *tendupatta* leaves and household stock of tobacco by the parents. Almost an equal proportion of boys and girls indulge in smokeless tobacco (*masheri/gul manjan*) consumption for cleaning their teeth every morning. Alcohol consumption starts early in tribal adolescents who routinely collect *Mahua* tree flowers for the preparation of country-made liquor, widely distilled at homes. Marijuana (*Ganja*) is also collectively consumed during religious festivals.

## Noncommunicable Diseases

It is a myth that tribal people are not as affected by noncommunicable diseases (NCDs) as the nontribal people. Several recent studies have demonstrated that NCD-related deaths are as high as 66–73% of all deaths across various tribal areas. Cardiovascular diseases, cancers, diabetes, and chronic respiratory diseases are attributed to high burden of risk factors such as poor dietary habits (high salt, nutrition deficient diet), tobacco and alcohol use, and stresses of a low level of subsistence and a hard life in tribal areas. These risk factors can be reduced if identified early in life when habits are still forming in adolescence, thus offering better health, more years of productivity, and a lesser cost of health care.

## Genetic Disorders

The incidence for sickle cell anemia has been estimated at >19% among 35 tribal population groups. 5 million are estimated to be carriers. The rural tribal population estimated to have glucose-6-phosphate-dehydrogenase (G6PD) deficiency is about 13 million, primarily residing in states of Madhya Pradesh, Maharashtra, Tamil Nadu, Odisha, and Assam (15%). The incidence is high in malaria zones. Screening kits are needed by health workers, to identify people and counsel high-risk families.

*Mental Health:* The lack of mental health support and the stressors associated with their environment can lead to mental health issues like depression and anxiety. There has been a recent upsurge in suicide in tribal adolescents.

## FACTORS CONTRIBUTING TO POOR TRIBAL ADOLESCENT HEALTH

### Socioeconomic Disparities

Poverty, limited access to clean drinking water, and sanitation contribute to the poor health of tribal adolescents.

### Cultural Practices

Traditional beliefs and practices, such as early marriage and home remedies, can hinder access to modern healthcare.

### Gender Disparities

Gender inequality within tribal communities can result in differential access to resources, education, and healthcare. However, in most tribal communities, gender discrimination causing female feticide, rape, and domestic abuse is almost absent.

### Lack of Awareness and Education

Limited health awareness and literacy among tribal adolescents and their families hinder preventive healthcare practices. As per Census 2011, the literacy rate of STs was 59% whereas the overall literacy rate was 73% at all-India level. Tribal girl children are enrolled in school but are withdrawn early due to lack of parental awareness, institutional support, girls who are the eldest in the family, irrelevant school curricula, and teaching in a language different from the child's spoken language.

### Limited Healthcare Infrastructure

Many tribal regions lack adequate healthcare facilities, qualified medical professionals, and essential medicines.

## KEY RECOMMENDATIONS

### Improved Access to Healthcare

Mere establishment of more health facilities, and ensuring access to essential services and medications, cannot overcome the poor health of tribal population. Considering the dearth of qualified medical staff in remote tribal regions, offering incentives like postgraduate seats and research fellowships to medical students serving the tribal population could be a gamechanger. The inclusion of traditional healers and local tribal peer educators in the overall health setup is important. Each state should act swiftly to assess the needs, priorities, and public health strategies of their own tribal population and set achievable targets.

## Health Education Programs

Implementing community-friendly health education programs through tribal schools and *gram sabhas* can raise awareness about nutrition, hygiene, and reproductive and sexual health. Popular folk art, songs, and dance-dramas can be innovatively used in impactful behavior change communications.

## Empowering Tribal Adolescents and Youth

Providing vocational training and skill development programs can empower tribal adolescents with income-generating opportunities. Life Skills Education programs specially designed for tribal adolescents with audiovisual aids and involvement of schoolteachers will be useful to prevent addictions and STDs and promote mental health, self-awareness, autonomy, and agency.

## Gender Sensitization

The workload of tribal women and girls is heavy, long, and increasing. Equal access to quality education contributes to their ability to make informed decisions about the well-being and empowerment of tribal women and subsequent better health outcomes.

## Mental Health Support

Mental health awareness campaigns and medical services are a key to preventing and treating often undiagnosed mental illnesses which are traditionally treated by faith healers for years together. The recent higher incidence of suicidal deaths in tribal youth needs door-to-door, small groups, and school-based community engagement for its prevention.

## Government Initiatives

Supporting and expanding excellent government schemes like RKSK, aimed at tribal development, healthcare, and informal education, should incorporate youth as mentors/peer educators to make it more relevant to tribal adolescents. Nutrition-dense, cereal-based MDM, and WIFS programs should become more inclusive for out-of-school tribal adolescents and also be better monitored for their outreach.

## Support to Nongovernmental Organizations (NGOs)

Many NGOs like SEARCH, MAHAN, Action against Hunger, Pratham, and others have excellent stakeholders' engagement in community-based work for health of tribal adolescents through programs like *Tarunyabhaan and SEHAT* (Strategic Enhancement of Health among adolescents in Tribal area). The government should work with academia as well as NGOs to tap their expertise in nutrition, diets, and agriculture and seek more private sector investment and engagement in adolescent health.

## Role of Indian Academy of Pediatrics (IAP)

Socially sensitive national medical associations like the IAP and its subchapter Adolescent Health Academy are working relentlessly in collaboration with government and NGOs to promote adolescent health. They should widen their purview and plan their interventions to reach out to these unreached tribal adolescents.

## ■ CONCLUSION

Addressing the health issues of tribal adolescents in India requires collaborative efforts between government agencies, NGOs, and the communities themselves through strategic, research-based interventions is essential to ensure the well-being and brighter future of these vulnerable adolescents.

## ■ KEY MESSAGES

- Tribal communities, constituting 9% of Indian adolescents, face unique challenges in remote areas with limited healthcare access.
- Key health issues include malnutrition, reproductive and sexual health concerns, infections, accidents, substance abuse, and mental health problems.
- Malnutrition is pervasive, leading to stunting and underweight issues among tribal adolescents.
- Early marriages, frequent pregnancies, and limited access to healthcare contribute to reproductive and sexual health challenges.
- Infections like malaria and TB, substance abuse, and NCDs pose significant threats.
- Socioeconomic disparities, cultural practices, and gender inequalities contribute to poor health outcomes.

- Recommendations include improved healthcare access, education programs, empowerment through vocational training, and mental health support.
- Collaborative efforts between government, NGOs, and communities are crucial for addressing these health challenges.
- The author stresses the importance of a holistic approach to ensure the well-being of tribal adolescents in India.

## ■ RECOMMENDED READING


1. Gunjal S, Borle A, Narlawar U, Ughade S, Chaudhari V, Humne A. Tobacco and Alcohol Use in Tribal School students from Central India. Int J Collab Res Intern Med Public Health. 2012;4(11):1852-7.
2. Gupta A, Sharma D, Thakur D, Thakur A, Mazta SR. Prevalence and predictors of the dual burden of malnutrition among adolescents in North India. Saudi J Obesity. 2014;2:63-79.
3. India State-Level Disease Burden Initiative Collaborators. Nations within a nation: variations in epidemiological transition across the states of India, 1990-2016 in the Global Burden of Disease Study. Lancet. 2017;390:2437-60.
4. International Institute for Population Sciences, and Macro International. National Family Health Survey (NFHS-4), 2015-16: India. Vol. 1. Mumbai: IIPS; 2016.
5. Ministry of Tribal Affairs, Government of India. ST statistical profile at a glance. New Delhi: MoTA, GoI. [online] Available from: https://tribal.nic.in/Statistics.aspx. [Last accessed March, 2024].
6. Rizwan SA, Kumar R, Singh AK, Kusuma YS, Yadav K, Pandav CS. Prevalence of hypertension in Indian tribes: a systematic review and meta-analysis of observational studies. PLoS One. 2014;9:e95896.
7. Sivagurunathan C, Umadevi R, Rama R, Gopalakrishnan S. Adolescent health: Present status and its related programmes in India? Are we in the right direction. J Clin Diagn Res. 2015;9:LE01-6.
8. Strategy Handbook. Rashtriya Kishor Swasthya Karyakram. (2014). Adolescent Health Division Ministry of Health and Family Welfare Government of India. [online] Available from https://nhm.gov.in/images/pdf/programmes/rksk-strategy-handbook.pdf [Last accessed March, 2024].
9. UNICEF. Progress for Children: A report card on adolescents. Adolescent Mortality, Morbidity and Health-Related Behaviours. Number 10 April 2012. Figure: 4.1; p. 18. [online] Available from https://www.unicef.org/media/86401/file/Progress_for_Children_-_No._10_EN_04272012.pdf [Last accessed March, 2024].
10. World Health Organization. (2020). Adolescent health and development. [online] Available from https://www.who.int/news-room/q-a-detail/adolescent-health-and-development [Last accessed March, 2024].


# 4E.4 Street Adolescents

*Nishikant Kotwal*

## ■ INTRODUCTION

In India, there are 18 million street children, out of which 11 million (almost 60%) are in urban areas. In urban areas also, they are more concentrated in metro cities. Whenever we stop at a signal, these children come to the car either to clean the glass or to beg for money. We do not like it, but we never think of their plight or illnesses.

I am quoting from an editorial published in Indian Pediatrics about street children: A window to the reality by Dr G R Sethi "STARE NOT AT THE TATTERED CLOTHES, BENEATH THEM LIE THEIR SHATTERED DREAMS."

We always think that these children miss love, protection, and warmth of parental care, but I am sorry to say that what they miss most is food for survival. This is the reason they are pushed to "child labor".

UNICEF has quoted them as children living in difficult circumstances and the most threatened population. A street child is a child "for whom the street has become his or her habitual abode or source of livelihood and who is inadequately protected, supervised or directed by responsible adults". There are different classifications of street children:

- Those who live on the street for work but have a family dwelling
- Those who live on the street, may be with their families
- Those who live on the street without family.

## ETIOPATHOLOGY

Poverty serves as the primary catalyst, exacerbated significantly by issues related to alcohol or drug dependency. These factors contribute to fostering an adverse environment within families. As a result, conflicts and violent outbursts may arise, prompting individuals to seek an exit from their familial settings. Due to the lack of access to adequate nutrition, a conducive environment, positive reinforcement, and compounded by instances of abuse, individuals perceive leaving their homes as both an opportunity and a necessity to improve their lives. Consequently, they find themselves on the streets, devoid of resources and susceptible to exploitation. Education is often absent, leading to a disdain for discipline, while the prevailing belief in this world propagates selfishness as a means of survival and accomplishment. The absence of basic amenities compels them to undertake personal hygiene activities, such as bathing and changing clothes, in public spaces. This unsanitary setting invites numerous physical ailments and diseases.

## COMMON PROBLEMS

These children suffer from physical, mental, psychological, and behavioral problems.

- *Malnutrition:* Residing in impoverished conditions, they face the challenges of rapid physical growth, necessitating a diet rich in carbohydrates, proteins, fats, minerals, micronutrients, and vitamins. Lacking the financial means to access proper nutrition and often unaware of the required nutrients, they subsist on insufficient or leftover food, which fails to meet their body's nutritional needs. Consequently, this inadequate diet can result in low body weight, reduced muscle mass, stunted growth, and the development of anemia.
- *Anemia:* Their diet lacks essential components such as iron, B12, and folic acid. Moreover, girls might experience menstrual irregularities, compounding the risk of anemia. While the primary cause of anemia is nutritional deficiencies, there might be instances where individuals also suffer from hemoglobinopathies.
- *Tuberculosis (TB):* TB is notably prevalent among individuals with low socioeconomic status, malnourishment, close contact with infected individuals, and those living in unhygienic conditions. Insufficient access to vaccinations further compromises their immunity. Additionally, the occurrence of multidrug-resistant TB is widespread due to improper and inadequate treatment, as well as noncompliance with prescribed medical regimens.
- *Sexually transmitted diseases:* The combination of poverty, sexual abuse, and the erosion of modesty renders them particularly vulnerable. This vulnerability exposes them to a high risk of sexual exploitation and engagement in prostitution. A survey conducted in Kolkata in 2002 revealed that 6 out of 554 street children were afflicted by HIV. Among the prevalent diseases in this demographic are gonorrhea, genital warts, pelvic infections, and HIV.
- *Gastrointestinal (GI) infection:* Consuming leftovers, drinking nonpotable water, and residing in unhygienic environments significantly heighten the risk of GI infections. Among the common infections prevalent in these conditions are acute gastroenteritis, typhoid, cholera, food poisoning, and worm infestations, which often lead to severe dehydration and, in extreme cases, fatalities.
- *Vector-borne diseases:* Due to their residence in roadside areas or in close proximity to drainage systems, these children are susceptible to a range of diseases, including malaria, dengue, chikungunya, scrub typhus, kala-azar, filariasis, and even rabies.
- *Skin infection:* Due to a lack of awareness regarding hygiene practices, inadequate skin care, and the exchange of unclean clothing, these individuals are more susceptible to skin fungal infections, scabies, eczema, and bacterial wound infections.
- *Environmental diseases:* Their increased exposure to various environmental pollutants such as benzene, carbon monoxide, dyes, fumes, smoke, industrial gases, and dust pollution heightens their susceptibility to respiratory tract illnesses and disorders. This elevated risk encompasses conditions like pneumonia, asthma, interstitial lung disease, and common occurrences of pneumonia resulting from exposure to chemical or hazardous gases.
- *Substance abuse:* Several factors contribute to this concerning issue, including peer pressure, the phase of experimentation, inadequate parental control and supervision, experiences of bullying, and a lack of self-esteem. Findings from focus group discussions on substance abuse highlight that 90% of individuals

are addicted to smoking, chewing tobacco, and gutka, with *ganja* being the second most prevalent substance of addiction. According to the magnitude of substance abuse in India report from 2019, inhalants are identified as the most commonly abused substance. An article in the International Journal of Community Medicine notes that substance abuse is more prevalent in rural areas compared to urban areas, with males exhibiting a higher prevalence than females.

- *Abuse:* This situation may involve mental, physical, or psychological abuse, which can take the form of verbal, physical, or sexual mistreatment. Insight from focus group discussions on sexual behavior revealed that many children engage in risky activities during their free time, such as gambling, teasing girls, watching pornography, and engaging in unprotected sexual encounters. Furthermore, these vulnerable individuals become targets for exploitation by pedophiles.
- *Road traffic accidents:* Living on the streets makes these children highly susceptible to road traffic accidents. Some of these children operate vehicles without proper control over speed, leading to significant issues and risks in road safety.
- *Interpersonal violence and gang war:* A significant number of these children experience injuries, disabilities, and even fatalities resulting from violent altercations. Consequently, this often leads to their involvement in legal conflicts or the juvenile justice system.
- *Low self-esteem and mental health issues including suicidal tendency:* Suicide stands as a major cause of death among adolescents, often attributed to a range of factors including abuse, poverty, drug addiction, diminished self-esteem, and depression. These issues contribute significantly to the occurrence of suicide in this age group.
- *Chronic conditions:* Street children often remain undiagnosed and endure chronic conditions such as epilepsy, hypertension, endocrine disorders like thyroid or diabetes, depression, and orthopedic problems. These persistent health issues often go untreated due to their circumstances.
- *Child labor:* The data from 2021 indicates that approximately 4.35 million children between the ages of 5–14 years are engaged in work to support their families. UNICEF statistics highlight that 12% of children in this age group are involved in child labor activities.

## MANAGEMENT

The comprehensive management for street children should encompass the following key elements:

- *Medical care:* Ensure access to medical assistance for diseases and health conditions. It is crucial to improve the percentage of street children receiving medical help, aiming for higher coverage. Only 33% of street children receive medical help.
- *Psychological counseling:* Provide mental health support and counseling to address the psychological challenges and traumas these children face.
- *Education:* Facilitate educational opportunities to ensure that these children have access to learning and skill development.
- *Substance-abuse management:* Develop programs and support systems to tackle and manage substance-abuse issues among street children.
- *Rehabilitation services:* Offer rehabilitation programs to reintegrate them into society and provide necessary support systems for their well-being.
- *Creating safe home environments:* Establish safe shelters or homes that provide a secure environment for these children.
- *Occupational therapy:* Introduce occupational therapy programs to help these children develop skills and abilities for future employment opportunities.
- *Vaccination:* Ensure access to essential vaccinations to protect them from preventable diseases.

The effective implementation of these management strategies would significantly improve the overall well-being and prospects of street children.

## PREVENTION AND PROTECTION

### Role of Government

*National Commission for Protection of Child Rights (NCPCR):* The Balswaraj Portal is a step in the right direction. It involves a systematic process for addressing issues related to children in street situations by collecting data, conducting social investigations, formulating individual care plans, and allocating resources for their welfare. The "PM CARES for Children Scheme," launched by Prime Minister Narendra Modi on May 29, 2021, is a notable initiative aimed at addressing the needs and welfare of children. This scheme consolidates and integrates multiple existing schemes related to child protection, ensuring a more cohesive and comprehensive approach to support and care for children in various vulnerable situations. The initiative aims to provide focused attention and resources toward safeguarding and enhancing the well-being of children, including those from challenging backgrounds such as street children and those in need of protection and care.

However, there is a noted gap between the laws enacted and the practical protection and support provided to street children.

## Role of Community

*Community involvement:* Societal involvement is crucial in supporting these children. Nongovernmental organizations (NGOs) and social organizations play a pivotal role in establishing homes and centers for street children and juvenile delinquents.

*Improving ground realities:* Although various homes and centers exist for street children and delinquents, the effectiveness of these setups needs significant improvement. Addressing the root causes, providing better facilities, care, and education, and creating a nurturing environment are essential.

Enhancing the collaboration and effectiveness of these initiatives, schemes, and efforts by the government, society, NGOs, and community members is vital to ensuring better protection and support for street children. This includes not only enacting laws and schemes but also implementing them effectively and ensuring their practical application for the well-being of these vulnerable children.

## Role of Society and NGOs

Though there are many homes opened for street children and juvenile delinquents, the ground reality is not satisfactory.

The oppression, suppression, and exploitation of street children is a great problem in India. The efforts are far from satisfactory. There is a need for a proper monitoring and rehabilitation system for these children which is honest, dedicated, focused, time-bound with a single goal of "zero street children".

## ◼ KEY MESSAGES

- Street children contribute to 18 million population.
- There are different categories of street children.
- Poverty and dysfunctional families are the main causes.
- They suffer from starvation, malnutrition, and anemia.
- They suffer from many physical illnesses without medical aid.
- They are sexually, mentally, physically, and psychologically abused.
- They fall prey to drugs, prostitution, illegal business and get sexually transmitted diseases (STDs).
- They are used in hazardous businesses as child labor.
- The government have many schemes but all do not reach the end person—the street child.
- A dedicated, honest machinery to give them shelter, food, skills, education, love, and medical aids to bring them to the main stream of society.

## ◼ RECOMMENDED READING


1. Agarwal R. Street Children, 1st edition. New Delhi: Shipra Publications; 1999.
2. Kliegman RM, St. Geme III JW. Nelson Textbook of Pediatrics, 21st edition. Philadelphia: Elsevier.
3. Kotwal N. Sexually transmitted diseases lecture on DIAP Platform. https://vimeo.com/436158655/137d1cb372.
4. Pagare D, Meena GS, Singh MM, Saha R. Risk factor of substance use amongst street children from Delhi. Indian Pediatr. 2004;41:221-5.
5. Saini N. Study of Health Profile and Morbidity Patterns of Street and Working Children. MD Thesis, Delhi University, 1997.
6. Sethi GR. Street Children: A Window to the Reality. Indian Pediatr. 2004;41:219-20.
7. Tomar SK. Shadows of the street: India's street children. J Sociol Social Anthropol. 2020;11(1-2):1-10.

# Part F: Drug Dosage in Adolescent Age Group

*Sub-section Editors:* **Shailaja Mane, Poonam Bhatia, Samir Shah**

## 4F.1 | Drug Dosage in Adolescent

*Jeeson C Unni*

### ■ INTRODUCTION

Childhood obesity is a growing public health concern in Indian children. Doses of various medications in these overweight/obese children could be at toxic levels if calculated according to total body weight. Hence, individualizing drug dosages for obese patients based solely on per kilogram criteria is not empirically viable.

Obese adolescents typically exhibit an expanded volume of distribution (Vd) for lipophilic medications. Conversely, the Vd for hydrophilic medications might fluctuate due to elevated lean body mass, blood volume, and reduced percentage of total body water. Additionally, they may encounter diminished hepatic clearance resulting from fatty infiltrates in the liver. Consequently, obesity can influence the loading dose, dosage interval, plasma half-life, and duration required to achieve steady-state concentration for various medications.

Drug and dosage selection may be influenced by the presence of obesity-related comorbidities, including metabolic syndrome (e.g., hypertension, hypercholesterolemia, and type 2 diabetes), fatty liver, obstructive sleep apnea, and polycystic ovary syndrome.

### ■ GENERAL PRINCIPLES

Weight-based dosing is recommended for patients aged <18 years weighing <40 kg.

- For children weighing ≥40 kg, weight-based dosing is typically utilized unless the prescribed dose or daily dosage surpasses the recommended adult dose for the particular indication.
- Clinicians should possess familiarity with adult dosage regimens to prevent exceeding the recommended maximum adult dose.
- When managing children with overweight or obesity, clinicians should consider potential alterations in pharmacokinetic parameters and adjust drug dosage accordingly whenever feasible, aiming for the most effective and safe regimen.

### ■ METHODS FOR DRUG DOSING APPLIED TO CHILDREN WITH OBESITY

The commonly used methods for drug dosing applied to children with obesity are as follows:

- Total body weight (TBW) is commonly used for determining drug dosage per kilogram and is universally applied for children up to 40 kg and 12 years of age. However, it is not recommended for lipophilic drugs. Lower doses are typically advised for lipophilic drugs and unfractionated heparins.
- Body surface area (BSA), calculated as the square root of [height (cm) × weight (kg)/3,600], is another method used for dosage calculation. This approach is utilized for both adults and children, particularly in dosing chemotherapy drugs.

*For children and adults:*

- Ideal body weight (IBW) is calculated as the 50th percentile weight (age)/height (cm). Accurate determination of IBW is crucial for proper medication dosing, including drugs like acyclovir, digoxin, and morphine. In children, there is no consensus on the most accurate calculation method. The Moore method, based on growth charts, determines IBW by aligning the child's weight percentile with their height percentile for that age.
- Clark's rule is an equation used to calculate pediatric medication dosage based on the known weight of a patient and a known adult dose of the medication.

*Equation:* Weight of pediatric patient in kg/68 kg × Adult dose = Pediatric dosage

*Note:* Adult dose refers to the recommended dosage for adult medication use.

Various drugs, their TBW dose for adolescents, and the maximum dose per day in children affected by obesity are given in **Table 1**.

*Ethinylestradiol and combined hormonal contraceptives:* Avoid if body mass index >35 kg/m$^2$ unless there is no suitable alternative.

**TABLE 1:** Common drugs that often require dosage adjustments in obese children.

| Drug | Total body weight (TBW) dose for adolescents | Maximum dose/day in children affected by obesity |
|---|---|---|
| *Antibiotics* | | |
| Amoxicillin | 40 mg/kg/day | 1 g, three times daily |
| Amoxicillin-clavulanic acid | 40 mg/kg/day of amoxicillin | 1 g of amoxicillin, three times daily |
| Azithromycin | 10 mg/kg/day | 1 g/day, given once daily |
| Cefazolin | 25–100 mg/kg/day | For obesity, no dose adjustment |
| Ceftriaxone | 1–2 g once daily | 4 g once daily |
| Ceftazidime | 50 mg/kg every 8 hours | 9 g/day |
| Clindamycin | 3.75–6.25 mg/kg 4 times a day, increased if necessary up to 10 mg/kg, four times a day | Maximum per dose 1.2 g |
| Trimethoprim–sulfamethoxazole | 160 mg trimethoprim and 800 mg sulfamethoxazole, two times daily | 480 mg trimethoprim and 2.4 g sulfamethoxazole |
| Vancomycin | 15–20 mg/kg, every 8–12 hours | Maximum per dose 2 g (no adjustment for obesity) |
| Meropenem | 0.5–1 g, every 8 hours | 2 g, every 8 hours |
| Linezolid | 10 mg/kg, every 8 hours | 600 mg, every 12 hours |
| *Analgesics and anesthetics* | | |
| Acetaminophen | 500 mg, every 4–6 hours | Maximum 4 g per day |
| Fentanyl | *Patch:* For 16–17 years, initially 12 µg/h every 72 hours; alternatively initially 25 µg/h every 72 hours | *Patch:* Maximum dose 300 µg/h |
| | *Intravenous (IV):* Initially 1–5 µg/kg, then 0–200 µg as required | IV maximum per dose 200 µg during surgery |
| Midazolam | Light sedation<br>*Oral:* 6 months to 16 years: 0.25–1 mg/kg orally once before the procedure | *Maximum oral dose:* 20 mg |
| | *Intramuscular (IM):* 0.1–0.15 mg/kg once, some require doses of 0.5 mg/kg | Maximum total dose 10 mg IM |
| | *IV:* 1–2.5 mg slow | Maximum total dose 10 mg IV |
| | *Epilepsy:* Initial dose, 5 mg (1 spray) intranasal, repeat if required after 10 minutes | Maximum 10 mg/day |
| Pethidine | 1 mg/kg, then 1 mg/kg after 1–3 hours, if required | Maximum 100 mg/dose, 400 mg/day |
| *Others* | | |
| Flecainide | *IV:* 0.2–2.0 mg/kg<br>*Cont.:* 0.2–0.5 mg/kg/h | *Maximum IV:* 200 mg/day |
| | *Oral:* 1–7 mg/kg | *Maximum oral:* 200 mg/day or 8 mg/kg/day |
| Atenolol | *Hypertension:* Oral, 25–50 mg once daily, dose may be given in two divided doses, higher doses are rarely necessary | Maximum 100 mg/dose |
| | *Arrhythmias:* Oral, 50–100 mg once daily, dose may be given in two divided doses | |
| Amlodipine (calcium channel blocker) | 0.1 mg/kg/day | TBW dosing |

*Contd...*

*Contd...*

| Drug | Total body weight (TBW) dose for adolescents | Maximum dose/day in children affected by obesity |
|---|---|---|
| Angiotensin-converting enzyme (ACE) inhibitor–ramipril | 0.05–0.15 mg/kg/day, maximum 40 mg/day | Empirically, a lower starting dose-based TBW can be employed [2, 32] |
| Antipsychotics (such as haloperidol, thioridazine, risperidone, and aripiprazole) | – | • Limited research exists regarding the appropriate dosing and therapeutic drug monitoring<br>• Recommended to begin treatment with a conservative dose and gradually increase it while closely monitoring the patient's metabolism. Discontinuation attempts following prolonged use may offer benefits |
| Fluvoxamine | 25–50 mg after food twice daily, could be increased to 100 mg OD | Increasing to maximum doses of 300 mg/day needs expert supervision |
| Antineoplastic medication | It depends on the drug and protocols | Drug dosage for chemotherapy is commonly calculated based on a patient's body surface area and doses are extrapolated from adult studies. Studies have shown that like in obese adults, TBW dosing in 7% of obese children with leukemia received less than the protocol-specified dose. Dosing using TBW is used in infants and children with weight <10 kg |
| Inhaled corticosteroids (beclomethasone, budesonide, flunisolide, fluticasone, etc.) | Depend on the drugs | Standard doses are not sufficient for obese children |
| Low molecular weight (LMW) heparin | Depends on the drug and indications | It is essential to adjust the dose of enoxaparin upon initiating therapy |
| Metformin (biguanide) | 500 mg/day | Maximum dose 2 g/day; for older children and adolescents with obesity, use adult doses of metformin |
| Proton-pump inhibitors (PPIs) (pantoprazole) | 10–20 mg/day | The dosing of PPI in obesity may be similar to that of normal-weight children |
| Steroids | Depends on indications | Standardizing drug-dosing guidelines for children with obesity is essential to mitigate the risk of harm |
| Vitamin D (25(OH)D) | 1,000 and 2,000 IU/day | The highest percentage of patients affected by obesity, with values ≥20 ng/mL, was observed solely among the 2000-IU group. This suggests the superiority in effectiveness of this dosage compared to lower ones |

## ■ KEY MESSAGES

- Dosing adjustments in obese adolescents should be meticulously tailored according to the provided chart.
- Ongoing research aims to assess medication dosing in obese or overweight adolescents.

## ■ RECOMMENDED READING


1. BMJ Group, Pharmaceutical Press. BNF for Children 2019-2020. London: BMJ Group, the Royal Pharmaceutical Society of Great Britain, and RCPCH Publications Ltd; 2019. [online] Available from https://www.arstapaligs.lv/wp-content/uploads/2021/04/BNF-for-Children-BNFC-2019-2020.pdf [Last accessed March, 2024].

2. Lin B, Hu Y, Xu P, Xu T, Chen C, He L, et al. Expert consensus statement on therapeutic drug monitoring and individualization of linezolid. Front. Public Health. 2022; 10:967311.

3. Matson KL, Horton ER, Capino AC; Advocacy Committee for the Pediatric Pharmacy Advocacy Group. Medication dosage in overweight and obese children. J Pediatr Pharmacol Ther. 2017;22(1):81-3.

4. Unni JC, Chatterjee P (Eds). IAP Drug Formulary 2024 with Recommendations for Drug Treatment for Pediatric Illness. Indian Academy of Pediatrics, Project of IAP CMIC, 6th edition. Kochi: Pixel Studio; 2024

# Nutrition

**Section Editor:** *Geeta Patil*

## 5.1 Adolescent Nutritional Requirements

*Elizabeth KE, Bindusha S*

### INTRODUCTION

Adolescence is considered as a nutritionally critical period in life, as it is the last and final chance for growth and development. Adolescence is the period of pubertal growth spurt, which increases the requirement of both macro- and micronutrients. A balanced diet containing appropriate amount of macronutrients and micronutrients is important to achieve full growth potential. The physique of an adolescent changes from that of a child to an adult, and this change is associated with increase in height, weight, body mass index, and changes in body proportion, body fat content, muscle and bone mass, blood volume, etc.

### GENDER-BASED DIFFERENCES

Nutritional requirement of adolescents varies as per gender. This difference in requirement is due to the difference in the rate of pubertal growth between boys and girls. Growth spurt starts and completes earlier in girls compared to boys. Thus, the protein requirement of girls aged 10–12 years is higher than boys of the same age group. Protein requirement of an adolescent girl aged 15–18 years is much lower than a boy of the same age group, as her adult height is already achieved. The energy requirement of adolescents also depends on physical activity in addition to growth. Adolescent boys are more active, and they require more energy than adolescent girls. Other factors such as differences in body composition and requirements of certain nutrients like iron also contribute to this differential recommendation.

### MACRO- AND MICRONUTRIENT REQUIREMENTS

Adequate energy intake during adolescence is needed to support linear and muscle growth. Around 4% of total energy requirement is spent to support growth during adolescence. Minimum daily carbohydrate intake of 100–130 g is recommended. This is the minimum intake needed to provide glucose for metabolism in the brain. Whole grains are preferred over processed cereals. Millets should contribute to 20–30% of cereal intake. Sugar intake should be limited to <5% of energy requirement.

Protein requirement of adolescents is almost equal to that for adults. Adequate intake of essential amino acids is critical during this period to support the pubertal growth spurt and development. Even if protein intake is adequate in quantity, protein deficiency can occur due to suboptimal quality of dietary proteins and poor utilization due to recurrent infections. Vegetarian sources are mostly incomplete with rate-limiting amino acids. If the calorie intake is suboptimal, proteins will be wasted for energy instead of tissue building; 1 g for just 4 kcal.

Requirements of calcium, phosphorous, and magnesium are the highest during adolescence, as these minerals are needed for bone growth, mineralization, and increase in the muscle mass. 40% of skeletal mass is added during adolescence. Lack of adequate dietary calcium can lead to low bone mineral density and osteoporosis during adulthood. Recommended dietary allowance (RDA) of calcium during early adolescence is 850 mg/day, which increases to 1,050 mg/day in late adolescence. The recommended calcium:phosphorus ratio in diet is 1:1. Zinc is a growth nutrient and is essential for linear growth, sexual maturation, and immunity.

Adequate intake of iron is essential for adolescents, girls to compensate for the menstrual blood loss, and boys to build up muscle mass, red cell mass, and blood volume. Infections and parasitic infestations can lead to iron loss from the body. Nonheme iron contributes to a major source of iron in Indian diet, which is less bioavailable due to antinutrients such as phytates, polyphenols, coffee, and tea. The absorption of iron depends on heme/nonheme iron, meal composition, and other dietary factors. Addition of fruits rich in ascorbic acid like guava and papaya has been found to increase iron absorption from plant sources. The desired ratio of vitamin C:iron is >4:1 and phytate:iron is <0.4:1.

Daily intake of sodium should be limited to 2 g/day, which is equivalent to salt intake of 5 g/day. The recommended sodium:potassium ratio is 1:1.

The requirements of key nutrients are summarized in **Tables 1 and 2**. The desirable amounts in a balanced diet are given in **Table 3** and tolerable upper limits of in **Table 4**.

## ACCEPTABLE MACRONUTRIENT DISTRIBUTION RANGE

Carbohydrates should make up 45–65% of energy intake; protein 5–15%; and fat 25–35%. In view of the obesity pandemic, carbs may be restricted to 50% and protein hiked to 20%. Dietary fat should come from sources of saturated:polyunsaturated:monounsaturated fatty acids in the ratio 10:10:10%. For reducing cardiovascular disease (CVD) risk, monounsaturated can be further hiked by

**TABLE 1:** Recommended dietary allowances (RDAs)* for energy, protein, and micronutrients: Indian Council of Medical Research (ICMR) 2024.

| Age group | Gender | Energy kcal/day | Protein g/day | Fiber g/day | Calcium mg/day | Magnesium mg/day | Iron mg/day | Zinc mg/day | Iodine µg/day |
|---|---|---|---|---|---|---|---|---|---|
| 10–12 years | Boys | 2,220 | 32 | 33 | 850 | 240 | 16 | 8.5 | 100 |
| | Girls | 2,060 | 33 | 30 | 850 | 250 | 28 | 8.5 | 100 |
| 13–15 years | Boys | 2,860 | 45 | 43 | 1,000 | 345 | 22 | 14.3 | 140 |
| | Girls | 2,400 | 43 | 36 | 1,000 | 340 | 30 | 12.8 | 140 |
| 16–18 years | Boys | 3,320 | 55 | 50 | 1,050 | 440 | 26 | 17.6 | 140 |
| | Girls | 2,500 | 46 | 38 | 1,050 | 380 | 32 | 14.2 | 140 |

*There is no RDA for energy. Instead, estimated average requirement (EAR) is given. EAR for energy is equivalent to estimated energy requirement (EER). Adequate intake (AI) is given for dietary fiber.
*Source:* Adapted from Revised Short Summary Report 2024, ICMR—NIN Expert Group on Nutrient Requirements of Indians, RDA and EAR 2020.

**TABLE 2:** Recommended dietary allowances for vitamins—ICMR 2024.

| Age group | Gender | Thiamine mg/day | Riboflavin mg/day | Niacin mg/day | Vitamin B$_6$ mg/day | Folate µg/day | B$_{12}$ µg/day | Vitamin C mg/day | Vitamin A µg/day | Vitamin D IU/day |
|---|---|---|---|---|---|---|---|---|---|---|
| 10–12 years | Boys | 1.5 | 2.1 | 15 | 2.0 | 220 | 2.2 | 55 | 770 | 600 |
| | Girls | 1.4 | 1.9 | 14 | 1.9 | 225 | 2.2 | 50 | 790 | 600 |
| 13–15 years | Boys | 1.9 | 2.7 | 19 | 2.6 | 285 | 2.2 | 70 | 930 | 600 |
| | Girls | 1.6 | 2.2 | 16 | 2.2 | 245 | 2.2 | 65 | 890 | 600 |
| 16–18 years | Boys | 2.2 | 3.1 | 22 | 3.0 | 340 | 2.2 | 85 | 1,000 | 600 |
| | Girls | 1.7 | 2.3 | 17 | 2.3 | 270 | 2.2 | 70 | 860 | 600 |

*Source:* Adapted from Revised Short Summary Report 2024, ICMR—NIN Expert Group on Nutrient Requirements of Indians, RDA and EAR 2020.

**TABLE 3:** Quantity of suggested food groups for a balanced diet to meet EAR for adolescents.

| Age | Gender | Cereals (g) | Pulses (g) | GLV (g) | Vegetables (g) | Roots and Tubers (g) | Fruits (g) | Nuts (g) | Milk (mL) | Fats and oils (g) |
|---|---|---|---|---|---|---|---|---|---|---|
| 10–12 years | Boys | 280 | 90 | 100 | 200 | 100 | 100 | 30 | 400 | 35 |
| 10–12 years | Girls | 250 | 85 | 100 | 200 | 100 | 100 | 30 | 400 | 30 |
| 13–15 years | Boys | 390 | 130 | 100 | 200 | 100 | 100 | 40 | 400 | 45 |
| 13–15 years | Girls | 300 | 100 | 100 | 200 | 100 | 100 | 35 | 400 | 40 |
| 16–18 years | Boys | 450 | 150 | 100 | 200 | 100 | 150 | 50 | 400 | 55 |
| 16–18 years | Girls | 315 | 105 | 100 | 200 | 100 | 150 | 40 | 400 | 40 |

(EAR: estimated average requirement; GLV: green leafy vegetables)
*Source:* Adapted from Revised Short Summary Report 2024, ICMR—NIN Expert Group on Nutrient Requirements of Indians, RDA and EAR 2020.

**TABLE 4:** Tolerable upper limit of nutrients for the adolescents.

| Age | Gender | Protein (PE ratio) | Calcium mg/day | Magnesium mg/day | Iron mg/day | Zinc mg/d | Iodine µg/day | Folate µg/day | Vitamin C mg/d | Vitamin A µg/day | Vitamin D IU/day |
|---|---|---|---|---|---|---|---|---|---|---|---|
| 10–12 years | Boys | <15% | 3,000 | 350 | 40 | 23 | 600 | 600–800 | 1,050 | 1,700 | 4,000 |
| 10–12 years | Girls | <15% | 3,000 | 350 | 40 | 23 | 600 | 600–800 | 1,300 | 1,700 | 4,000 |
| 13–15 years | Boys | <15% | 3,000 | 350 | 45 | 34 | 900 | 600–800 | 1,550 | 2,800 | 4,000 |
| 13–15 years | Girls | <15% | 3,000 | 350 | 45 | 34 | 900 | 600–800 | 1,800 | 2,800 | 4,000 |
| 16–18 years | Boys | <15% | 3,000 | 350 | 45 | 34 | 1,100 | 600–800 | 1,950 | 2,800 | 4,000 |
| 16–18 years | Girls | <15% | 3,000 | 350 | 45 | 34 | 1,100 | 600–800 | 2,000 | 2,800 | 4,000 |

*Source:* Adapted from Revised Short Summary Report 2024, ICMR—NIN Expert Group on Nutrient Requirements of Indians, RDA and EAR 2020.

reducing saturated fat. Omega-6 polyunsaturated fatty acid (PUFA) should contribute to 4–10% and omega 3 PUFA to 0.5–1% of energy. Omega 6:omega 3 ratio of 5–10:1 is desirable. Trans fats that are solid at room temperature, found in animal fat, hydrogenated oils, frozen desserts, and bakery products, should be avoided as they increase serum low-density lipoproteins. Ghee has only 4% trans fats.

## ■ KEY MESSAGES

- Adolescence is a nutritionally critical period. Nutritional requirement of adolescents varies as per gender and stage of adolescence.
- Around 4% of total energy requirement is spent to support growth during adolescence.
- The energy requirement of adolescents also depends on physical activity in addition to growth.
- A balanced diet containing appropriate amount of macronutrients and micronutrients is important to achieve full growth potential.
- Carbohydrates should make up 45–65% of energy intake; protein 5–15%; and fat 25–35%.
- Minimum daily carbohydrate intake of 100–130 g is recommended. Sugar intake to be limited to less than 5% of energy requirement.
- Millets should contribute to 20–30% of cereal intake.
- Adequate intake of high-quality protein is needed for optimal growth during adolescence.
- Requirements of iron, calcium, phosphorous, and magnesium are highest during adolescence.
- In view of the obesity pandemic, carbs may be restricted to 50% and protein hiked to 20%.

## ■ RECOMMENDED READING

1. Christian P, Smith ER. Adolescent Undernutrition: Global Burden, Physiology, and Nutritional Risks. Ann Nutr Metab. 2018;72(4):316-28.
2. Elizabeth KE (Ed). Nutrition and Child Development, 6th edition. Paras Medical Publisher; 2022.
3. Norris SA, Frongillo EA, Black MM, Dong Y, Fall C, Lampl M, et al. Nutrition in adolescent growth and development, Adolescent Nutrition Series. Lancet. 2022;399(10320):172-84.
4. Revised Short Summary Report 2023, ICMR—NIN Expert Group on Nutrient Requirements of Indians, RDA and EAR 2020.

# 5.2 Undernutrition Among Adolescents

*Elizabeth KE, Bindusha S*

## ■ INTRODUCTION

Adolescence is a period of transformative growth. 15–20% of final adult height and 50% of adult weight is gained during adolescence. The "Triple burden" of malnutrition, namely undernutrition, micronutrient deficiency, and overweight/obesity during adolescence can have lasting effects, as they affect the maturation of multiple biological systems. Thinness during adolescence is associated with a higher risk of infectious diseases, delayed puberty and maturation, reduced muscular strength, and work capacity and bone density later in life. In addition, thinness in adolescent girls is associated with adverse pregnancy outcomes, intrauterine growth retardation, and transgenerational malnutrition.

Nutritional status affects both the onset of puberty and its duration. Puberty occurs earlier in children who are overweight, and may be delayed in underweight children. Different studies have shown that higher intake of animal proteins, carbohydrates, and fats during early adolescence is associated with earlier onset of puberty.

## ■ ASSESSMENT OF UNDERNUTRITION AMONG ADOLESCENTS

The World Health Organization (WHO) recommends the use of body mass index (BMI) for age and height for the assessment of adolescent growth patterns **(Table 1)**. The terms thinness and underweight are often used interchangeably when making reference to adolescents' low BMI-for-age, <3rd percentile. For Indian children and adolescents, it is recommended to use BMI cut offs of >23 adult equivalents and >27 adult equivalents for overweight and obesity, respectively. This recommendation takes into account the difference in the body composition of Indians compared to westerners.

## ■ PREVALENCE OF UNDERNUTRITION AMONG ADOLESCENTS

Global prevalence of underweight among adolescents is 8.4% among girls and 12.4% among boys. Despite the current interventions, the prevalence has not declined over the last three decades. There is significant difference in the prevalence of thinness, stunting, and overweight among different nations. The prevalence of moderate and severe thinness among adolescents is highest in South Asia.

Undernutrition among adolescents in India is a public health issue, which is often overlooked by the researchers and health planners. Even the National Family Health Survey 5 (NFHS-5) groups all individuals above 15 years among adults. Data from the Comprehensive National Nutrition Survey 2018 (CNNS 2018) points to high prevalence of malnutrition among adolescents **(Box 1)**.

**TABLE 1:** Assessment of abnormal growth patterns among adolescents.

| | |
|---|---|
| Stunting | Height for age <2 SD below the WHO child growth reference median |
| Thinness | BMI for age <2 SD below the WHO growth reference median |
| Overweight | BMI for age >1 SD above the WHO growth reference median |
| Obesity | BMI for age >2 SD above the WHO growth reference median |

(BMI: body mass index; SD: standard deviation)

Comprehensive National Nutrition Survey found that prevalence of stunting at 18 years was 30%. Prevalence of underweight was higher among out of school adolescents (45%) than those in school (34%). Prevalence of underweight was higher among adolescents from households with low wealth (43%) and it was found to decrease steadily as household wealth increased. Prevalence of underweight among adolescents from the highest wealth quintile was 21%.

Twenty-four percent of adolescents aged 10–19 years had low BMI (BMI for age <–2 SD). Boys (29%) had a higher prevalence of low BMI compared to girls (19%) during adolescence. The prevalence of low BMI declined slowly through adolescence to a prevalence of 12% by age 19 years. Another finding which raises high concern is that 6.5% of adolescents aged 10–19 years had BMI <–3 SD. 8% of adolescents aged 10–19 years had triceps skinfold thickness below –2 SD.

---

**BOX 1:** Key findings of CNNS 2018 regarding malnutrition among adolescents aged 10–19.

- 24% of adolescents were thin for their age (BMI-for-age <–2 SD)
- 5% of adolescents were overweight or obese (BMI-for-age >+1 SD)
- 4% of adolescents were overweight as measured by triceps SFT (TSFT-for-age >+1 SD)
- 6% of adolescents were overweight as measured by subscapular SFT (SSFT-for-age >+1 SD)
- 2% of adolescents had abdominal obesity (waist circumference-for-age >+1 SD)

(BMI: body mass index; CNNS 2018: Comprehensive National Nutrition Survey 2018; SD: standard deviation; SFT: skinfold thickness)

---

The double burden of malnutrition is described by the coexistence of undernutrition along with overweight, obesity, or diet-related noncommunicable diseases (NCDs). CNNS found that while 26.4% of adolescents were stunted and 6.1% overweight, 0.8% of adolescents suffered from the double burden of both stunting and overweight. While the percentage appears to be low when compared to stunting and undernutrition, the actual number of Indian adolescents experiencing dual burden of malnutrition is large enough to be of public health concern. The magnitude of micronutrient deficiencies like iron poses a huge public health burden. **Table 2** depicts the data from various studies.

## DIETARY PATTERNS AMONG ADOLESCENTS

Many studies have pointed out that dietary intake of nutrients is inadequate during adolescence. This inadequacy in diet is more among adolescents from the low- and middle-income countries (LMICs). Dietary habits play an important role in ensuring adequate nutrient intake. Dietary patterns of adolescents have changed over the years, as a result of urbanization and industrialization. This change in the dietary pattern is more pronounced among the urban adolescents. Adolescents of the current decade have become more independent in their food choices. This can be attributed to the easy availability of different types of food items.

Diet of Indian adolescents is mainly composed of cereals and pulses. Consumption of other food items such as milk and milk products, nonvegetarian items, fruits, and vegetables are inadequate.

---

**TABLE 2:** Data on prevalence of adolescent undernutrition.

| Author and Year | Country | Findings |
| --- | --- | --- |
| Sushama S Thakre et al.; 2020 | Adolescent girls, Nagpur, India | • 36% of adolescent girls were underweight<br>• 80% of adolescent girls were anemic |
| Amitava Pal et al.; 2016 | Rural adolescents, West Bengal, India | 54% of adolescents were stunted and 49% were thin |
| Vikram Patel et al.; 2010 | Adolescents rural, Goa, India | 38% of boys and 28% girls were underweight. 59% reported experiencing hunger due to inadequate food |
| Handiso YH et al.; 2021 | Adolescent girls, Southern Ethiopia | Thinness (27.5%) and stunting (8.8%) among adolescent girls were found to be public health problems |
| Segni Mulugeta Tafasa; 2022 | Adolescent girls, Central Ethiopia | Stunting was 15.4% [95% confidence interval (CI): 12–18] and thinness was 14.2% (95% CI: 11–17) |
| Temam Beshir Raru; 2010–2016 | Late adolescent girls, East Africa | The overall magnitude of undernutrition was 16.50%. The overall magnitude of obesity was 2.41% |

## FACTORS AFFECTING DIETARY HABITS IN ADOLESCENTS (FIG. 1)

### Sociodemographic Factors

Age, gender, and demographic factors such as location and urbanization affect the eating habits of adolescents. Girls are more prone to undernutrition. They usually eat last and least in many families. Girls tend to prioritize body image over health. Dieting, lack of exercise, and food fads all contribute to poor eating habits and hence undernutrition.

### Behavioral Factors

Behavioral factors such as skipping meals, irregular meal times, and dieting will lead to undernutrition, whereas eating in front of TV, large portion sizes, and high intake of sweetened beverage will lead to overweight. Snacking is an integral part of adolescent eating behavior. Snacks can provide up to one quarter of daily energy requirement. Snacking will reduce appetite during regular meal times. Regular physical activity is essential for normal growth. Adolescents who eat with their family usually have a diet rich in varied nutrients.

### Environmental Factors

The availability of food at home is the most important factor, which decides the food intake of adolescents among the LMICs. Undernutrition is more prevalent among adolescents from lower socioeconomic status and large families. Adolescents may miss meals due to lack of time as they are engaged in academic and social activities. Ability to buy snacks and frequency of eating out/take out dinners will also affect the dietary pattern. Parental diet is another important factor, which affects the adolescent eating habits. Adolescents from families in which the parents follow healthy and balanced eating pattern are more likely to have balanced diet. Peer pressure and advertisements also decide the food preference. Discriminative cultural and gender norms also affect the eating habits of adolescent girls.

### Health-related Factors

Infections and illnesses during adolescence will affect the food intake. Adolescents suffering from some illnesses may have to follow a restricted dietary pattern. Infections and infestations affect the appetite also. Infections and inflammatory diseases can affect the growth despite adequate food intake.

### Education and Knowledge

Knowledge about the nutritive content of the food will also affect the diet. Habits which are acquired during adolescence often last throughout the adult life. This is true for the eating/dietary habits also. Adolescents, who later become the parents, decide the dietary pattern of next generation. This stresses the importance of nutritional education to adolescents and nurturing a healthy eating behavior among adolescents.

## CHRONIC HEALTH ISSUES ASSOCIATED WITH ADOLESCENT UNDERNUTRITION

Undernutrition during childhood and adolescence is associated with decrease in the number of beta cells in pancreas and decreased insulin production. It is compensated during adolescence by higher number of peripheral insulin receptors. This compensation can lead on to adiposity in later life. Stunted children and adolescents are at a higher risk to develop hypertension and coronary arterial diseases in later life. Undernutrition is also associated with increased physiological and psychological stress. The stress hormones can decrease the secretion of thyroxine and insulin-like growth factor 1 (IGF-1).

Undernutrition in adolescent girls has intergenerational effect. Infants of mothers who were underweight or stunted during adolescence are more likely to be borne with low birth weight.

Prolonged periods of undernutrition result in reduction of grey and white matter, especially in the frontoparietal network. Frontoparietal network controls

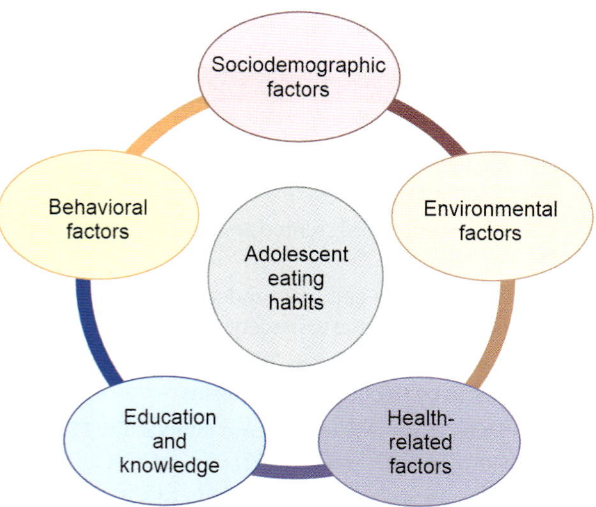



**Fig. 1:** Factors affecting adolescent dietary habits.

the higher executive functions and abnormalities in its maturation result in poor emotional intelligence and poor processing of social cues. Micronutrient deficiency, which is more prevalent among undernourished children, is also associated with long-term consequences. Iron deficiency anemia is associated with low mental performance, inattention, and lower learning capacity. Iron deficiency is associated with memory problems and also leads to long-term deficits in cognitive function. Iodine deficiency is associated with impaired concentration and poor social and cognitive performance. The mild forms of vitamin A deficiency cause impaired immune function and an increased risk of morbidity from infectious diseases.

## KEY MESSAGES

- About 15–20% of final adult height and 50% of adult weight is gained during adolescence.
- The "Triple burden" of malnutrition, namely undernutrition, micronutrient deficiency, and overweight/obesity during adolescence can have lasting effects, as they affect the maturation of multiple biological systems.
- Global prevalence of underweight among adolescents is 8.4% among girls and 12.4% among boys.
- CNNS observed that 24% of adolescents were thin for their age (BMI-for-age <-2 SD).
- Dietary patterns of urban adolescents have changed over the years, as a result of urbanization and industrialization.

- Adolescent malnutrition is multifactorial.
- Sociodemographic, environmental, behavioral, and health-related factors play an important role in adolescent nutrition.
- The double burden of malnutrition is described by the coexistence of undernutrition along with overweight, obesity, or diet-related NCDs.
- Stunted children and adolescents are at a higher risk to develop hypertension and coronary arterial diseases in later life.
- Prolonged periods of undernutrition result in reduction of grey and white matter, especially in the frontoparietal network.

## RECOMMENDED READING


1. Christian P, Smith ER. Adolescent Undernutrition: Global Burden, Physiology, and Nutritional Risks. Ann Nutr Metab. 2018;72(4):316-28.
2. Elizabeth KE (Ed). Nutrition and Child Development, 6th edition. Paras Medical Publisher; 2022.
3. Madjdian DS, Azupogo F, Osendarp SJM, Bras H, Brouwer IB. Socio-cultural and economic determinants and consequences of adolescent undernutrition and micronutrient deficiencies in LLMICs: a systematic narrative review. Ann NY Acad Sci. 2018;1416(1):117-39.
4. Norris SA, Frongillo EA, Black MM, Dong Y, Fall C, Lampl M, et al. Nutrition in adolescent growth and development, Adolescent Nutrition Series. Lancet. 2022;399(10320):172-84.


# 5.3 Nutritional Hunger and Increasing Incidence Among Adolescents

*Elizabeth KE, Gibby Koshy*

## INTRODUCTION

The term "nutritional hunger" has been proposed to describe micronutrient deficiencies which include essential minerals and vitamins. These deficiencies when termed "hidden hunger" can often go unrecognized and unsuspected. However, often these are recognizable if there is a high index of suspicion. The four major micronutrient deficiencies—iron, iodine, vitamin A, and zinc—are considered of highest public health concern globally because of their increasing prevalence and related developmental and health consequences. Nutritional hunger affects more than 2 billion individuals, or one in three people, globally. Its effects can be devastating, leading to mental impairment, poor health, low productivity, and even death. The National Family Health Survey (NFHS) 4 and 5 and the Comprehensive National Nutrition Survey (CNNS) of India have identified very high burden among adolescents. As per the Global Hidden Hunger Index

# 5.4 Undernutrition Special Reference with Girls

*Elizabeth KE, Bindusha S*

## INTRODUCTION

Undernutrition, especially among girls, is a significant global health concern. Undernutrition refers to a condition in which a person's nutritional intake is insufficient to meet their dietary needs, resulting in various health problems and stunted growth. Special attention to addressing undernutrition in girls is crucial, because it can have long-lasting effects on their physical and cognitive development.

## PREVALENCE

The United Nations Children's Fund (UNICEF) estimates that one billion adolescent girls suffer from undernutrition and micronutrient deficiencies. Despite the multiple interventions, there is no decline in the prevalence of underweight among the adolescent girls for the past 20 years. Global prevalence of undernutrition among adolescent girls is 8%. Prevalence of anemia is 30% and micronutrient deficiencies is 69% among adolescent girls. Majority of girls with undernutrition (68%) and anemia (60%) reside in South Asia and Sub-Saharan Africa.

Girls, particularly during their adolescence, have unique nutritional requirements that need special attention. Adequate nutrition is needed to meet the demand during rapid growth and sexual maturation during adolescence. The onset of menstruation increases the requirement of iron. Inadequate nutritional intake compounded by increased nutritional needs related to menstruation, pregnancy, and lactation increases the risk of undernutrition and micronutrient deficiency among adolescent girls. Studies have pointed out the higher prevalence of anemia among adolescent girls, especially in developing countries. The prevalence of anemia among adolescent girls in India is 59% as per the National Family Health Survey 5 (NFHS-5).

## UNIQUENESS OF GIRLS

Many of the adolescent girls in the developing countries are expected to undertake adult responsibilities, which are far beyond their physical, emotional, and psychological development. Early marriage and pregnancy is common among adolescent girls from Asia. Worldwide, 16 million girls aged 15–19 years give birth every year. Adolescent pregnancies contribute to 20% of all births in Sub-Saharan Africa. In absolute numbers, Bangladesh, India, and Nigeria contribute to 30% of adolescent pregnancies. Adolescent pregnancies are more common in poor, uneducated, and rural communities. Pregnancy occurring in a state where the girl herself is still growing will further increase the nutritional demands. The resulting competition between the needs of the developing fetus and the growing young mother will result in high-risk pregnancy. Pregnancy can halt linear growth of the adolescent mother. Prevalence of adverse pregnancy outcomes and low birth weight babies is higher following adolescent pregnancy.

An important aspect of undernutrition in adolescent girls is its effect on the next generation. Undernutrition is perpetuated through life cycle. Babies who are born with low birth weight grow up to be stunted adolescent girls and stunted women. These women gain inadequate weight during pregnancy resulting in fetal malnutrition. This problem is worsened in adolescent pregnancies. The babies of undernourished women are born with lower birth weight, thus perpetuating the "intergenerational cycle of growth failure" **(Fig. 1)**. Recent research shows that

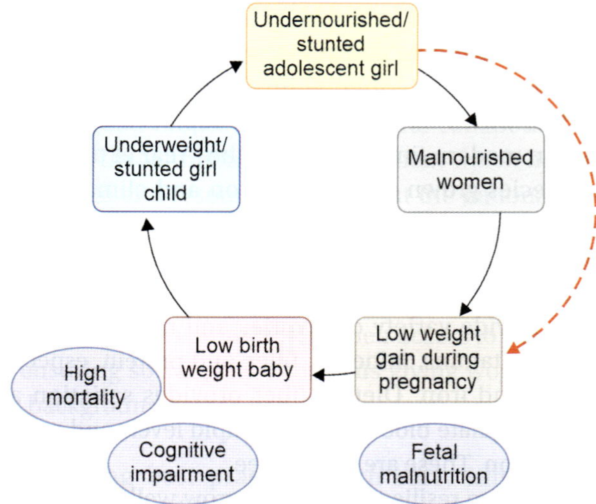


**Fig. 1:** Intergenerational cycle of growth failure.

this phenomenon can span more than two generations through epigenetic changes. Children of undernourished mothers are more likely to have short stature, cognitive impairment, increased risk of infections, and are at a higher risk of diseases and mortality throughout their life.

Another factor that contributes to undernutrition among girls is discrimination in access to food and nutrition. Discriminatory norms and practices limit their access to nutritious diets. In many societies, girls may receive less food or lower quality food than boys. In some household, women and girls are expected to eat last or eat least. Longitudinal survey in India shows that dietary diversity of girls and women is less when compared to boys and men.

Undernutrition, micronutrient deficiencies, and anemia further increase the gender inequalities by lowering learning potential, opportunities, and wages of young women. Undernutrition will also weaken their immune system, making them more prone to infections. Frequent infections and other morbidities further lower their earning abilities, perpetuating the social factors behind the undernutrition.

Adolescence is the period in life during which many lifestyle habits develop. Unhealthy habits like smoking, drinking, substance abuse, unhealthy eating habits, and lack of exercise will affect the health of adolescents. Since most of the habits developed during adolescence persist throughout life, developing good health and dietary and exercise habits during adolescence will lead to a healthier life.

Adolescence is the age in which the girls attain at least partial dietary independence. The adolescent is the one who decides what to eat and how much to eat, though the availability and selection of food available may vary between households. Likes and dislikes to certain food groups is very common in this age group. Adolescents are the major consumers of the unhealthy, ultra-processed junk food and beverages. Unhealthy habits and behaviors started during adolescence are major contributors to the lifestyle diseases in adults. Nutritional education imparted to adolescent girls can improve the dietary habits of her future family and children.

Food fads and eating disorders can also prevent girls from taking a balanced diet. Adolescent girl may have altered perception of body image and may want to remain slim by limiting the amount of food intake or avoiding certain food groups. Eating disorders such as anorexia nervosa, bulimia, and avoidant/restrictive food intake disorder will interfere with healthy eating pattern. These disorders have to be considered when evaluating girls with severe undernutrition and multiple micronutrient deficiencies.

## IMPROVING NUTRITION AMONG ADOLESCENT GIRLS

Addressing the specific nutritional needs of girls is crucial for their growth, development, and overall well-being. Addressing undernutrition among girls is not only a matter of public health but also one of social justice. It requires a multifaceted approach that involves governments, nongovernmental organizations (NGOs), healthcare providers, community, and families working together to ensure that every girl has the opportunity to grow up healthy and reach her full potential. Adolescents require special attention due to the following reasons mentioned further.

## KEY CONSIDERATIONS FOR ADDRESSING UNDERNUTRITION IN GIRLS

- *Adequate caloric intake:* Ensure that girls receive sufficient calories to meet their energy needs. This is especially important during growth spurts, puberty, and menstruation, as these periods require additional energy. Nutritional needs of girls may vary based on factors such as age, physical activity level, and overall health. It is essential to tailor dietary recommendations to individual needs and consult with healthcare professionals or nutritionists for personalized guidance.
- *Balanced diet:* Promote a balanced diet that includes a variety of foods from all food groups, such as fruits, vegetables, grains, proteins, and dairy products. This helps provide essential nutrients for growth and development. Studies have found that most adolescents have inadequate vegetable and fruit intake.
- *Iron and anemia prevention:* Girls are at a higher risk of iron deficiency and anemia, particularly due to menstruation. Encourage the consumption of iron-rich foods such as lean meats, beans, fortified cereals, and leafy green vegetables. Consider iron supplementation if necessary and under the guidance of a healthcare professional. Ensure weekly supplementation with iron and folic acid tablets through the Intensified National Iron Plus Initiative.

- *Calcium for bone health:* Adequate calcium intake is essential for building strong bones. Encourage the consumption of dairy products such as milk, yogurt, and cheese, as well as calcium-fortified foods.
- *Folate and vitamin $B_{12}$:* These vitamins are important for girls, especially during adolescence. They play a crucial role in cell division and preventing birth defects. Foods such as leafy greens, legumes, fortified cereals, and animal products are good sources.
- *Protein:* It is vital for growth and development. Include sources of lean protein like poultry, fish, beans, and nuts in their diet. Despite adequate intake, protein inadequacy can occur due to poor quality of protein and poor utilization of proteins due to infection.
- *Hydration:* Ensure girls drink an adequate amount of water throughout the day, as dehydration can affect their health and well-being.
- *Education and awareness:* Promote healthy eating habits and portion control. Multiple communication channels can be used to impart nutrition education. Adolescent girls, women, and their family members should have access to counseling, so that they can take informed decisions and take actions to improve nutrition. Adolescent girls and their caregivers should be told about the importance of a nutritious diet and the consequences of undernutrition.
- *Access to healthcare:* Regular check-ups with healthcare providers can help identify and address any nutritional deficiencies or health issues early.
- *Food security:* Address issues related to food insecurity, as access to an adequate and nutritious food supply is fundamental to combating undernutrition. Supply and affordability of nutritious foods should be ensured by the governments. Mandatory food fortification of staple foods is to be ensured where nutrient deficiencies are common. Policies to limit the sales of unhealthy, ultra-processed junk food, especially near the educational institutions will protect young people from the adverse health effects of these food items.
- *Empowerment:* Promote gender equality and empower girls to make informed decisions about their nutrition and health. This includes educating them about their nutritional needs and reproductive health.
- *Community support:* Engage communities in efforts to combat undernutrition among girls. This can involve community-based nutrition programs, support groups, and awareness campaigns. Addressing undernutrition in girls is not only a matter of nutrition but also involves addressing social, economic, and cultural factors that may contribute to their vulnerability to undernutrition. Gender transformative policies and legal measures should be implemented to strengthen the empowerment of girls and women. Discriminatory gender and social norms have to be eliminated, so that the adolescent girls and women can realize their rights to food and nutrition.

Addressing undernutrition in girls should begin during pregnancy and infancy. Proper maternal nutrition during pregnancy and breastfeeding is essential for the healthy growth of the baby. Early life interventions can have a significant impact on a girl's future health and development. Ensure that girls have access to a diverse and balanced diet that provides essential nutrients. This may involve improving food security, promoting home gardening, and increasing the availability of nutritious foods in local markets.

## ■ KEY MESSAGES

- Girls have unique nutritional requirements during adolescence.
- Inadequate nutritional intake and increased nutritional needs are related to menstruation, pregnancy, and lactation, which increase the risk of undernutrition and micronutrient deficiency among adolescent girls.
- The prevalence of anemia among adolescent girls in India is 59%.
- Prevalence of adverse pregnancy outcomes and low birth weight babies are higher following adolescent pregnancy.
- Undernutrition is perpetuated through life cycle.
- Children of undernourished mothers are at a higher risk of diseases and mortality throughout their life.
- Addressing undernutrition in girls is not only a matter of nutrition but also involves addressing social, economic, and cultural factors that may contribute to their vulnerability to undernutrition.
- Addressing undernutrition in girls should begin during pregnancy and infancy.
- Promoting gender equality and empowering girls to make informed decisions about their nutrition and health are essential to improve their health.
- Nutrition education of adolescent girls shall facilitate healthy eating habits in their future family.

## ■ RECOMMENDED READING

1. Christian P, Smith ER. Adolescent Undernutrition: Global Burden, Physiology, and Nutritional Risks. Ann Nutr Metab. 2018;72:316-28.
2. Handiso YH, Belachew T, Abuye C, Workicho A, Baye K. Undernutrition and its determinants among adolescent girls in low land area of Southern Ethiopia. PLoS ONE. 2016;16(1):e024067.
3. Patil A, Patel N. Challenges in Nutrition of Adolescent Girls Indian. J Trauma Emerg Pediatr. 2017;9(1):4-55.
4. United Nations Children's Fund (UNICEF). (2023). Undernourished and Overlooked: A Global Nutrition Crisis in Adolescent Girls and Women. UNICEF Child Nutrition Report Series, 2022. New York: UNICEF. [online] Available from https://www.unicef.org/reports/undernourished-overlooked-nutrition-crisis [Last accessed March, 2024].

# 5.5 Therapeutic Nutrition

*Elizabeth KE, Gibby Koshy*

## ■ INTRODUCTION

Therapeutic nutrition is a modified form of regular diet used as part of treatment of a medical condition controlling the intake of certain foods and nutrients. This has to be customized to suit the changing nutritional requirements of individual and is used as part of medical treatment for improving the health condition.

Therapeutic nutrition forms an essential part of adolescent growth and development because of their unique nutritional needs along with rapid transition phase from childhood to adulthood, which is characterized by important social and psychological changes in this group and when there is increased demand for nutrient needs. Adolescent nutrition is also influenced by behavioral, sociodemographic as well as environmental factors.

The adolescents need more nutrients when compared to adults as they gain at least 40% of their adult weight and 15% of their adult height during this period and any inadequate intake of these essential nutrients could lead to delayed sexual development and slower linear growth. Growth spurt triggered by puberty increases the demand for macro- as well as micronutrients including iron, calcium, zinc, folate, and increased calories, which need to be provided during this critical phase of rapid growth. This is further affected by the higher incidence of anorexia and bulimia along with effects from environmental endocrine disruptors on pubertal development among adolescents, which imposes a nutritional risk on pubertal development.

Therapeutic nutrition or nutritional therapy follows a diet plan, which helps in controlling lifestyle diseases, such as diabetes mellitus, obesity, cardiovascular diseases by improving the therapeutic effects of specific foods for specific health conditions. It gives more importance to preventive care for specific diseases and helps in preventing further progression through modified diet specific for the health condition.

Benefits of therapeutic nutrition includes stress reduction, improving hormonal imbalance, increasing energy levels and immunity, improving well-being and digestion process, reducing high blood pressure and high cholesterol levels, and also cutting down the risk of some functional disorders like diabetes, stroke, cancers, osteoporosis, and allergies. It also helps to create a personalized treatment for a balanced diet by reducing the harmful substances which could result in chronic illnesses.

Therapeutic diets could be modified depending on the food allergy status, nutritional intolerance, and food texture. Different types of therapeutic diets include diabetic diet, renal diet, low cholesterol diet, fat-restricted diet, salt and sugar restricted diet, etc.

## ■ KEY MESSAGES

Therapeutic nutrition forms an essential part of adolescent growth because of the rapid transition phase from childhood to adulthood.

## ■ RECOMMENDED READING

1. Elizabeth KE (Ed). Nutrition and Child Development, 6th edition. Paras Medical Publisher; 2022.

# 5.6 | Nutritional Anemia in Adolescents

*Chandrika Rao*

## ■ INTRODUCTION

Adolescence is the formative period of life when the maximum amount of physical, psychological, and behavioral changes take place, setting the foundation of adulthood. Changing behavior and liking of JUNCS (Junk foods, Ultra-processed foods, Nutritionally inappropriate foods, Caffeinated/colored/carbonated foods/beverages, and Sugar-sweetened beverages) is commonly. Food containing micronutrients are less liked by them. Most of the time there is gap between demand and supply, which increases deficiency states like nutritional anemia. Anemia is common in adolescents, and affects their physical growth and well-being and may have long-standing consequences as cognitive changes and poor academic performance. All the changes put acute stress on erythropoiesis during adolescent age group. Hence, iron and folic acid prophylaxis is part of the national program.

Anemia may be due to both nutritional and nonnutritional factors, of which iron deficiency is overwhelmingly the most prevalent cause.

## ■ DEFINITION

Anemia is present when there is decreased oxygen-carrying capacity of blood due to deficiency of hemoglobin (Hb) in the red blood cells (RBCs) for particular age and sex **(Table 1)**.

*Anemia is defined as blood Hb levels <120 g/L (i.e., <12 mg/dL) in adolescents.*

During adolescence, the adequate level of Hb depends on age and sexual maturity **(Table 2)**.

## ■ ETIOLOGY OF ANEMIA IN ADOLESCENCE

### Nutritional Causes

- *Iron deficiency:*
  - *Decreased intake:*
    - A high-carbohydrate diet rich in phytates, with minimal intake of fruit/dark green leafy vegetables/meat
    - Strict vegetarian diet has low bioavailability of iron
    - Routine intake of junk food low in iron
    - Dieting and meal-skipping
    - Absence of absorption enhancers like vitamin C
    - *Presence of inhibitors:* Tea and coffee consumed along with meals
  - *Increased loss:*
    - Menstruation, especially menorrhagia
  - *Increased requirement:*
    - The pubertal growth spurt increases lean body mass, blood volume, and red cell mass, which

**TABLE 1:** Cut offs for Hb level for anemia in adolescents.

| Age group | No anemia | Mild | Moderate | Severe |
|---|---|---|---|---|
| 10–11 years | >11.5% | 11–11.9 | 8–10.9 | <8% |
| 12–14 years | >12% | 11–11.9 | 8–10.9 | <8% |
| Nonpregnant women 15 years and above | >12% | 11–11.9 | 8–10.9 | <8% |

*Source*: WHO. Nutritional Anemia: Tools for Effective Prevention and Control, 2017.

**TABLE 2:** Criteria for diagnosis of anemia (Hb levels—WHO).

| NFHS | Girls aged 15–19 years, anemic <12 g/dL | Boys aged 15–19 years, anemic <13 g/dL | Pregnant women age 15–49 years, anemic <11 g/dL |
|---|---|---|---|
| NFHS 5 | 59.1% | 31.1% | 52.2% |
| NFHS4 | 54.1% | 29.2% | 50.4% |

(NFHS: National Family Health Survey; WHO: World Health Organization)
*Source*: WHO. Nutritional Anemia: Tools for Effective Prevention and Control, 2017.

increase iron needs for myoglobin in muscles and Hb in the blood.

- Teenage pregnancy
- *$B_{12}$ deficiency:* Vegetarian diet, malabsorption due to intestinal parasites.

## Nonnutritional Causes

- *Malaria: Plasmodium falciparum* and *vivax* rupture RBCs, and suppress production of RBCs in the bone marrow
- *Helminthiasis:* Hookworm causes chronic blood loss; roundworm and whipworm cause malabsorption.
- Inherited genetic disorders, e.g., sickle cell anemia, thalassemia, hereditary spherocytosis, and glucose-6-phosphate dehydrogenase (G6PD) deficiency
- Autoimmune disorders [systemic lupus erythematosus (SLE) and autoimmune hemolytic anemia]
- Involvement of bone marrow in viral infections such as cytomegalovirus (CMV), human immunodeficiency virus (HIV), and infiltration with malignancy
- Chronic inflammatory diseases.

## ■ CLINICAL FEATURES

*History taking:* Most patients with mild anemia are asymptomatic. There may be a lack of interest in play and studies, poor concentration, leg cramps, and increased susceptibility to infections. Adolescents with severe anemia may complain of dizziness, tiredness, fatigue, exertional tachycardia and dyspnea, and frequent headaches.

A HEEADSSS screen is informative:

- Home—family history of blood transfusions, anemia, or jaundice
- Education—poor scholastic performance
- Eating—detailed nutritional history, e.g., routine intake of cereals/fruits/vegetables/pulses/nuts, whether they are strict vegetarians, dieting, skipping breakfast, frequency of junk food consumption, eating out, consuming tea or coffee with meals, bingeing and purging, body image concerns, and recent weight gain or loss.
- Activities—involvement in games and sports, fatigue
- Sexuality—menstrual history, pregnancy.

*Examination:* The major signs are pallor noted in the eyes, tongue, nail and palms, glossitis, angular cheilitis, and koilonychia. There may also be features of the disease that caused anemia, like hepatosplenomegaly.

*Investigations:* The initial investigation consists of a complete hemogram, which would reveal a microcytic hypochromic picture in iron deficiency anemia (IDA), and normal white blood cell (WBC) and platelet counts and morphology. Based on the clinical picture, one might decide on a thick smear for malaria parasite, stool examination for occult blood, serum iron studies to confirm iron deficiency, serum $B_{12}$ levels, serum electrophoresis, a bone marrow examination, etc.

## ■ TREATMENT

Treatment depends on the severity of anemia and rapidity of its development and etiology. Clinical examination and complete blood count (CBC) with peripheral smear examination are likely to provide enough clues.

- The cause of the anemia should be treated. $B_{12}$ supplementation is essential in $B_{12}$ deficiency. Folic acid supplementation is required in hemolytic anemias with high serum iron.
- Treatment of iron deficiency consists of proper diet, oral iron administration, and if necessary intravenous iron therapy, and packed cell transfusion.

### Dietary Modifications

Advice against junk food, a monotonous high-carbohydrate diet, and dieting. Promote intake of:

- Iron-rich foods like meat, chicken, eggs, fish, pulses, groundnuts, ragi, dark green leafy vegetables, and jaggery.
- Vitamin C-rich foods like lime and oranges
- Vitamin $B_{12}$-rich foods like eggs, fish, mutton, chicken, mushrooms, milk, and dairy products.

### Iron Therapy—Oral

- 3–6 mg/kg/day of elemental iron in two doses, up to a maximum of 150–200 mg daily. (e.g., ferrous sulfate/fumarate)
- Folic acid and vitamin $B_{12}$ supplementation (1,000 µg of $B_{12}$ stat, followed by 250–500 µg weekly for 3 months). Some of them may require monthly injection of vitamin $B_{12}$ 1,000 µg in case of poor absorption.
- Check Hb and reticulocyte count at the end of 1 week; Hb remains the same while reticulocyte count responds by 3–5 days, and peaks by 7 days.
- Repeat Hb at 1 month to confirm rise in Hb; Hb normalizes by 3 months. If no response, consider other causes, like thalassemia minor or anemia of chronic infection.

- Continue iron for another 3 months after Hb normalizes to replenish stores and thereafter give weekly prophylaxis to prevent anemia.

## Intravenous Iron Therapy

It is useful in:
- Reduced patient compliance to oral iron due to side effects
- Ineffective oral iron therapy when the gut is impaired, due to diseases like coeliac disease
- Severe iron deficiency.

## Blood Transfusion

Blood transfusion may be required when there is severe or continuous blood loss, as in menorrhagia or gastro-intestinal (GI) bleeding. The World Health Organization (WHO) recommends blood transfusion if Hb <4g/dL, or Hb is 4–6 g/dL associated with cardiac failure. Transfuse 5–10 mL/kg of packed red blood cells (PRBC) over 4 hours with close cardiac monitoring and administration of furosemide.

## PREVENTION OF IRON DEFICIENCY ANEMIA

- *Dietary modifications:* As mentioned earlier
- *Oral iron supplementation:* Weekly iron folate supplementation (WIFS) with 1 blue tablet (containing 60 mg of elemental iron and 500 µg of folic acid), which is given by the teacher in school every Monday to every adolescent aged 10–19 years. Out-of-school adolescent girls 10–19 years will be provided the tablets through the quarterly Adolescent Health Day component of the Rashtriya Kishore Swasthya Karyakram (RKSK) program at Anganwadi centers **(Table 3)**.
- *Twice-yearly deworming* on 10 February and 10 August.

## ANEMIA MUKT BHARAT

This campaign specifies six interventions:
- Prophylactic iron folic acid supplementation
- Bi-annual deworming
- Intensified year-round behavior change communica-tion campaign (Solid Body, Smart Mind) focusing on four key behaviors:
  - Improving compliance to iron folic acid supplementation and deworming
  - Appropriate infant and young child feeding practices

**TABLE 3:** Prophylactic dose and regime for iron folic acid supplementation.

| Age group | Dose and regimen |
|---|---|
| Children 6–59 months of age biweekly, 1 mL iron and folic acid syrup | Each mL of iron and folic acid syrup containing 20 mg elemental iron + 100 µg of folic acid bottle (50 mL) to have an "autodispenser" and information leaflet as per MoHFW guidelines in the monocarton |
| 5–9 years of age | Weekly, 1 iron and folic acid tablet. Each tablet containing 45 mg elemental iron + 400 µg folic acid, sugar-coated, pink color |
| Children school-going adolescent girls and boys, 10–19 years of age out-of-school adolescent girls, 10–19 years of age | Weekly, 1 iron and folic acid tablet. Each tablet containing 60 mg elemental iron + 500 µg folic acid, sugar-coated, blue color |

(IFA: iron folic acid; MoHFW: Ministry of Health and Family Welfare; SAM: severe acute malnutrition)
*Note 1:* Prophylaxis with iron should be withheld in case of acute illness (fever, diarrhea, pneumonia, etc.), and in a known case of thalassemia major/history of repeated blood transfusion.
In case of SAM children, IFA supplementation should be continued as per SAM management protocol.
*Source:* Age group and dose and regime—Anemia Mukt Bharat Portal.

  - Increase in intake of iron-rich **(Table 4)**, protein-rich, and vitamin C-rich food through diet diversity/quantity/frequency and/or fortified foods with focus on harnessing locally available resources
  - Ensuring delayed cord clamping after delivery (by 3 minutes) in health facilities
- Testing of anemia using digital hemoglobinometers, and point-of-care treatment for adolescent anemia with two blue tablets once daily after food for 3 months. If Hb levels have normalized, continue with weekly prophylaxis. If no response, or in all adolescents with Hb <8, refer to the FRU (first referral units)
- Mandatory provision of iron folic acid fortified food in public health programs.
- Intensifying awareness, screening, and treatment of nonnutritional causes of anemia in endemic pockets, with special focus on malaria, hemoglobinopathies, and fluorosis.

## KEY MESSAGES

- Anemia is common in adolescents, and iron deficiency is the most common cause.

| **TABLE 4:** Best vegetarian sources of iron. | |
|---|---|
| *Leaves* | *Per 100 g serving* |
| Curry leaves | 8.7 mg |
| Mint leaves | 8.6 mg |
| Beet greens | 5.6 mg |
| Fenugreek leaves | 5.6 mg |
| Parsley | 5.5 mg |
| Drumstick leaves | 4.6 mg |
| Radish leaves | 3.8 mg |
| Spinach leaves | 2.9 mg |
| Mustard leaves | 2.8 mg |
| *Nuts and fruits* | *Per 100 g serving* |
| Gingelly seeds | 14.9 mg |
| Pistachios | 7.3 mg |
| Cashews | 5.9 mg |
| Dried apricots | 4.4 mg |
| Dried figs | 3.2 mg |
| Almonds | 3.6 mg |
| *Pulses* | *Per 100 gm serving* |
| Horse gram | 8.2 mg |
| Soyabean | 8.2 mg |
| Moth beans | 7.9 mg |
| Bengal gram (whole) | 6.8 mg |
| Rajma | 6.3 mg |
| Black gram (whole) | 6.0 mg |
| Green gram | 3.9 mg |
| Red gram | 3.9 mg |
| *Grains and cereals* | *Per 100 g serving* |
| Bajra | 6.4 mg |
| Ragi | 4.6 mg |
| Rice flakes | 4.5 mg |
| Whole wheat atta | 4.1 mg |
| Jowar | 3.9 mg |
| Brown rice | 1.02 mg |
| Tofu | 2.8 mg |

*Source*: Taneja DK, Rai SK, Yadav K. Evaluation of promotion of iron-rich foods for the prevention of nutritional anemia in India. Indian J Public Health. 2020;64.3:236.
InformedHealth.org [Internet]. (2006). How can I get enough iron? Available from Cologne, Germany: Institute for Quality and Efficiency in Health Care (IQWiG). [online]. https://www.ncbi.nlm.nih.gov/books/NBK279618/ [Last accessed March, 2024].

- Hb should be at least 12 g from 12 years onward.
- Iron deficiency in adolescents is due to low intake of iron-rich food, loss through menstruation, and increased requirement for pubertal body growth and increased blood volume and muscle mass.
- Other important causes include malaria, helminthiasis, sickle cell anemia, and thalassemia.
- Mild anemia is asymptomatic or associated with nonspecific symptoms like tiredness, lethargy, and poor concentration.
- Treatment of IDA includes nutritional advice about iron-rich food, oral iron supplementation, and occasionally intravenous iron therapy or blood transfusion.
- The Anemia Mukt Bharat campaign focuses on six interventions.
  - Weekly iron folate supplementation to all adolescents every Monday
  - Bi-annual deworming
  - Behavioral change educational campaign to promote WIFS, deworming, proper weaning and infant feeding, consuming the right food, and delaying cord clamping
  - Iron folate fortified food in public health programs
  - Detection and treatment of nonnutritional causes of anemia like malaria, hemoglobinopathies, and fluorosis.

## ■ RECOMMENDED READING


1. Chandra J, Dewan P, Kumar P, Mahajan A, Singh P, Dhingra B, et al. Diagnosis, Treatment and Prevention of Nutritional Anemia in Children: Recommendations of the Joint Committee of Pediatric Hematology-Oncology Chapter and Pediatric and Adolescent Nutrition Society of the Indian Academy of Pediatrics. Indian Pediatr. 2022;59(10): 782-801.
2. Operational Guideline. [online] Available from https://anemiamuktbharat.info/resources/home#Operational%20Guideline. [Last accessed March, 2024].
3. Upadhye JV, Upadhye JJ. Assessment of anaemia in adolescent girls. Int J Reprod Contracept Obstet Gynecol 2017;6:3113-7.
4. World Health Organization. Regional Office for South-East Asia. (2011). Prevention of iron deficiency anaemia in adolescents. WHO Regional Office for South-East Asia. [online] Available from https://iris.who.int/handle/10665/205656 [Last accessed March, 2024].

<table><tr><td>**5.7**</td><td># Adolescent Obesity</td></tr></table>

*Jugesh Chhatwal, Geeta Patil*

## INTRODUCTION

Obesity has been classified as a chronic, relapsing, multifactorial disease by the International Classification of Diseases 10 (ICD-10). Obesity often starts early in life and tracks into adulthood. The concerns relate not only to the occurrence of obesity per se but also as a risk factor for occurrence of many comorbidities, long-term morbidity, and early mortality.

Childhood obesity is a growing public health problem in many countries of all levels and is rising fastest in emerging economies. The increase in spending power, marketing, and easy availability of calorie-dense foods in combination with declining open cityscapes for physical movement, increasing screen time, and the academic achievement pressures on children have all been contributing to what is now comprehensively termed as "The Obesogenic environment." The net effect of this is a positive balance of calories leading to adiposity.

## PREVALENCE

Obesity has been considered as a global health problem for all age groups, from early childhood to adults. Once obesity was considered as a problem of higher income countries but now has reached epidemic proportions even in middle and low income countries. Considering the global increasing trend, the World Health Organization (WHO) formed the commission on "Ending Childhood Obesity" in 2014, which has developed a comprehensive, integrated package of recommendations to address childhood obesity. In 2019, the World Obesity Federation estimated there would be 206 million children and adolescents aged 5–19 years living with obesity in 2025. The annual increase in child obesity from 2010–2030 is projected as 10.8%, which is very high. Of the 42 countries estimated to have more than one million children with obesity in 2030, the top ranked are China, followed by India and the USA. In India, various studies from different parts of the country from year 2003–2021 have given a wide range of prevalence for overweight as 3–35.8% and obesity as 2–24.6%. The Comprehensive National Nutrition Survey (CNNS) (2016–2018) has given much lower rates.

## DEFINITIONS

The American Heart Association (AHA) defines pediatric overweight and obesity as below:

- *Overweight:* Body mass index (BMI) is ≥85th percentile but <95th percentile for age and sex (corresponding with an adult BMI of 25 kg/m$^2$).
- *Obesity:* BMI is ≥95th percentile (corresponding with an adult BMI of 30 kg/m$^2$).

Indian Academy of Pediatrics (IAP) guidelines 2023 using IAP 2015 BMI charts for age 5–18 years defines them as below:

- *Overweight:* BMI cut offs equivalent to adult BMI of 23 kg/m$^2$
- *Obesity:* Equivalent to adult BMI of 27 kg/m$^2$

Obesity has been categorized as exogenous (primary) or endogenous (secondary).

- *Exogenous or primary obesity:* The primary causes of exogenous obesity are factors outside the body and a net positive balance of calories, most often related to lifestyle. This is the major category seen in clinical practice (90%).
- *Endogenous or secondary obesity:* This is secondary to conditions within the body related to underlying genetic, endocrine (1%), or other conditions, and is much less common **(Table 1)**.
  - *Neurological/hypothalamic causes:* Space occupying lesion (SOL) like craniopharyngioma, glioma, hamartoma, histiocytosis, tuberculoma, trauma, radiotherapy, ROHHAD (rapid-onset obesity, hypothalamic dysregulation, hypoventilation, and anatomic dysregulation)
  - *Drug-induced:* Glucocorticoids, antipsychotics, and antiepileptics
  - Psychological depressive disorders and eating disorders
  - Emotional deprivation, neglect, abuse, and over-protective parents.

## RISK FACTORS

There are a number of risk factors that are considered important and significant for development of obesity.

**TABLE 1:** Causes of endogenous obesity.

| Genetic | Endocrine | Syndromic |
|---|---|---|
| Leptin or leptin receptor gene deficiency | Cushing syndrome | Alstrom syndrome |
| Melanocortin-4 receptor gene mutation | Growth hormone deficiency | Bardet–Biedl syndrome |
| Deletion 9q34 | Hyperinsulinism | Carpenter syndrome |
| *ENPP1* gene mutations | Hypothyroidism | Down syndrome |
| Pro-opiomelanocortin deficiency | Pseudohypo-parathyroidism | Prader–Willi syndrome |
| | Cushing syndrome | • Turner syndrome<br>• Froehlich syndrome |

A comprehensive socioecological framework of the associations and risk factors as shown in **Table 2** is useful to understand the diverse nature of the influences on development and progression of obesity.

Obesogenic environment refers to a setting, such as a home, school, and community, that encourages weight gain and is not supportive of weight loss.

## ■ CLINICAL WORK-UP

The clinical work-up for an adolescent with obesity must be comprehensive, which will identify the etiology of obesity and associated comorbidities.

Investigations and structured management strategies for sustained weight loss and no relapse should be planned accordingly.

## History

*History of present illness:* Obtain weight trajectory from prenatal period, maternal weight gain, and onward. A weight or BMI charts are preferable. A system review includes the symptoms as seen in **Table 3**.

- *Birth history:* Maternal weight, birth weight, and perinatal complications
- *Family history:* Parent health status, viz. obesity and related illnesses
- *Medication history:* Corticosteroids, antipsychotics, and antiepileptics
- *Social and psychosocial history:* Family routines, neighborhood, school, and friends
- *Dietary history:* 24-hour recall; outside foods, sugar-sweetened beverages, eating habits, portion size, fruit/vegetable consumption, snacking, and bingeing

**TABLE 2:** Socioecological influences and risks for exogenous obesity.

| Individual factors | Family- and peers-related factors |
|---|---|
| • Nonmodifiable biology (e.g., genes)<br>• Race or ethnicity<br>• *Early life factors*: Maternal obesity, excessive gestational weight gain, gestational diabetes, high birth weight, early complementary feeding, lack of breastfeeding, nonresponsive infant feeding, exposure to smoke, antibiotic exposure, and early life events<br>• Psychosocial health | • Family socioeconomics and structure<br>• Family food security<br>• Family modeling of healthy eating, recreation, screen behaviors, and sleep<br>• Parental weight status<br>• Family feeding and parenting practices<br>• Peer support for healthy lifestyles<br>• Family psychosocial stress |
| **School factors** | **Community factors** |
| • School food and activity patterns<br>• Family involvement<br>• Bullying/stigmatization | • Safe walking spaces and recreation areas<br>• Availability of healthy foods in local market and fast food outlets<br>• Food marketing practices |
| **Society factors** | **Policy level factors** |
| • Media food marketing policies<br>• Cultural norms on food, weight, physical activity, and screen viewing | *At all levels, policies on:* Agriculture and food, transport, food marketing and labeling, media advertisements of HFSS (high in fat, salt, and sugar), and paucity of public grounds and gardens |

**TABLE 3:** Symptom review.

| System | Symptoms |
|---|---|
| Respiratory | Shortness of breath, snoring, apnea, and disordered sleep—OSA |
| GIT | Abdominal pain, heartburn, dysphagia, chest pain, regurgitation, encopresis, anorexia, constipation, and hyperphagia |
| Endocrine | Polyuria and polydipsia |
| Orthopedic | Pain in the hip, thigh, groin, knee, foot or back; painful or uneven gait; muscle wasting |
| CNS | Morning headaches, persistent headache, and daytime sleepiness |
| Skin | Intertrigo, darkened skin, pustules/abscesses, hirsutism (girls), and striae |

(CNS: central nervous system; GIT: gastrointestinal tract; OSA: obstructive sleep apnea)

- *Development/school history:* Delayed development and school grades
- *Activity history and sleep:* 24-hour recall (school and home), nonexercise activity thermogenesis (NEAT, i.e., activity other than exercise or sleeping, like walking to school, house work, going shopping, and climbing the stairs); sleep duration and pattern, and hours/day of total physical activity
- *Media habits:* Type of media screens used (computer/TV, etc.), type of programs, duration, and total screen time in hours/day
- *Menstrual history (for girls):* Menarche age, menstrual pattern, and dysmenorrhea.

## ■ EXAMINATION

**Table 4** depicts the general and systemic examination. Some of the markers of endogenous obesity are shown in **Box 1**.

*Measurements:* Accurate anthropometric measurements are essential. The measurements must include weight (in kg), standing height (in cm), and calculation of BMI by using the formula: Wt in kg/(Ht in m)$^2$. Midparental height should also be estimated. All measurements should be plotted on the IAP 2015 growth charts (ages 5–15 years).

The waist circumference (WC) [cut off value is 70th percentile for metabolic syndrome (MS)] is a defining factor for MS in children and adolescents 10–16 years of age, and is a finding of concern in children 6–10 years old. It should be measured in the standing position at the level of the iliac crest. WC is an important predictor of visceral obesity which is associated with MS.

Recently, measures such as wrist circumference are used to identify metabolic risk as it is easy to measure and more socially acceptable. More studies are required to validate the cut offs.

## ■ COMPLICATIONS

- *Pulmonary:* Sleep abnormalities—OSA and hypoventilation syndrome—asthma
- *Neurological:* Pseudotumor cerebri and migraine
- *Orthopedic:* SCFE (slipped capital femoral epiphysis), osteoarthritis, and Blount disease
- *Mental health:* Low self-esteem, depression, anxiety, and poor school performance
- Body image issue and eating disorders
- *Endocrinological:* Insulin resistance + type 2 diabetes mellitus (DM), pubertal advancement, menstrual abnormalities, and polycystic ovarian disease (PCOD)

**TABLE 4:** General and systemic examination.

| | |
|---|---|
| General | Dysmorphic features, developmental delay, skin tags, extreme acne, hirsutism in girls, edema, and thyroid examination |
| Vital signs | *Blood pressure:* SBP or DBP >95th percentile, on at least three readings, using height/age/sex percentile normalized tables to interpret; heart rate |
| HEENT (head, eyes, ears, nose, and throat) | Papilledema, dental caries, and periodontal disease |
| Chest | Gynecomastia >2 cm of breast tissue in boys and cervicodorsal hump |
| Cardiorespiratory | Asthma, obstructive sleep apnea, impaired exercise tolerance, sleep disorders, and hypoventilation syndrome |
| Gastrointestinal | Liver enlargement, abdominal tenderness (gallstones/liver tenderness) fecal masses (constipation), and GERD |
| Genitourinary | *Buried penis:* Suprapubic fat accumulation leading to the appearance of a shortened penile shaft |
| Musculoskeletal | Gait, hip pain and/or limp, knee pain, bowlegs or knock knee, flat feet, tibial bowing, and impaired balance and coordination |
| Skin | *Acanthosis:* Thickened, darkened skin at the nape of neck (99%), axillae (73%), less commonly groin, eyelids, and hands. Hirsutism, acne, striae, intertrigo, and pannus (excess skin and subcutaneous fat below the umbilicus) |
| Mental health issues | Depression and body image issue |

(DBP: diastolic blood pressure; GERD: gastroesophageal reflux disease; SBP: systolic blood pressure)

**BOX 1:** Common features in genetic syndromes.

- Hypotonia
- Hyperphagia
- Failure to thrive in infancy followed by weight gain
- Short stature and hypogonadism
- Skeletal defects
- Renal abnormalities/impairment
- Frequent infections
- Obsessive behaviors
- Neurobehavioral abnormalities
- Autistic behavior and hyperactivity
- Impaired olfaction, retinal dystrophy or pigmentary retinopathy, and deafness
- Autonomic dysfunction
- Speech and language delay
- Sleep disturbances

- *Cardiovascular:* Hypertension, MS, dyslipidemia, and coronary artery disease
- *Nonalcoholic fatty liver disease (NAFLD)/metabolic dysfunction-associated steatotic liver disease (MASLD)* (34% in obese children) and gallbladder disease
- *Malignancy:* Breast, uterus, prostrate, and colorectal.

Obesity is associated with *chronic inflammatory process* characterized by the increase in circulating levels of proinflammatory cytokines, such as interleukin 6 (IL-6), tumor necrosis factor alpha (TNF-$\alpha$), and C-reactive protein (CRP) in healthy obese people by white adipose tissue. This makes them prone for infections.

## POINTERS TO COMPLICATIONS WHICH REQUIRE IMMEDIATE ATTENTION

Headache, hypertension—benign raised intracranial tension (pseudotumor cerebri), especially in:
- Obese girls
- Daytime somnolence—OSA
- Abdominal pain—gallstone, renal stones, and DM
- SCFE
- Osteoarthritis and Blount disease
- Cutaneous acanthosis—insulin resistance

*Staging of obesity:* As per Pediatric Endocrine Society and American Academy of Pediatrics (AAP) guidelines for childhood obesity, the staging can be done as follows: *Class 2 obesity:* ≥120 to <140% of 95th percentile or BMI ≥35 kg/m$^2$ to <40 kg/m$^2$ whichever is lower, based on age and gender. *Class 3 obesity:* ≥140% of the 95th percentile or BMI ≥40 kg/m$^2$ whichever is lower, based on age and gender. Classes 2 and 3 are considered as Severe Obesity (refer to IAP Extended BMI Charts 1 and 2 in *Annexure*).

## INVESTIGATIONS

Investigations are required either for etiology or for screening comorbidities. For etiology, they are indicated only when physical growth or velocity of growth is affected or there are specific markers on history and physical examination. Routine endocrine or genetic work-up is not required. All overweight (BMI ≥85th percentile to <95th percentile) children 10 years and older should be evaluated for lipid abnormalities. Adolescents with obesity (BMI ≥95th percentile) or WC >70th centile need evaluation for lipid abnormalities, abnormal glucose metabolism, and liver function. See **Table 5** for investigations cutoffs.

Children and adolescents with obesity are at the higher risk for hypertension (5–30%) and dyslipidemia.

**TABLE 5:** Cutoffs for metabolic comorbidities.

| Investigations | Levels of concern | Pathological level |
|---|---|---|
| Fasting blood sugar | 100–125 mg/dL | ≥126 mg/dL |
| Blood sugar >2 hours after glucose | 140–199 mg/dL | ≥200 mg/dL |
| HbA1c | 5.7–6.4% | ≥6.5% |
| Total cholesterol | 170–199 mg/dL | ≥200 mg/dL |
| LDL | 110–129 mg/dL | ≥130 mg/dL |
| Triglyceride | 90–129 mg/dL | ≥130 mg/dL |
| HDL | 40–45 mg/dL | <40 mg/dL |
| ALT (SGPT) | >26 IU/L (boys) >22 IU/L (girls) | ≥60 IU/L |

(ALT: alanine aminotransferase; HbA1c: hemoglobin A1c; HDL: high-density lipoprotein; LDL: low density lipoprotein; SGPT: serum glutamic pyruvic transaminase)

Prevalence of MS is 13.6% in overweight and 46.4% in obese Indian children. Indians are likely to develop MS at lower BMI and WC.

In obese adolescent girls, evaluation for PCOD is indicated if, 2 years after menarche, she has hyper-androgenemia (hirsutism and acne) along with ovarian dysfunction (irregular menstrual cycles <20 or >45 days). (Refer for the details to PCOS Guidelines in Endocrinology chapter)

Other causes should be ruled out. Possible investigations include 17-hydroxyprogesterone, total and free testosterone, dehydroepiandrosterone sulfate, androstenedione, luteinizing hormone, follicle-stimulating hormone, estradiol, prolactin, thyroid function tests, and insulin.

In obese children thyroid functions should be carefully interpreted. The mild thyroid-stimulating hormone (TSH) elevation is due to peripheral resistance to thyroid hormone as well as due to increased hypothalamic thyrotropin-releasing hormone (TRH) drive caused by increased leptin levels.

*Inference:*
- Tall and fat—usual cause is exogenous and requires lifestyle modifications.
- Short- and fat-endogenous, requires to be investigated.

## MANAGEMENT

The goals of treating adolescent obesity are:
- Reduce adiposity
- Prevent or improve and monitor-related physical comorbidities

- Prevent or improve psychosocial complications
- Prevent the development of chronic diseases
- Improve lifestyle pattern for lifelong prevention/relapses
- Provide ongoing medical support.

Treatment must be tailored to the severity of the obesity, age, and developmental stage of the adolescent, and needs and preferences of the patient and family. Integration of multiple components, viz. nutrition, exercise and psychological therapy, pharmacotherapy, and surgical procedures is required. Providing behavioral support and nonstigmatizing, nonjudgmental communication is essential. The stage-wise treatment as shown in **Table 6** is useful for a comprehensive approach. For overweight and obese adolescents, Stage 1 or Prevention Plus is appropriate to begin with whereas those with class 2 or 3 obesity can be started with Stage 2, if willing.

*Intensive health behavior lifestyle:* Lifestyle modification includes dietary management, enhancement of physical activity, and restriction of sedentary behavior. The treatment must be focused, goal-directed, and patient-centered.

*Dietary interventions* should focus on decreasing consumption of fast foods and processed foods and elimination of sugar-sweetened beverages including fruit juices. Dietary interventions also include portion control education, timely regular meals, and avoiding constant "grazing" during the day, especially after school. Limit snacking. Recognize eating cues in the adolescent's environment, such as boredom, stress, loneliness, or screen time. Encourage mindful eating. The principal of 5-2-1-0 must be followed. Avoid fourth meal (midnight) meal.

Use of recommended daily allowances (RDA), the estimated average requirement (EAR), and tolerable upper limits tables to be done (refer to *Chapter 5.1*).

Many obese adolescents are prone for iron, vitamin $B_{12}$, zinc, and vitamin D deficiency and should be addressed timely.

Traffic light approach is very effective and is one of the sustainable intervention. My plate approach to be adapted to different cultures.

Schools should not serve ultra-processed foods and teaching staff should educate the teens and parents.

*Physical activity* as per age, gender, socioeconomic status, disability/fitness level 60 min/day and 6–7 days/week includes vigorous muscle and bone-building activity 3–4 times/week, minimum for 20 minutes. Physical activity can be different on different days of the week, e.g., skipping, jogging/running, swimming, dancing, football, hockey, tennis, squats, weight lifting, and push-ups. Allow the adolescent to make a choice.

**TABLE 6:** Staged treatment for obesity.

| | |
|---|---|
| *Stage 1:* Prevention Plus (PP) | • At the primary care office<br>• Promote a healthy "5-2-1-0" lifestyle (eat 5 fruits and vegetables daily, limit screen-time to ≤2 h/day, ≥1 hour of physical activity, and 0 sugary drinks)<br>• The expected outcome is reduced BMI<br>• Monthly follow-up of child and family<br>• Failure to respond after 6 months of this strategy indicates an intensification of intervention to Stage 2 |
| *Stage 2:* Structured Weight Management (SWM) | • In the primary care office with support<br>• Focus on target behaviors such as structured daily meals, healthy snacks, reduced screen time, and physical activity<br>• The goal is weight loss of no more than $1/_2$ kg per month for children 2–11 years of age and no more than 1 kg per week for adolescents<br>• If there is no change in BMI after 6 months, management should move to Stage 3 |
| *Stage 3:* Comprehensive Multidisciplinary Intervention (CMI) | • At a pediatric weight management center with a multidisciplinary team<br>• Focus on a structured behavior modification program that includes a "short-term" diet plan, physical activity as per individually set goals, and parental involvement, especially if the child is 12 years or younger<br>• The outcome expected is weight loss or reduction in BMI with a goal of BMI maintenance below the overweight cut off<br>• Frequent office evaluation visits for a minimum of 8–12 weeks<br>• Failure to achieve these goals will need Stage 4 care |
| *Stage 4:* Tertiary Care Intervention (TCI) | • In a tertiary care center<br>• The child may have significant comorbidities requiring hospitalized care<br>• Focus is on continued diet and physical activity counseling<br>• May be offered a very low-calorie diet and medications in some cases of severe obesity when there is no response to behavioral interventions |

*Sedentary behavior:* Screen time should be ≤2 hours. Limit nonacademic screen time, take breaks every 20 minutes of sitting time, increase active time by helping in house/using stairs/walking to the nearby shops, etc. Maintaining sleep hygiene is also very important.

*Motivational interviewing:* Behavior change is an implicit underlying requirement for successful treatment of obesity and it is critical for behavior change that the motivation must come from the patient. Motivational interviewing is helpful for approaching behavioral change.

*Pharmacotherapy:* Limited use in clinical practice and requires careful assessment for indication as well as close monitoring for adverse effects. It must always be instituted with lifestyle modifications. Adjunct use of pharmacotherapy to a comprehensive lifestyle modification program may be recommended in adolescents ≥12 years of age having Class 2 obesity with immediate or life-threatening comorbidities or Class 3 obesity with or without comorbidities. There are a few drugs that are approved for use in adolescents, viz. liraglutide and orlistat and phentermine for >16 years.

*Surgical management:* Metabolic and bariatric surgery is only considered for BMI ≥35 kg/m$^2$ or 120% of the 95th percentile for age and sex, whichever is lower; with comorbidities and BMI ≥40 kg/m$^2$ or 140% of the 95th percentile for age and sex, with or without comorbidities, completion of linear growth. The types of surgery usually done are sleeve gastrectomy or Roux-en-Y gastric bypass.

## ■ PREVENTION

*Preventing relapses:* Relapses are a frequent occurrence as up to 90% regain weight in the coming years. Sustained weight loss is mainly seen with bariatric surgery. Causes of weight regain are poorly understood. There are multiple challenges to weight maintenance: Easily available calorie-dense foods are a big temptation, physiologically the food deprived has increased sensitivity, and neuroendocrine mechanisms promote eating. In addition, physical activity is not sustained due to factors like lack of time, decreased confidence, motivation, and energy levels over a period of time.

*Preventing obesity:* Prevention of obesity requires a multi-level and multisectoral approach as there are many stake-holders involved. The socioecological influences as shown in **Table 2** need to be addressed at all levels, starting from the mother to the level of the policy makers, for any significant impact.

## ■ KEY MESSAGES

- Obesity is a chronic disease and requires long-term (usually lifelong) management.
- Early, regular screening of weight and weight trajectory is essential for early intervention. WC should be measured in all overweight and obese children to assess metabolic risk.
- A multidisciplinary approach is necessary with primary focus on lifestyle and behavior modification.
- Management (screening and treatment) of obesity-associated complications is essential.
- A developmentally appropriate approach, support for long-term behavioral change, and long-term weight maintenance strategies should be used.
- Obesity is often a multigenerational disease and requires a family-focused approach.
- Obese adolescents should be approached in a positive and compassionate manner without stigmatizing.
- Pharmacotherapy and bariatric surgery are the last resort.

## ■ RECOMMENDED READING

1. Barlow SE, Expert Committee. Expert committee recommendations regarding the prevention, assessment, and treatment of child and adolescent overweight and obesity: summary report. Pediatrics. 2007;120(Suppl 4): S164-9217.
2. Hall K, Gibbie T, Lubman DI. Motivational interviewing techniques—facilitating behaviour change in the general practice setting. Aust Fam Physician. 2012;41(9):660-7.
3. Hampl SE, Hassink SG, Skinner AC, Armstrong SC, Barlow SE, Bolling CF, et al. Clinical Practice Guideline for the Evaluation and Treatment of Children and Adolescents with Obesity. Pediatrics. 2023;151(2):e2022060640.
4. Jebeile H, Kelly AS, O'Malley G, Baur LA. Obesity in children and adolescents: epidemiology, causes, assessment, and management. Lancet Diabetes Endocrinol. 2022;10(5): 351-65.
5. Khadilkar A, Ekbote V, Chiplonkar S, Khadilkar V, Kajale N, Kulkarni S, et al. Waist circumference percentiles in 2–18-year-old Indian children. J Pediatr. 2014;164(6): 1358-62.
6. Khadilkar V, Lohiya N, Chiplonkar S, Khadilkar A. Body mass index quick screening tool for Indian Academy of Pediatrics 2015 growth charts. Indian Pediatr. 2020;57:904-6.
7. Khadilkar V, Yadav S, Agrawal KK, Tamboli S, Banerjee M, Cherian A, et al. Revised IAP growth charts for height,

weight and body mass index for 5- to 18-year-old Indian children. Indian Pediatr. 2015;52:47-55.

8. Kirk SF, Penny TL, McHugh TL. Characterizing the obesogenic environment: the state of the evidence with directions for future research. Obes Rev. 2010;11: 109-17.

9. Madhu SV, Nitin K, Sambit D, Nishant R, Sanjay K (on behalf of the Endocrine Society of India). ESI clinical practice guidelines for the evaluation and management of obesity In India. Indian J Endocr Metab. 2022;26:295-318.

10. Obesity data: NCD Risk Factor Collaboration projections by World Obesity NCD premature deaths: World Health Organization Global Health Observatory Obesity—NCD preparedness calculated from multiple metrics (Appendix 1, World Obesity Atlas 2022).

11. Styne DM, Arslanian SA, Connor EL, Farooqi IS, Murad MH, Silverstein JH, et al. Pediatric Obesity—Assessment, Treatment, and Prevention: An Endocrine Society Clinical Practice Guideline. J Clin Endocrinol Metab. 2017;102(3):709-57.

# 5.8 JUNCS, Fad Diets, Supplements, and Energy Drinks for Adolescents

*C P Bansal, Geeta Patil, Ranjith P*

## INTRODUCTION

The acronym JUNCS refers to Junk food, Ultra-processed food, Nutritionally inappropriate foods, Caffeinated/colored/carbonated foods/beverages, and Sugar-sweetened beverages. It attempts to encompass almost all foods that are considered undesirable, whether due to inappropriate nutrient content, method of preparation, addictive palatability, or content of potentially toxic additives or flavors.

## EXAMPLES OF JUNCS

"*J*unk food" refers to foods that are inappropriately high in calories but poor in nutritional value as they are high in fats, sugar, and/or salt but have low content of proteins, vitamins, and minerals.

"*U*ltra-processed foods" are commercially prepared by mixing several ingredients and adding additives such as sugars, flavors, and colors. They are usually nutritionally poor, or high in sugar, salt, or fat, for example, packaged breakfast cereals, ready bread, instant noodles, commercial ice creams and flavored yogurts, margarine, milk supplements, and packaged snacks and chips.

"*N*utritionally inappropriate foods" include snacks like chips and *samosas*, and restaurant foods like pizzas, burgers, French fries, noodles, and pasta.

"*C*affeinated/colored/carbonated foods/beverages" include carbonated drinks and energy drinks.

"*S*ugar-sweetened beverages" include fruit drinks (packaged juices with added sugar) and flavored drinks.

These foods are addictive, as the high levels of sugar and fat trigger the release of dopamine, resulting in a craving for them. In recent years, there has been a noticeable increase in their consumption among adolescents, attributable to taste, free availability, convenience, peer influence, increased purchasing power, and aggressive marketing.

Children and adolescents should limit consumption of these foods at home or outside to not more than one serving per week, the serving not exceeding 50% of the total daily calorie requirement for that age.

## HARMFUL EFFECTS

The harmful effects of JUNCS are as follows:

- Most of these foods are energy-dense due to a disproportionate content of sugar and fats, resulting in excessive weight gain.
- The high sugar, fat, and salt content increases the risk of diabetes mellitus, hypercholesterolemia, and hypertension, and later heart attacks and stroke.
- The high sugar content may lead to dental caries.
- Microbial contamination due to poor hygiene in preparation can lead to gastrointestinal infections such as diarrhea, typhoid, and hepatitis.
- Food additives and coloring agents may cause allergies.
- Some of the additives used in ultra-processed foods may increase the risk of cancer.
- Caffeinated drinks often cause sleep disturbance and irritability. In excess, they may cause arrhythmias, violent behavior, and even psychiatric illness.

## ■ BALANCED DIET FOR ADOLESCENTS

A balanced diet should include all food groups daily. An adolescent boy should eat as much as his father (2,400–2,800 kcal) and a girl more than her mother (2,100–2,400 kcal), depending on whether they are sedentary or into active sports. Carbohydrates should make up 50–65% of energy intake, protein 10–30%, and fat 25–35%. They should avoid skipping meals and eat three major meals (breakfast, lunch, and dinner) daily. They should try to consume a mix of Go, Grow, and Glow foods at every meal.

*Go foods (energy-giving foods) include:*
- *Cereals:* 240–450 g of wheat, rice, maize, jowar, etc.
- *Sugars:* 20–30 g/day
- *Fats and oils:* 35–50 g/day; preferably 10–15 g each of
  - Desi ghee/butter and palm oil
  - Mustard/sesame/groundnut/olive/coconut oil
  - Sunflower/safflower, soyabean, and canola

*Grow foods (growth-promoting foods) include:*
- *Pulses:* 2–3 servings of 30 g each about 2 cooked katori of variety of dal, beans, lentils, etc. For nonvegetarians, one serving of pulses may be replaced by one serving (50 g) of eggs/meat/fish/chicken, etc.
- *Milk and milk products:* 5 servings of 100 mL each. It includes low fat milk, butter milk, curd, cottage cheese, and vegetable milk such as soya, almond and tofu, etc.

*Glow foods (protective foods) include:*
- *Fruits:* Two servings of 80 g each; one medium-sized apple/banana/orange/mango or two small kiwi/plums/apricots or 250 mL of fresh fruit juice. Whole fruits are preferred over fruit juices; avoid packaged fruit juices
- *Green leafy and other vegetables:*
  - 80 g of green leafy vegetable (about 1 cup of green vegetables)
  - One *katori* of other colored vegetables (brinjal, capsicum, pumpkin, tomato, peas, etc.).
  - One serving of tubers, radish, cucumber, etc.

*Others include:*
- 30 g of nuts (a handful of groundnut, cashew, almonds, or walnuts)
- *Fiber:* 15–25 g from fruits, vegetables, whole grain (like whole wheat bread, etc.) is important for bulk, satiety, and prevention of constipation
- *Water:* 1.5–2 L/day

To simplify matters, the US Food and Nutrition Department has come up with "Choose My Plate." In India, the National Institute of Nutrition has introduced an Indian version, the "*Thali*" **(Fig. 1)**. They recommend that half the plate should be filled with fruits and vegetables, while the remaining half should have more of cereals and some proteins (pulses/nonveg foods). It should be accompanied by low-fat milk (200–250 mL) or buttermilk/fresh juice/fresh lime/kanji, etc., Girls need extra iron and calcium.

## ■ FAD DIETS IN ADOLESCENTS

Statistics reveal that >50% of adults in the USA are overweight and have tried dieting at some time. Being

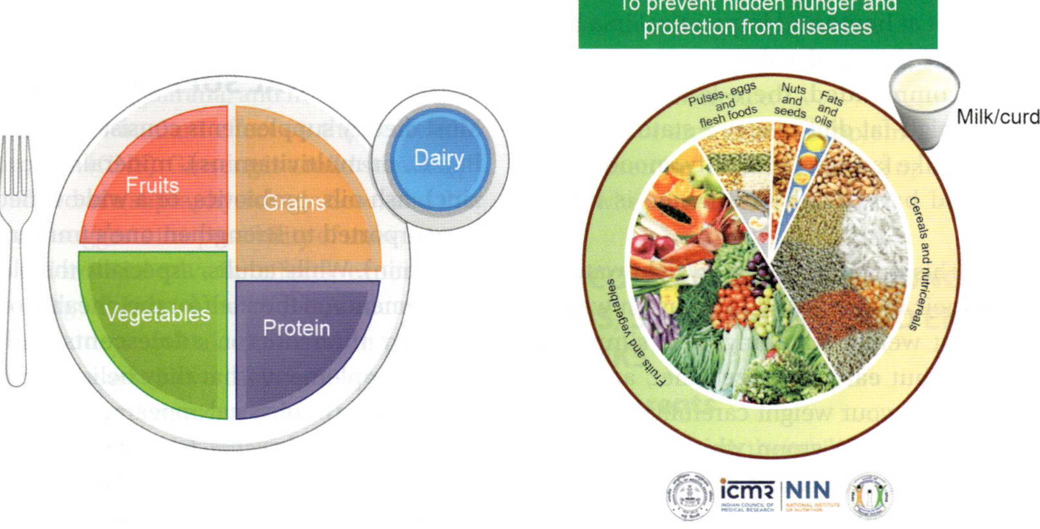


**Fig.1:** A balanced plate recommended by the National Institute of Nutrition (the *Thali*).

video games, and mobile phones should be restricted to <2 hours a day.

- *Use of tobacco, alcohol, and illicit drugs* should be managed by creating awareness and counseling.
- *Health education* in schools and communities should emphasize the importance of a balanced diet, regular exercise, and avoidance of tobacco and alcohol. Adoption of Sankalp Swasthya Sampoorna (SSS) program is an excellent initiative of the Indian Academy of Pediatrics (IAP) in schools for awareness on healthy lifestyle in adolescents.
- *Mental health awareness:* Implement school-based programs, digital resources, and family education.
- *Regular health screening:* Early detection can lead to timely interventions, preventing complications.
- *Policy interventions:* Governments can play a crucial role. Some ideas are as follows:
  - Raise taxes on alcohol and tobacco and enforce the ban on surrogate advertising.
  - Public promotion of balanced diet.
  - Make food labels compulsory.
  - Manage food taxes and subsidies.
  - Promote healthy eating in schools and workplaces.
  - Create safe spaces for physical activities.
  - Restrict marketing of junk food and sugary beverages to children and adolescents.
  - Provide incentives for the food industry to prepare foods with less sodium, trans-fat, and saturated fat.

## INNOVATIONS IN HEALTHCARE DELIVERY

The coronavirus disease 19 (COVID-19) pandemic accelerated the adoption of telehealth, offering opportunities for better NCD management in adolescents. Digital platforms with wearable devices, mobile applications, and online resources provide real-time monitoring and education.

## CONCLUSION

Noncommunicable diseases are a significant concern in adolescents, setting them on a trajectory for lifelong health issues, and require urgent multidimensional interventions. We must recognize the challenges and approach them proactively and holistically, combining advanced medical care, public health strategies, and community engagement, for a healthier future generation.

## KEY MESSAGES

- The four main NCDs are cardiovascular diseases (such as heart attacks and stroke), cancers, chronic respiratory diseases (such as chronic obstructive pulmonary disease and asthma), and diabetes mellitus, and they account for over 70% of all deaths globally.
- Recent studies have shown a rising trend of NCDs among adolescents and young adults in India, and approximately 50% of them have elevated risks of diabetes mellitus, cardiovascular diseases, and hypertension.
- The four major modifiable behaviors that lead to NCDs are tobacco use, unhealthy dietary choices, physical inactivity, and harmful use of alcohol.
- Adolescents consume fried and sugary foods and salt in excess.
- Exposure to pollution, urbanization, and environmental toxins like pesticides increase the risk of NCDs.
- Adolescents with a family history of CAD, diabetes mellitus, or any other NCD should be regularly screened for the same.
- A detailed HEEADSSS screening is essential to pick up the multiple factors associated with NCDs.
- Regular screening and early diagnosis are important for timely management of NCDs.
- Parents should be positive role models on a healthy lifestyle.
- Government policies can restrict use of tobacco, alcohol, and drugs; discourage advertising of harmful substances and unhealthy foods; and create open spaces for physical activity.

## RECOMMENDED READING


1. Abarca-Gómez L, Abdeen ZA, Hamid ZA, Abu-Rmeileh NM, Acosta-Cazares B, Acuin C et al. Worldwide trends in body-mass index, underweight, overweight, and obesity from 1975 to 2016: a pooled analysis of 2416 population-based measurement studies in 1289 million children, adolescents, and adults. Lancet. 2017;390(10113): 2627-42.
2. Dabelea D, Mayer-Davis EJ, Saydah S, Imperatore G, Linder G, Divers J, et al. Prevalence of type 1 and type 2 diabetes among children and adolescents from 2001 to 2009. JAMA. 2014;311(17):1778-86.
3. Ekelund U, Luan J, Sherar LB, Esliger DW, Griew P, Cooper A. Moderate to vigorous physical activity and sedentary time and cardiometabolic risk factors in children and adolescents. JAMA. 2012;307(7):704-12.

4. Flynn JT, Kaelber DC, Baker-Smith CM, Blowey D, Carroll AE, Daniels SR, et al. Clinical practice guideline for screening and management of high blood pressure in children and adolescents. Pediatrics. 2017;140(3): e20171904.

5. Hanson MA, Gluckman PD. Early developmental conditioning of later health and disease: physiology or pathophysiology? Physiol Rev. 2014;94(4):1027-76.

6. Ministry of Health and Family Welfare (MoHFW), Government of India, UNICEF and Population Council. New Delhi. (2019). Comprehensive National Nutrition Survey (CNNS) National Report. [online] Available from https://nhm.gov.in/WriteReadData/l892s/1405796031571201348.pdf. [Last accessed March, 2024].

7. Patton GC, Sawyer SM, Santelli JS, Ross DA, Afifi R, Allen NB, et al. Our future: a Lancet commission on adolescent health and wellbeing. Lancet. 2016;387(10036): 2423-78.

8. World Health Organization. (2023). Noncommunicable diseases. [online] Available from https://www.who.int/news-room/fact-sheets/detail/noncommunicable-diseases. [Last accessed March, 2024].

### Fashion Bullying

This kind of bullying has reached sky-high after the launch of clothing brands targeted toward children and teens. Nearly 83% of teens get bullied due to physical appearance, clothing, and weight. The problem is that what we see is only the tip of the iceberg as most teens fail to report this type of bullying.

### Role of School Uniforms

There are variable reports of the positive connection between school uniforms and bullying. In some studies, 95% of the teachers and parents felt that uniforms help teens play on level ground and reduce bullying based on clothing, appearance, and socioeconomic status; 7 out of 10 children also felt the same.

### Body Image, Media and Cosmetic Procedures

The explosion of media has a profound effect on an adolescent's body image. This has resulted in younger adolescents between 13 and 18 years seeking cosmetic surgery. Constant comparison in the media and focus on physical appearance leads to bullying, poor self-esteem, anxiety, depression, and body dissatisfaction. India ranks among the top 5 countries in the world for cosmetic surgeries and there is a 30% increase in plastic surgery under the age of 18 years.

## HOW TO HELP ADOLESCENTS NAVIGATE THIS CHALLENGE?

- *Promoting media literacy:* Empower adolescents with the ability to critically evaluate media portrayals of beauty. Teaching them to discern between reality and digitally altered images fosters a more realistic self-perception.
- *Reframe toxic vocabulary on media:* Look at what the teens are watching on social media and ask them to show you. Media exerts a subtle and subconscious pressure. Content that promotes harmful eating habits like skipping meals, drinking coffee, and smoking to reduce weight should be avoided. Teens internalize these messages and are, hence, more vulnerable. The focus must be shifted to maintaining a healthy body rather than appearance only.
- *Encouraging self-expression:* Advocate for individuality and self-expression in fashion choices. Helping adolescents discover and embrace their unique style can contribute to a positive self-image.
- *Open communication:* Create a supportive environment where adolescents feel comfortable discussing their concerns about body image. Open dialogue allows professionals to provide guidance tailored to individual needs.
- *Educating on healthy habits:* Emphasize the importance of adopting healthy lifestyle habits, including balanced nutrition and regular exercise. Focusing on overall well-being rather than unrealistic beauty standards promotes a positive body image.

## ROLE OF PEDIATRICIANS IN PROMOTING POSITIVE BODY IMAGE IN ADOLESCENTS

- *Screening:* Every adolescent visit should be treated like an opportunity. Body image concerns are an integral part of HEADSSS (home, education/employment, peer group activities, drugs, sexuality, suicide/depression/self-image, and safety) assessment in outpatient practice.
- *Parental guidance:* Parents are role models. Studies indicate that mothers with body image issues and weight loss obsession have a great impact on teens and unconsciously promote negative body image and poor self-esteem. If they model healthy eating behaviors and physical activity as means to having a healthy body, then the focus shifts away from appearance. Parents should be taught to also look out for signs of body image and eating disorders that may manifest as anxiety, depression, and aggression.
- Pediatricians should check during assessment for offline and online bullying that the adolescent might be experiencing as this may be directly connected to body image problems.
- A quick way of screening for eating disorders is using the SCOFF questionnaire.
- Pediatricians can guide adolescents with resources for healthy eating and adequate physical activity.
- Mobile apps like BodiMojo can help adolescents build self-compassion and positive body image.
- Teens are increasingly looking at cosmetic procedures to improve their appearance. Pediatricians should counsel them on the pros and cons of these procedures and explain the difference between reconstructive and cosmetic surgery and who is eligible for the same.
- Referring adolescents with serious body image and eating disorders to mental health professionals is another responsibility of pediatricians.

## ■ KEY MESSAGES

- Addressing fashion, cosmetics, and body image apprehensions in adolescents requires a comprehensive approach that considers the multifaceted influences at play.
- By understanding the data, identifying contributing factors, acknowledging the impact on adolescents, and implementing strategies for support, pediatricians and professionals can play a pivotal role in guiding the youth toward a healthier and more positive self-perception.

## ■ RECOMMENDED READING


1. Morgan JF, Reid F, Lacey JH. The SCOFF Questionnaire: A new screening tool for eating disorders. West J Med. 2000;172(3):164-5.
2. Sharon. Clothing as a Factor in Bullying. www.southern-earlychildhood.org/clothing-as-a-factor- in-bullying/.
3. Shetty KJ, Kotian S. Psychological & social impact of fashion on young adolescents-A case study. IRJMETS. 2022;4(8):11-5.
4. Yoo JJ, Kim HY. Use of beauty products among U.S. adolescents: An exploration of media influence. J Glob Fash Mark. 2010;1(3):172-81.


# 6.3   Peer Influence

*M Vijayarani*

## ■ INTRODUCTION

Adolescence is a part of growing into adulthood that mainly constitutes the transition phase, changes taking place physically, mentally, and psychosocially. The psychosocial transformation is of great significance and has gained more importance with the better understanding of the changes taking place in the brain and its neural connectivity.

One of the major tasks of adolescence is to gradually transition from the dependence of childhood to the independence of adulthood. They must use their burgeoning intelligence to think out issues independently and try to develop their own opinions, ideas, and values. They must also stop clinging to their parents for emotional support and try to become emotionally independent. As part of their efforts in this direction, they may deliberately keep away from family activities, demand more privacy, and talk less openly about their friends and about what is happening in school and their lives.

But having distanced themselves deliberately and conspicuously from their parents, they realize that on many occasions, they are simply not capable of standing on their own feet. Desperate for support, they are forced to turn to their peers, and henceforth they will be strongly influenced by them. To prove their loyalty to the peer group, they may sometimes defy their parents and teachers, even when this defiance is traumatic.

Additionally, there is a shift during adolescence from activities that are closely monitored by parents at home and teachers at school to unsupervised online and offline leisure activities typically involving minimal adult contact. Adolescents quickly learn to depend on peers for companionship, protection, and guidance as they navigate this transition period. They adopt the norms established and enforced by the peer group.

At this stage, they may hero-worship a particular friend who has strong leadership qualities, or an older colleague, a teacher, an uncle, or even a film star. If the "hero" has a violent or negative personality, this may have a bad influence, but a suitable hero may have a positive influence. As they reach young adulthood, they become more mature and gain confidence in themselves as independent individuals. They respect themselves and no longer feel the need to be uncommunicative, rebellious, or assertive toward their parents.

## ■ DEFINITIONS

*Peer influence* is when one chooses to do something one might not otherwise do because one wants to feel accepted and valued by friends. Peer influence occurs when an individual is affected by, or affects, one or multiple others who are of similar age. It is not always about doing something against your will. *Peer pressure* has a negative connotation that implies compulsion by peers of the same age group. Peer pressure has a forcible element, whereas peer influence is letting the peers influence them because they want to feel they belong to the group of friends or peers.

## FACTORS THAT PROMOTE PEER INFLUENCE DURING ADOLESCENCE

Adolescence is a period of heightened conformity. The desire to be part of a group who are similar to them starts in early adolescence and peaks in midadolescence. This enhances the vulnerability to peer pressure during this period. Peer influence wanes in late adolescence and early adulthood.

As the influence of the home goes down in midadolescence, peers play a crucial role in determining the standards of appearance and behavior. Conformity is a necessary prerequisite to peer group membership and the process of identity formation. The peer group also serves as the hub for experimentation and new life experiences. Neurologically, adolescents are primed to monitor input from their peers.

The presence of friends and peers activates the reward processing center in the brain. While the limbic system is highly sensitive to emotional input, the prefrontal areas responsible for cognitive control like decision-making are yet to complete the maturational process. Hence, both prosocial and risk-taking behaviors can be rewarding, depending upon the reinforcement of the friends or peers. The tasks that are rewarded can be anything—a positive behavior like participating in a beach cleaning group activity or a negative activity like substance abuse or unprotected sex.

## EFFECTS OF PEER INFLUENCE

Peer influence not only affects the behavior of an adolescent but also the way they feel. Generally, adolescents feel happy when they are with friends; they share their feelings and experiences and do fun activities. It is also observed that the quantity of peer relationships is not important; rather, it is the quality that matters. High-quality friendships provide understanding, support, self-worth and are linked to better mental health. They also help nurture healthy habits and are protective against risk-taking behaviors.

Low-quality friendships are detrimental and fraught with conflicts, criticism, and aggression. The adolescent may want to let go of the friendship. Low-quality friendships or peer group relationships are associated with poor scholastic performance and behavioral issues.

In some peer relationships, talking excessively about negative happenings, how everything is wrong, and how one feels bad can affect the mood of the group or an individual. It can depress an adolescent as the focus is only on negative things. This is called co-rumination.

## Positive Peer Influence

The most important influence peers can do is to help make healthy choices like eating healthy, getting into physical activities, and taking part in group activities like volunteering. Trying new things along with peers needs courage and confidence. It can be inspirational and also overcome fears. Stage activities and leading a school activity help adolescents boost their self-worth.

Adolescents become more assertive as they get involved in more academic work, sports, seminars, discussions, and other activities along with their peers. There is no pressure but an untold influence of the high-quality peer group. These activities also bring happiness and lessen stress.

When adolescents try to support each other during tough times, it builds their inner strength and resilience. When they are in distress, peers are there to give emotional support and this becomes a coping mechanism for life.

Adolescents learn to indulge in romantic relationships from peers and as a part of their biological needs. Curiosity and the feeling of excitement encourage them to indulge in these relationships. They also are very happy to share their experiences with their peers. They learn to talk, socialize, and maintain friendship with the opposite sex.

Music, art, media knowledge, dress sense and style, watching TV and movies, language of the teens, following role models of the present generation, following trends with social media, social activism, all can be in a very positive manner whenever there is a limitation and self-control among the peers.

Social media can help positively when used appropriately. It is the medium of communication for all adolescents today, where they can share ideas and creativity, explore options, search for solutions, seek help in choices, and many more. It can be particularly helpful for teens who are isolated but can find peers with similar interests or struggles. It can be a space for their voice to be heard.

## Negative Peer Influence

Although there are a lot of positive effects of peer influence, the negative effects easily surpass the positive ones. Some of the negative effects are drinking alcohol, smoking, substance abuse, driving bikes at high speed, unprotected sexual activity, violence, watching adult content, anxiety, depression, eating disorders, and obesity followed by their lifelong consequences. Depression is a leading mental health issue in adolescents and peer pressure is one of its several causes.

Some of the major negative peer influences are as follows:

- *Cell phone addiction and social media addiction:* Cell phones have become an integral part of modern-day life irrespective of age, gender, and socioeconomic status. During the coronavirus disease (COVID) pandemic, it universalized its necessity for academic learning and communication. It also progressed to various applications and platforms developed for learning purposes and widely available. Unsupervised learning using cell phones has led to dependency. Here, the peer influence is initially to possess a cell phone, and later to be constantly in communication with peers through social media platforms. Along with this, DSM-5 now defines an "internet gaming disorder", and internet addiction disorder.
- *Smoking and drinking alcohol:* Smoking is one of the greatest preventable health threats, with onset in adolescence. Peers play a vital role in initiating this lifestyle choice, considering it a sign of maturity. Peer pressure is an important factor for substance abuse among adolescents.
- *Skipping classes and hanging out with peers:* Occasional skipping classes is simply a sign of the rebellious nature of adolescents. When this turns into a frequent habit, the reason can be multifactorial. When peers skip classes and hang out it affects their academic performance, and they often indulge in antisocial activities.
- *Having unprotected sex with many and multiple dating friends:* Some adolescents start having sex due to peer influence, thinking it is fashionable to have friends of the opposite sex and indulge in physical intimacy. Many girls are coerced to have sexual intercourse to retain their boyfriends. Some indulge under the influence of drugs or alcohol.
- *Watching adult content videos:* Unsupervised cell phone usage has led to many adolescents watching pornography, aggravated by alcohol and substance abuse. These lead to aggression and violence.
- *Conflict with parents and teachers beyond the normal level:* Parents and teachers often have conflicts with their adolescents once they know the adolescent is in the company of friends with negative influence, falling grades in school, and has behavioral issues in school and outside.

- *Anxiety, depression, and suicidal ideation:* These increase when the adolescents try to keep up with the expectations of the peers against their own wishes or capability.
- *Bullying and eve-teasing:* Many learn this behavior from their peers.
- *Delinquency:* Socially unacceptable behaviors such as stealing, cheating, and destruction of public property are a growing concern, which are often learned from peers.

Consequences of negative peer pressure include poor academics, low self-esteem, conflict with parents and family, high-risk behavior, aggression, violence, antisocial behavior, depression, self-harm, and suicidal ideation.

### Helping Adolescents Overcome Negative Peer Pressure

- Being nonjudgmental
- Active listening
- Reasoning with scientific details
- Guiding and supporting to overcome difficulties
- Inculcating acceptance and self-esteem
- Gatekeepers themselves have to be a role model to emulate.
- To engage adolescents in organized group activities like sports, events, and clubs
- Set limits whether at school or home
- Being firm but not punitive
- To know the friends of adolescents
- Activities involving long periods must be supervised.

## TEACH HOW TO SAY "NO" TO PEER PRESSURE

Young children and adolescents must be taught and encouraged to say "no" to undesirable coercive acts by known or unknown individuals—peer or adult. They must also say "no" if it is something not to their liking or if they think it is harmful or dangerous to themselves or others. For example, most adolescents know that smoking and alcohol are injurious to health, but they take it when pressurized by peers as they lack the skill to say no.

The following are the steps to be taught to the adolescents. If the first step is ineffective, progress to the next step, and so on.

- Say "no thanks" with a smile
- Give a reason or excuse
- Repeat the reason firmly and refuse
- Walk away

## ■ KEY MESSAGES

- Recognizing the challenges faced by adolescents in managing their time, the role of pediatricians emerge is pivotal.
- Through the establishment of trusting relationships, screening for time-related stressors, and educational interventions, pediatricians become advocates for holistic well-being.
- The concept of "Me time"—deliberate moments of personal rejuvenation and self-care—is particularly important.
- Pediatricians, understanding its significance, guide adolescents in integrating these practices into their lives.
- This intentional pause amid life's demands is not a luxury but a prescription for resilience.
- There are societal pressures and guilt associated with "Me time", emphasizing its importance for mental health.

## ■ RECOMMENDED READING


1. American Academy of Paediatrics. Communication in the Paediatric Office: A Snapshot of Paediatricians and Parents. Paediatrics. 2019;144(2):e20183129.
2. Blakemore SJ, Choudhury S. Development of the adolescent brain: implications for executive function and social cognition. J Child Psychol Psychiatr. 2006;47(3-4): 296-312.
3. Eccles JS, Roeser RW. Schools as developmental contexts during adolescence. J Res Adolesc. 2011;21(1):225-41.
4. Hsin Y, Xie Y. Sleeping their way to the top? Education, social networks and status attainment. Social Forces. 2018;96(2):619-50.
5. Owens J. Insufficient sleep in adolescents and young adults: an update on causes and consequences. Paediatrics. 2014;134(3):e921-32.
6. Steinberg L (Ed). Adolescence. McGraw-Hill Education; 2017.


---

# 6.7   I had a Breakup and I am very Stressed about It

*Afreen Khan*

## ■ INTRODUCTION

The adolescent phase is characterized by a range of psychosocial and developmental hurdles, including navigating intense emotions and experiencing "first loves." Research increasingly emphasizes the pivotal role of romantic relationships during adolescence, shedding light on the behavioral, emotional, and psychosocial outcomes associated with these experiences. Considerable evidence supports the idea that adolescent romance serves as a crucial developmental milestone, influencing self-identity, overall functioning, and the ability to form intimate connections. However, the dissolution of these relationships, commonly known as breakups, can induce significant stress among adolescents.

## ■ CAUSES OF ADOLESCENT BREAKUPS

Affiliation-, intimacy-, autonomy-, infidelity-, and status-related concerns have been identified by youths as key factors explaining the breakdown of their romantic unions.

## ■ IMPACT OF BREAKUPS ON ADOLESCENTS

Most romantic unions of adolescence are mere infatuations, "love at first sight," shallow to start with, and they almost always breakup within months, with not much mental trauma. The adolescent feels sad, but depression is rare. Time heals, and they learn from the experience. The next infatuation is not too far away.

Nevertheless, romantic relationship concerns were the fifth most common reason for seeking help, comprising 8.7% ($N = 4,019$) of all counseling contacts. Breakups were identified as the most common among the eight specific romantic concern types, representing a third of all romance-related counseling sessions across both genders. The data indicate that breakups are a common challenge for adolescents, with similar impact irrespective of age or gender. The emotional aftermath of a breakup can manifest as a significant psychological burden during adolescence. The dissolution stage of a relationship (breakup) is significantly associated with mental health issues, depression, self-harm, suicidal ideation, and suicidal attempts. Researchers found that teens had a 41%

increase in insomnia if they had started a relationship, a 35% increase if they had experienced a breakup, and a 45% increase if they had both in the previous year.

## MANAGEMENT OF BREAKUP-RELATED STRESS

Teenage breakups present significant emotional challenges, necessitating parental support even in the face of resistance. Romantic relationships in adolescence offer valuable learning experiences, fostering communication, and empathy skills. However, not all relationships endure, and the mental health impact of breakups depends on factors such as the quality and duration of the relationship, as well as the age of the adolescent. Younger teens, in particular, may face more pronounced effects due to ongoing cognitive and emotional development. Breakups are influenced by attachment styles formed during childhood interactions with caregivers. Teens with secure attachments tend to cope better, keeping self-confidence and openness to new relationships. Insecure attachment styles, including avoidant, anxious, or disorganized subsets, may affect how teens navigate breakups, potentially influencing their approach to future relationships. Understanding these dynamics provides insights into diverse coping mechanisms among adolescents in the aftermath of romantic relationship challenges.

Recognizing the psychological toll of breakups on adolescents, it is imperative to provide targeted psychological support. Adolescents receive help from a supportive environment that encourages emotional expression, guidance, and the development of coping mechanisms. Scientifically validated approaches, such as cognitive behavioral therapy (CBT), can be instrumental in assisting individuals in navigating the emotional challenges associated with breakups.

## ALARMING SIGNS

- Withdrawal from friends, family, and once-enjoyed activities, as isolating themselves and avoiding social interactions could be indicative of emotional turmoil.
- Sudden shift in their social circle, potentially avoiding old friends and associating with different peers
- Changes in online behavior, as an increase or decrease in time spent online, may expose them to risky online activities or bullying.

- Heightened instances of crying or anger, which could be emotional symptoms of depression.
- Significant and unexpected decline in school performance, alterations in eating habits such as reduced meal times or binge eating, and disruptions in their sleeping routine—excessive sleep or insomnia—indicating potential emotional struggles.
- Identifying and addressing these warning signs promptly is essential for providing necessary support to adolescents navigating the challenges of a breakup.

## PARENTAL SUPPORT

- *Availability and presence:* Parents should ensure their availability by offering to talk or simply being in the same space. Acknowledge the emotional weight of heartbreak and refrain from downplaying it, recognizing it as akin to physical pain.
- *Express love through actions:* Demonstrate love and support through thoughtful actions like preparing their favorite food together, or engaging in activities like a nature walk or cycling.
- *Attentiveness to nonverbal cues:* Pay attention to nonverbal cues to gauge their emotional needs. Offer a hug if they seem receptive, or provide space if they indicate a preference for solitude.
- *Encourage peer support:* Recognize the importance of peer relationships in emotional expression. Consider allowing additional time with friends to facilitate interaction and sharing of feelings.
- *Professional intervention:* If the adolescent continues to struggle with the aftermath of a breakup, consider seeking professional help from a counselor to provide targeted support and guidance.

## COUNSELING AND THERAPEUTIC INTERVENTIONS

Scientifically informed counseling and therapeutic interventions tailored to the unique developmental needs of adolescents are crucial for managing breakup-related stress. Evidence-based techniques, including *CBT* and *mindfulness-based interventions*, have demonstrated efficacy in helping individuals navigate the emotional aftermath of a breakup. These interventions target maladaptive thought patterns and promote emotional regulation, fostering resilience in the face of relationship challenges.

## EDUCATIONAL PROGRAMS AND RELATIONSHIP EDUCATION

Integrating relationship education into educational curricula is a proactive step toward equipping adolescents with the skills needed to navigate romantic relationships and cope with breakups effectively.

## KEY MESSAGES

- Though adolescent romance is a crucial developmental milestone in the ability to form intimate relationships, breakups are the norm, and can cause significant stress.
- Breakups are significantly associated with mental health issues like insomnia and rarely depression, self-harm, suicidal ideation, and suicidal attempts.
- The mental health impact of breakups depends on factors such as the quality and duration of the relationship, the age of the adolescent, and the strength of childhood attachment to parents.
- Red flags suggesting the onset of depression include withdrawal from friends, family, and once-enjoyed activities, avoiding old friends and associating with different peers, an increase or decrease in time spent online, heightened instances of crying or anger, significant and unexpected decline in school performance, alterations in eating habits such as reduced meal times or binge eating, and excessive sleep or insomnia.
- Parents should offer support by being present, available for a talk, acknowledging the emotional pain, demonstrating love and support through thoughtful gestures, offering a hug if receptive, encouraging peer support, and arranging professional intervention if needed.
- CBT and mindfulness-based interventions are the effective therapeutic options.
- Relationship education should be introduced into the educational curricula.

## RECOMMENDED READING

1. Bravo V, Connolly J, McIsaac C. Why did it end? Breakup reasons of youth of different gender, dating stages, and ages. Emerg Adulthood. 2017;5(4):230-40.

# Substance Use Disorder

***Section Editor:*** *Newton Luiz*

## 7.1 Substance Abuse: Evolution and Current Scenario

*Mothi SN, Manini Moudgal*

*"Teenage is a vulnerable period wherein they are curious to explore different experiences while trying to discover their own identity".*

## ■ INTRODUCTION

Teenage is a vulnerable period wherein they are curious to explore different experiences while trying to discover their own identity. Doing so, they tend to push boundaries and experiment. With the advent of the internet and social media, teens get easy access to information. In turn, they also become easy targets for drug traffickers. In the absence of proper guidance, they tend to fall prey to drugs and other risky behaviors.

## ■ DEFINITION OF SUBSTANCE ABUSE

The World Health Organization defines substance abuse as "harmful or hazardous use of psychoactive substances, including alcohol and illicit drugs." Licit drugs fall within the law and are regulated. They include alcohol, nicotine, caffeine, and pharmaceutical agents, to be used as intended. Illicit drugs, e.g., Cannabis products, opiates, amphetamine-like substances, and cocaine, are illegal to possess. Both forms of drugs, especially when the former is abused, are hazardous to life.

## ■ BRIEF HISTORY AND EVOLUTION

Ancient Indians were privy to the mind-altering effects of several compounds. The earliest reference to cannabis comes from the Atharvaveda around 1500 BCE wherein it is described as an anxiolytic. By 8–3 BCE it was mentioned in the Sushruta Samhita as a cure for catarrh and diarrhea. Its use as an anesthetic and painkiller was also known. Cannabis in several forms was, and continues to be, a socially acceptable calming substance and pharmacologic agent.

Datura, a hallucinogen, is known from the Vedic times to be Shiva Shikhara or crown of Lord Shiva, who used it to calm the effects of Halahala, the legendary poison from the Churning of the Ocean. It is still used as an offering to Lord Shiva in temples. Somarasa, the Divine Elixir, mentioned in the Rigveda 1500–1200 BCE, was thought to be the extract of the Somalata plant and presumed to grant immortality to the consumer. It was later speculated to be either an extract of cannabis or ephedra plant or psilocybin from mushrooms.

In more modern times, Sadhus continue to smoke chillums of weed as part of their religious practices. India's foodscape also includes sweets made of poppy seed and nutmeg to provide the calming end to a large meal. The use of Bhang (Cannabis) laced edibles during Holi is the norm. Khaini, Gutkha, and certain Paan Masalas are popular tobacco preparations that are extensively chewed in India. Urban rave parties in clubs and farmhouses with use of ecstasy and lysergic acid diethylamide (LSD) are frequented by the upwardly mobile. These days hookah bars in neighborhoods and at social gatherings are all too common. Smoking in its myriad forms has always been glamorized in the Indian film and media, and continues to remain so.

Given this background, the opportunity for youngsters to experiment is omnipresent.

## DISTRIBUTION PATHWAYS

In order to fathom the extent of drug addiction in India, one needs to understand how the illegal drugs reach the users.

India's geographic location places it at an ideal juncture for major drug smuggling routes. It is sandwiched between The Golden Triangle (Thailand—Laos—Myanmar) and the Golden Crescent (Afghanistan—Pakistan—Iran), which are the world's largest opium producers. Drug trafficking occurs via India in either direction to reach markets in Asia, Africa, and the Americas and vice versa. 70% of drugs enter India via containers in ports. The border with Pakistan is especially vulnerable via land, especially into the northern states of Punjab, Haryana, and Delhi. The northeastern Indian states are equally badly hit due to porous and poorly policed borders.

Additionally, India itself is a major producer of pharmaceutical agents. This allows for easy access to drugs and their precursors. Many such drugs can be purchased without prescriptions. Parts of Madhya Pradesh, Rajasthan, and Uttar Pradesh also have legal opium farms.

Suppliers obtain the drugs from larger dealers and the chain of distribution then gets ramified. Teenagers generally obtain drugs through contacts in their educational institution, peers, or even family members who are users. Many get their supply via post or private couriers.

Nowadays, most young people have a phone with internet access. With the advent of social media, illegal websites, the dark web, cryptocurrency, etc., obtaining illegal substances has become easier than ever.

## MODALITIES OF ABUSE

There are many routes by which drugs are abused:

- *Ingestion:* Alcohol, prescription tablets, marijuana-laced edibles, MDMA (3,4-methylenedioxymethamphetamine), ecstasy, etc.
- *Injection:* Cocaine, heroin, methamphetamine, benzodiazepines, steroids, etc.
- *Insufflation (snorting):* Heroin, MDMA, stimulants, and other medicines in pill form that can be crushed

- *Smoking:* Marijuana, tobacco, crack, phencyclidine (PCP), etc.
- *Inhalation:* Paint thinners, glues, petroleum, nail polish remover, etc.
- *Rectal:* Benzodiazepines, alcohol, and opioids
- *Transdermal:* Fentanyl, nicotine, and methylphenidate.

## CURRENT SCENARIO IN INDIA

India is the world's most populous country at 1.43 billion people per the United Nations Population Fund 2023 data. Even though the population involved is substantial, there have not been many comprehensive studies from India to help quantify the problem of substance abuse among children.

In 2016, a survey was conducted by the National Commission for Prevention of Child Rights with 4,000 respondents, all less than 18 years of age, from 100 cities across India. They reported tobacco, alcohol, cannabis, and opiates as the major substances abused with progression from licit toward illicit drugs. More males reported use than females. It is not just an urban phenomenon but fairly widespread in the rural areas. The average age of initiation was lowest for tobacco at 12.3 years versus 15.1 years for injectables. Street children also initiated use 1–1.5 years earlier than those living at home. Tobacco and inhalant users reported near daily use. Familial stressors including a using family member and peer pressure were major risk factors. Around 70% never sought treatment or support. The Understanding the Lives of Adolescents and Young Adults (UDAYA) survey also that year added that substance abuse was significantly higher in adolescent boys who were school dropouts.

The National Survey on Extent and pattern of Substance use in India 2019 is one of the most recent and comprehensive studies. This survey included 473,569 individuals aged 10–75 years from all states and Union Territories. It is the only recent study in India wherein data from the 10–17 age group is presented separately. Interestingly, inhalants are the only category wherein the prevalence in 10–17-year-olds is higher than in adults! Among those children, 0.09% show a dependent pattern of use.

These numbers have, for the first time, helped quantify the extent of the problem nationwide among the youth in particular. In 2019, the National Consultation on Drug/Substance conference saw 26 States and 3 Union Territories participating. A comprehensive plan to combat pediatric and adolescent drug use, including legislation, access to treatment and deaddiction, and rehabilitation was put forth.

## EMERGING TRENDS

Substance use has evolved various trends over time and a fancy name adds to the allure. A few examples include:

- *Vaping or pen-hookah*, even though it has been illegal in India since 2019, is on the rise among youth these days. Misinformation that these e-cigarettes do not contain nicotine has been the primary cause.
- The *CK1 pill* is made in Goa. It contains a combination of cocaine and the anesthetic ketamine. Its street names are Blizzard or Calvin Klein.
- A *California Drop* is LSD that is put on a stamp, which is then chewed.

Coronavirus disease 2019 (COVID-19) added to the burden wherein people sought solace from isolation and depression by using drugs procured online or via couriers. According to the UN Office on Drugs and Crime World Drug Report 2022, cannabis legalization in parts of the world appears to have accelerated daily use and increased related health impacts. The war in Ukraine has displaced traditional cocaine and heroin routes. There are signs that manufacturing of drugs like methamphetamines and fentanyl will go up. These sociopolitical scenarios are bound to have an impact in India sooner or later.

## KEY MESSAGES

- Substance abuse is common among teens, both urban and rural.
- Several forms of habit-forming substances have been socially acceptable in India for centuries.
- India is uniquely positioned geographically along with major drug routes.
- Vulnerable youth have easy access to drugs with the advent of the internet and social media.
- Tobacco, alcohol, cannabis, and inhalants are the most common abused substances.
- Comprehensive national data regarding substance abuse among children in India is lacking.
- Modalities of drug use are constantly evolving.
- Further research, constant surveillance, and active enrolment into rehabilitative programs are the need of the hour.

## RECOMMENDED READING


1. Childline India. Child Drug Addiction In India. [online] Available from https://www.childlineindia.org/a/issues/addiction [Last accessed March, 2024].
2. Dhawan A, Pattanayak RD, Chopra A, Tikoo VK, Kumar R. Pattern and profile of children using substances in India: Insights and recommendations. Natl Med J India. 2017;30:224-9.
3. Nadeem A, Rubeena B, Agarwal VK, Piyush K. Substance Abuse In India. Pravara Med Rev. 2009;4:4-6.
4. NCB. [online] Available from https://narcoticsindia.nic.in/ [Last accessed March, 2024].
5. NCPCR. (2021). Joint action plan on prevention of drugs and substance abuse among children and illicit trafficking. [online] Available from https://ncpcr.gov.in/uploads/165650396962bc3ea1e5141_joint-action-plan-on-prevention-of-drugs-and-substance-abuse-among-children-and-illicit-trafficking-2021.pdf. [Last accessed March, 2024].
6. Parmar A, Bhatia G, Sharma P, Pal A. Understanding the epidemiology of substance use in India: a review of nationwide surveys. Indian J Psychiatry. 2023;65(5):498-505.
7. Remesh KR. Substance Use: Focus on Adolescent Health. Indian Pediatr. 2022;59(2):103-4.
8. Singh J, Gupta PK. Drug Addiction: Current Trends and Management. Int J Indian Psychol. 2017;5(1):2348-5396.


# 7.2   Substance Use Disorders

*Narmada Ashok, Newton Luiz*

## INTRODUCTION

The Diagnostic and Statistical Manual of Mental Disorders, 5th edition (DSM-5) discusses 11 classes of pharmacological agents: Alcohol, amphetamines, caffeine, cannabis, cocaine, hallucinogens, inhalants, nicotine, opioids, phencyclidine (PCP) and similar agents, and prescription drugs such as sedatives, hypnotics, and anxiolytics. Alcohol and nicotine are discussed in individual chapters.

## TERMINOLOGY

The term substance use disorder (SUD) has replaced the former terms "substance dependence" and "substance abuse" in DSM-5.

Nevertheless, the following words continue to be in popular use:

- *Substance misuse:* Use of a prescribed drug for a medically unacceptable purpose
- *Substance abuse:* The use of a drug in a socially disapproved manner. (Used even when it prevents the person from fulfilling responsibilities, or creates social problems, or in physically hazardous situations).
- *Substance dependence/addiction:* The repeated, uncontrollable, and often increasing use of a substance, the deprivation of which leads to a craving for it, often associated with considerable physical and mental distress. "Addiction" is not preferred as it does not recognize dependence as a medical disorder, and sounds derogatory.

## EPIDEMIOLOGY

The most common substances used in India, in decreasing order of frequency, are nicotine, alcohol, marijuana, and inhalants, followed by opioids, heroin, and sedatives. Substance use is higher in adolescents than in the general population due to their inherent inquisitiveness and experimentation.

Substance use peaks at 18–25 years of age, when adolescents and young adults enjoy maximum freedom and experimentation, and then gradually declines with increasing responsibility and maturity. Though it is common in adolescents, it is mostly experimental or recreational. Intoxication may occur following binge drinking among peers. Chronic uncontrolled substance use is fortunately infrequent.

Adolescents with SUD may acquire the money to buy drugs by stealing from their own homes, or by robbery, drug dealing, or prostitution. They are more likely to have unprotected sex to catch a sexually transmitted infection (STI) [including human immunodeficiency virus (HIV)], to get infected with hepatitis C virus (HBV) or HCV through infected needles, and to experience violence.

## ETIOLOGY OF SUBSTANCE USE

The important factors for initiation to substance use are affordability, availability, peer pressure, and social acceptability. There may be multiple factors for persistent

---

**BOX 1:** Factors causing substance use.

- *Biologic factors* include genetic predisposition, and psychological factors include conduct disorder and antisocial personality disorders
- *Behaviors* such as rebelliousness, poor school performance, delinquency, criminal activity, and personality traits with lack of self-control
- *Psychological factors:* Teens with depression, anxiety, eating disorders, and schizophrenia are more vulnerable
- *Social factors:*
  - *Family:* Familial conditions include parental substance use, intrauterine exposure, and family dysfunction. The presence of a first-degree relative with alcohol use disorder increases the risk of alcoholism sevenfold. The increase in the family economy and reduction in the time spent as a family has contributed to the children having economic freedom and personal space not monitored by elders
  - *Peer pressure:* This may be from a desire to fit into a group or avoid being bullied. In a study from Chandigarh, 45.6% attributed their use to peer pressure. Children are also lured by friends who have become drug carriers
  - *Media*: In recent years, reports of youth icons indulging in substance use and the growing trend of celebrity drug scandals have had an impact on adolescent minds
  - *Social:* Low socioeconomic status aggravates the problem
  - *Education:* The undue pressure on children to excel academically and socially has led to substance use as a coping mechanism
  - *Mental disorders:* Comorbid psychiatric disorders and stressful life events are major factors. The scale of mental disorder in India is huge and largely not addressed

---

**BOX 2:** Protective factors.

- Strong bond with parents and siblings
- Adequate parental supervision
- Stable daily routine
- Good peer group
- Enjoys going to school
- Aware of the dangers of substance use
- Trained in life skills (assertiveness, stress management, etc.)
- Actively participates in sports, games, and cultural activities
- Spiritual inclination

---

use, and they are similar irrespective of the class or type of drugs **(Box 1)**.

These factors act on adolescent minds that are vulnerable due to their experimental risk-taking behavior and hormonal mood disturbances **(Box 2)**.

## PSYCHOPATHOLOGY

- A drug may be used voluntarily for its beneficial effect (opioid to reduce pain, euphoriant when depressed, and alcohol to control anxiety) until they get accustomed to it.

- Drug use may be considered a learned behavior. When initial use results in a social reward (approval of peers) or an alleviation of suffering (reduction in feelings of depression or anxiety), it is reinforced. Eventually environmental stimuli like the sight of the paraphernalia (bottle, cigarette pack, and needle) create an emotional craving. This is worsened if a peer lights a cigarette, opens a bottle, or offers a drug.
- Once tolerance develops, a higher dose is needed, which then causes physical dependence.
- Once physical dependence develops, the withdrawal symptoms are themselves an adequate motive for drug use.
- Voluntary drug use may become compulsive drug abuse when the drug brings about changes in the structure and chemistry of the brain. Dopamine, norepinephrine, gamma-aminobutyric acid (GABA), and endorphins are the part of the reward circuitry of the brain, especially the limbic system that facilitates addiction; and many drugs excite these pathways.
- Most substance abusers have a psychiatric comorbidity, such as major depressive disorder or antisocial personality disorder.
- Twin studies suggest that there may be a small genetic predisposition to drug use.

## STAGES OF ADOLESCENT SUBSTANCE ABUSE

Stages of adolescent substance abuse are mentioned in **Box 3**.

> **BOX 3:** Stages of adolescent substance abuse.
>
> - *Curiosity about the substance:* Common in adolescence
> - *Experimenting:* Uses it with friends; usually tobacco and alcohol; may become a weekend habit; and few consequences and minimal changes in behavior
> - *Seeking it:* Looks for opportunities to use it; mostly with friends but sometimes alone; significant behavioral changes and some consequences occur; may try more potent drugs
> - *Preoccupied with the substance:* Uses it daily; cannot control use; time spent on getting and using it prevents the adolescent from fulfilling responsibilities and may distance him from family and friends
> - *Dependence:* Needs to take the drugs to feel normal; uses multiple drugs; may be expelled from school; and guilt and shame lead to depression and occasionally suicide

## SUBSTANCES COMMONLY USED

### Cannabis (Marijuana and Ganja)

Cannabis is obtained from the plant *Cannabis sativa*. The euphoriant and hallucinogenic effects are primarily derived from 9-tetrahydrocannabinol (9-THC). It is usually available as a cigarette in which the tobacco has been replaced with marijuana leaves. Hashish is concentrated marijuana in the form of sticky black oil. There is increasing use of the substance, especially in those countries where use of marijuana is legally permitted. In India, it is legally permitted as bhang in some situations but is otherwise illegal. It is prescribed along with anticancer therapy for its antiemetic action, in some countries.

Marijuana usually produces elevated mood for a few hours, during which time there is poor memory (interfering with studies) and poor concentration (which increases the risk of driving). A mentally stressed person who takes marijuana may occasionally experience a panic attack caused by frightening hallucinations.

With heavy and prolonged use, there may be:
- Decreased testosterone levels and spermatogenesis, which may potentially interfere with pubertal development.
- Prone to bronchial asthma, pharyngitis, sinusitis, and chronic bronchitis, due to heavy smoking.
- An amotivational syndrome.
- Subtle cognitive deficits that interfere with learning.
- Precipitation of anxiety, depression, and psychosis in those who are prone to it.
- Episodes of hyperemesis.
- A withdrawal syndrome, with irritability, agitation, insomnia, and malaise, which may last for a fortnight.

The active ingredient, 9-THC, can be detected in urine assay. To escape detection, synthetic marijuana is now being used increasingly, which consists of various herbs sprayed with chemicals that have a similar effect as THC, such as carboxamides.

### Inhalants

Inhalant abuse is the deliberate inhalation of volatile substances to produce an altered mental state. A wide variety of readily accessible products such as glue, correction fluids, petrol, shoe polish, spray paint, paint thinners, and polish removers are used. The abusers are mainly early adolescents from a poor background who are attracted by the easy availability, low cost, and rapid action. It is most common in street children, and peaks at 13–15 years before tapering off. Inhalation may be by sniffing (direct inhalation of fumes), bagging (from a plastic or paper bag), huffing (from a chemical-soaked cloth), gliding (from air freshener aerosols), or dusting (direct spraying of an aerosol cleaner into the mouth or nose). As the effect is brief, the abuser repeatedly inhales it every few minutes for a few hours. Rebreathing from the bag can cause intense headache due to hypercapnia and hypoxia.

As the chemicals are highly varied, the effects and adverse effects vary a lot. The general effect is usually like that of alcohol intake, with initial euphoria, progressing with intense use to loss of self-control, and later slurring of speech, ataxia and drowsiness, and finally seizures and coma. Toluene, present in some glues, is a euphoriant and hallucinogen. Nitrites, present in room fresheners, are euphoriants and are said to increase enjoyment of music and physical sex **(Box 4)**.

Chronic abuse of inhalants leads to irreversible neurological and psychological effects, producing irritability, tremors, ataxia, nystagmus, slurred speech, and decreased visual acuity.

## Sedatives and Hypnotics

*Benzodiazepines* and *barbiturates* are medications prescribed for insomnia, anxiety, seizure control, and

> **BOX 4:** Some hazards of common inhalants.
>
> - *Toluene*, common in correction fluid, paint remover, paint thinner, petrol: Brain damage resulting in poor memory and decreased learning ability, ataxia, vertigo, and hearing and vision loss
> - *Nitrites:* Immunosuppression. "Sudden sniffing death syndrome", due to cardiac arrhythmia, which is the leading cause of death among inhalant abusers. As nitrites are vasodilators, they often cause headache, fainting, and cutaneous flushing
> - *Benzene*, in petrol: Damage to the bone marrow, decreased immunity, and decreased reproductive function
> - *Butane*, in paint spray and lighter fluid: Sudden sniffing death syndrome, burns from inflammability
> - *Freon*, an aerosol propellant: Respiratory obstruction, death due to sudden airway cooling and injury, sudden sniffing death syndrome, and liver damage
> - *Methylene blue*, found in paint thinners and removers: Methemoglobinemia and myocardial injury
> - *Trichloroethylene*, found in spot removers and degreasers: Sudden sniffing death syndrome, cirrhosis, hearing and vision problems, and decreased fertility

alcohol withdrawal. Occasionally, the adolescent may take them off-prescription to reduce social anxiety and mental stress, as they create a sensation of calmness, relaxation, and euphoria. Barbiturates (e.g., phenobarbitone) are addictive. During withdrawal it may cause tremors and agitation. In high doses, the patient may go into a fatal coma.

Flunitrazepam is a benzodiazepine that causes amnesia, loss of inhibitions, and muscle weakness. It acts 1–2 hours after ingestion, and the effects last for 8–12 hours. Being tasteless and odorless, it can be added to a drink to make the victim incapable of resisting rape, or even wanting to resist. It is the best-known of the date-rape drugs. GHB (gamma-hydroxy butyrate) has a similar action that lasts 3–6 hours. Other examples are ketamine and chloral hydrate. To avoid becoming a victim, one would have to pour one's own drink, and never leave it unattended even to visit the bathroom or talk to a friend across the room.

## Hallucinogens

They attract adolescents in search of novelty. They are believed to act by their structural similarity to serotonin. Methylene-dioxy-methamphetamine (MDMA) and lysergic acid diethylamide (LSD) are being increasingly used in India.

- MDMA is a synthetic compound that is related to amphetamine and is highly addictive. It is very popular at "raves" (all-night dance parties), as its effects include euphoria, sharpened senses, and high energy. It can occasionally cause panic attacks. MDMA disturbs temperature regulation, resulting in hyperthermia during vigorous and prolonged dancing, which may cause permanent damage to the brain, kidneys, or liver. Chronic use damages cognition and memory.
- LSD is a highly potent hallucinogen that is absorbed onto small pieces of paper. Its action peaks at 3 hours and lasts 12 hours. It distorts perceptions and causes hallucinations. Rarely, it can cause psychotic delusions, disorganized speech and severe agitation, and frightening flashbacks, and the adolescent may have to be calmed with benzodiazepines. It is not addictive.
- PCP is a synthetic drug that is comparatively easy to produce. It is sold as a liquid or a white powder than can be dissolved in water or alcohol. It causes immediate euphoria on smoking. The adolescent experiences pleasant hallucinations but may become

anxious, confused, and amnesic. Adverse physical effects include fever, tachycardia, and blurred vision. In high doses, it can cause seizures, hypertension, and cardiac arrhythmias, which may rarely be fatal.

## Stimulants

Stimulants make the person feel powerful, confident, and energetic. They are called "uppers" as they keep people awake and have the opposite effect of depressants. However, when their effect wears off, they tend to produce extreme feelings of malaise and loss of energy. Stimulants such as cocaine and methamphetamine trigger release of norepinephrine, resulting in increased heart rate and blood pressure (BP), and increased motor activity, but simultaneously cause vasoconstriction. This can cause a heart attack or a stroke.

- *Cocaine:* It is a powerfully addictive stimulant made from the leaves of the coco plant native to South America. It is a fine white crystal powder. Generally, adolescents snort cocaine powder through the nose or rub it on the gums. It causes euphoria and energy, mental alertness, and hypersensitivity to sight, sound, and touch.

  It may also cause restlessness, irritability and paranoia, dilated blood vessels, nausea, raised body temperature, and irregular heartbeat. Snorting cocaine for long periods can result in loss of smell. Smoking can lead to lung problems. Withdrawal symptoms include depression, fatigue, unpleasant dreams, insomnia, and slowed thinking. Death from overdose can occur unexpectedly, even on the first use of cocaine, due to arrhythmia, seizures, and strokes.

- *Amphetamines:* Dextroamphetamine and methamphetamine are generally available as tablets, as they are sympathomimetic amines that are prescribed for attention-deficit hyperactivity disorder (ADHD). These tablets are often diverted to substance users for nonprescription use. Acute intoxication can cause behavioral problems such as agitation, confusion, paranoia, impulsivity and violence, and rarely fatal cardiac events. Adolescents are unaware that chronic usage leads to deficits in memory and verbal reasoning, and use it to keep awake while preparing for examinations.

## Opioids

Opiates are prized medically for their powerful analgesic properties. *Morphine* is a natural opioid obtained from the poppy plant and prescribed for relief of severe pain, especially in patients with incurable cancer. Today the synthetic opiates *fentanyl* and *oxycodone* are preferred, but they have become a major cause of death from drug overdose in developed nations. *Codeine* is used as a cough syrup and mild painkiller.

*Heroin* is a highly addictive synthetic opiate made from morphine, and has no medical use. It is usually taken intravenously, and it causes euphoria and pinpoint pupils. Constipation and loss of libido are common adverse effects. Withdrawal symptoms are intense, with lacrimation, sneezing, sweating, abdominal cramps, diarrhea, pupil dilatation, elevated BP, and severe agitation. Naltrexone can be used for acute withdrawal symptoms and has been used to block the euphoric effects. Heroin intoxication is the leading cause of death from drug use in the USA. Treatment is by administering naloxone.

## ASSESSMENT OF DRUG ABUSE AMONG THE ADOLESCENTS

The clinician should assess how many substances are used, the chronicity and severity of use, the problems associated with use at home, school and in society, physical and psychological consequences of use, and whether there is comorbidity.

### History Taking

The clinician's primary role is to identify users early and intervene early. Every adolescent who visits a clinic should routinely be screened for substance use, as it is so common and generally offers no clinical clues. A successful interview with an adolescent starts by assuring confidentiality and privacy. The clinician should take time to establish a rapport and avoid judgmental statements. The HEEADSSS (Home, Education and employment, Eating, Activities, Drugs, Sexuality, Suicide and depression, and Safety) screen is a good starting point. The clinician should be familiar with one of the numerous well-researched screening questionnaires, such as the CRAFFT tool (see the article on alcohol) or SBIRT (Screening, Brief Intervention, and Referral to Treatment). The parents too should be interviewed.

Screening is especially important when there is a history of falling school performance, poor family relationships, change in friends, spending less time on favorite activities such as meeting friends or playing football, change in mood, appetite or sleep patterns, and loss of weight—though all these symptoms are also features of depression. More specific features are spending too much time in the bedroom or bathroom, secrecy about social plans, missing school, frequent accidents, or loss of money or valuables from the home.

Clinical signs include a decrease in personal hygiene or careless grooming. Heavy users of marijuana often smell of it, and so do their clothes and their bedrooms. There may be nasal mucosal damage from drug snorting, bloodshot eyes, or pinpoint pupils. The intravenous (IV) drug abuser has "tracks," hypertrophic linear scars following the paths of large veins. Unsterile technique often results in skin abscesses and occasionally septicemia. Some patients take it subcutaneously, resulting in local fat necrosis. Inhalant users may leave high-risk products or a chemical-soaked cloth in their room, or have chemicals on their hands or mouth.

## DIAGNOSIS OF DRUG ABUSE ACCORDING TO DSM-5 CRITERIA

Diagnosis of drug abuse according to DSM-5 criteria is by a cluster of cognitive, behavioral, and physiologic symptoms that indicate that the adolescent is using the substance even though it is harming him/her. SUD is diagnosed based on 11 criteria that should be met within a 12-month period. The SUD is classified as mild if 2–3 criteria are met, moderate if 4–5, or severe if 6 or more criteria are met. Thus "Moderate Alcohol Use Disorder" indicates that the person meets 4–5 criteria for alcohol use **(Box 5)**.

## INVESTIGATIONS

- Urinary drug screening may be useful in select circumstances, such as unexplained psychiatric symptoms, significant changes in behaviors or school performance, frequent respiratory issues or accidents, evaluation of serious motor vehicle accidents, and as a monitoring procedure in recovery programs. It may reveal the presence of benzene or toluene in inhalant use.
- Blood tests may pick up high levels of substances, such as alcohol, heroin, or barbiturates.
- Complete blood counts, liver and renal function tests, and imaging modalities when needed.
- Tests for HIV, hepatitis B and C in case of injectable drug usage or when sexual abuse is suspected.
- Tests for pregnancy and sexually transmitted infections if the adolescent has had unprotected sexual activity.

---

**BOX 5:** Criteria for diagnosis of substance use disorder.

*Impaired control:*
- The substance is often taken in larger quantities and for longer duration than intended
- There is a persistent desire or recurrent attempts to control substance use
- Much time is spent on procuring the substance, using it, and recovering from it
- Craving for it

*Social impairment:*
- Recurrent failure to fulfil major obligations at work, school, or home
- Persistent social or interpersonal problems
- Gives up important social, occupational, or recreational activities

*Increased risk:*
- Substance use continues despite awareness of the problems it causes
- Use in hazardous situations, e.g., when driving a car or operating machinery

*Pharmacological response:*
- Tolerance develops, resulting in a marked need for higher amounts of the substance
- Typical withdrawal symptoms on stopping

## TREATMENT

Treatment should be accessible and affordable. Detoxification may require in-patient care. Some detoxification programs include the use of drugs: Nicotine replacement therapy or bupropion for nicotine and disulfiram or naltrexone for alcohol. Heroin deaddiction requires opioid substitution therapy, replacing heroin with buprenorphine or methadone, which are longer-acting but less euphoric and addictive, and are given under medical supervision. Specific treatment is not available for inhalants.

Treatment should simultaneously offer counseling and pharmacotherapy of psychiatric comorbidity, such as depression, anxiety, conduct disorder, and ADHD.

After detoxification, treatment should aim to educate the patient and family about the specific drug, and to manage the mental, emotional, and psychiatric factors that influence substance use. Multiple modalities, such as individual therapy, family therapy, and group therapy, are used. Self-help groups like alcoholics anonymous have proved their usefulness. Treatment is multidisciplinary, and may require the combined efforts of a pediatrician, a psychiatrist, a psychologist, and a social worker.

Multiple relapses are common, especially with brief interventions; treatment generally lasts 3 months or more.

CBT is important in relapse prevention. Exercise, yoga, and mindfulness are potential adjunctive therapies. Consistent physical exercises can improve sleep, establish structure, strengthen relationships, and improve self-perception. Digital interventions that offer automated feedback, tailored messages and assessing outcomes, motivation, and self-efficacy are being explored. Episodic urine drug testing may be required.

The prognosis depends greatly on parental influences, peer use patterns, and personal psychosocial factors. The management of those who are addicted to nicotine, alcohol, and cannabis is much easier than that of other drugs.

## ■ PREVENTION OF SUBSTANCE ABUSE

Prevention of substance abuse requires adolescent and parental commitment.

### The Adolescent

- Get sufficient knowledge of the ways in which substance abuse develops.
- Avoid temptation and peer pressure by developing healthy friendships and relationships.
- Avoid peers who use substances.
- Seek help for mental stress promptly.
- Examine the risk factors in the biological and environmental surroundings.
- Live a well-balanced life focused on your goals.

### The Family

- Regularly monitor adolescent activity.
- Establish limits on screen time and social time.
- Limit monetary privileges in a friendly manner.
- Have open-ended discussions about studies and career options.
- Get to know the adolescent's peers.
- Be involved in the activities of the adolescent.
- Resolve parental and family conflicts.
- Parents who suspect that their adolescent may be experimenting with drugs should talk to them openly, encourage honesty, focus on the behavior and not the person, and get professional help if needed.

### The Government

The Narcotic Drugs and Psychotropic Substances Act, 1985 (NDPS Act) makes it illegal for a person to produce/manufacture/cultivate, possess, sell, purchase, transport, store, or consume any narcotic or psychotropic substance. In 2015, new rules were added, whereby the state drug controller has to approve recognized medical institutions to stock and dispenses these drugs, while the institutions have to maintain proper records of use.

The Social Justice Ministry has recommended that the NDPS Act should be modified to make it more compassionate and understanding. Persons apprehended with small quantities of drugs should be considered as victims rather than culprits. They should be labeled as drug users rather than addicts. Rather than being jailed, they should have to undergo a mandatory period of at least 30 days at a rehabilitation or deaddiction facility, followed by a year of community service.

Some possible governmental interventions are:

- As alcohol and tobacco are gatekeepers to the use of other substances, the Government may restrict their sale to adolescents, tax them maximally, and ban the advertising of tobacco and alcohol. Surrogate advertising is still permitted in India. In the USA, 97% of drug abusers also use alcohol, while marijuana use is the strongest predictor of future cocaine use.
- Notices discouraging substance use (usually alcohol or smoking) are now compulsory in movie scenes depicting their use.
- Fund awareness programs in schools
- Use the mass media to build up social disapproval of drug use, and project positive role models who reject substance abuse.
- Provide adolescents with healthy alternate sources of entertainment, e.g., adequate facilities for sports, games, yoga, and cultural facilities.
- Random roadside testing to reduce alcohol use.

The Ministry of Social Justice and Empowerment launched Nasha Mukt Bharat Abhiyaan (NMBA) in 2020, in the 272 districts most vulnerable to substance abuse. It intends to reach out to the masses and spread awareness about substance abuse with the active participation of youth, women, and the community. Some programs are:

- Awareness generation programs, especially in educational institutions, university campuses, and schools.
- Involvement of youth groups such as NYK (Nehru Yuva Kendra Sangathan), NSS (National Service Scheme), and NCC (National Cadet Corps)
- Reaching out into the community and identifying dependent population groups.

Most nicotine addicts are strongly desirous of stopping smoking, as it immediately reduces all the risks and discomforts associated with smoking. Most smokers repeatedly attempt to stop smoking by themselves. However, powerful withdrawal symptoms develop, peak at 24–48 hours, and can last for weeks. The common symptoms are an intense craving for tobacco; tachycardia, tremors, sweating, and dizziness; feeling stressed, irritable, and restless; anxiety or depression; headache and poor concentration; insomnia or drowsiness; and increased appetite. Consequently, success is usually achieved only after multiple attempts at quitting.

### Quitting: Pediatrician's Role

- Ask every adolescent at every visit about smoking.
- Advise the adolescent to quit.
- Congratulate them on their adult resolve to do so. Decide mutually on a quit date. Ask about the high-risk situations in which they are most likely to smoke, and advise them to strictly avoid such situations. Mention the withdrawal symptoms, and encourage them to stand firm. Success doubles with pediatrician's support.
- Review after 2 days, as failure is highest in the first 2 days.
- Consider the need for nicotine supplements, medication, and cognitive behavior therapy, all of which significantly increase the success rate.

*Nicotine replacement therapy* is started immediately on quitting smoking to prevent nicotine withdrawal symptoms. It is used immediately on awakening and continued throughout the day.

- Nicotine 14 mg transdermal patch is used every morning. It may occasionally cause a local rash. After 6 weeks, a 7 mg patch is used for 2 weeks.
- Nicotine 2 mg gum should be chewed hourly for 6 weeks and then with decreasing frequency for another 6 weeks. Side-effects are a bad taste and jaw soreness. It is less effective if tea, coffee, or juices are taken.
- Nicotine lozenge is sucked (not swallowed) every 1–2 hours.
- Nicotine nasal spray may be needed frequently every hour and causes rhinorrhea, coughing, and watering of the eyes in the majority of patients.

*Medication:* It should be started 1 week before the quit date. Bupropion 150 mg twice daily stimulates dopaminergic and adrenergic receptors and is an effective anti-depressant, and doubles quit rates. Varenicline is effective, but not yet approved in adolescents. Nortriptyline has shown promise.

### ▪ PREVENTION

Creating awareness in schools is only mildly effective in the individual adolescent, but it is an essential component as it gradually builds up social disapproval of smoking, which is essential in the long run **(Box 2)**.

### ▪ GOVERNMENT ROLE

- *The Cigarette and Other Tobacco Products Act, 2003 (COTPA-2003):*
  - Prohibits advertisement of tobacco products
  - Prohibits smoking in public spaces (buses, shops, restaurants, etc.)
  - Prohibits sale to persons below 18 years, and in places within 100 meters of an educational institute, but with a trivial fine of ₹ 200 for breaking the law.
  - Where tobacco products are sold, messages should be displayed stating that "tobacco causes cancer"

---

**BOX 2:** What to tell adolescents about smoking.

*Immediate ill-effects:*
- Bad breath
- Staining of teeth
- Reduction in stamina in sports
- Costly
- Temporary erectile dysfunction
- Irritant cough
- Precipitates wheezing

*Long-term effects:*
- Reduces sexual potency and sperm count
- *Causes early aging:*
  - Wrinkling of the face
  - Loss of teeth
- *High risk of:*
  - Heart attacks
  - Strokes
  - Cancer
  - Chronic lung disease with cough and mucus

*Social aspects:*
- Girls disapprove of it
- More common in those who are less educated, poor, or suffering from depression or anxiety
- 75% of adult smokers repeatedly try to stop smoking due to its ill effects, but only half of them succeed. Why start?
- Smoking is gradually becoming unpopular

and "sale of tobacco products to a person below 18 years of age is a punishable offense".
- *Prohibition of e-cigarettes Act, 2019:* Production, manufacture, import, export, transport, sale, distribution, storage, and advertisement of e-cigarettes are prohibited.

## ■ KEY MESSAGES

- Nicotine is the most common substance abused by Indian adolescents.
- Nicotine use starts early, and 90% of chronic adult smokers start in adolescence.
- Tobacco use is the single largest preventable cause of death in the world today.
- Nicotine is a gateway to the use of alcohol, cannabis, other drugs, and other risky behaviors.
- Vaping devices are becoming increasingly popular in developed nations, and have contributed to an uptick in the use of tobacco.
- Adolescents consider smoking an "adult" behavior, an act of rebellion, or a glamorous act.

- Smoking is encouraged by parental smoking, peer pressure, easy availability and affordability, and media glorification of smoking.
- Nicotine is highly addictive, and smoking cessation may require multiple attempts, but success is significantly increased by pediatrician support, nicotine supplementary therapy, medication, and cognitive behavior therapy.

## ■ RECOMMENDED READING


1. Henssen BP. Tobacco and electronic nicotine delivery systems. In: Kliegman RM, St Geme JW, Blum NJ, Shah SS, Tasker RC, Wilson KM, Behrman RE, Nelson WE (Eds). Nelson Textbook of Pediatrics, 21st edition. Philadelphia: Elsevier; 2020. pp.1049-51.
2. Narain R, Sardana S, Gupta S, Sehgal A. Age at initiation & prevalence of tobacco use among school children in Noida, India: A cross-sectional questionnaire based survey. Indian J Med Res. 2011;133(3):300-7
3. Sadock BJ, Sadock VA, Ruiz P. Kaplan and Sadock's Synopsis of Psychiatry, 11th edition. Philadelphia: Wolters Kluwer; 2015. pp. 680-5.


<table>
<tr><td>**7.4**</td><td><h1>Alcohol Use Disorder</h1></td></tr>
</table>

*Sulbha Amol Pawar*

## ■ INTRODUCTION

Alcohol use by adolescents and young adults has serious short-term and long-term consequences for the individuals, their families, the community, and society. It contributes to academic problems, mental health disorders, road traffic accidents, unprotected sex, human immunodeficiency virus (HIV), rape, violence, and suicide. It is a gateway to the use of tobacco and drugs of abuse.

## ■ EPIDEMIOLOGY

The legal age for alcohol consumption varies from state to state in India but is generally around 21 years, yet alcohol use is typically initiated during adolescence. Data on prevalence of alcohol use in adolescents is difficult to interpret, as it varies according to many factors such as age, gender, urban versus rural, cultural factors, and

financial and educational status. Locally brewed alcohol is initiated at a younger age compared to commercially available alcohol, especially in rural areas, often at home during a cultural event.

Adolescent use is likely to be recreational when it occurs occasionally, on a weekend, in a male, in late adolescence, in a social group, and the substance used is comparatively mild (e.g., beer) and limited in quantity. It is riskier when it occurs in early adolescence, in a female, on weekdays, in an adolescent who is sad, is not doing well in studies, takes it alone or in large quantity, takes stronger substances, and drives after the drink.

Alcohol use in moderation is socially accepted. Nevertheless, alcohol use disorder (AUD) is a major issue in late adolescence and young adults. Even among recreational drinkers, binge drinking with peers occasionally results in intoxication.

## ALCOHOL METABOLISM

Ethanol (ethyl alcohol) is commercially available in various preparations (e.g., rum, brandy, beer, wine, whiskey, and gin), each of which comes in a wide variety of flavors, and their alcohol content varies a lot. Despite commercial claims to the contrary, the effects of alcohol are almost entirely due to the quantity of alcohol consumed and is practically unaffected by the formulation or by the additional flavoring substances in it. One "drink" contains 12 g of ethanol and is contained in an average 300 mL can of beer, 120 mL of wine, or 30 mL of 40% rum or brandy.

Alcohol is rapidly absorbed from the stomach and is transported into the liver, where it is metabolized by alcohol dehydrogenase into acetaldehyde, which is then metabolized to acetic acid by aldehyde dehydrogenase. Women and Asians have lower levels of alcohol-metabolizing enzymes, and hence become intoxicated at lower levels of alcohol intake. Peak blood concentration is attained about 45–60 minutes after the drink, or faster if the drink is taken rapidly on an empty stomach. 90% of the alcohol is metabolized by the liver, while the remaining 10% is excreted unchanged by the kidneys and lungs. It takes over 1 hour to metabolize 30 mL of brandy.

## EFFECTS OF ALCOHOL ON THE CENTRAL NERVOUS SYSTEM

It is not known how alcohol affects brain function, though there are various hypotheses regarding its effect on neuronal membranes, serotonin and NMDA (N-methyl-D-aspartate) receptors, etc.

- It is a central nervous system (CNS) depressant and acts not by creating feelings of euphoria but by suppressing restraint and judgement even at low levels. The adolescent becomes disinhibited, gregarious, and talkative and is more likely to try out other drugs or be sexually promiscuous.
- At higher levels it affects motor ability, slows reactivity time, and impairs clarity of thought. As a result, the adolescent is prone to a road traffic accident. Some adolescents ingest caffeine (coffee) before driving, which combats the drowsiness caused by alcohol but does not improve motor reactivity.
- Alcohol may help an insomniac adolescent to fall asleep, but it reduces both deep sleep and rapid eye movement (REM) sleep, resulting in very poor quality of sleep, waking up the next day with a headache, feeling lethargic and irritable, and with poor concentration.

- Though alcohol temporarily suppresses feelings of sadness, frequent use causes depression by making the person less competent at study and work and in social interactions. AUD is associated with a high risk of depression and suicide in young adults.
- As levels increase further, there is ataxia, progressive emotional lability and cognitive dysfunction, slurring of speech, memory impairment, a confusional state or, stupor. The CNS depressant action may be dramatically increased if the adolescent deliberately takes a sedative like diazepam or even an antihistamine along with the alcohol.
- Chronic alcohol use alters brain metabolism in unexplained ways, resulting in poor memory and concentration in the short term, and early dementia in the long term.

## EFFECTS OF ALCOHOL ON OTHER SYSTEMS

- Alcohol increases the desire for sex by reducing inhibitions but simultaneously reduces sexual ability. It reduces testosterone levels, and persistent use causes atrophy of the testes.
- When pregnant women take alcohol regularly, there is a 35% chance that the child will have a birth defect. Alcohol causes fetal alcohol syndrome, which is the leading cause of intellectual disability in countries like the USA where a high percentage of women consume alcohol. The child may have intrauterine growth restriction, microcephaly and lowered IQ, craniofacial anomalies, and limb and heart defects.
- It increases the risk of heart attacks and strokes.
- It increases the risk of cancer, especially of the esophagus, stomach, liver, pancreas, colon, head and neck, and lungs.
- Blood pressure is raised.
- It causes fatty liver, hepatitis, and cirrhosis.
- It causes peptic ulcers and pancreatitis.
- There is often reduced food intake, poor digestion, and poor absorption of B-complex vitamins.

## WHY ADOLESCENTS START USING ALCOHOL?

- Curiosity and thrill-seeking behavior.
- Recreational; believes the risk is low.
- Peer pressure, especially at parties.

- Enjoys it; it helps with shyness and when depressed or worried.
- Role modeling by heroes.

## RISK FACTORS FOR DEVELOPING ALCOHOL USE DISORDER

- *Genetic vulnerability:* Twin studies, adoption studies, and analysis of family relationships suggest that up to 60% of the tendency to AUD may be genetically determined.
- *Family environment:* Parental substance abuse, poor parental supervision, poor parental communication, severe or inconsistent discipline, family conflicts, and child sex abuse.
- *Underage drinking:* Teens who start drinking before the age of 15 years may be five times more likely to develop AUD. Given the widespread use of alcohol, parents may not be able to prevent their children from social drinking, but they should attempt to discourage it until they are 21 years of age.
- Adolescents with mood disorders, and less commonly attention-deficit hyperactivity disorder (ADHD), conduct disorder, and antisocial personality disorder are prone to AUD.
- Those who say they drink to cope with stress, worry, and anxiety are at higher risk. They may be using alcohol as a self-medication to combat depression by its euphoric effect, and to relieve anxiety, especially social phobia. The risk may be lower in persons who take low doses of alcohol to help them relax after a tough day.

## PREVENTION: WHAT THE PEDIATRICIAN CAN DO?

- *Anticipatory guidance:* Educating parents and adolescents about the ill effects of alcohol use, via community and school programs. Helping adolescents develops life skills, especially self-assertive skills.
- *Screening for alcohol use:* HEEADSSS (Home, Education and employment, Eating, Activities, Drugs, Sexuality, Suicide and depression, and Safety), SBIRT (Screening, Brief Intervention, and Referral to Treatment), and CRAFFT are some useful tools.
- Referral of adolescents with serious issues to the psychiatrist
- Advocacy for government initiatives to discourage availability and advertising of alcohol

## Screening

Every adolescent should be screened routinely for alcohol use. The general format of screening questionnaires is that the adolescent is asked, one by one, about whether he has used nicotine, alcohol, cannabis, or other drugs anytime in the last 12 months. If all answers are negative, he is commended: "You are a mature and independent person, and you are not excessively influenced by your peers." If he has occasionally used a risky substance, he is asked about it in further detail, and the benefits of not using it are touched upon briefly, along with the difficulty associated with stopping it later. If use has been more regular, specific and detailed advice is given; for example, "My recommendation is not to use any alcohol, marijuana, or other drug, because they can harm your developing brain, interfere with learning and memory, and put you in embarrassing or dangerous situations." Advice treatment.

One well-known standardized screening questionnaire is the CRAFFT tool, which can be administered by the clinician or self-administered (refer to Annexure). This questionnaire is available on *https://crafft.org/get-the-crafft/* in many languages, including Hindi, Chinese, and Arabic. The original tool did not enquire about nicotine, but this deficit has been corrected in the CRAFFT-N version. There is an additional query on risky driving under influence of substance use, and risk counseling is given if there is a positive history, e.g., "Road traffic accidents are the leading cause of death for young people. Do take care." One weakness is that it specifies driving a car, whereas most adolescents in developing countries like India use a two-wheeler, which is associated with much higher accident and fatalities than a car. The clinician should clarify that it applies to all vehicles.

## PREVENTION: ROLE OF THE GOVERNMENT

- Routine education of adolescents in schools on the evils of all types of substance abuse, through inclusion in the syllabus and/or awareness programs.
- Enforce the legal age of drinking, at least in public spaces. In Indian studies, the mean age for initiation of drinking ranged from 14.4 to 18.3 years. AUD is highest at 18–25 years, and then gradually decreases with age.
- Strict restrictions on advertisement of alcohol.
- Restrict number of sales outlets; none should be permitted near educational institutions; none should open on the first day of a month.

- The maximum punishment for public drinking when followed by creating nuisance in the public place is imprisonment of 3 months and fine of ₹10,000.
- The maximum punishment for drunk driving is now increased to imprisonment up to 4 years and fine up to ₹10,000; it depends on the blood alcohol levels and the consequences.

## MANAGEMENT OF ALCOHOL USE DISORDER

- *Motivate* the adolescent to stop the habit. They are often in denial, and claim that their problem was initiated by depression, anxiety, an accident, or a life stress, but usually the alcohol use precedes and causes the depression or life stress. Instead of asserting the diagnosis, the clinician should be nonjudgmental and focus on troublesome physical health issues, and state repeatedly that they can be eradicated by abstaining from alcohol.
- *Detoxification* usually requires good nutrition, vitamins (especially thiamine), and propranolol or a benzodiazepine for a brief period.
- *Benzodiazepines* are effective in controlling severe withdrawal symptoms. In severe symptoms like seizures and delirium, diazepam 5–20 mg intravenous (IV) may be given and repeated every 30 minutes if needed.
- *Psychological counseling:* The counselor or therapist should teach skills to:
  - Change the behaviors that make the person want to drink.
  - Deal with stress and other triggers.
  - Set goals and reach them.
  - Bring about healthy lifestyle changes.
- *Family counseling:* The family should accept the diagnosis, stop trying to protect the adolescent from the consequences, and focus on helping him overcome the problem.
- Treat psychological problems
- Treat associated health conditions
- *Oral medications:*
  - Disulfiram inhibits aldehyde dehydrogenase, resulting in toxic levels of acetaldehyde when alcohol is consumed. This causes highly distressing symptoms, and can occasionally be fatal. It is only used to discourage alcohol intake in highly motivated adults, and is not recommended in adolescents.
  - Naltrexone shows promise to reduce alcohol craving.
  - *Acamprosate:* It has been found to reduce relapse of drinking behavior.
- Enlist help of *alcoholics anonymous (AA)*, a self-help group that has been found to be highly beneficial in encouraging the reformed alcoholic from relapsing, and in supporting and guiding the other family members.

## PROGNOSIS

According to the Global Burden of Diseases (GBD) study 2019, alcohol is the second highest risk factor contributing to disability-adjusted life years among adolescents and young adults aged 10–24 years.

At least 10% of adult men in the USA have had features of AUD at some time in their lives. Their life expectancy is reduced by 10 years. The common causes of death are suicide, cancer, heart disease, and cirrhosis.

When AUD is an isolated event, the prognosis for recovery with treatment is good. When it is associated with the use of other substances, with psychiatric illness, or with an unfavorable family atmosphere, the prognosis is poor.

## KEY MESSAGES

- Alcohol consumption is typically initiated during adolescence. Delaying first use beyond adolescence is highly protective against future AUD.
- It is socially approved in moderation, despite having serious short-term and long-term consequences.
- The CNS depressant action results in a reduction in self-restraint and judgment even at low doses, resulting in risky behavior. At slightly higher doses, it reduces motor ability, contributing significantly to adolescent deaths from road traffic accidents. Regular use is associated with depression and even suicide.
- Fetal alcohol syndrome is a leading cause of intellectual disability in societies where alcohol consumption is common among young women.
- It reduces sexual potency and fertility.
- It is a major contributor to cirrhosis, heart attacks, strokes, hypertension, and cancer.
- Risk factors for AUD include a genetic predisposition, a toxic family environment, parental alcohol use, depression, and alcohol intake for stress management.
- The pediatrician's primary role is screening and preventive counseling.

- Appropriate government policies have a major role in reducing the prevalence of alcohol use.
- Management should include detoxification and simultaneously tackle associated psychological issues and health-related problems.

## ■ RECOMMENDED READING


1. Breuner CC. Alcohol. In: Kliegman RM, St Geme JW, Blum NJ, Shah SS, Tasker RC, Wilson KM (Eds). Nelson Textbook of Pediatrics, 21st edition. Philadelphia: Elsevier; 2020. pp. 1048-9.
2. CRAFFT. [online] Available from www.crafft.org [Last accessed March, 2024].
3. Jaisoorya T, Beena K, Beena M, Ellangovan K, Jose DC, Thennarasu K, et al. Prevalence and correlates of alcohol use among adolescents attending school in Kerala, India. Drug and Alcohol Review. 2016;35:523-9.
4. Nadkarni A, Tu A, Garg A, Gupta D, Gupta S, Bhatia U, et al. Alcohol use among adolescents in India: a systematic review. Global Mental Health. 2022;9:1-25.
5. Sadock BJ, Sadock VA, Ruiz P (Eds). Kaplan and Sadock's Synopsis of Psychiatry, 11th edition. Philadelphia: Wolters Kluwer; 2015. pp. 624-39.

# Adolescent Reproductive and Sexual Health (ARSH)

**Section Editors:** *Vaishali Deshmukh, Deepa Janardhanan*

## 8.1 Evolution of Sexuality during Growing Years

*MKC Nair*

### ■ INTRODUCTION

Way back in 1898, Sigmund Freud had cautioned that children's sexual lives started before puberty and that this was a fact that one should not overlook. Freud seemed to be mentioning Albert Moll when he said, "Children are capable of every psychical sexual activity, and many somatic sexual ones as well," although he did not name him. However, Freud went on to say, "the organization and evolution of the human species strives to avoid any great degree of sexual activity during childhood". The hormonal fluctuations that lead to the commencement of puberty are a major factor in the determination of biological sex, with development of secondary sexual traits and psychological sex, with development of attitude toward their sexuality, further influenced by psychological characteristics such as temperament and personality.

Freud's stages of psychosexual development, which he delineated in his psychoanalytic theory, provide insight into his perspective on sexuality—oral, anal, phallic, latent, and genital stages, all having direct or indirect relationship to development of adolescent sexuality.

### Phallic Stage

Approximately between the ages of 3 and 6 years, the phallic stage is most closely linked to Freud's concept of adolescent sexuality. Children learn about their own bodies at this age, as well as the distinctions between males and girls. Freud's theories regarding this stage revolve around the Oedipus and Electra complexes. Oedipus complex—Freud postulated that boys experience sexual impulses for their mothers and regard their fathers as competitors. The process of identifying with the father helps to address this problem. The term "Electra complex" refers to Freud's theory that girls have feelings for their fathers and feel competition and jealousy toward their mothers. By identifying with the mother, this issue will overcome.

### Genital Stage

This is the last stage, which lasts from the start of puberty as an adult until maturity. Healthy adult sexuality was seen as the result of earlier stages being successfully resolved, according to Freud. Though revolutionary at the time, Freud's theories regarding teenage sexuality have since been criticized for a number of reasons:

- *The emergence of interest in childhood sexuality:* Before the seventeenth century, the general consensus was that children were inherently sinful, corrupt, and wicked because of original sin. Teachers advocated a rigorous upbringing in the eighteenth century to shape youngsters into morally upright adults. The risks associated with youngsters masturbating particularly worried theologians, clergy, pedagogues, and doctors. These discourses presented the masturbating child as morally depraved, physically and mentally ill, and ultimately hopeless. Therefore, by alerting young people to the risks associated with masturbation and requiring them to exercise extreme self-control, anti-masturbation campaigns throughout the Enlightenment in the eighteenth century sought to safeguard children's sexual innocence. The recognition of sexuality as a crucial component in the formation of human identities in the latter part of the 1800s contributed to the surge in interest in childhood sexuality concerns. The development of a person's sexual identity was eventually seen as a component of their personal history, dating back to their early years. At the start of the twenty-first century, discussions about pedophilia and the numerous instances of child sexual abuse that have been documented by the media and by survivors in the wildly popular "misery literature" have also increased interest in child sexuality and its past.

- *Lack of scientific rigor:* Science found it difficult to examine Freud's theories since they were dependent on clinical observations and interpretations rather than factual study.
- *Limited attention to biological factors:* The contributions of biology and hormones to teenage sexuality are mainly disregarded in favor of psychological and psychoanalytic aspects in Freud's theories.
- *Heteronormativity:* Freud's theories assumed heterosexual development and were founded on a binary conception of gender. The variety of gender identities and sexual orientations is not sufficiently addressed by them.

Although Freud's theories about teenage sexuality served as a springboard for discussions in this field, they are no longer accepted as the only or ultimate explanation for the intricacies of adolescent sexual development. In the current globalized and digitalized era, online platforms are a major source of sexual behavior modeling.

## EVOLUTION OF SEXUALITY

From an evolutionary point of view, there are some critical information, that may not be connected; (1) sexual reproduction in animals and plants is far more prevalent than asexual reproduction, (2) even bacteria and viruses, which reproduce by cloning, engage in promiscuous horizontal gene exchange (parasexual reproduction), (3) there is a jungle of diverse courtship and mating strategies that we find in nature, and (4) the phenotypic plasticity of sex determination in animals suggests that the central nervous system and reproductive tract may not reach the same endpoint on the continuum between our stereotypic male and female extremes.

## EVOLUTION AND DEVELOPMENT OF PRIMATE FEMALE SEXUALITY

Trying to understand sexuality invoking evolutionary theory concepts, it may be stated that; (1) in contrast to nonprimate mammals, hormones do not regulate the capacity to engage in sex in female anthropoid primates, uncoupling fertility and the physical capacity to mate, (2) instead, in primates, sexual motivation has become the primary coordinator between sexual behavior and fertility, (3) this dependence upon psychological mechanisms to coordinate physiology with behavior is possibly unique to primates, including humans, and allows a variety of nonphysiological influences, particularly social context, to regulate sexual behavior, and (4) the independence between hormonal state and sexual behavior allows sex to be used for social purposes. It is understood that this complex regulation of sexuality of primates develops during adolescence, as female monkeys show both hormonally influenced sexual motivation and socially modulated sexual behavior.

From a biological point of view, the transition to adolescence occurs when children sexually mature and become capable of reproduction, after a series of early stages of sexual development in childhood. On the other hand, development beyond childhood is completely different, with no generally achieved biological or psychological milestones or scientific evidence that differentiates a state of maturity as adolescents progress through development into young adulthood.

A systematic review examining physiological influences of adolescent sexual behavior, including associated psychosocial factors, highlighted hormonal and gender differences with (1) females appearing to be more influenced by psychosocial aspects, including the effects of peers, than males, (2) males may be more inclined to engage in unprotected sex with a greater number of partners, and (3) early maturing adolescents are more likely to be sexually active at an early age and hence hormonal, psychosocial context, and sexual preference need to be acknowledged in intervention package development.

## PUBERTY AND ADOLESCENT SEXUALITY

The adolescent sexuality is not only seen as immature, but also as being qualitatively distinct from the sexuality of adults, the hallmarks of which are; sexual desire, sexual arousal, sexual behaviors, and sexual function. A critical lacuna exists in the understanding of continuum of sexuality development through the lifespan. Sexuality development is mediated by cognitive development and emotional development. Understanding sexuality through developmental lens suggest that development of adolescent sexuality is a complex dynamic evolution, involving different domains of development—progressive, extended, qualitative, and self-regulated **(Fig. 1)**.

Many elements of sexual experience are assumed to be inappropriate for adolescents and preserved for adults, and from this perspective, sexual experiences such as coitus are seen as fundamentally transformative, thus marking an irreversible status boundary between adolescence and adulthood. Whereas, adult sexuality is seen as a domain requiring maturity to experience and express, adolescent sexuality is portrayed as tentative, experimental, confused, inept, and innately dangerous, with focus on risk-taking, needing broad social efforts to suppress or control the same. On the other hand, it is also true that throughout the sexual lifespan; (1) essential elements of adult sexuality identifiable in early adolescence are relatively continuous, (2) sexual anatomy, hormonal underpinnings of sexuality remain relatively intact, and (3) subjective interpretations of the experiences of sexuality almost certainly change over the life course.

## ■ SELF-STIMULATION/MASTURBATION

In 1909, Still documented instances of childhood masturbation. Usually starting in infancy or early childhood, it is characterized by self-stimulation of the genitalia, which is often linked to abnormal posture and movement, sweating, flushing, and tachypnea. Unusual postures and movements that take place during masturbation in newborns and early children can be mistaken for convulsions, movement abnormalities, colic, abdominal pain, or other neurological or medical issues. It is possible to conduct lengthy and unnecessary inquiries. On the other hand, it is also true that 50–60% of girls and 90–94% of boys engage in masturbation at some time in their life and the activity is predisposed by the maturation of sex hormones. There are few previous reports on infants and early childhood masturbation that do not try to pinpoint the impact of sex hormones, despite data linking sex hormones to an increased risk of teenage masturbation behavior.

Despite the stigma and social disapproval that surround it, the medical community views it as a natural part of development. The literature does not provide a clear definition for when masturbation starts. According to retrospective research, it should be on an average 15 years for girls and 13 years for boys. There is a connection between other adolescent sexual behaviors and masturbation. It might offer a way to become more at ease and familiar with one's genitalia and sexual responses.

Adolescents may experience low self-esteem and socially undesirable avenues for expressing their sexual needs and desires due to internalizing ideal standards from incorrect body image representation and overly ambitious sexual activity demonstration. Thus, this might lead to a vicious cycle of acceptable social and sexual disengagement due to expectations of perceived preset and unachievable ideal standards.

Behavior problems exhibited at school entry predicts early sexual activity and those who initiate sexual intercourse in early adolescence experience various risks such as concurrent adjustment problems and high-risk sexual practices. A longitudinal sample of 694 boys and girls with data collected from kindergarten through high

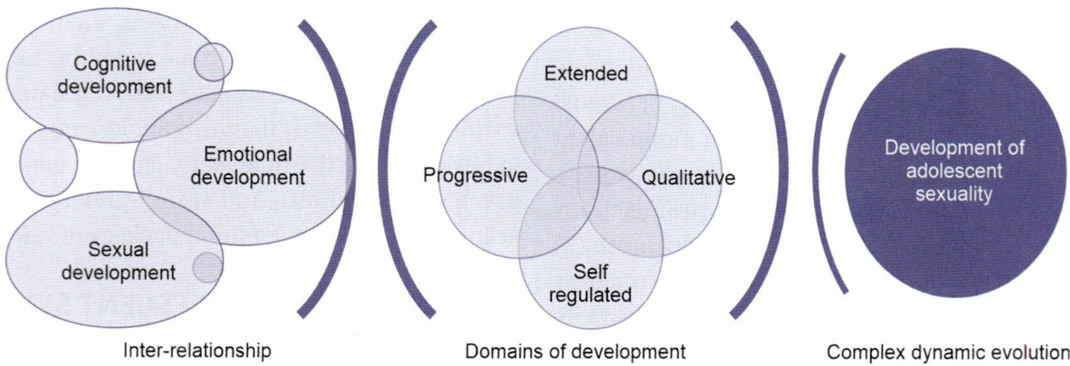


**Fig. 1:** Understanding sexuality through developmental lens.

school, showed that; (1) irrespective of gender or race, high rates of aggressive disruptive behaviors, (2) attention problems at school entry increased risk for a constellation of problem behaviors in middle school, and (3) those with school maladjustment, antisocial activity, and substance use which, in the school, promoted the early initiation of sexual activity.

## FACTORS AFFECTING ADOLESCENT SEXUALITY

The factors that may directly affect adolescent sexuality are:

- *The parental and familial roles:* As per studies, young people with poor interpersonal relationships and a dysfunctional family structure typically have negative attitudes about sexuality. The adolescent's perspective on sexuality is significantly influenced by the interaction between the child and parent. Social sexualization, which involves parents, siblings, friends, and significant other adults, starts in late childhood and lasts until adolescence. Any child's primary source of information regarding sexuality is their parents. The topic of sexuality is rarely discussed in the family in the majority of conservative nations. There are a number of reasons why parents are reluctant to give their kids the right sex education. Gender attitudes, parental relationships, discussions about age appropriate sexual and reproductive health, good touch and bad touch within the family, and standards for dyadic relationships are a few elements of family sexual culture that impact adolescents' understanding of sexuality.
- *The friendship and peer role:* If parents avoid adolescents from educating and discussing regarding sexuality development, it is sure that their classmates and friends will have an influence in them. However, for better or worse, gathering sources from the surroundings is very important, peers might serve as the right and wrong source of information regarding the sex and sexuality.
- *Gender differences in sexuality:* Gender can be broadly defined as a multidimensional construct that encompasses gender identity and expression, as well as social and cultural expectations about status, characteristics, and behavior as they are associated with certain sex traits. There are gender disparities in the feelings associated with having sex. After having sex, boys stated they felt prouder, while girls said they felt ashamed and "dirty". It also highlights how virginity

is perceived through a sexual double standard. Most girls saw being a virgin as a gift to give to a beloved spouse, but more boys saw it as a stigma and a lack of sex possibilities. Boys are typically expected to be more outspoken and take proactive roles in determining the boundaries of sexual encounters, whereas females adopt a reactive one, given the sexual behavior of teenagers. Mid- and late-adolescent years saw a progressive rise in the prevalence of partnered sexual behaviors. Things have changed a lot, but only in selected urban pockets.

- *Genetic and environmental influences:* A review of relevant behavioral genetic studies, taken from a developmental perspective in a sample of 3,762 adolescent twins suggested that behaviors that are more common and socially sanctioned like dating were more heritable than behaviors that are less common and socially acceptable like sexual intercourse.

Finally, a systematic review suggested that the following factors affect the sexual self-concept:

- Biological—age gender, marital status, race, disability, and sexual transmitted infections
- Psychological—impact of body image, sexual abuse in childhood, and mental health history
- Social factors—the roles of parents, peers, and the media.

## KEY MESSAGES

- Essential elements of adult sexuality identifiable in early adolescence are relatively continuous.
- Sexual anatomy and hormonal underpinnings of sexuality remain relatively intact.
- Subjective interpretations of the experiences of sexuality almost certainly change over the life course.
- Biological, psychological, and social factors affect the sexual self-concept.
- Masturbation is a normal part of development of sexuality.

## RECOMMENDED READING

1. Ajlouni HK, Daoud AS, Ajlouni SF, Ajlouni KM. Infantile and early childhood masturbation: sex hormones and clinical profile. Ann Saudi Med. 2010;30(6):471-4.
2. Bates N, Chin M, Becker T. Measuring Sex, Gender Identity, and Sexual Orientation. Washington (DC): National Academies Press; 2022.
3. Boislard MA, Bongardt DV, Blais M. Sexuality (and lackthereof) in adolescence and early adulthood: a review of literature. Behav Sci (Basel). 2016;6:8.

4. Clark DA, Durbin CE, Heitzeg MM, Iacono WG, McGue M, Hicks BM. Sexual Development in Adolescence: An Examination of Genetic and Environmental Influences. J Res Adolesc. 2020;30(2):502-20.

5. Dimijian GG. Evolution of sexuality: biology and behavior. Proc (Bayl Univ Med Cent). 2005;18(3):244-58.

6. Drury KM, Bukowski WM. Sexual development. In: Bromberg DS, O'Donohue WT (Eds). Handbook of Child and Adolescent Sexuality, 1st edition. Cambridge: Academic Press Publications; 2013. pp. 113-44.

7. Ferreira M, Nelas P, Duarte J, Albuquerque C, Grilo C, Nave P. Family culture and adolescent sexuality. Aten Primaria. 2013;45(Suppl 2):216-22.

8. Fortenberry JD. Puberty and adolescent sexuality. Horm Behav. 2013;64(2):280-7.

9. Hegde A, Chandran S, Pattnaik JI. Understanding Adolescent Sexuality: A Developmental Perspective. J Psychosexual Health. 2022;4(4):237-42.

10. Pinkerton SD, Bogart LM, Cecil H, Abramson PR. Factors associated with masturbation in collegiate sample. J Psychol Hum Sex. 2002;14:103-121.

11. Potki R, Ziaei T, Faramarzi M, Moosazadeh M, Shahhosseini Z. Bio-psycho-social factors affecting sexual self-concept: a systematic review. Electron Physician. 2017;9(9):5172-8.

12. Pringle J, Mills KL, McAteer J, Jepson R, Hogg E, Anand N, et al. The physiology of adolescent sexual behaviour: a systematic review. Cogent Soc Sci. 2017;3(1): 1368858.

13. Schofield HL, Bierman KL, Heinrichs B, Nix RL; Conduct Problems Prevention Research Group. Predicting early sexual activity with behavior problems exhibited at school entry and in early adolescence. J Abnorm Child Psychol. 2008;36(8):1175-88.

14. Wallen K, Zehr JL. Hormones and history: the evolution and development of primate female sexuality. J Sex Res. 2004;41(1):101-12.

<table>
<tr><td>**8.2**</td><td></td></tr>
</table>

# Sexual Behaviors in Teens and Youth: Changing Trends

*Ritu Gupta, Abheet Gupta*

## ■ INTRODUCTION

Adolescence and young age is a time of new opportunities as well as great risks. During this time, a young person's future begins to develop and take shape according to their values, attitudes and behaviors. According to the World Health Organization (WHO), 70% of health-related issues in adults are largely due to behaviors that began during adolescence. Sexual debut starts at an early age, yet there is a dearth of knowledge on sexuality.

In India, the population aged between 10 and 24 years accounts for 373 million of 1,210 million of the nation's population with every third person in our country belonging to this age group. They are not a homogenous group; their needs vary enormously by age, gender, region, socioeconomic condition, cultural context, etc. Similarly, their sexual and reproductive health needs vary considerably across different groups, cultures, and religion.

The emerging trends of sexual activities of adolescents and young people are a cause of great public health concern. Secondary sexual growth, spurt in hormones, and cognitive, emotional, and psychosocial development result in sexual curiosity and experimentation, often in situations of little reproductive health information or services.

There is a consensus that adolescents and young adults engage in high-risk sexual behaviors that predispose them to reproductive health issues. This is a result of physiological and psychological changes that cause them to desire sexual intercourse and take risks, leading to unfavorable sexual and reproductive health indices. Although sexual behaviors are a normative and physiological component of adolescent development, risky sexual behaviors including early age of sexual debut, having multiple sexual partners, and non-use of condoms are of significant public health concern among adolescents due to their potentially detrimental effects on later sexual and reproductive health.

Although sexual debut does not determine later sexual activities and risks, sexual intercourse initiated at an earlier than normative age, i.e., 15 years or younger exposes adolescents, particularly adolescent girls, to a variety of risks such as human immunodeficiency virus (HIV) infection and other sexually transmitted infections (STIs). Girls who indulge in sex early were found to be at higher risk of unintended pregnancies and STIs than those who delay intercourse until late adolescence. In addition, early sexual intercourse has been associated with reporting negative social and psychological outcomes (such as suicidal behaviors) and subsequent condom use and forced sex.

Having multiple sexual partners is another common risky behavior among young people that increases the risk of HIV and STI. A review of data from the Global School-based Student Health Survey (GSHS) in 21 countries between 2010 and 2016 found that 53.1% of sexually active adolescents aged 12 years to 15 years reported having multiple sexual partners.

## ■ PREVALENCE

The recent global prevalence of adolescents who have ever had sexual intercourse was 6.9% and was higher among boys (10%) than girls (4.2%) and among those aged 14–15 years (8.5%) than those aged 12–13 years (4%).

According to two rounds of Indian demographic health survey, the National Family Health Survey (NFHS)-3 (2005–06) and NFHS-4 (2015–16), overall high-risk sexual behavior has increased among adolescent boys (64–70%) and young men (18–27%) from 2005–06 to 2015–16.

The trend of live-in relationship has increased among adolescent boys in rural areas (0.6–6%) as well as urban areas (3.1–10.9%) over the last 10 years. Adolescent boys having 10th and above years of schooling, residing in urban areas and belonging to affluent class of households were more likely to engage in high-risk sexual activities than young men in India.

The chances of high-risk sexual behavior were higher among adolescent boys and young men consuming alcohol (2015–16).

Early sexual debut is seen in:
- Adolescent boys (9%) more than girls (4%)
- School dropouts—both boys (17.2%) and girls (6%)
- Boys who had rare or frequent media exposure
- Exposure to pornography
- Those with moderately severe/severe depressive symptoms
- Living in an unsafe community or a high poverty neighborhood.

According to ncbi.nlm.nih.gov, the reported age at the first sexual intercourse ranged from 9 to 24 years with an average age estimated at 14.75 ± 2.18. Male teenagers initiated themselves at an earlier age 14–27 years, compared to the females 15–38 years ($p < 0.000$).

Approximately 31.66% of the respondents in a survey of girls and boy (10–24 years of age) had sex before the age of 15. The prevalence of early sexual intercourse was significantly higher ($p < 0.000$) for male teenagers and young adults (41.11%) than for those of girls (20–24%).

## ■ FACTORS AFFECTING THE CHANGING TRENDS IN SEXUAL BEHAVIOR

Sexuality is a fundamental quality of human life, important for health, happiness, individual development and indeed, for the preservation of the human race. During adolescence, when transitioning from childhood to adulthood takes place, sexuality takes on new dimensions; attraction toward the opposite sex, intense feelings, and complex relationships mark this period. The patterns of sexual behavior have changed in the contemporary world. The sexual attitudes of young people are shaped by their parents, parenting styles, peer groups, media, and teachers. The place where one is born and brought up, parents, family, culture, religion, and social construct will all have a profound influence on sexual attitudes.

Various environmental, interpersonal, and individual factors influence sexual behaviors.

## ■ RISK FACTORS/PREDISPOSING FACTORS

In general, early puberty, later marriage, an altered family system with less control and more autonomy, increased exposure to sexual stimuli through mass media, and travel across cultural boundaries have made early sexual activity in adolescents more common.

### Environmental Factors

#### *Media and Neighborhood*

Increased sexual activity and permissive attitudes about sex during adolescence are significantly caused by exposure to media content through the internet, television, movies, and magazines. Adolescents are easily influenced by all the glamor around romantic relationships and premarital sex being portrayed by the celebrities and the influencers on the social media and, get easily carried away. Dating Apps attract and allure the young people to explore the world of romantic dating. The use of or exposure to internet pornography is associated with numerous sexual risk outcomes, including increased risk of having recent sex partners, engaging in anal sex, and an increased risk of using alcohol and other drugs with sex. Neighborhoods with high rates of violence, hunger and/or substance abuse tend to have poor sexual health outcomes among youth. In today's late night party culture where the use of alcohol and drugs is high, the risk of unhealthy sexual behaviors increases multifold.

## Interpersonal Factors

### Parents, Family, Peers, and Partners

Having grown up in an insecure environment and little nurturing from parents or caregivers and a history of abuse or neglect is associated with an increased number of sexual partners and a probability of engaging in sexual behavior with casual acquaintances and not a romantic partner. In the families where there is lack of communication and a disconnect between the parents and children, adolescents who experience an emotional void are vulnerable and more prone to indulge in unhealthy sexual behaviors. Overcontrolling/authoritarian and neglectful parenting styles can also push the adolescents away from the parents and can predispose the young people to risky sexual behaviors. Lack of parental monitoring and guidance is also a significant risk factor.

Fear of missing out, a want to ape and experience the latest sexual trends, pressure from peers and increased opportunities to mingle increase the incidence of sexual contact. Nuclear families, single parent families, and no families are replacing the extended multigenerational families of traditional societies. The traditional institution of marriage is contrasted with the Western system of unparalleled freedom to make decisions.

Peers play a major role in influencing youth's decision-making and behaviors related to sexual risk. Risky peer behavior, such as alcohol or drug use, and permissive peer sexual norms can increase the probability of youth's susceptibility to engaging in unsafe sexual behavior including sex without a condom and sex while using drugs.

Romantic involvement and expectations of the sexual partner also influence sexual risk related outcomes. Chances of engaging in sexual activity increase when one is in a steady or serious relationship.

## Individual Factors

### Biological and Psychological Characteristics, Along with Behaviors, Intentions, and Beliefs

Adolescence is the transition phase from childhood to adulthood when the limbic system of the brain is driving the behavioral and emotional responses. The prefrontal cortex of the brain which is responsible for analytical thinking and rational behavior is not fully developed till the age of 24 or 25 years. During this phase, the young people are commonly driven by their emotions and there is great curiosity to explore, experiment, and experience new things. Their desire to seek pleasure and instant gratification makes them easy prey to fall for sexual encounters, even with strangers and random people. Adolescents who are low on self-confidence and self-esteem often get validation, false appreciation, and a transient boost in confidence during these experiences which encourages and reinforces the sexual behavior. The dating Apps often attract the youngsters and make it easy for them. Also, in today's world, youth often stay away from family in paying guest (PG) accommodation, rented apartments, etc., and have more freedom than ever before to venture out in the world of sexual relationships. Moreover, having romantic relationships right from school time is considered trendy and cool. Everyone wants to have a romantic partner and it has become like a status symbol. Also, being older increases the risk of recent sexual activity among those who had already initiated sex with increased frequency of sexual activity and pregnancy.

Adolescent males are more likely than females to be sexually active. However, female adolescents are more susceptible to sexual coercion and harassment. Feelings of sexual desire, i.e., excess interest in and thoughts about sex and reporting high levels of pleasure from having sex, is a risk factor for continued engagement in sexual activity.

Negative self-perception or body objectification is a risk factor.

- Drug or alcohol use is associated with elevated risk of having had two or more sexual partners and having sex at an early age.
- Being lesbian, gay, or bisexual is associated with an increase in risky behaviors.
- Gang involvement, fighting, and violence are associated with risky sexual behavior.

## ■ PROTECTIVE FACTORS

## Environmental Factors

### Community or Neighborhood Factors

- The incidence of risky sexual behaviors and pregnancy among young people is low in communities with high levels of trust, harmony, and social capital. Such neighborhoods are also supportive of positive and attentive parenting styles.

- Neighborhoods that offer opportunities such as after-school programs, sports, and job training to their youth, support positive sexual health including decreased teen pregnancy.

### School Factors

- Sex education and awareness programs in school
- School connectedness—involvement in school activities, liking school and finding it important, bonding with teachers and peers, feeling safe and fairly treated—protects against sexual risk taking
- Academic achievement and aspirations lead youth to make healthy decisions about sex.

## Interpersonal Factors

### Family Factors

- Young people raised with supportive and responsive parenting styles feel safe and secure and are more likely to plan positively for their future. This, in turn, prevents youth from indulging in high-risk behaviors.
- Parental monitoring—if it is not overcontrolling → helps youth maintain health and safety.
- Family connectedness and open parent—child communication, including conversations about sex, condoms, and contraception, help young people achieve positive sexual health outcomes.
- Youth who live with both parents are less likely to indulge in risky sexual behaviors.
- Youth are more likely to act on family values, e.g., disapproval of adolescent sex by parents or support for contraception if a teen does have sex, acts as a protective factor.
- Higher levels of parents' education and higher family income are protective factors.

*Peer factors:* Social norms followed by peers tend to be reflected in youth and can be a protective factor. For example, if the peers disapprove of early sex, others are also less likely to become sexually active.

*Relationship factors:* If the sexual partners have good and open communication, there is a higher likelihood of using contraception.

## Individual Factors

- Young people who are self-aware and have a positive self-image, high self-esteem, and self-confidence are less likely to indulge in risky sexual behaviors.
- Having a clear vision for one's future and believing in one's ability to control one's own life act as a protective factor.
- Practicing spirituality and one's religion helps youth avoid risky sexual behavior.
- Initiating sex at an older age is associated with better sexual health.
- Beliefs and attitudes about sex, condoms, and contraception can be protective. For example, a positive attitude toward condoms is protective.
- Having the skills and intention to use condoms and contraception, as well as belief in one's own ability to successfully use those skills protects young people against early pregnancy and STIs/HIV.

## ■ PREVENTION OF UNHEALTHY AND RISKY SEXUAL BEHAVIORS IN YOUNG PEOPLE

### The Way Forward

As a society, we need to learn how to intervene to improve the protective factors and reduce the risk factors. The focus needs to be on improving the health-seeking behavior of teens and youth through access to adolescent-friendly services and an enabling environment in the community.

Multiple players other than the health sector, such as education, media, and social agencies need to work in unison to promote the factors that prevent unwanted health outcomes due to unsafe and unhealthy sexual behaviors.

The intervention programs should target the multifaceted factors affecting the adolescent's sexual behaviors, from the individual to the societal level. Allowing parents, teachers, and adolescents to work together could help reduce the sociocultural and personal barriers that prevent effective communication about sexuality. Furthermore, schools can play a key role in reducing risky sexual behaviors and STI acquisition rates in adolescents by promoting sex education in school curricula and encouraging adolescents to engage in extracurricular activities and awareness campaigns. The taboo around communication about sexuality and STIs needs to be dropped in our conservative society and, we need to open up.

Parents need to sensitize their children about this topic and have open communication with their adolescent children to educate and guide them appropriately. Parents play a major role in monitoring and supervising their children. Through social media, the Government can play a big role in raising awareness and protecting young people from risky behaviors through social media.

Sociocultural norms at the societal level such as strong religious and moral beliefs among adolescents can prevent adolescents from engaging in risky sexual behaviors, as the ethical considerations enable them to distinguish healthy from unhealthy behaviors.

## ■ KEY MESSAGES

- Adolescents and youth constitute a major part of our population, and their sexual health is critical. Healthy adolescent sexual development involves not only bodily changes, sexual behaviors, and new healthcare needs, it also involves building emotional maturity, relationship skills, and healthy body image.
- Sexual health requires a positive and respectful approach to sexuality and sexual relationships, as well as the possibility of having pleasurable and safe sexual experiences, free of coercion, discrimination, and violence.
- It is important to understand the changing trends of sexual behavior among the teens and youth and the risk and protective factors underlying the unhealthy and risky sexual behaviors.
- Multiple players other than the health sector, such as education, media, and social agencies need to work in unison to promote protective factors that prevent unwanted health outcomes due to unsafe and unhealthy sexual behaviors.
- Parents, teachers, and adolescents must join hands in developing and implementing effective interventions that address and reduce identified facilitators of risky behavior, particularly working to lift sociocultural and personal barriers that prevent effective communication between adolescents and adults and providing adequate sex education for both parents and adolescents.

- Schools can be an effective setting for reducing risky sexual behaviors in adolescents by providing sexuality education in the school curriculum, perhaps through reinforcement of our moral beliefs related to sexual behavior and teaching communication and life skills.
- The engagement of adolescents in extracurricular activities can improve confidence and help teens makes healthy decision.
- The policymakers must contribute to reduce these risks among adolescents by creating cultural and supportive facilities that enable adolescents to make good use of their leisure time and develop their communication and life skills.
- Media should also contribute by broadcasting messages to teens not to engage in risky sexual practices and by blocking pornographic sites.
- The Adolescent Health Experts and pediatricians can play an important role in bringing the adolescents and young adults, parents, and teachers together, toward having sexually healthy youth population.

## ■ RECOMMENDED READING

1. El Kazdouh H, El-Ammari A, Bouftini S, El Fakir S, El Achhab Y. Perceptions and intervention preferences of Moroccan adolescents, parents, and teachers regarding risks and protective factors for risky sexual behaviors leading to sexually transmitted infections in adolescents: qualitative findings. Reprod Health. 2019;16(1):1-7.
2. Hegde A, Chandran S, Pattnaik JI. Understanding adolescent sexuality: a developmental perspective. J Psychosexual Health. 2022;4(4):237-42.
3. Joshi B, Chauhan S. Determinants of youth sexual behaviour: program implications for India. Eastern J Med. 2011;16(2):113.
4. Suarez L. Risk and Protective Factors in Romantic and Sexual Relationships: Findings from a National Survey of Transgender and Non-Binary Youth. Doctoral dissertation, Harvard University; 2020.

# 8.3  Protecting Self and Others: Decent Expression of Sexuality

*R N Sharma*

## ■ INTRODUCTION

Sexuality is the total expression of who we are as human beings. It includes physical, emotional, and spiritual part of our being and encompasses our personality, value, attitude, gender, race, thoughts, feelings, and sexual behaviors. Human sexuality is not just the act of sex but it involves the personal concept of his/her own body image, sexual identity, role at home, and socially personal feeling and self-esteem.

Sexuality comprises of the following concepts:
- Anatomical and biological sex
- Gender and sexual identity
- Sexual orientation and behavior.

Adolescents express their sexuality by one's behavior, mannerisms, interests, and appearance that are socially associated with gender, namely femininity or masculinity. Gender expression can also be defined as the external manifestation of one's gender identity through behavior, clothing, hairstyles, voice, or body characteristics. Sexuality can be expressed in thoughts, fantasies, desires, beliefs, attitudes, values, behaviors, practices, roles, and relationships. Sexual interests can be expressed in a number of ways verbal and nonverbal that can be flirting, kissing, masturbation, or having sex with partner.

## ROLE MODEL OF EXPRESSION OF SEXUALITY FOR ADOLESCENTS

Development of sexuality begins at birth and ends at death. Parents are the first role model of expression of sexuality in adolescents. Parents' attitude, parenting style, cultural influence, social factors, and peer relationship are the important factors that facilitate and decide the sexual learning and sexual attitude of the adolescents. Later, peers take over the developing brain of adolescents. As they grow, they use and search online media for sexually-related material.

Media (print, broadcast, internet, and out of home) and Internet, social media, over-the-top (OTT) platform, and dating play a huge role today. The depiction of sexuality here is quite crude, and mostly age-inappropriate; leading to conflicts, confusion, and defiance in the minds of adolescents.

The sexually-related topics, pornography, and sexual violence in media affect the adolescents' attitude and perception toward their sexuality. Adolescents are at risk because of their immature and developing brain. They are unable to perceive and analyze the messages from media correctly.

The adolescent risk taking behavior and experimentation also makes them vulnerable for sexual abuse.

Due to hormonal changes in adolescence, they want to express and explore the physical aspect of sexuality. At the same time, the need for intimacy and love with opposite gender increases. Adolescents start exploring different aspects of love. It is the role of gatekeepers to facilitate this expression with dignity. Adolescents need to know how to handle this emerging sexuality using emotional quotient, while understanding consequences.

## Decent Ways of Expressing Sexuality

- Sexuality can be expressed in body, clothes, behavior, verbal and nonverbal communication, and online communication.
- Being respectful, mindful, and empathetic toward the other person.
- Style is one of the ways of sexual expression. It depends upon how they dress? How they present physically to the society? Wearing clothes that are comfortable and appropriate for the place and occasion, are culturally and socially acceptable.
- How they communicate? Do they use socially appropriate language? Do they listen?
- Nonverbal communication is powerful. The body language, facial expressions, and tone can signify the real intent behind a person's behavior.
- The way one conducts himself or herself in public, the clothes, attitude, and behavior reflects aspects of a person's sexual self.

### Indecent Ways of Expressing Sexuality

- Unwanted touching, hugging, or kissing.
- Improper dressing, piercings, tattoos, and weird hairstyles because of peer- or media-pressure.
- Sexually offensive intrusive, explicit, and lewd comments, questions, words, songs, or sexual remarks on one's body or clothes.
- Expressing yourself in socially and sexually offensive way through writings, poems, or art; or under influence of addictive substances.
- Touching others without permission with sexual intent.
- Masturbation in inappropriate places, indecent exposure/flashing of private parts.
- Pornographic interest or sending explicit images online including child abuse images (it can be from websites, through messaging, or social media forums).
- Degradation/humiliation of others using sexual themes.
- Stalking a person, connecting electronically, or contacting physically despite disinterest.
- Written or verbal sexual threats.
- Sexual interest in children (pedophilia).

### Consequences of Indecent Expression of Sexuality

Adolescents are ill equipped to foresee the consequences due to their mostly concrete thinking and poor decision-making skills. This can lead to:

- Rape, unwanted pregnancies, abortion, and psychosexual disorders.
- Watching porn may lead to body image disorders, and sexual performance.
- Formation of weak relationships or inability to create meaningful relationships.
- These behaviors may constitute criminal offences in terms of law.
- Such behaviors in public may lead to physical harm and assault by mobs.

### ■ ROLE OF PEDIATRICIANS

- Pediatrician should have adolescent friendly clinics and supportive office staff. They should encourage adolescents to talk about sexual behavior in a nonjudgmental way.
- It is necessary to discuss about abstinence, contraceptives, consent, substance abuse, Protection of Children from Sexual Offences (POCSO), life skills, and safe sex.
- Dating violence and sexual abuse to be discussed.
- Listen carefully for hidden feelings. Adolescents sometimes have trouble saying exactly what they mean, especially when it comes to sex.
- Let the adolescent express their feelings freely. Listen to what they have to say in a nonjudgmental way.
- Avoid over/under answering of the questions. Answer questions directly, in words that the adolescent understands.
- Parents should be counseled that the adolescents' interest in one's own body may be natural. It does not indicate that they are involved in sexual activities. Parents can also be educated about how to give scientific sexuality education at home.

### Parental Education

- Keep reminding your child that you are in his/her corner every step of the way. Try to exhibit unconditional love and affection.
- Empower your child with knowledge, information, and values so that they do not indulge in the sexual risk-taking behavior and can overcome the peer pressure, etc.
- Develop media literacy among adolescents.
- Talk about ethics, values, and morals.

### Schools and Teachers

- Giving sexuality education in schools is a priority.
- Treat students and their emerging sexuality in a respectful and nonjudgmental way.
- Impart scientific knowledge about sex, gender, and anatomy.
- Teach life skills such as delayed gratification, responsibility, saying, and accepting "no", handling peer pressure, and effective communication.

### ■ KEY MESSAGES

- Sexuality is multi-dimensional in nature including anatomical and biological sex, sexual identity, gender identity, sexual orientation, sexual behavior, attraction, fantasies, and affiliation.
- Pediatrician have key roles to play in sexually related issues in adolescents as a counselor, educator, and healer.
- We must respect feelings of one another empathetically while communicating.

## ■ RECOMMENDED READING

1. Byron P. Troubling expertise: social media and young people's sexual health. Commun Res Pract. 2015;1(4):322-34.
2. Choudhary KC, Kumari S. Effect of Media on Sexual Behaviour: A Study of two Generations. Int J Indian Psychol. 2021;9(4):93-115.
3. Healthychildren.org. (2009). Adolescent Sexuality: Talk the Talk Before They Walk the Walk. [online] Available from https://www.healthychildren.org/English/ages-stages/teen/dating-sex/Pages/Adolescent-Sexuality-Talk-the-Talk-Before-They-Walk-the-Walk.aspx. [Last accessed March, 2024].
4. Jones K, Williams J, Sipsma H, Patil C. Adolescent and emerging adults' evaluation of a Facebook site providing sexual health education. Public Health Nurs. 2019;36(1):11-7.
5. Khubchandani J, Clark J, Kumar R. Beyond Controversies: Sexuality Education for Adolescents in India. J Family Med Prim Care. 2014;3(3):175-9.
6. Ministry of Health and Family Welfare. (2014). Strategy Handbook: Rashtriya Kishore Swasthya Karyakram. [online] Available from http://nhm.gov.in/images/pdf/programmes/rksk-strategy-handbook.pdf. [Last accessed March, 2024].
7. United Nations Population Fund–India. (2014). A Profile of Adolescents and Youth in India. [online] Available from https://india.unfpa.org/sites/default/files/pub-pdf/AProfileofAdolescentsandYouthinIndia_0.pdf. [Last accessed March, 2024].

# 8.4 Self-stimulation

*Deepa Janardhanan*

## ■ INTRODUCTION

Self-stimulation or masturbation is a process designed to derive sexual pleasure through any means other than sexual intercourse. It involves touching and playing with the genitals and stimulating them to get pleasure. Masturbation and self-examination are typical developmental processes. Research indicates that most kids will partake in some form of sexual exploration prior to reaching puberty, and this habit becomes even more prevalent following puberty. According to an Indian study, 45.9% of teenage boys and 12.7% of teenage girls masturbate. In another report, 90–94% of men and 50–60% of women recalled masturbating at some point in their childhood. Pediatricians must be able to distinguish between normal behavior and pathological behavior that may indicate an alternative medical diagnosis or abuse.

## ■ MASTURBATION: BIOLOGICAL AND DEVELOPMENTAL PERSPECTIVE

Masturbation normally begins in infancy and is a healthy part of development. Both boys and girls masturbate and it is a normal behavior. At the beginning of puberty, sex hormones, thoughts, and curiosity increase, which increases body awareness and sexual tension. Masturbation is a normal developmental process in adolescence. Most teenagers find self-exploration sexually pleasurable and understand that it is an expression of their own developing sexuality.

## ■ MYTHS AND FACTS ABOUT MASTURBATION

There are lots of myths surrounding masturbation, though they have been scientifically dispelled. Many of these myths persist. Many cultures still actively discourage masturbation, may be because of the general moral constraints often placed on sexual behavior.

Certain myths and facts about masturbation are given in **Table 1**.

## ■ INDICATORS OF CONCERN: POTENTIAL CAUSES AND RESPONSES

When masturbation is excessive or happens in public, it may indicate a more serious psychological or personal problem.

- It may be because the child is preoccupied with sexual thoughts, fantasies, or urges.
- The child may be overly stressed or not receiving adequate attention at home.
- Masturbation could even be a tip-off to sexual abuse; children who are being sexually abused may become overly preoccupied with their sexuality, suggesting the need for further investigation.

**TABLE 1:** Masturbation.

| Myth | Fact | Explanation |
|---|---|---|
| Self-stimulation (masturbation) is wrong or unhealthy | Self-stimulation is a normal and healthy part of human sexuality | It is a way for people to explore their own bodies, and thus they learn what feels good to them. It can also have health benefits such as reducing stress and helping with sleep. It also curtails unsafe sexual experimentation by adolescents |
| Self-stimulation can cause blindness and other health problems | Self-stimulation is a safe and healthy activity for most people | There is no scientific evidence to prove these claims |
| Only single people can masturbate | People in relationships also self-stimulate | It can be a way to explore one's own sexuality and learn what one likes and dislikes. It can also be a way to enhance sexual pleasure with one's partner |
| Self-stimulation is addictive | Most people are able to self-stimulate in a healthy and balanced way | Though it is possible to develop a compulsive masturbation habit, this is rare |
| Masturbation can cause hairy palms | Masturbation cannot cause hairy palms | Hair follicles are not present in the palms, and therefore no hair |
| Only men masturbate. | People of all ages, genders, and sexual orientations self-stimulate | Many may not reveal it |
| Masturbation can make erection impossible | Masturbation cannot cause erectile dysfunction | There is no relationship between masturbation and erectile dysfunction |
| Masturbation can cause infertility | Masturbation does not lead to infertility in men or women | It is a way for people to explore their bodies and learn what feels good to them |
| Self-stimulation is a sign of loneliness or sexual problems | Self-stimulation is not a sign of loneliness or sexual problems | Many people in healthy relationships masturbate regularly |

When parents of school-age children discover their child's masturbatory play or activity, some react with embarrassment, anger, and even moral outrage; others take it in stride and recognize it as developmentally normal behavior. Ideally, this discovery provides a wonderful opportunity for teaching children about their own sexuality and about the differences between public and private activities.

## ■ WHEN TO SEEK PROFESSIONAL HELP?

In certain situations, children require professional help by a behavioral pediatrician, psychiatrist, or psychologist. These include:

- Frequent excessive daily self-stimulation, both at home and in public.
- Public masturbation that continues even after the parents have talked about it with their child.
- Masturbation that takes place in conjunction with other symptoms of behavioral or emotional difficulty, including social isolation, aggression, destructiveness, sadness, withdrawal, bed-wetting, or soiling (encopresis).

- Sexual talk that is inappropriate or other sexual activity.
- Suspicion of sexual abuse.

## ■ ROLE OF PORNOGRAPHY

The portrayal of sexual subject matter for the purpose of sexual arousal is called pornography. These days, it has become widespread and easily accessible due to easy availability of the internet.

Adolescents are among the most frequent users of porn. They often believe what they see in the media is true. Teenagers commonly combine pornography with masturbation. The first externally stimulated sexual experiences of many teenagers may be watching and masturbating to porn. Initiation of sex at a younger age has been associated with negative outcomes in adulthood. Studies have shown that sexual development may be accelerated by exposure to pornography.

## ■ ROLE OF SEXUALITY EDUCATION

Comprehensive sexuality education (CSE) does not promote masturbation. The World Health Organization (WHO) observes that children start to explore their bodies through sight and touch at a relatively early age. Teenagers need to be provided up-to-date information related to sexuality, which is appropriate to their stage of development. CSE includes correcting misperceptions relating to masturbation, and teaching them about their bodies, boundaries, and privacy in an age-appropriate and nonjudgemental way. To prevent the development of wrong notions about sexuality among adolescents, sex education needs to be inculcated into the curriculum.

## ROLE OF PARENTS

The changing dynamics of family relationships during adolescence often create turbulence in both adolescents and their parents. But adolescents need their parents for critical support during this turbulent phase of their life.

What can parents do?
- Help their teenager anticipate changes in his or her body.
- Start early conversations about topics like healthy relationships, sex, sexuality, consent, and safety.
- Keep conversations with your child positive. Point out strengths. Celebrate successes.
- Emphasize normalcy. Reassure them that the acts of self-stimulation are normal, not deviant, and that they are doing nothing wrong by exploring what makes them feel good.
- Set Boundaries. Remind them of the boundaries and expectations, both within the household and society, that accompany exploring one's sexuality. Although everyone has a right to privacy and quiet contemplation of their mind or of their body, there are limits here.
- Be supportive and set clear limits. Parents need to communicate clearly reasonable expectations for curfews, media use, and behavior. At the same time, more independence needs to be given over time as your child takes on responsibilities.
- Honor independence and individuality. This is all part of moving into early adulthood. Always remind your child that you are there to help when need arises.

## SELF-STIMULATION AND ITS EXPRESSION IN SPECIAL CHILDREN

Children and teenagers with autistic spectrum disorder (ASD) frequently engage in self-stimulation, also referred to as stimming; although, children with other developmental disabilities may also exhibit this behavior. Stimming behaviors come in a variety of forms. A few instances are pacing, rocking, licking, biting oneself, rubbing objects, staring at lights, bouncing, twirling, jumping, and repetitive noises like humming or clicking.

Some adolescents with developmental disabilities start engaging in inappropriate sexual behaviors, like getting undressed and masturbating in public, and inappropriately touching people. Given the taboo nature of such behaviors and the possibility of serious negative outcomes, including injury, legal repercussions, and restricted community access, such acts are problematic.

To some children, stimming behaviors like masturbation can be beneficial in different ways. It may help some kids communicate or express themselves, self-regulate sensory input, or control emotions like excitement or anxiety. As a matter of fact, stimming is a harmless coping mechanism for a lot of kids. Nonetheless, efforts to lessen or control such behaviors might be required if they are impeding a child's capacity to learn or carry out daily tasks or causing social problems. While treating inappropriate sexual behavior in people with developmental disabilities can be difficult, research suggests that behavioral treatment and parental education can effectively lessen or even completely eradicate this type of problematic behavior.

## KEY MESSAGES
- Self-stimulation or masturbation is a process designed to derive sexual pleasure through any means other than sexual intercourse.
- Self-exploration and masturbation are a normal part of development.
- There are many myths about masturbation, though they have been scientifically dispelled.
- Excessive and socially inappropriate masturbation requires professional help.

## RECOMMENDED READING

1. Acred C (Ed). Adolescent Health. United Kingdom: Independence Educational Publishers; 2013.
2. Adarsh H, Sahoo S. Pornography and its impact on adolescent/teenage sexuality. J Psychosex Health. 2023;5(1):35-9.
3. Nair MKC, Babu G, Deepa SC. Sexual and reproductive health. In: Bhave SY, Parthasarathy A, Nair MKC, Menon PSN, Greydanus Donald E (Eds). Bhave's Textbook of Adolescent Medicine, 1st edition. New Delhi: Jaypee Brothers Medical Publishers (P) Ltd; 2006. pp. 160-6.
4. World Health Organization. (2023). Comprehensive sexuality education. [online] Available from https://www.who.int/news-room/questions-and-answers/item/comprehensive-sexuality-education. [Last accessed March, 2024].

# 8.5 Trans and Gender Divergent Adolescents: Pediatrician's Perspectives

*Harish Pemde, Tanu Shree*

## INTRODUCTION

Self-identity is a critical milestone for adolescents. Although this relates mainly to the identity different than "the child of parent", it also extends to self-development and recognition as a sexual being. Some children may experience a gender identity (GI) that is not aligned to the sex assigned at birth. Such children are considered sexual or gender divergent or transgender children.

Sexual orientation means choice of a sexual partner in fantasy or in real practice. Although most individuals are heterosexual (i.e., the partner is of opposite sex), some are homosexuals (i.e., they like a partner of the same sex; and are also known as gay, lesbian, etc.), and some may identify as asexual or their orientation may vary over time. The SO may vary irrespective of the GI viz. a cisgender person may be heterosexual or homosexual or asexual and similarly a transgender person may also be heterosexual or homosexual or asexual. Various terminologies are used to describe transgender and gender-diverse (TGD) individuals **(Box 1)**.

## DEVELOPMENT OF GENDER IDENTITY

Children discover their genitals during infancy. According to Gender Role Development Theory by Kohlberg, labeling occurs by 3–4 years of age, when children can label their own gender and recognize phenotypic differences between genders. They begin to separate out as "boy" versus "girl" activities. Gender stability occurs between age 4 and 6 years with development of an understanding that gender will not change over time. By school age children achieve gender constancy and the understanding that gender does not change despite changes in appearances and activities.

All children participate in games and play role of a different gender. However, gender diversity during prepubertal years is something more that the gender play. Some children exhibit play, dresses, attributes, and activities of other gender in consistent, persistent, and insistent manner well over a period of 2 years. These children are likely to develop as gender diverse or transgender individuals.

Thus, the GI is established before puberty begins. This brings onus of identifying and managing these children on pediatricians. Some of these TGD children experience distress (or dysphoria) regarding their genitalia or express mild to intense discomfort and dislike of their sex assigned at birth. GI has a spectrum covering binary, nonbinary, asexual, variable, and other descriptions. No clinician should take a risk of assuming GI by name, appearances, clothing, and mannerisms but should always ask about it. Methods of asking for GI are described in the later sections.

People often wonder if this diverse GI be aligned to the sex assigned at birth. Landmark research by Giordano (2019) demonstrated that the efforts, time, and opportunities for TGD children being supported and living in their *asserted gender* (at birth) do not appear to change their GI. The study also established that being responsive and supportive to a child's gender expression and needs does not push children toward adopting a TGD identity, and that children follow their internal cues and grow into a GI that make sense internally for them, something like their *cisgender peers* do. Evidences are strong against any kind of conversion therapy to change transgender persons to cisgender persons **(Fig. 1)**.

## DEVELOPMENT OF SEXUAL ORIENTATION

The SO refers to a pattern of physical, emotional, sexual, and romantic attraction to others, which may or may not be acted upon. The attraction may be toward a person of a different sex (heterosexual) or same sex (homosexual) or both sexes (bisexual) or none (asexual) or not sure (questioning), etc.

The SO develops around the time puberty begins, i.e., around 13 years of age. Thus, we can bring the issue of SO in discussion with adolescents while discussing sexuality issues. It is believed that the development of homosexuality goes through four stages.

1. *Stage 1—feeling different:* Adolescent develop feeling of being different than other peers and feel attracted to same sex individuals. This often occurs during middle teenage years.
2. *Stage 2—identity confusion:* While reaching physical maturity adolescents realize that they are attracted to

---

**BOX 1:** Understanding LGBTQ+ terminology.

- **Agender:** Term for individuals who do not identify as any gender at all
- **Ally:** Term for individuals that support and rally the rights of LGBTQIA+ even though they do not identify within the community
- **Androgynous:** Term for individuals with both male and female traits
- **Cisgender:** A term for individuals whose experienced and expressed gender is congruent with their gender assigned at birth, that is, those who are not transgender
- **Coming out:** The act of sharing one's sexual orientation or gender identity with loved ones
- **Crossdresser:** These terms generally refer to those who may wear the clothing of a gender that differs from the sex which they were assigned at birth for entertainment, self-expression, or sexual pleasure, aka drag queen or drag king
- **Eunuch:** An individual assigned male at birth whose testicles have been surgically removed or rendered nonfunctional and who identifies as a eunuch
- **Gender:** A person's social status as male (boy/man) or female (girl/woman), or alternative category
- **Gender diverse:** People who do not conform to their society or culture's expectations for males and females
- **Gender Dysphoria (GD) (capitalized):** A diagnostic category in DSM-5, with specific diagnoses defined by age group-specific sets of criteria
- **Gender dysphoria (not capitalized):** The distress caused by the discrepancy between one's experienced/expressed gender and one's assigned gender and/or primary or secondary sex characteristics
- **Gender expression:** Refers to how a person enacts or expresses their gender in everyday life and within the context of their culture and society, in the form of one's name, clothing, behavior, hairstyle, or voice, and which may or may not fit the usual frame of socially defined behaviors and characteristics associated with being either masculine or feminine
- **Gender identity disorder (GID):** A diagnostic category in DSM-III and DSM-IV that was replaced in DSM-5 by GD
- **Gender identity:** One's identity as belonging or not belonging to a particular gender, whether male, female, or a nonbinary alternative, aka experienced gender
- **Gender incongruence (capitalized):** A diagnostic category (analogous to GD in DSM-5) proposed for ICD-11
- **Gender incongruence (not capitalized):** Incongruence between experienced/expressed gender and assigned gender, and/or psychical gender characteristics
- **Gender role:** Cultural/societal definition of the roles of males and females (or of alternative genders)
- **Gender transition:** The process through which individuals alter their gender expression and/or sex characteristics to align with their sense of gender identity
- **Gender-affirmation procedures:** Procedures that help an individual affirm their gender identity including social (clothes, name, and pronouns), medical (hormone, laser, and surgery), and legal (changing their name, and gender on identification documents), aka gender reassignment
- **Intersex conditions:** A subset of the somatic conditions known as "disorders of sex development" or "differences of sex development" in which chromosomal sex is inconsistent with genital sex, or in which the genital or gonadal sex is not classifiable as either male or female. Some individuals who report their identity as "intersex" do not have a verifiable intersex condition
- **Lesbian:** Term for women sexually and romantically oriented toward other women
- **LGBTQIA+:** Term used to collectively refer to lesbian, gay, bisexual, transgender, questioning, queer, intersex, and asexual; and the plus sign (+) denotes inclusivity to cover all different sub-sects such as allies, pansexual, non-cisgender, and non-heterosexuals, aka LGBT, LGBTQ, or LGBTQ+
- **Sex:** An individual's categorization as biologically male or female, usually based on the genitals and reproductive tract
- **Sexual orientation:** An individual's pattern of sexual attraction and physiological arousal to others of the same (homosexual), other (heterosexual), both (bisexual), all (pansexual) or neither sex (asexual)
- **They/them/their:** Neutral pronouns used by some who have a nonbinary or nonconforming gender identity
- **Trans:** More recent umbrella term being increasingly used to avoid distinguishing between transgender and transsexual individuals
- **Transgender:** An umbrella term usually referring to individuals whose experienced or expressed gender does not conform to normative social expectations based on the gender they were assigned at birth
- **Transgender man:** A term to describe an individual who was assigned female at birth who identifies as a male, aka transman, female-to-male (FTM), transgender male, or man of trans experience
- **Transgender woman:** A term to describe an individual who was assigned male at birth who identifies as a female, aka transwoman, male-to-female (MTF), transgender female, or woman of trans experience
- **Transsexual:** A term often reserved for the subset of transgender individuals who desire to modify, or have modified, their bodies through hormones or surgery to be more congruent with their experienced gender

(DSM: Diagnostic and Statistical Manual of Mental Disorders; ICD-11: International Classification of Diseases, 11th Revision; LGBTQ: lesbian, gay, bisexual, transgender, and queer; LGBTQIA: lesbian, gay, bisexual, transgender, queer, intersex, and asexual)

provide confidence to the client in gender-neutrality and gender-friendly policies and approaches in the facility.

## COMPREHENSIVE CLINICAL EVALUATION IS NECESSARY

For comprehensive clinical evaluation, one can follow the following given processes:

- Provide audio and visual privacy
- Establish rapport by asking presenting complaints and general questions
- Declare the policy of confidentiality (and associated riders)
- Behave in nonjudgmental and culturally appropriate manner
- Use patient's chosen name and pronouns [telling your (physician's) name and pronouns will help]
- Begin with presenting complaints
- Conduct Home, Education/Employment, Eating, Activities, Drugs, Sexuality, Suicidal ideation and Safety (HEEADSSS) assessment; evidence of resilience (e.g., connectedness and positive social network), and risk (e.g., victimization, isolation, suicidality, housing access, food availability, and financial or safety concerns)
- Obtain other relevant history and conduct physical examination
- Evaluate for mental health issues and especially the gender dysphoria and the need for gender affirming care
- Enlist the issues, concerns, and diagnosis, if any
- Plan for investigations, treatment, and follow-up (and referral, prognosis, etc.).

These may require several visits to complete the process. Family support and social environment also warrant evaluation. Legal formalities related to consent and assent should be completed properly.

The examination of the transgender patients should be tailored as they may have discomfort during physical examination because of on-going dysphoria or negative past experiences. The process of examination should be explained well, chaperoned, and be stopped if patient finds any discomfort with it.

Screening for mental health of various disorders/conditions should be done, and these disorders are depression, anxiety, post-traumatic stress disorder, eating disorder, substance abuse, self-harm, bullying, truancy, homelessness, intimate partner violence, high risk sexual behaviors, and suicidality.

## MANAGING TRANSGENDER CHILDREN AND ADOLESCENTS

Like any other child or adolescent, the transgender persons also need treatment of common concurrent illnesses.

Mental health needs to be dealt with care and an experienced Psychiatrist should be involved in the care. Counseling and psychotherapy should be provided as needed.

### Gender Affirmative Care and Treatment

Thorough psychological evaluation should be done and documented for readiness of gender affirmative care.

Assent of the patient and consent of the caretakers (parents, guardian, or other legal guardian) should be documented for both agreement and denial of gender affirmative care at that age.

Prepubertal children need routine care for gender dysphoria or other mental health concerns or diagnosis. The clinician needs to counsel and guide parents and other caretakers to provide general affirmative care at home, assess for safety of affirmation environment at home and school, to prepare for supporting their child during adolescence and later adult life, and desist from any kind of conversion therapy. A policy of "wait and see" should be adopted and follow the transgender child carefully for future need of gender affirmative care.

Early puberty [sexual maturity rating (SMR) 2 or 3] is the time where hormonal therapy for pubertal suppression may begin. Shared care approach along with pediatric endocrinologist is desirable. Only reversible care (hormonal therapy) should be offered during adolescence. Irreversible surgical affirmation is considered when the individual is able to provide legal consent, i.e., as an adult.

The care during early puberty may also continue to the late puberty (SMR 3 or 4) **(Table 1)**.

## TRANSGENDER PERSONS (PROTECTION OF RIGHTS) ACT AND RULES, INDIA

Government of India passed Transgender Persons (Protection of Rights) Act 2019 (TPA) in August 2019 and it was brought into effect in January 2020.

### Provisions of the Transgender Persons (Protection of Rights) Act and Rules

This act provides a certificate of identity, underlines the rights and entitlements (regarding discrimination,

**TABLE 1:** Gender affirming treatment of TGD adolescents.

| Essential requirements for gender-affirming treatment | • Diagnosed as gender incongruence as per the ICD-11<br>• The experience of gender diversity/incongruence is marked and sustained over time<br>• Gender dysphoria worsened with the onset of puberty<br>• Demonstrates the emotional and cognitive maturity required to provide informed consent/assent for the treatment<br>• Mental health concerns (if any) that may interfere with diagnostic clarity, capacity to consent, and gender-affirming medical treatments have been addressed<br>• Informed of the reproductive effects, including the potential loss of fertility and the available options to preserve fertility<br>• Reached Tanner's stage 2 of puberty |
| --- | --- |

(ICD-11: International Classification of Diseases, 11th Revision; TGD: transgender and gender-diverse)

residence, employment, education, healthcare, and awareness).

It also makes indicates that the government will constitute National Council for Transgender Persons; and creates provisions for penalties for offenses against transgender persons.

## KEY MESSAGES

- Pediatricians should empower themselves to provide primary care to TGD children and adolescents.
- GI develops early in childhood and SO develops in early puberty. Thus, the pediatricians should be able to recognize gender incongruence.

- Gender friendly services should be provided and routine care should be extended to TGD children and adolescents without any discrimination.
- Gender affirmative care and treatment should be offered by pediatricians.
- Only reversible treatment (puberty suppression) should be offered during adolescence.
- Partially irreversible (feminizing and masculinizing hormonal therapy) and irreversible treatment (affirmative surgery) should be discussed during late adolescence preparatory to these treatments when the person becomes an adult.
- Pediatricians should be aware of ethical and legal aspects of gender friendly care including Transgender Persons (Protection of Rights) Act (2019) and Rules (2020).

## RECOMMENDED READING


1. Georgetown University. (2008). Adolescence. [online] Available from https://www.brightfutures.org/development/adolescence/sexual-identity.html. [Last accessed March, 2024].
2. Herman JL, Flores AR, O'Neill KK. (2022). How Many Adults and Youth Identify as Transgender in the United States? [online] Available from https://williamsinstitute.law.ucla.edu/publications/trans-adults-united-states/. [Last accessed March, 2024].
3. Levine DA; Committee on Adolescence. Office-based care for lesbian, gay, bisexual, transgender, and questioning youth. Pediatrics. 2013;132(1):e297-313.
4. Pemde HK, Bansal U, Bhattacharya P, Sharma RN, Kumar S, Bhatia P, et al. Adolescent Health Academy Statement on the Care of Transgender Children, Adolescents, and Youth. Indian Pediatr. 2023;60(10):843-54.


# 8.6 Same-sex Attractions

*Ashok Banga*

## INTRODUCTION

Growing up is a demanding and challenging period for every adolescent. One important aspect is forming one's sexual identity. All children explore and experiment sexually as part of normal development.

Researchers have found that over 95% of individuals are mainly attracted to individuals of the opposite sex and identify as heterosexual. The rest are either attracted toward same sex or both.

People who are homosexual are romantically and physically attracted to people of the same sex. It is part of the range of sexual expression. Homosexuality has existed throughout history and across cultures. Females who are attracted to other females are lesbian; males who are attracted to other males are often known as gay. (The term gay is sometimes used to describe homosexual individuals of either sex.)

## CAN YOU REALLY FALL IN LOVE WITH THE SAME GENDER?

It is possible that a teen might experience same-sex attraction, but might not necessarily ultimately identify as gay or even bisexual. Letting adolescents know that sexual attraction is normal and healthy, and that it is what we do with that attraction that gives sex its power—or diminishes it—can help them understand the power of attraction and create healthy sexual meanings. An adolescent might have a passing curiosity about the same sex, or a moment of arousal that confuses her or him. Parents can help teens understand that they are normal and not alone, and that sexual identity might be very clear early on or it might be something that unfolds more slowly.

## AM I GAY? AM I BISEXUAL?

Some people know they are same-sex attracted from a very young age. However, for others, there is a period of uncertainty or questioning. Not everyone who questions their sexuality ends up identifying as lesbian, gay, bisexual, transgender, queer, intersex, and asexual (LGBQTIA+). Many young people have sexual experiences with their own sex or "feelings" toward someone of the same gender at some point; this is a normal part of exploring their sexuality. They may come to realize that this is their preferred form of sexual expression.

Labels such as "gay", "bi", "queer", or "straight" are just the labels. They help to place people into easily understood categories. Getting hung up on defining their sexuality before they are ready can cause a lot of unnecessary angst. If they are unsure what to call themselves at this point, a better approach might be just to think of themselves as a sexual being. In time, they may find a label that feels right.

## IS SAME-SEX ATTRACTION NORMAL?

Same-sex attraction is in no way unusual, immoral, abnormal, or sick. It does not need to be cured or fixed. There are thousands of people going through the same situation at this moment. In fact, one in four families will have a family member who is gay or lesbian.

## COMING OUT

Coming out is the process of telling friends, family members, or others about their same-sex attraction. Many people fear negative reactions when they disclose their sexuality. Sometimes this fear is justified, as while attitudes are much more accepting than they once were, it is still possible that some people will react badly. On the other hand, many young people are often surprised by very supportive, accepting responses.

Coming out can be a huge relief. It may ease the feelings of isolation. The adolescent may feel like he/she can finally be themselves, and not have to lie anymore. However, it is extremely important that they do this only when they feel comfortable with the situation.

## WHAT IS HOMOPHOBIA AND WHY?

Homophobia is an attitude of irrational fear or hostility toward gays and lesbians. It can take a subtle form, such as put-downs or "jokes", or be expressed in overt discrimination, harassment, or violence. Most gays and lesbians will experience homophobic attitudes at some point, and it is often very distressing.

It is important to remember that just because you are attracted to the same sex does not mean you lose any of your rights as a human being. Harassment and violence are unacceptable regardless of whom they are directed at.

## WHAT IS SEXUAL ORIENTATION?

*Sexual orientation* is a term used to refer to a person's pattern of emotional, romantic, and sexual *attraction* to people of a particular gender (male or female).

Sexuality is an important part of who we are as humans. Beyond the ability to reproduce, sexuality also defines how we see ourselves and how we physically relate to others.

Sexual orientation is usually divided into these categories:
- *Heterosexual:* Attracted to people of the opposite gender
- *Bisexual:* Attracted to genders the same as themselves or different than themselves
- *Homosexual:* Attracted to people of one's own gender
- *Pansexual:* Attracted to people of any gender identity
- *Asexual:* Not sexually attracted to other people.

Sexual orientation involves a person's feelings and sense of identity; it is not necessarily something that is noticeable to others. People may or may not act on the attractions they feel.

## WHAT DETERMINES SEXUAL ORIENTATION?

Most scientists agree that sexual orientation (including homosexuality and bisexuality) is the result of a combination of environmental, emotional, hormonal, and biological factors. In other words, many things contribute to a person's sexual orientation, and the factors may be different for different people.

Homosexuality and bisexuality are not caused by the way children were reared by their parents or by something that happened to them when they were young. Also, being homosexual or bisexual does not mean the person is mentally ill or abnormal in any way. They may face burdens caused by other people's prejudices or misunderstandings.

Scientists know very little about this process, which usually takes place between the ages of 14 and 21 years. For example, it is not clear whether bisexual identity is more or less stable over time than a gay or straight identity. Neither do we know for sure whether men or women report greater changes in their sexual attraction over time.

## HOW DO PEOPLE KNOW THEIR SEXUAL ORIENTATION?

Many people discover their sexual orientation as teens or young adults, and in many cases without any sexual experience. For example, someone may notice that their sexual thoughts and activities focus on people of the same gender or both genders. But it is possible to have fantasies or to be curious about people of the same sex without being homosexual or bisexual. And they may not pursue those attractions.

For adolescents who do feel same-sex attraction, the typical time-period children report feeling a sense of same-sex attraction is at about 10 years old, with usually about 3 more years passing before adolescents' act on that attraction.

## CONCERNS OF ADOLESCENTS WITH SAME-SEX ATTRACTION

Despite increased knowledge and information, gay, lesbian, and bisexual teens still have many concerns. These include:

- Feeling different from peers
- Feeling guilty about their sexual orientation
- Worrying about the response from their families and loved ones

- Being teased and ridiculed by their peers
- Worrying about acquired immunodeficiency syndrome (AIDS), human immunodeficiency virus (HIV) infection, and other sexually transmitted diseases
- Fearing discrimination when joining clubs, sports, seeking admission to college, and finding employment
- Being rejected and harassed by others.

## HOW DO I TALK TO MY CHILD ABOUT THIS ISSUE?

Parents need to clearly understand that sexual orientation is not a mental disorder and the cause(s) of homosexuality or bisexuality are not yet fully understood. A relationship of love and trust between parent and child is of utmost importance whenever parents talk to children about sexuality. Children need to know that they can ask a parent any questions they have, and that their concerns will be accepted and answered in an atmosphere of love and safety.

Same-sex attraction is a topic that parents are sometimes hesitant to discuss with their children. Some parents' worry they will give teens ideas they otherwise would not have had. It is important to remember that talking about same-sex attraction is not going to influence a child to "choose" to be gay or not gay, because that is not a choice that individuals make. However, talking to adolescents about same-sex attraction in open and loving ways can help both parents and children navigate these waters, as can talking to other parents or support groups if needed. Perhaps reassuring them that transitory same-sex attraction is common might be helpful as they work through their questions about sexual identity and attraction. Creating this loving environment will benefit the relationship and establish a pattern for continued discussions. And in the end, the best thing we can do as parents is assure our children that we love them exactly as they are.

### ■ COUNSELING

Counseling may be helpful for teens who are uncomfortable with their sexual orientation or uncertain about how to express it. They may benefit from support and the opportunity to clarify their feelings. Therapy may also help the teen adjust to personal, family, and school-related issues or conflicts that emerge.

### ■ CONCLUSION

Sexuality can be confusing at the best of times. Discussing how feeling unsure about your sexual orientation, or unable to reveal your sexual identity for fear of rejection or discrimination can be a difficult experience.

If you are in this situation, remember that it gets better with time. You will find your sexual place in the world and have people around you who support and accept you for who you are.

As you move through this process, we would advise you to look closely at your life, your identity, and your sexuality in terms of the following four categories:

1. *Values:* Decide what is most important to you. What is the guiding "polestar" of your life? Think about your personal belief system. Remember that it is never wise to give greater weight to *feelings* than to rational conclusions.

2. *Behavior:* We understand that feelings are difficult, if not impossible, to control. They can blind-side you and take you by surprise. Fortunately, the same thing cannot be said about actions. There is such a thing as self-control, and it is possible to subject your behavior to your will regardless of what your emotions are saying. It takes discipline, determination, and a community of support.

3. *Attractions:* Sexual attraction is a complex subject. The origins of sexual feelings often lie deeply hidden within the individual psyche. They are frequently well-explained and understood in terms of developmental psychology and trait development, and there is no single "one-size-fits-all" theory to account for them. Despite this, it is feasible, with the help of a counselor, to gain valuable insights into some of the factors that may have contributed to the shaping of your present situation. In turn, these insights can be useful in freeing you from emotional bondage and enabling you to live according to your consciously chosen values, no matter how much the attractions come or go over the course of your life.

4. *Identity:* Remember that human identity—*who* and *what* we are in terms of our essential humanity—does not depend upon feelings, behavior, or attractions. We are free to accept or reject this idea as we fit. We can elect to self-label or self-identify in any way.

Though we may not be able to control our feelings willfully or directly, but we can decide how to respond to them, what we will believe about them, and how to will seek help and direct them into our future.

Many healthcare professionals provide medical care to teenagers who are gay, lesbian, and bisexual (GLB) far more often than they realize. The practitioner's knowledge and sensitivity regarding sexuality issues strongly influences the patient's comfort level in seeking optimal health care in the future.

## ■ KEY MESSAGES

- Growing up is a demanding and challenging period for every adolescent and one important aspect of this process is forming one's sexual identity.
- Over 95% of individuals are mainly attracted to individuals of the opposite sex and thus identify as heterosexual.
- Sexual identity might be very clear early on or it might unfold more slowly.
- Same-sex attraction is in no way unusual, immoral, abnormal, or sick. It does not need to be cured or fixed.
- Coming out can be a huge relief.
- We need to learn it first because treating doctor's knowledge and sensitivity regarding sexuality issues strongly influences the patient's comfort level in seeking healthcare in the future.

## ■ RECOMMENDED READING


1. American Academy of Child and Adolescent Psychiatry. (2013). Gay, Lesbian and Bisexual Adolescents. [online] Available from https://www.aacap.org/AACAP/Families_and_Youth/Facts_for_Families/FFF-Guide/Gay-Lesbian-and-Bisexual-Adolescents-63.aspx. [Last accessed March, 2024].
2. Burriss R. (2015). How Same-Sex Attraction Changes During Adolescence. [online] Available from https://medium.com/@RobertBurriss/how-same-sex-attraction-changes-during-adolescence-cd2ddf393be1. [Last accessed March, 2024].
3. Busseri MA, Willoughby T, Chalmers H, Bogaert AR. Same-sex attraction and successful adolescent development. J Youth Adolesc. 2006;35(4):563-75.
4. Clarke RW. Talking to Teens About Same-Sex Attraction. [online] Available from https://www.chelomleavitt.com/talking-to-teens-about-same-sex-attraction/. [Last accessed March, 2024].
5. Reitman DS. (2019). Sexual Orientation. [online] Available from https://emedicine.medscape.com/article/917792-overview#a1?form=fpf. [Last accessed March, 2024].

# 8.7 Decisions Regarding Marriages in Today's Adolescents and Young Adults

*Kalyani Patra*

## INTRODUCTION

In the rapidly evolving sociocultural landscape of India, the decision-making process regarding marriage among today's adolescents and young adults (AYAs) has undergone significant changes. This chapter aims to delve into the intricacies of these changes, exploring the factors that influence marital decisions and the implications they have on the individuals involved and society at large. Traditionally, marriage in India has been a familial affair, with elders predominantly steering the decision-making process. However, with increasing globalization, urbanization, and the advent of digital technology, young adults in India are now more exposed to diverse cultures and ideologies. This exposure has led to a shift in their perspectives on marriage, relationships, and personal autonomy.

This understanding is crucial for policymakers, educators, parents, and the youth themselves as they navigate these changing tides.

## FACTORS INFLUENCING DECISIONS

The decision-making process is influenced by a complex interplay of various sociocultural, economic, and psychological factors.

Some key factors are:

- *Cultural traditions and family expectations:* India has a rich cultural heritage. Family expectations, cultural traditions, and societal norms play a pivotal role in shaping the marriage decisions of AYA. Pressure from parents and relatives to adhere to traditional practices, such as arranged marriages or caste-based alliances, often affects the choices of individuals.
- *Education and career aspirations:* With the increasing emphasis on education and career opportunities, many Indian AYAs are prioritizing their professional aspirations over early marriages. As the youth become more career-oriented, they tend to delay marriage to focus on achieving their educational and professional goals.
- *Changing gender roles and women empowerment:* The evolving dynamics of gender roles and the empowerment of women have influenced marriage decisions significantly. More women are now actively participating in the workforce and seeking financial independence, leading to a desire for partnerships based on mutual respect, shared responsibilities, and decision-making equality, fostering a more balanced and collaborative approach to marriages. As a result, young women in India are increasingly asserting their right to choose a life partner.
- *Urbanization and global influences:* Exposure to diverse cultures, lifestyles, and ideologies through media, the internet and social interactions have led to a broader perspective on relationships, and have encouraged individuals to seek partners who align with their personal beliefs and values, irrespective of traditional customs and societal pressures.
- *Socioeconomic background and financial stability:* This is considered a crucial factor in ensuring a secure future for the couple. Young adults often prioritize finding a partner who can contribute equally to the financial well-being of the household and support their aspirations for a comfortable lifestyle.
- *Individualistic values and compatibility:* Today's AYA place a strong emphasis on emotional and intellectual compatibility, shared interests, and mutual understanding in their prospective partners. This shift reflects a desire for companionship and emotional fulfilment in marital relationships.
- *Individual autonomy:* As Indian society progresses toward a more inclusive and liberal mindset, young adults are asserting their independence and seeking to make decisions based on their own aspirations, values, and preferences, signifying a departure from the historically prevalent familial and societal influences, underscoring the growing recognition of personal choice as a fundamental tenet in the pursuit of fulfilling and meaningful relationships.

- *Influence of peer group and media:* Peer groups play a significant role in shaping individual perceptions of relationships, love, and marriage, which can impact their preferences and expectations. Additionally, the pervasive influence of media, including television, films, and social media platforms, contributes to the formation of idealized notions of love and relationships. The portrayal of diverse romantic narratives and modern relationship dynamics in media often serves as a catalyst for redefining traditional notions of marriages, encouraging young adults to seek partners who align with their contemporary ideals and aspirations.
- *Changing attitudes toward love and relationship:* Traditionally, marriages in India were often arranged, and love was perceived through a lens of duty and commitment. However, the current generation is increasingly embracing a more liberal and individualistic perspective on love and relationships. There is a departure from the purely practical and duty-bound approach that historically characterized Indian marriages.

## TRADITIONAL VERSUS MODERN PERSPECTIVE OF MARRIAGES IN CONTEMPORARY INDIA

Traditionally, marriages are perceived as a union not just between two individuals but between two families, symbolizing the continuity of lineage and cultural traditions. Conversely, the modern perspective of marriages in India is shaped by a paradigm shift toward individual autonomy, egalitarian values, and personal choice. There has been an increasing inclination toward love marriages, intercaste unions, and partnerships based on emotional compatibility and shared values.

The coexistence of these contrasting viewpoints signifies the intricate tapestry of Indian culture, and underscores the ongoing evolution of Indian society, as the youth strive to strike a balance between honoring their cultural heritage and embracing the ethos of individualism and personal choice in their pursuit of marital happiness.

## EARLY MARRIAGES

India is home to the largest number of child brides in the world. While it is illegal for girls under the age of 18 years to marry in India, estimates suggest that at least 1.5 million girls under age 18 years get married in India each year. Nearly 16% of all adolescent girls aged 15–19 years are currently married. Early marriages are often a result of parental and familial expectations, as well as economic considerations.

Early unions have negative consequences that can:
- Curtail educational and career opportunities
- Perpetuate gender inequalities
- Cause adverse physical and psychological consequences, impacting the overall well-being of the individuals involved
- Contribute to health and social challenges.

## DOWRY PRACTICES

Despite legal interventions and societal awareness campaigns, the custom of dowry remains deeply entrenched in certain communities. However, empowered by education and a desire for more equitable relationships, many young adults are actively advocating against dowry. This shift in mindset reflects a progressive stance toward creating more inclusive and respectful marital relationships in contemporary India.

## CHANGING PARENTAL PERSPECTIVE: THE SHIFT TOWARD SUPPORTIVE AND COLLABORATIVE MARITAL DECISION-MAKING IN INDIA

There is a discernible transformation in the parental perspective on marriage decisions, reflecting a departure from the traditional norms of parental control and authoritative decision-making. Parents are increasingly embracing a more supportive role in the decision-making process, prioritizing open communication, mutual understanding, and the empowerment of their children in choosing life partners, at least in the urban, higher socioeconomic strata.

## IMPACT OF MODERNIZATION ON TRADITIONAL PRACTICES IN MARRIAGES AMONG INDIAN AYA

One significant impact is the gradual shift from arranged marriages toward a greater acceptance of love marriages. While many young adults continue to honor traditional ceremonies, there is a discernible trend toward more personalized and intimate wedding celebrations, reflecting a blend of traditional customs and modern sensibilities.

## Increase in Intercaste and Inter-religion Marriages

- There has been a notable rise in the prevalence of intercaste and inter-religion marriages, reflecting a shift in societal attitudes and a growing acceptance of diversity within the institution of marriage.
- By transcending caste boundaries, young couples are challenging age-old prejudices and advocating for a more inclusive and harmonious society. Inter-religion marriages, similarly, demonstrate a willingness to embrace religious diversity and foster communal harmony.
- However, despite the progressive outlook, these marriages in India often encounter societal resistance, familial opposition, and at times, even legal and communal challenges which can sometimes pose significant obstacles for couples seeking to marry outside their caste or religion.

## Embracing Online Matrimonial Platforms: A Shift in Marriage Decision-making

- In the digital era, online platforms have emerged as powerful tools for individuals seeking compatible partners, offering a diverse array of profiles and filtering options that cater to specific preferences, including education, profession, and lifestyle choices.
- The convenience and accessibility of online matrimonial platforms have revolutionized the traditional matchmaking process, transcending geographical boundaries, fostering an environment that promotes open communication, transparency, and informed decision-making.
- Furthermore, it has facilitated conversations about personal preferences, values, and life goals before committing to a marital relationship, thereby fostering a more informed and thoughtful approach to the decision-making process.
- While it has streamlined the search for compatible partners, it also raises concerns regarding privacy, authenticity of profiles, and the potential for misrepresentation. As a result, it is essential for users to exercise caution and employ critical judgment.

## CHANGING TRENDS IN MARRIAGE PATTERNS AMONG TODAY'S AYA IN INDIA

The prominent shifts in marriage patterns are increasing prevalence of love marriages, delaying marriages—as more young adults prioritize their education, career aspirations, and personal development, nuclear family units and a more egalitarian distribution of household responsibilities, intercaste and inter-religion marriages.

The changing trends in marriage patterns reflect the evolving mindset of today's AYA in India.

## CHALLENGES AND BENEFITS OF RECENT TRENDS IN MARRIAGE

### Challenges

- *Societal acceptance:* Despite the increasing acceptance of these trends, societal approval remains a significant challenge. Many young adults face resistance from their families and society, particularly in rural areas with conservative values.
- *Legal recognition:* Living-in relationships and prenuptial agreements are not legally and widely recognized in India. This can lead to complications regarding property rights and child custody.
- *Emotional challenges:* Young adults may face stress and anxiety due to societal pressure, the fear of being ostracized, and adjustment issues.

### Benefits

- *Autonomy in decision-making:* Young adults now have more autonomy in choosing their life partners based on their personal preferences rather than societal norms.
- *Better understanding:* Trends like living-in relationships allow couples to understand each other better before marriage.
- *Breaking stereotypes:* These trends are helping break stereotypes related to caste, religion, and gender roles in marriage promoting equality and mutual respect among couples.
- *Convenience and wider choices:* Online matrimonial platforms provide convenience and a wider range of choices.

## EMPOWERMENT AND AGENCY: A TRANSFORMATIVE FORCE IN CONTEMPORARY MARITAL DECISION-MAKING FOR INDIA'S AYA

The empowerment of women has played a pivotal role in reshaping gender dynamics within marital relationships. Women are increasingly asserting their rights, advocating for equitable partnerships, and challenging societal norms that perpetuate gender-based inequalities, thus fostering a more balanced and progressive marital environment.

## FUTURE OUTLOOK FOR MARRIAGES AMONG INDIA'S AYA

- A promising shift toward greater individual empowerment
- Technological integration particularly the utilization of online matrimonial platforms and integration of artificial intelligence and advanced matchmaking algorithms
- A more inclusive and progressive societal mindset, underscoring the potential for fostering harmonious and resilient marital relationships.

### LGBTQ+ Marriages: A Shift toward Inclusivity and Legal Recognition in India's Changing Social Landscape

In recent years, there has been a significant shift in societal attitudes toward lesbian, gay, bisexual, transgender, and queer (LGBTQ+) marriages in India, reflecting a growing recognition of the need for inclusivity and equality within the institution of marriage. While the legal landscape is gradually evolving, with the decriminalization of same-sex relationships and the recognition of transgender rights, the issue of legalizing same-sex marriage remains a topic of ongoing debate and advocacy. While progress is being made, challenges persist, including societal prejudice, discrimination, and a lack of comprehensive legal protection for LGBTQ+ individuals. The future outlook for LGBTQ+ marriages in India holds the promise of a more inclusive and accepting society, one that values and celebrates the diversity of love and relationships, irrespective of gender identity or sexual orientation.

## EXPECTED ROLE OF NATION, SOCIETY, AND FAMILY: NURTURING INCLUSIVE AND PROGRESSIVE MARITAL CHOICES FOR TODAY'S AYA IN INDIA

The nation plays a pivotal role in enacting and enforcing laws that promote gender equality, protect individual rights, and ensure the legal recognition of diverse marital partnerships. Comprehensive legal frameworks that safeguard the rights of women, LGBTQ+ individuals, and marginalized communities are essential for creating a more equitable and inclusive societal landscape.

*Society*, on the other hand, has the responsibility of fostering a culture of acceptance, tolerance, and inclusivity, one that celebrates diversity and promotes open dialogue about progressive marital norms. Educating the public, challenging discriminatory attitudes, and providing support for individuals, navigating nontraditional marital choices are integral in building a more compassionate and understanding social fabric.

*Families*, as primary social units, play a crucial role in nurturing an environment of mutual respect, understanding, and support for the marital choices of their members. Encouraging open communication, respecting individual autonomy, and fostering an environment that values emotional well-being and personal growth are essential in nurturing healthy and fulfilling familial relationships.

As the nation, society, and family collectively strive to play their respective roles in fostering an environment conducive to inclusive and progressive marital choices, the future outlook for Indian marriages holds the promise of greater mutual understanding, respect, and emotional fulfilment for all individuals, underscoring the importance of collaborative efforts for generations to come.

## KEY MESSAGES

- The decision-making process regarding marriage among today's AYAs has undergone significant changes.
- It is influenced by a complex interplay of various sociocultural, economic, and psychological factors.
- The modern perspective of marriages in India is shaped by a paradigm shift toward individual autonomy, egalitarian values, and personal choice.
- The parental perspective has shifted toward more supportive and collaborative marital decision-making.
- The roles of nation, society, and family are important in nurturing inclusive and progressive marital choices for today's AYA in India.

## RECOMMENDED READING

1. Alexander M, Garda L. Marriage Related Decision Making among Young People: What Influences Their Involvement and Why should Young People be Involved-Evidence from Community Based Survey in Rural and Urban Pune District, India. [online] Available from https://ipc2009.popconf.org/papers/91390. [Last accessed March, 2024].
2. Bhakat P. Involvement of youth in marriage related decision making in India. Eur Sci J. 2015;11(10):178-90.

3.  McDougal L, Jackson EC, McClendon KA, Belayneh Y, Sinha A, Raj A. Beyond the statistic: exploring the process of early marriage decision-making using qualitative findings from Ethiopia and India. BMC Womens Health. 2018;18(1):144.
4.  Moore AM, Singh S, Ram U, Remez L, Audam A. Adolescent Marriage and Childbearing in India: Current Situation and Recent trends. [online] Available from https://www.guttmacher.org/report/adolescent-marriage-and-childbearing-india-current-situation-and-recent-trends. [Last accessed March, 2024].
5.  Singh M, Shekhar C, Shri N. Patterns in age at first marriage and its determinants in India: A historical perspective of last 30 years (1992-2021). SSM Popul Health. 2023;22: 101363.

<table>
<tr><td>

**8.8**

</td><td>

# The Married Adolescent

*Sushma Desai, Newton Luiz*

</td></tr>
</table>

## ■ INTRODUCTION

Adolescent marriage is illegal in India, as the legal age of marriage is 18 years for a girl and 21 years for a boy. A marriage below the age of 18 years is called a "child marriage", or "early marriage". Parents who get their adolescents married are denying them the basic right to decide whether, when, and whom to marry. This chapter focuses on the adolescent girl, as early marriage has severe consequences for them, and is five times more common in them than in adolescent boys.

Occasionally, the adolescent girls themselves decide to get married, because they love someone or to leave the homes where they are considered a burden and treated with a gender bias. In such cases, they generally forfeit the support of their family and society.

## ■ HOW SERIOUS IS THE PROBLEM?

- Globally, approximately one in five girls gets married before attaining adulthood.
- According to the 2019–2021 National Family Health Survey-5 (NFHS-5), 14.7% of urban and 27% of rural women in India get married before the age of 18 years. This is a major decline from the 2005–2006 NFHS data, which indicated that 47% of married women aged 20–24 had got married before their 18th birthday.
- Another 40% of females get married soon after reaching the legal age of marriage, i.e., at 18–20 years.
- *In India, over half the married girls live in five states:* Uttar Pradesh, Bihar, West Bengal, Maharashtra, and Madhya Pradesh.
- 3.8% of urban and 7.9% of rural women aged 15–19 years are mothers.

- The younger a girl is at marriage, the longer her period of fertility. On average adolescent brides in India have one child more than adult brides, and their first child is born earlier.

## ■ THE IMPACT ON THE MARRIED ADOLESCENT

Marriage has a profound impact on adolescents. It curtails their education, compromises their health, exposes them to violence, and traps them in poverty, undermining their prospects and potential.

### Health Issues

- Early marriages may result in early pregnancy. Pregnancy is the number one cause of death in adolescent girls, who are less likely to receive adequate antenatal care, and more likely to be undernourished, anemic, and to develop pregnancy-induced hypertension, than adult women. Early childbearing is associated with a higher maternal mortality and morbidity. They need their husbands' permission to use contraception. Often there is parental pressure to conceive within a year of marriage.
- Children born to adolescent girls have higher neonatal and infant mortality and morbidity, mainly due to prematurity, asphyxia, birth trauma, and sepsis.
- As the introitus is narrower in adolescents compared to adults, there is a higher chance of local trauma, which increases their risk of human immunodeficiency virus (HIV) and sexually transmitted infections (STIs). Married adolescent girls are at higher risk for HIV than unmarried girls, despite having a single regular partner, because they have sex frequently, without a condom.

- There is a higher risk of mental health disorders such as depression and anxiety disorders in both boys and girls. Girls may experience post-traumatic stress disorder due to domestic violence or sexual abuse. Early marriage is a major risk factor for suicidality.

## Other Issues

- An adolescent has not attained intellectual or emotional maturity. Despite their fierce desire for independence, adolescents need parental support and guidance. An adolescent marriage takes away the right of the adolescent girls to benefit from their parents' presence.
- The married girl is frequently not permitted by her husband or his family to continue with her studies. This affects her future, limiting her career options, her financial security, and her ability to contribute to society. She becomes an unpaid worker in her husband's house.
- As she stays with her in-laws, she often lacks status and influence in the house. She is isolated from her family and friends, and cannot visit a friend or go to the market without her husband's permission. Her husband believes that he has a right to sex, and does not need her consent. She is at risk for domestic violence and sexual abuse.
- If a married couple stays apart from their parents, an unexpected pregnancy frequently compels the girl to drop out of her studies or her job. The husband too may find that his mobility and opportunities are restricted as he must stay with his wife.
- A young married couple may not have the emotional maturity required to adjust to the ups and downs of a marital relationship.
- Marriage brings with it financial burdens, which were until then borne by the parents. Married adolescents with limited educational qualifications will have difficulty finding a satisfactory job. Even if the parents are willing to support the couple, there is a stigma attached to their lack of financial independence.
- Young, poorly educated couples are less likely to have children who will pursue higher education, leading to a cycle of poor literacy and scarce job possibilities.

## WHY DO PARENTS MARRY OFF THEIR DAUGHTERS IN ADOLESCENCE?

- *Gender inequality:* As the girl is expected to leave her family after marriage her parents consider her as someone else's property, whereas the son is one's own wealth, and is expected to look after the parents in their old age and perform their last rites when they die. Hence, spending money on feeding and educating the girl is considered a waste of money.
- *Protecting the girl's virginity:* The parents consider it a disgrace if a daughter has premarital sex. Marrying her off at puberty relieves the family of the responsibility of keeping her pure.
- *Tradition:* Getting the daughter married is considered a major duty of parents. Low life expectancy in the past pressurized parents to get their daughters married early, thus fulfilling their dharma.
- *Poverty:* Dowry increases with the age of the girl. Once the girl leaves her parental home, there is one less mouth to feed, and one less person to educate.
- *Limited job opportunities:* Where job opportunities are limited, it is considered unprofitable to educate a girl, who is destined to be housebound. More importance is placed on teaching her to do housework. There may also be reluctance to send the girl child to school, due to security concerns, if there is no school nearby.

## WHAT ARE THE LAWS REGARDING ADOLESCENT MARRIAGE?

- *The Child Marriage Restraint Act,* amended in 1978, makes it illegal for a girl to be married before the age of 18 years and for a boy to be married before the age of 21 years. Unfortunately, the Act has no teeth: It does not consider a child marriage null and void, but merely permits a sentencing of 15–90 days imprisonment, and even this is optional.
- *The Prohibition of Child Marriage Act (2006)* states that a marriage will be void if the child decides that she does not want to continue with it. The adolescent may not feel competent to make such a decision, nor does she have the power to take care of herself if the marriage is nullified. (In Karnataka, from 2017 onward, a child marriage is null and void, irrespective of whether the child asks for an annulment or not.) In addition:
  - The solemnization of child marriages is a nonbailable offence, and punishment is meted to the parents or organizations that conduct the marriage.
  - It provides for maintenance and residence of the child bride.
  - It gives a legal status to all children born from child marriages and makes provisions for their custody and maintenance.

## WHAT IS OUR COUNTRY DOING TO ELIMINATE CHILD MARRIAGE?

- India has committed to eliminate child marriage by 2030.
- "Beti Bachao, Beti Padhao" is a campaign that aims to improve the public perception of the importance of daughters. Keeping girls in schools is recognized as one of the best ways to delay marriage. The government has also used cash incentives (Dhan Laxmi scheme) and adolescents' empowerment programs (Kishori Shakti Yojana) to improve awareness and bring about behavior change.
- The registration of births and deaths, and of marriage, is mandatory in India.
- There is a controversial proposal to increase the minimum age of marriage to 21 years for girls too. Rights activists strongly oppose it, stating that it would lead to an increase in premarital sex, elopement, honor killings, and cases of kidnapping filed against innocent boys.

## KEY MESSAGES

- In India, the legal age of marriage is 18 years for a girl and 21 years for a boy.
- Most adolescent marriages are forced by parents upon their daughters.
- Adolescent marriages are declining steadily, but still constitute one-fifth of all marriages.
- Adolescent marriage curtails the girl's education, compromises her health, exposes her to violence, and traps her in poverty.
- Childbirth is associated with higher maternal, neonatal, and infantile mortality and morbidity. The girl is prone to STIs including HIV, and to mental illnesses and suicide.
- Parents marry off their adolescent daughters due to poverty, the pressure of tradition, to safeguard them from premarital sex, and because daughters are less valued than sons.
- The Prohibition of Child Marriage Act (2006) makes child marriage a nonbailable offense, and the marriage will become void if the girl states that she does not want to continue with it.
- The "Beti Bachao, Beti Padhao" campaign aims to improve the public perception of the importance of daughters.
- The compulsory registration of births and deaths, and of marriage, should be implemented strictly.

## RECOMMENDED READING


1. Haberland N, Chong E, Bracken. (2003). Married Adolescents: An Overview, Paper prepared for the WHO/UNFPA/Population Council Technical Consultation on Married Adolescents WHO, Geneva. [online] Available from https://knowledgecommons.popcouncil.org/cgi/viewcontent.cgi?article=2505&context=departments_sbsr-pgy. [Last accessed March, 2024].
2. Jejeebhoy SJ. (2019) Ending Child Marriage in India: Drivers and strategies. New Delhi: UNICEF. AKSHA Center for Equity and Wellbeing. [online] Available from chrome-extension://efaidnbmnnnibpcajpcglclefindmkaj/https://www.unicef.org/india/media/2556/file/Drivers-strategies-for-ending-child-marriage.pdf [Last accessed March, 2024].
3. Luiz N. Rights of the Girl Child. In: Ashok K. Handbook of Child Rights. Cochin: Indian Academy of Pediatrics, Kerala; 2020. pp. 59-63.
4. WHO. (2006). Married adolescents: no place of safety. [online] Available from https://www.who.int/publications/i/item/9241593776. [Last accessed March, 2024].


# 8.9    Adolescent Pregnancy

*Sucheta Kinjawadekar, Krutika Arunachalam*

## INTRODUCTION

The World Health Organization (WHO) defines an adolescent as a person between the age of 10 and 19 years. This is the transition phase of psychological and physical changes that occur from a child to an adult.

An adolescent pregnancy or a teenage pregnancy is termed when the woman is pregnant between the ages of 10 and 19 years. Adolescent pregnancy remains a global concern, with approximately 14 million girls under the age of 19 years becoming pregnant worldwide in 2021.

In Maharashtra, 10.6% of rural women aged 15–19 years initiated childbearing, thus exceeding the state average of 7.6%. Similarly, in Tripura and West Bengal, where socioeconomic challenges persist, adolescent pregnancy rates were 22% and 16%, respectively.

Adolescent pregnancy holds risks for maternal, fetal, neonatal, and infant morbidity and mortality compared to the older reproductive age period.

Adolescent fertility rate (births per 1,000 women ages 15–19 years) in India was reported at 17.23% in 2021, according to the World Bank collection of development indicators, compiled from officially recognized sources.

At birth, the length of the cervix is approximately 4 cm which is 2–2.5 times longer than the length of the uterine corpus. As the girl enters her adolescent age, there is an increase in the uterine volume and endometrial thickness as puberty progresses. During adolescence the corpus grows relatively more than the cervix and this growth continues through adolescence until early adulthood.

It is around this time that the uterus begins to respond to hormones and ovulatory maturation of the hypothalamus pituitary ovarian axis (HPO axis).

The ongoing uterine growth and the maturation of the HPO axis makes the adolescent liable to a pregnancy in a vulnerable situation in a still immature size uterus.

## ■ CAUSES FOR ADOLESCENT PREGNANCY

- *Economic hardships:* Poverty plays a major role in the advent of teenage marriages leading to adolescent pregnancy. Illiteracy among young girls brings about a lack of job opportunities compelling the parents of many to consider early marriage as a course of action for a propitious future.
- *Social norms and expectations:* Many times teenage marriages are also accepted in the name of tradition and culture. Social causes such as concern regarding safety over the girl child and the parents often grant marriage at an earlier age as even by law, the legal age for marriage for girls in India is 18 years.
- On several occasions adolescent pregnancy is a result of rape due to lack of respect for the girl and the law of the state.
- Experimentation and unsafe sexual encounters.

## ▌ RISKS ASSOCIATED WITH ADOLESCENT PREGNANCY

### Anemia

There is an increase in plasma volume and decrease in the hemoglobin concentration in the normal pregnancy. The WHO defines the minimum hemoglobin concentration in normal pregnancy as 11.0 g/dL. Anemia in pregnancy is often caused by nutritional deficiencies, especially folic acid and iron. A large number of adolescents suffer from nutritional anemia. If a pregnant adolescent does not receive adequate antenatal care, the preexisting anemia could worsen in the postpartum period.

## Ramifications of Emotional Immaturity

An adolescent just coming to terms with the physical body changes after puberty now has to deal with the physical changes that would occur in pregnancy to her body and may lack the emotional maturity to do so; leading to poor self-esteem, depression, and may even resort to self-harm.

If this pregnancy is a consequence of a failure of consent, she may develop a tendency to neglect this pregnancy and may even harbor infanticidal tendencies.

## Obstetric Outcome

One of the important physiological changes that occur during placentation is the spiral artery remodeling. This takes place in two phases, phase one in which the trophoblast invades the decidual portion of the spiral arteries, (by 10–12 weeks). The phase two takes place at around 16 weeks, the tertiary villi invade the myometrial portion of the spiral arteries. During the trophoblastic invasion, the elastic and the muscular layers of the spiral arteries are replaced by hyaline material and the endothelial layer is replaced by trophoblast.

When there is a defect in this deep placentation, trophoblastic invasion, the pregnancy is associated with complications like the *great obstetrical syndrome* which include the likes of gestational hypertension, preeclampsia, eclampsia, fetal growth restriction (FGR), and prelabor/premature rupture of membranes.

## Preterm Labor

In an adolescent pregnancy, preterm labor could mainly occur because of two reasons. One is a result of defective placentation resulting into conditions such as preeclampsia and eclampsia where preterm delivery would warrant a better outcome for the neonate (iatrogenic preterm birth) and the other is the result of low gynecological age (gynecological age = chronological age – age of menarche). It was found that when the pregnant adolescent has a gynecological age of <2 years, there is increased chances of preterm labor and delivery.

## Inadequate Pelvis

The growth of the pelvis continues even after the age of sexual maturity both the total superior inferior length and lateral breath of the pelvis continues to grow after puberty and they reach adult proportion beyond the age of 21 years.

This often leads to complications like prolonged labor and increased incidences of operative delivery and cesarean section.

## Sexually Transmitted Diseases

The pregnant adolescent is susceptible to various sexually transmitted diseases, especially if there is an older partner, failure to use any form of barrier contraception, or multiple partners.

## Unsafe Abortion

In order to avoid any form of social stigma, especially in the case of an unmarried adolescent pregnant woman (PW), many may resort to seeking help from less skilled professionals, thereby putting their lives in danger.

## Neonatal Outcome

### Small for Gestational Age Babies

Babies with birth weight below the 10th percentile for gestational age are termed as small for gestational age (SGA) babies. There is a higher incidence of SGA babies in pregnant adolescent mothers as compared to the all the mothers.

### Prematurity

Premature birth due to medical causes of pregnancy (iatrogenic prematurity) or due to poor gynecological age of the adolescent mother makes it rather difficult for her to carry a full-term pregnancy. Higher incidence of spontaneous birth is noticed with lesser maternal age.

### Neonatal Mortality and Stillbirths

Teenage per say is not risk factor for stillbirth. However poor antenatal, intrapartum, and postnatal care may contribute to various poor neonatal outcomes. Difficulty in breastfeeding leading to health issues in the neonate.

## MANAGEMENT OF A PREGNANT ADOLESCENT

The management of a pregnant adolescent depends on the choice she makes with regards to this pregnancy.

- If the pregnant adolescent opts for termination of pregnancy the caregiver must be empathetic and accept the decision without any judgment. The caregiver must share all the safe options that can be provided for their termination of pregnancy.
- Alternatively, if the adolescent chooses to continue with the pregnancy the caregiver must ensure a safe, secure, and supportive environment. A detailed history for medical and surgical illness must be taken. Any relevant family history is noted along with her daily habits. She is supplemented with folic acid, iron, and calcium in this pregnancy.

Importance of a nutritional diet is explained. She is requested to consume a well-balanced diet containing proteins, carbohydrates, and fats.

The need for regular antenatal checkups is explained and investigations to rule out any associated conditions such as hypothyroidism, diabetes, and anemia. Tests to rule out serological diseases and asymptomatic bacteriuria are conducted with the intention to keep her antenatal period uneventful.

Tests like hemoglobin and albuminuria are checked in every trimester. Blood pressure (BP) check is carried out more frequently in last trimester (every 15 days).

Antenatal immunization is given [flu vaccine and injection tetanus-diphtheria (Td) two doses 4–6 weeks apart).

She is informed about the changes that her body may experience in the course of 9 months. At term she is explained about the process of labor so as to have a positive birthing experience.

## ■ CARE DURING LABOR

As an adolescent pregnancy is considered high risk, it is advisable to conduct this delivery in a well-equipped hospital with 24 hours operation theater (OT) availability.

The caregiver must practice respectful maternal care. Give her privacy in the delivery room and respect her choice of having a birth companion during labor. Attention to be paid toward nutrition, hydration, and ambulation during labor. Give her as much information and explanation as she chooses to know.

The caregiver needs to observe the labor and monitor the fetal well-being with the use of a partograph which works as a decision-making tool.

## ■ POSTNATAL CARE

Within the first 2 hours the condition of the mother and the baby should be evaluated and corrective measures should be taken when necessary.

Breastfeeding should be initiated within 1 hour of delivery. She must be counseled about the importance of breastfeeding and taught the correct technique.

During the hospital stay in the postnatal period the caregiver must examine for signs of physical and mental signs of well-being. A counselor must be engaged if there are signs of postpartum depression.

## POSTPARTUM CONTRACEPTION

The adolescent mother must be encouraged to accept postpartum contraception. It not only will help her for spacing between children but also give her adequate time to regain and build her health. Various contraceptive options such as lactational amenorrhea method (LAM), progesterone only pills, depot medroxyprogesterone acetate (DMPA) injection, and intrauterine contraceptive device (IUCD) should be offered.

Emphasis on nutrition with extra caloric intake during lactation must be explained to the adolescent mother.

## MANAGEMENT OF UNMARRIED AND ADOLESCENT PREGNANCY

In this scenario, if the teenage PW chooses to keep the child, then after delivery as per the Indian law, she becomes the sole guardian of the child.

In cases where the woman chooses to give the child up for adoption, she is permitted to do so under the provision called safe surrender of the child. The Juvenile Justice Act of India allows the parents and the guardian to legally surrender the child without any consequences. The adolescent mother can safely and legally surrender the child at the nearest specialized adoption agency registered with the government terminating their parental rights and letting the child enter the legal adoption process.

## ADOLESCENT PREGNANCY AND THE PROTECTION OF CHILDREN FROM SEXUAL OFFENCES ACT 2012

This Act stipulates a child friendly, judicial process with the aim to encourage children who have been victims of sexual abuse to report the offence and seek justice.

This Act recognizes almost every known form of sexual abuse against children as a punishable offence, where the child is defined as a person below 18 years of age.

As a caregiver, the following points must be noted:

- Section 27 of the Protection of Children from Sexual Offences (POCSO) Act states that medical examinations must be carried out. Even if first information report (FIR) or complaint has not been registered.
- Rule 5(3) of POCSO rules categorically bars doctors and hospitals from demanding legal documents before conducting medical examination.
- The Act mandates reporting all sexual offences that come to the notice of health service providers after careful history and examination.
- As per section 21, any individual who knowingly withhold such information and fails to report the case can be punished with up to 6 months in prison or with a fine.
- Although this is the Act for children with respect to sexual abuse, it is also applicable for married pregnant teenager under the age of 18 years who has reported for care during pregnancy and not for any sexual offence as under the POCSO Act, a minor is unable to consent to sexual intercourse and hence a pregnant minor (married/unmarried) will be considered a victim of sexual assault and mandates illegal action to be taken by the healthcare provider which is to file FIR.
- According to the POCSO Act, it is not mandatory for reporters to inform the adolescent teenager or her parents or guardians about the fact that they would be reporting to the authorities.
- The documentation should be complete with a thorough medical report with diagnosis and recommendation for treatment.
- Testifying in court of law when required.
- If she is uncertain of her age, then it is advised to report the pregnancy as per the legal requirement under POCSO Act and allow the authorities to decide what action needs to be taken.

## CONCLUSION

Although it is a declining trend, adolescent pregnancy still is a global concern and these pregnancies must be considered high risk. It is necessary to implement holistic prenatal care for these pregnant adolescent girls. To avoid such situations in future, it is crucial to counsel the parents to educate the girl child, so it can bring about job opportunities thereby improving her health, economic and social situations, and ultimately giving her the option to choose the path of her life.

## KEY MESSAGES

- Adolescent pregnancy remains a global concern and carries significant risk.
- Adolescent pregnancy holds risks for maternal, fetal, neonatal, and infant morbidity and mortality compared to the older reproductive age period.
- Ignorance, sexual assault, and a lot of socioeconomic and cultural factors are responsible for it.
- The complications are due to the physical, cognitive, and emotional immaturity.
- Special care needs to be taken during the antepartum, partum, and postpartum period.
- The POCSO Act plays an important role in adolescent pregnancy, for married as well as unmarried adolescents.

## RECOMMENDED READING


1. Brosens I, Pijnenborg R, Vercruysse L, Romero R. The "Great Obstetrical Syndromes" are associated with disorders of deep placentation. Am J Obstet Gynecol. 2011;204(3): 193-201.
2. Fraser AM, Brockert JE, Ward RH. Association of young maternal age with adverse reproductive outcomes. Engl J Med. 1995;332:1113-18.
3. Gibbs CM, Wendt A, Peters S, Hogue CJ. The impact of early age at first childbirth on maternal and infant health. Paediatr Perinat Epidemiol. 2012;26 Suppl 1(01): 259-84.
4. Holm K, Laursen EM, Brocks V, Muller J. Pubertal maturation of the internal genitalia: an ultrasound evaluation of 166 healthy girls. Ultrasound Obstet Gynecol. 1995;6:175-81.
5. International Institute for Population Sciences (IIPS) and ICF. (2021). National family health survey (NFHS-5), 2019–21: India Report. [online] Available from https://dhsprogram.com/pubs/pdf/FR375/FR375.pdf. [Last accessed March, 2024].
6. Moerman ML. Growth of the birth canal in adolescent girls. Am J Obstet Gynecol. 1982;143(5):528-32.
7. Press Information Bureau, Government of India. POCSO Act–Providing Child-Friendly Judicial Process. [online] Available from https://pib.nic.in/newsite/efeatures.aspx.?relid=86150. [Last accessed March, 2024].
8. UNICEF. (2024). Early childbearing. [online] Available from https://data.unicef.org/topic/child-health/adolescent-health/#:~:text=Globally%20in%202021%2C%20an%20estimated,their%20education%2C%20livelihoods%20and%20health. [Last accessed March, 2024].
9. Zlatnik FJ, Burmeister LF. Low 'gynecologic': an obstetric risk factor. Am J Obstet Gynecol. 1977;128(2):183-6.


# 8.10 Contraception

*Chandrika Rao, Newton Luiz*

## NEED FOR CONTRACEPTION IN ADOLESCENCE

Adolescent sexual activity may be associated with unintended pregnancy and sexually transmitted infections (STIs). Worldwide, adolescent mothers make up 11% of births, and most adolescent pregnancies are unintended. In most developed countries, the median age of first intercourse is around 17 years. Adolescents who give birth must often give up their studies, and face significant socioeconomic challenges. The greatest risk of unintended pregnancy is in those who are poor, less educated, and marginalized. Complications from pregnancy and childbirth are the leading cause of death for girls aged 15–19 years.

Use of contraceptives is lowest at first intercourse and is very inconsistent thereafter. Adolescents have very low level of contraceptive knowledge and use. They need a range of contraceptive methods and information on the effectiveness, risks, and benefits of these methods.

## LEGAL ASPECTS OF CONTRACEPTION AMONG ADOLESCENTS

The Government of India has removed legal barriers for unmarried adolescents to access sexual reproductive and health services. Currently, family planning services are being provided in India under the Reproductive Maternal Newborn Child and Adolescent Health (RMNCH + A) program. The Government of India is taking steps to designate one trained Adolescent Reproductive and Sexual Health counsellor per facility.

## BARRIERS TO ADOLESCENT CONTRACEPTION

Barriers to accessing contraceptive information and methods include social or culture taboos, legal restrictions, healthcare provider (HCP) attitudes, and healthcare systems.

- The acceptability and availability of contraception for adolescents varies by region and even by countries in the same region.
- Adolescents may experience barriers like inconvenient clinic hours, financial restrictions, lack of confidentiality, and lack of provider training.
- HCPs may act as barriers by imposing their own personal values and moralistic beliefs on the adolescent, by applying inappropriate medical contraindications to contraceptive use, by delaying initiation of contraception unnecessarily (e.g., waiting until the next menses or until STI screening results are available), by requiring unnecessary investigations prior to contraceptive initiation (e.g., erroneously insisting on a Pap smear prior to starting contraception), or by perpetuating unfounded myths about contraceptive use.

## METHODS OF CONTRACEPTION

*Coitus interruptus:* Withdrawal of the penis just before ejaculation is a common contraceptive method among adolescents, but has a failure rate of 27 pregnancies per 100 women in one year (27/HWY), as the adolescent male often does not have sufficient self-control and cannot withdraw in time; also, precoital secretions may contain sperm. It is often the only method available to adolescents at sexual debut, which is often unplanned.

*Male condom:* This is the contraceptive method most adolescents depend upon during a planned sexual encounter, as it is easily available, cheap, and simple to use. It also protects against STIs. It has a high failure rate of 15/HWY, as it may accidentally slip off or break during coitus. The male may refuse to use it as it reduces sensation.

*Other barrier methods:* The female condom is difficult for adolescents to insert. So too the diaphragm, which must be introduced up to 3 hours before intercourse and kept for 6 hours after coitus. Their failure rate is as high as the male condom. They can be combined with spermicides for extra protection.

## Fertility Awareness-based Methods ("Rhythm Method")

These methods are based on identification of the approximate time of ovulation of a menstrual cycle and abstaining from sexual intercourse during that period. They require that the girl has a regular menstrual cycle, undergoes several months training to use these methods reliably, keeps a regular record, and is willing to be abstinent during the unsafe period. Unsurprisingly, the failure rate is 20–30/HWY.

The methods include:
- Noting the basal body temperature chart (*temperature rhythm*). There should be abstinence until the third day of the rise of temperature.
- Noting excessive mucoid vaginal discharge (*mucus rhythm*). This requires abstinence on all days of noticeable mucus and for 3 days thereafter.

### Long-acting Reversible Contraception

Implants and intrauterine devices (IUDs) are safe long-term reversible contraception methods. They have the highest efficacy and acceptance among adolescents and young adults who have tried them out. The American Academy of Pediatrics (AAP) and the American College of Obstetricians and Gynecologists (ACOG) support the use of long-acting reversible contraception (LARC) by adolescents.

### Implants

A radiopaque closed capsule, 40 × 2 mm, is inserted under the dermis in the inner aspect of the nondominant arm, 6–8 cm above the elbow fold, between the biceps and triceps muscles, under local anesthesia. It contains 68 mg of etonogestrel (a progesterone), and provides reversible contraception for 3 years by inhibiting ovulation. It is removed after 3 years, and return of fertility is immediate. Failure rate is <1%. Side-effects are absent, decreased or irregular menstruation. Local side-effects such as infection, bleeding, scar formation, and migration of the device are rare.

### Intrauterine Devices

Intrauterine devices are safe and reversible long-term contraceptive devices. Their advantages are:
- *Inexpensive:* The Copper-T is distributed free of cost through government channels.
- Technique of insertion is simple.

- Prolonged contraceptive protection of 5–10 years.
- Systemic side effects are nil.
- The failure rate is only 0.1–2/HWY.

A pelvic examination is required to insert the IUD. IUDs are usually inserted 2–3 days after the period is over, but can be inserted at any time in a nonpregnant adolescent. They can also be inserted immediately after termination of pregnancy by suction evacuation or dilation and evacuation (D&E), or following a spontaneous abortion. Contrary to common myths, the IUD can be used in adolescents, and fertility returns promptly on removing the IUD.

- *Copper-containing IUDs:* The IUD acts as a foreign body and prevents implantation. The copper additionally prevents implantation through enzymatic interference. Duration of action is 10 years. It acts as an emergency contraception after unprotected sex if inserted within 5 days. Heavy bleeding and dysmenorrhea are adverse effects.
- *Progesterone-containing IUDs* are costly. Their duration of action is about 5 years. The hormone induces strong and uniform suppression of the endometrium. There may be less dysmenorrhea, hypomenorrhea, and occasionally amenorrhea.

## Injectable Progestins

Like all progestin contraceptives, they act by causing inhibition of ovulation, thickening of cervical mucus, and atrophy of endometrium.

- Depot medroxyprogesterone acetate (DMPA) is given deep intramuscular (IM) in the deltoid or gluteus maximus in a dose of 150 mg every 3–4 months or 300 mg every 6 months within 5 days of the cycle.
- Norethisterone enanthate (NET-EN) is given similarly in a dose of 200 mg every 2 months.

They are useful in adolescents who are poorly compliant, have physical or intellectual disability, or cannot use estrogen. 50% of them develop amenorrhea within a year, which may be an advantage in adolescents who have menorrhagia, dysmenorrhea, chronic anemia, or impairments that make hygiene difficult. There is temporary loss of bone mineral density until this treatment is stopped. Weight gain may occur.

## Combined Oral Contraceptives

These are combinations of an estrogen and a progesterone, and they act mainly by inhibiting ovulation, though there may be other significant effects like thickening of the cervical mucus, making it less penetrable to sperm. They are to be consumed once a day at the same time, following a simple regime of "3 weeks on and 1 week off" irrespective of cycle. The dose of estrogen and type of progesterone vary among brands. In India, the government supplies Mala-N free of cost.

*Advantages:* They are low-cost, reversible, highly effective, and well tolerated in the majority. Mala-N is supplied free of cost by the government.

*Disadvantages:*
- Combined oral contraceptives (COCs) may cause nausea and vomiting, abdominal cramps, weight gain, fluid retention, headache, depression, and irregular menstruation, which discourage adolescents, but these side-effects are usually short-lived.
- Adolescents find it inconvenient to take a pill daily. While the theoretical failure rate is only 0.3% in a year, in practice it is as high as 7% in adolescents as they frequently forget to take the pill regularly, or willfully skip it. They should be advised to keep a reminder on their mobile.
- If one pill is late in the last 24 hours, or missed in the last 48 hours, they should take it at once, and the next dose at the usual time, even if they must take two tablets on the same day. If they have skipped two pills in a row, they need to avoid sexual intercourse until they have taken seven consecutive doses.

*Contraindications* to COCs are many in adults, but rare in adolescence. They include past thromboembolism, significant cardiovascular disease, diabetes with vascular complications, severe hypertension, hyperlipidemia, cancer, major surgery or prolonged immobilization, migraine with aura, liver disease, and unexplained genital tract bleeding. A girl with any significant major illness, past or present, should consult a physician before starting COCs.

## Progesterone-only Pills

It works mainly by making cervical mucus thick and viscous, thereby prevents sperm penetration. The endometrium becomes atrophic, which hinders blastocyst implantation. The first pill must be taken on the first day of the cycle and then continuously, with no break between the packs. They are generally safe in adolescents.

*Disadvantages:*
- The pill must be taken at the same time every day; a delay of >3 hours may result in an unintended pregnancy. Adolescents have difficulty in taking the pill so regularly, and the POP failure rate is about 7%.
- Acne, mastalgia, headache, breakthrough bleeding, or at times amenorrhea in about 20–30% cases.
- Simple cysts of the ovary may be seen.

## Emergency Contraception

*Indications of emergency contraception:*
- Unprotected intercourse, condom rupture, missed pill, delay in taking POP for more than 3 hours, sexual assault or rape, and unplanned first time intercourse
- Risk of pregnancy following a single act of unprotected coitus around the time of ovulation is 20%.

*Emergency contraceptives:*
- *Levonorgestrel:* 0.75 mg stat and after 12 hours
- *Ulipristal acetate:* 30 mg stat within 5 days
- *Copper IUDs (gold standard):* Within 5 days
- *Mifepristone:* 100 mg single dose
- *Ethinyl estradiol:* 2.5 mg BD for 5 days
- *Ethinyl estradiol 50 µg + norgestrel 0.25 mg:* Two tablets stat and after 12 hours.

## ■ KEY MESSAGES

- Sexual intercourse is often initiated during adolescence. Adolescents have a right to information on contraceptive methods, including their effectiveness, risks, and benefits.
- Their low level of awareness and skills place them at high risk of unwanted pregnancy, unsafe abortion, and STIs.
- The Government of India has removed legal barriers that prevent unmarried adolescents from accessing sexual reproductive and health services.
- Coitus interruptus and the male condom are the two most commonly used contraceptive methods used by adolescents, and both have a high failure rate.
- Implants and IUDs are safe, highly effective and reversible long-term contraception methods for adolescents and young adults.
- Injectable progestins are highly effective and safe, but require an injection every 3 months.
- COCs are effective if taken daily, at a fixed time.
- Emergency contraception should be offered when needed, e.g., in unprotected intercourse, condom rupture, missed pill, delay in taking POP for more than 3 hours, rape, and unplanned first time intercourse.

## ■ RECOMMENDED READING

1. Konar H (Ed). DC Dutta's Textbook of Obstetrics. New Delhi: Jaypee Brothers Medical Publishers Pvt. Ltd.; 2021.
2. Todd N, Black A. Contraception for adolescents. J Clin Res Pediatr Endocrinol. 2020;12(Suppl 1):28.
3. Shukla A, Kumar A, Mozumdar A, Acharya R, Aruldas K, Saggurti N. Restrictions on contraceptive services for unmarried youth: a qualitative study of providers' beliefs and attitudes in India. Sex Reprod Health Matters. 2022;30(1):2141965.

# 8.11 | Sexual Abuse in Teens and Youth

*Atul Kanikar*

## HANDLING INAPPROPRIATE GESTURES AND UNWANTED TOUCH

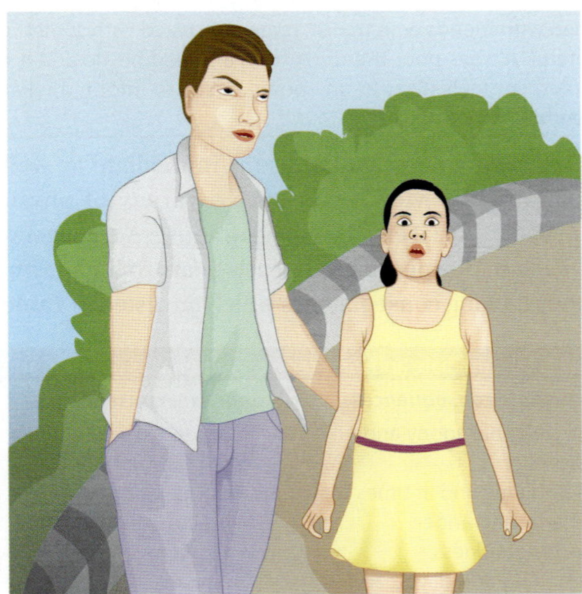


Over 80% girls and women and nearly 40% boys have experienced some form of humiliation or disgrace from *a known or unknown sick and coward person* at least once in their lifetime.

Any attempt to ridicule, humiliate, feel ashamed, or embarrassed is taken as an offense and becomes punishable by law. Even staring at a teenager in an insanitary way for >15 seconds is a crime. Sexual pestering also covers cyber harassment by "predators" and revenge porn.

In countries like India where many teenager girls are married by the age of 16; abuse by the husband is very common, especially in the rural and tribal area. A recent order by the supreme court of India mentions sex with a wife who is <18 years be considered as a sexual assault. Laws like these may prevent early marriages of girls and help improve their physical and mental health.

Sexual abuse is a worldwide phenomenon happening in all races and religions, socioeconomic classes, and developed and underdeveloped nations since the evolution of mankind. The age of the victim, choice of fashion, type of clothing, time of the day, academic skills, etc., have no role in causation or prevention of abuse. It affects girls more than boys and is many times caused by a person *known* to the child.

A person in authority (office boss), fatherly figures like uncle, teacher, cousin, neighbor, and respectable visitor known to the family are all capable of misbehaving. The so-called sugar dads or chocolate uncles may oblige the family and expect returns in the form of physical pleasures from the dependent and defenseless teenager. Many times, the victim is pressurized not to disclose the "secret" to anyone. A few unfortunate victims may have experienced bad touch from their first-degree relationships (brother, father, etc.).

Girls may disclose such incidences with their mothers but alas may be asked to "forget" the incidence and keep quiet. Boys may as such are unlikely to notice such advances and may not talk to anyone and suffer in solitude. A few of such victims project their frustration on to the weaker ones by abusing them.

The perpetrator (abuser) is an adult male in majority of the cases. At times it could be an adult woman, teenager girl, or a juvenile male also. On many occasions, the teenager is innocent and timid. It is the abuser who is unlawful.

Many adults put the blame on teen fashions and body revealing trends. The outgoing, franker and extrovert teens tend to get labeled as "easily available". However, abuse also occurs in modest, fully dressed, and "well behaved" teens. Hence, it can be concluded that the fashion styles or clothing does not necessarily make the teenager more vulnerable for abuse. The trends of adults need to be changed and not teenager's trends/choice of fashion. This education is vital for boys and men too.

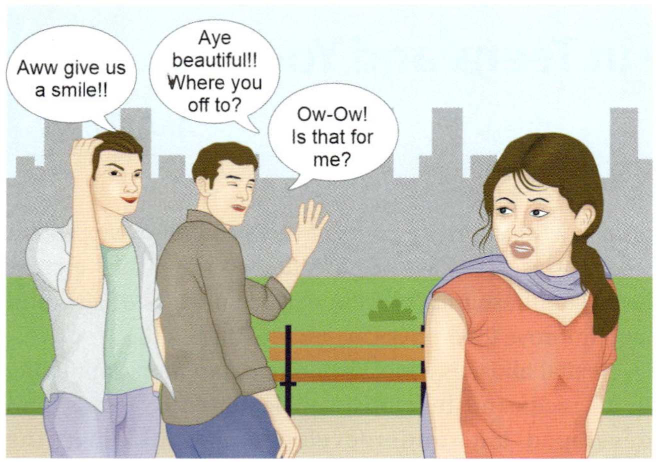


Apart from the abuser's hideous mindset, the other predisposing factors for teenage sexual abuse are:

- Evolving sexual urges of growing teens.
- Early maturation of teens (especially girls). Physical maturity but with a child's mind and innocence are peculiar to early bloomers.
- Ignorance of the teenager and parents toward possibility and management of abuse.
- Tendency to disregard and hide the mishap. *This gives perpetrator a chance to continue abusing further which he may continue doing to other innocent victims also.*
- Economic dependence on the abuser.
- Too many opportunities these days for convenient isolation of victim and abuser.
- Parental conflicts and neglect.
- Changing social norms and family structure (latch key parenting or education away from the safety of home).
- Media influence through depiction of plans and plots for abusing and all-time display of girls/women as objects for entertainment.
- Peer acceptance and pressure both for causing and tolerating abuse.

- Victim may be labeled as being easily "available".
- Influence of date rape drugs.
- Increasing incidence of drug abuse in teenagers as well as adults which reduces inhibitions and civic sense.
- Poor attachment with the parents and family and a feeling of "loneliness".
- Street children and children in institutes and residential schools.

> Never accept a drink/snack from anyone known or unknown when with friends or in transit. It may be mixed with something spiteful. Always pour the drink from a sealed bottle and if the adolescent feels dizzy at any point, needs to inform a reliable friend/family immediately.

The sequel of sexual abuse is immediate as well as persistent. The victim can have a variety of physical, mental, and social effects following abuse. A teenager who has such bad experiences in early years of life may have serious lifelong consequences which are listed in **Table 1**.

**TABLE 1:** Immediate and long-term consequences of sexual abuse.

| Immediate consequences | Long-term consequences |
|---|---|
| • Unbearable agony and disbelief | • Poor self-esteem |
| • Self-blame and at times guilt | • Lack of confidence |
| • Shame and anger | • Social isolation |
| • Revengefulness | • Migraine like headaches |
| • Planning and daydreaming about revenge on the perpetrator | • Unexplained body aches |
| | • Drug abuse |
| • Poor sleep and appetite | • High-risk sexual experimentations |
| • Horrid dreams | • Depression |
| • Depression and suicidal ideation | • Anxiety disorders |
| • Anxiety about consequences | • Fear about the future of married life |
| • Worry about possible recurrence | • Academic underachievement |
| | • Vulnerability to abuse by others |
| • Post-traumatic stress disorder | • Inclination to abuse the weaker people |
| • Tendency to over generalize | |

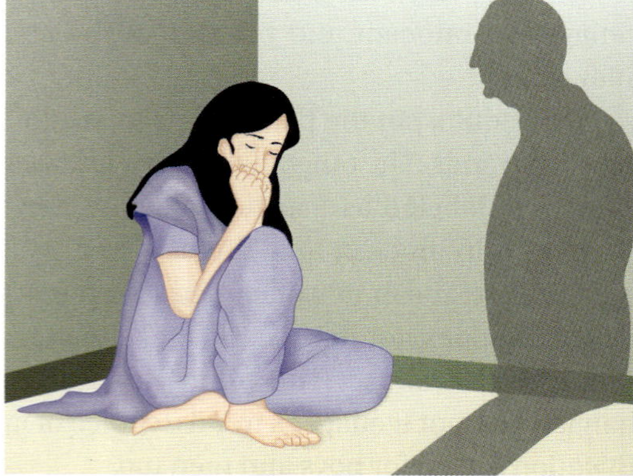

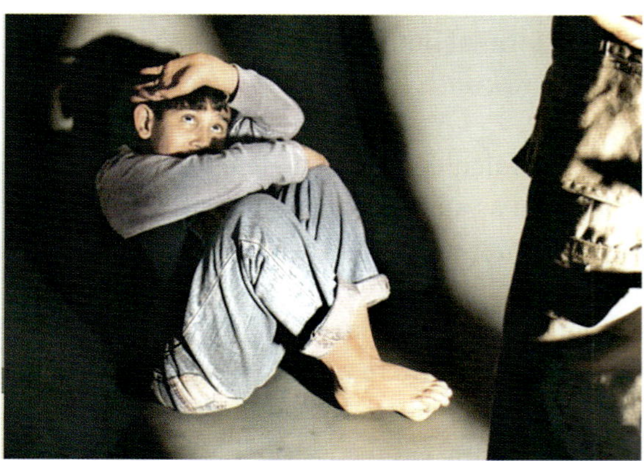

Before they turn 18......

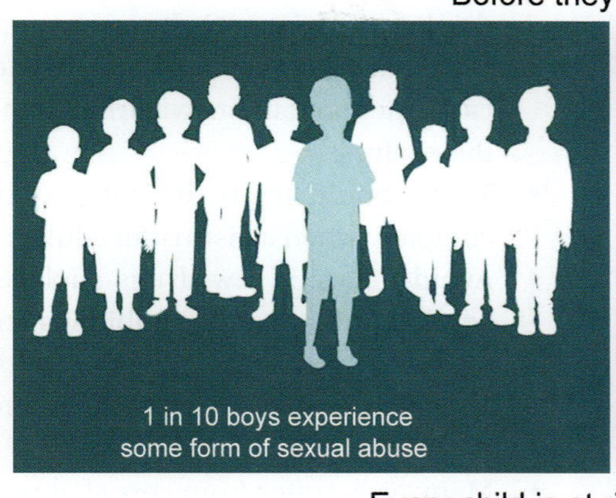


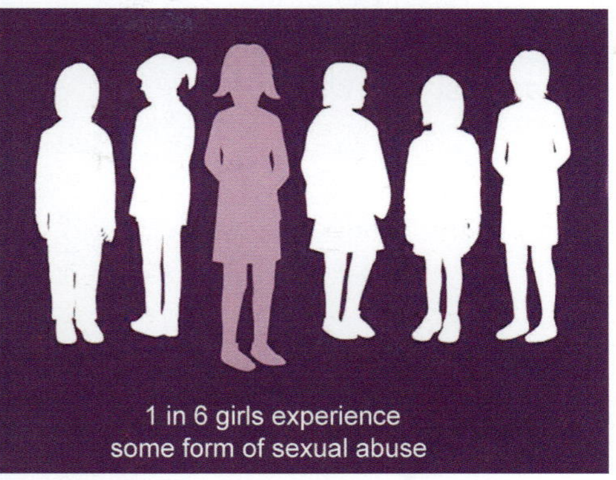


Every child is at risk, regardless of
nationality or religion

*Source:* https://twitter.com/sianystarr/status/1051106619457724417.

## PAINFUL FACTS ABOUT CHILD AND ADOLESCENT SEXUAL ABUSE

- <10% cases are reported to the authorities.
- The parents/guardians may know about the abuse but many times ignore the issue and even ask the child to ignore.
- In >90% cases the perpetrator (abuser) is known to the child and family.
- The innocent victim alone suffers from physical, mental, and social trauma.
- Abuse may be repeated by the same or different perpetrators.
- Many children do not receive any information on prevention and handling of abuse. Many parents do not know how to teach their children ahead of time.
- The consequences of the abuse may be devastating and lifelong. Many victims are compelled to leave education and may be forced to marry early, especially in the rural area.
- Many girls as well as boys experience some form of abuse at least once. Girls have an innate skill to identify bad intentions. Boys may not identify them till late. Moreover, a boy may find it difficult to share the problem with anybody. A girl at least can complain to her mother occasionally. A few unfortunate children may not find a trustworthy listener due to shame, threat by abuser or poor communication skills.
- Unless exposed or punished, the perpetrator may continue to abuse the victim or new victims.
- Many children and teenagers are innocent not to notice several other less severe forms of abuse.

## FORMS OF SEXUAL OFFENSES

- Word, gesture, or act intended to outrage the modesty of a teenager
- Trailing a teenager, attempting to contact, and obtain personal information
- Monitoring teenager's use of mobile/internet
- Watching or capturing a teenager engaging in private act
- Blackmailing a teenager after video/voice recording her/his private chats/acts
- Assault or use of criminal force to teenager with intent to disrobe
- Physical contact and advances involving unwelcome and explicit sexual overtures
- A demand or request for sexual favors
- Showing pornography against the will of a teenager
- Making sexually colored remarks
- Giving drugs to a teenager to obtain sexual pleasures
- Assault or criminal force intending to outrage the modesty of teenager
- Rape (nonpenetrative or penetrative sexual act with or without consent)
- Sexting (sending sexually explicit messages or images).

There are cases reported where innocent boys/men were falsely victimized with the intention to extract money.

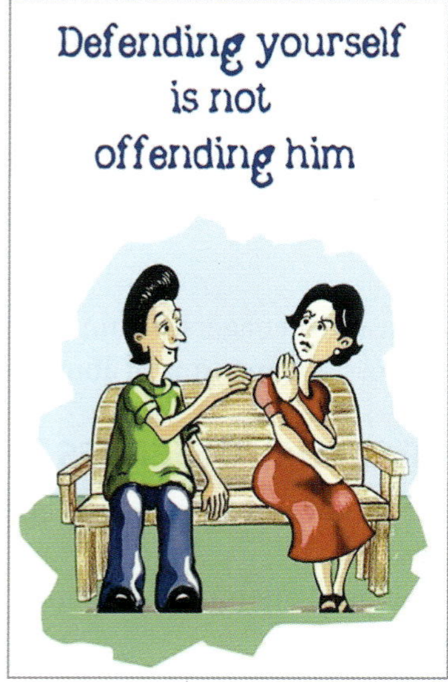



## ■ WAYS TO RESIST HUMILIATION



*Source:* Poster by WHO on adolescent health.

- ■ *Avoid the situation:*
  - Adolescents should be made aware of the following preventive strategies beforehand:
    - ◆ Not to be extra friendly with strangers or newly introduced persons. Maintain formalities till they know someone's background and vested interests. Even smiling, giggling, casual touching, hand shake, or friendly hug may be wrongly taken as a clue by a few people.
  - Teenagers should be careful while going to a friend's home who is not trustworthy when he/she is alone. Care should be taken to keep the doors and windows open if no third person is in the house. Many times, sexual abuse is perpetrator's planned activity.
  - Adolescents should be warned against late night parties. They need to inform their parents about their expected time of return, the venue, and their friends. Give contact numbers of at least two close friends and their parents. It is better to be safe than sorry.
  - Teenagers need to think before blindly identifying with their friends and take the risk.

- They should be cautioned against accepting any drink from strangers. It may contain a date rape drug that causes memory loss for a few hours. They can better pour their own drink from a sealed bottle themselves.
- They should try to be with some dependable company when a distrustful adult is around.
- Avoid drugs. A few drugs such as alcohol and amphetamine reduce inhibitions and increase the desire for physical and sexual acts. Some drugs also lead to aggression and violence which can precipitate sexual crimes.
- Many girls suffer from sexual abuse and violence in relationships. Emotional blackmailing and threat to abandon pushes many girls to surrender and compromise. Girls need to be firm about the boundaries if they are in a relationship and the boy/man must be informed in advance about the same. They must never compromise for his/her satisfaction. Learning to say "No" is many times useful. Girl's safety and future stands much before his/her fun and satisfaction. Sacrifice must be mutual.
- Be cyber-literate. Have a cautious online activity.
- Call "1098" (toll free number) if the girl smells trouble. Help should arrive immediately. For cyber harassment a teenager may call 1098 or 1931. The identity of the child and family is kept confidential.

- ■ *Resist the actual act:*
  - Be bold at least outwardly.
  - Forget about the status and authority of perpetrator. He may be anyone. Right now, he is an unlawful person trying to harm you.
  - Look into the perpetrator's eyes and shout *"No"*.

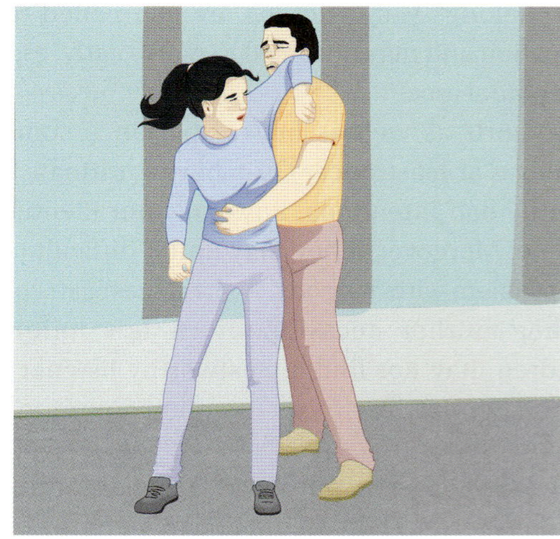

- Say, *"Go away, I do not like this."*

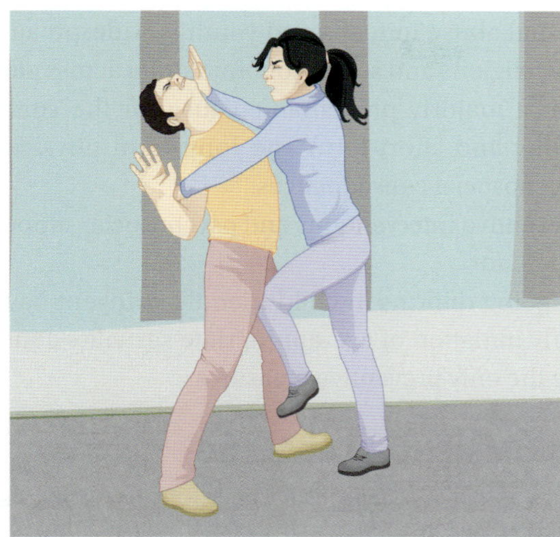

- Use your right knee and elbow to crush the perpetrators vital area between his legs with all your strength.
- Aim your nails into the abusers' eyes.
- Bend his right thumb firmly backward.
- Push him using your both hands.
- Hit him hard with any object which comes to your rescue.
- Call for help *loudly.*
- *Things to do immediately, if such incidence has already occurred:*

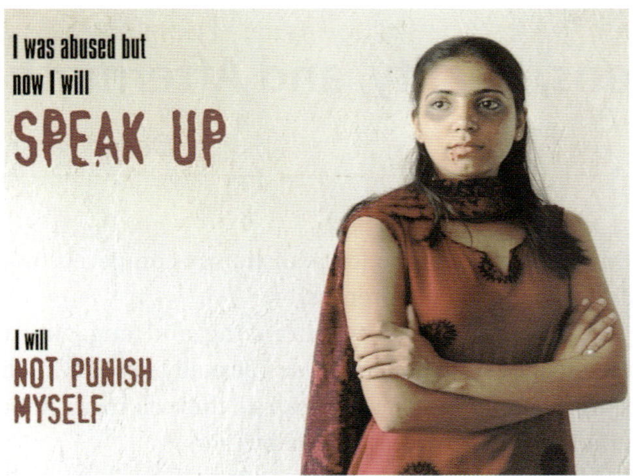


*Source:* Poster by WHO on adolescent health.

- *Counseling of victims of sexual abuse:* The following points may help in counseling a victim of sexual abuse:
  - Do not blame yourself for the act. Try to remain confident. You are the survivor of abuse and it was never *your* fault at all.

- Be realistic and rational, not revengeful. Let the law and sensible parents take care of the situation.
- Report to some trustworthy person immediately. It may be your parent, teacher, doctor, or relative. If this "trustworthy" person asks you to ignore and you still are not comfortable, contact 1098 (toll free) and report the matter. Call your best friends immediately.

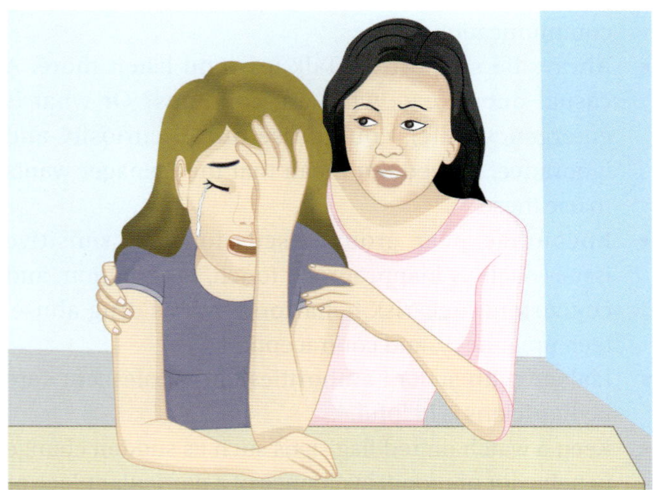

- Try to preserve as much evidence of the mishap as possible. (It could be a phone call in mobile memory, message, used contraceptive or a glass of drink.) This may be needed for legal purpose, just in case. Avoid taking bath and cleaning yourself till the legal formalities are over. This is extremely essential in cases of rape victims.
- If a mishap in the past is hindering your progress, affecting your academics or causing physical symptoms like unknown aches or sleep disturbances, talk to someone. Do not suffer alone. Take professional help. Counseling and/or medications prescribed by a healthcare professional may help you elbow out these symptoms. Always remember that it was never your fault and no one has a right to spoil your entire existence and purpose of life.

## ROLE OF GATEKEEPERS

- Age-appropriate sexuality education beginning at an early age is necessary.

- Encouraging child's queries and making use of TV ads and newspaper stories to initiate open discussion definitely helps.
- Consult a healthcare personnel or counselor if there are any hindrances or doubts.
- Be comfortable with yourself and the topic and ask what the child already knows. Imbibe values at the end of discussion. Avoid lectures and ideologies.
- Ask open-ended questions which give descriptive answers with maximum use of nonverbal communication.
- Always be supportive. Talk less and listen more. A casual query (e.g., what are condoms? Or what is emergency pill?), could arise out of curiosity and ignorance. It need not mean that the teenager wants to use these.
- Encourage peer group discussions on sensitive issues such as inappropriate touch, molestation, and concurrent high-risk behaviors such as drug abuse, teen pregnancy, and contraception.
- Liaison with school authorities and adolescent care pediatricians is helpful.
- Keep a watch on red flag signs such as sudden change in behavior or mood, avoidance of a particular place or person, and sudden academic deterioration.

## ■ KEY MESSAGES

- Sexual abuse in teens and youth is widespread in all the religions and socioeconomic strata across globe.
- It is a majorly preventable cause for the survivor's agony and short-term and long-term physical and psychosocial consequences.
- Preventive interventions and psychosocial support are mandatory.
- Ongoing reforms in child friendly stringent laws and early initiation of age-appropriate sexuality education are the only preventive measures.

## ■ RECOMMENDED READING

1. Deshmukh V. Teenage Dot Com #1. Maharashtra: Rajhans Prakashan; 2017.
2. Deshmukh V. Teenage Dot Com #2. Maharashtra: Rajhans Prakashan; 2020.
3. Kanikar A. Nature's gift, my responsibility. In: Kanikar A (Ed). From Terrible to Terrific Teens, 1st edition. Chandigarh: White Falcon Publishers; 2019.
4. Nair MKC, Kamath SS. Sex, Sex, sexuality and sexual behavior, AFSI Manual, 2007.
5. Parthasarathy A, Nair MKC. Sexual Reproductive Health of Young People, 1st edition. New Delhi: Jaypee Brothers Medical Publishers (P) Ltd.; 2006.

# 8.12 Pornography: Depictions, Reality, and Aftermath

*Deepa Passi*

## ■ INTRODUCTION

The recent augmentation of internet-enabled technology has significantly altered the way adolescents come upon and devour sexually explicit material. Internet offers more pervasive access to pornography. Adolescence is defined by sexual development, increasing romantic relationships, and initiation of sexual activity. Adolescents are exposed to pornography more frequently due to a variety of factors, including the normal development of sexuality that peaks during adolescence, sexual exploration (a growing need for sexual knowledge during puberty), ineffectual parent–child sexuality communication, and a paucity of formal sex education. Pornographic practices or messages could seem more pragmatic to a young adolescent who has not developed a prototype for realistic sex compared to an adult with greater matureness.

Pornography is both entrancing and engaging to many teenagers. They have used sexually explicit media to stimulate themselves and satiate their curiosity about nudity and sexual activity for many years.

Adolescents' exposure to pornography has raised concerns in the light of potential risks to adolescent development. Pornography affects the three responses: *Cognitive, behavioral, and emotional.* The very quality that makes teens resilient is, however, what makes them vulnerable. At the onset of puberty, adolescents' brain is moldable—an increased likelihood to rewire. Driven to seek out novelty and risks, teenagers have flexible neural circuits that help them adapt to environments as they make decisions and learn. As they enter adulthood, the window where connections between brain structures are formed starts to close, crystallizing their behaviors. Any experience they have during the time when the brain is malleable has the potential to affect it.

## DEFINITION OF PORNOGRAPHY

The word *pornography*, derived from the Greek terms *porni* ("prostitute") and *graphein* ("to write"), was originally defined as any work of art or literature depicting the life of prostitutes.

The term "pornography" can be defined as the reporting or portrayal of sexual actions in order to produce sexual excitement through books, pictures, gestures, films, or other media. Pornographic websites and material created using computers, and the use of the internet to download and transmit pornographic films, texts, photographs, and photos, among other things, fall under this category.

## HISTORY

In most of the historical societies, be it ancient Greece, Rome, and India, pornographic representations in the form of statues, carvings, phallic imagery, and depictions of orgiastic scenes were widely present.

The Indian Sanskrit text *Kama Sutra* (3rd century CE) contained prose, poetry, and illustrations regarding sexual behavior. British English text *Fanny Hill* (1748), considered "the first original English *prose* pornography", has been one of the most prosecuted and banned books.

In the 19th century, with the inventions of photography and later of motion pictures pornography was used. Pornographic films were widely available no later than the 1920s, and in the 1960s, their popularity enjoyed a massive uptrend. Then came, the era of the internet in 1990s. Cooper (1998) described three factors, usually referred to as "the triple-A engine", that combine to make the internet a powerful force regarding sexuality. These factors are affordability (low cost), accessibility (easy to get), and anonymity (belief that one is unknown). Pornographic websites are called an "erotic engine". The internet also increased the availability of child pornography.

## PREVALENCE OF PORNOGRAPHY

Adolescent pornography use has continuously increased over time and the age of first exposure to sexually explicit materials has also been getting younger. The prevalence rates have varied but nationally representative surveys of adolescents in the United States of America (USA) have found that 68.4% reported exposure to online pornography.

Gender is also an important factor to account for when considering the prevalence of pornography use, with males more likely to report pornography use.

## Predictors of Adolescents' Pornography Use

*These are:*

- *Demographics:* Males use pornography more than females. Bi-or homosexual male adolescents use internet pornography more often than heterosexual male adolescents. Pubertally more advanced teens, sexual sensation-seeking youth are more prone to pornography.
- *Personality characteristics:* Thrill-seeking adolescents who have lower self-control consumed more internet pornography.
- *Norm-related variables:* Adolescents who break rules and delinquents substance abuse in the form of gateway drugs like tobacco and alcohol.
- *Sexual interest:* Adolescents who have more sexual interest and greater exposure to sexual media.
- *Internet behavior:* Violent sexually explicit sites.
- *Social predictors:* Poor family emotional bond and no parental control leads to excessive use of pornography. At the individual level, those who have experienced child abuse and have poor self-concept and self-esteem tend to use pornography excessively.
- *Organizational and institutional settings (such as schools):* Poor academic performance, noncaring school climate, gangs, not participating in extra-curricular activities, etc.
- *Community contexts:* Availability of pornographic materials, economic deprivation, neighborhood attachment/disorganization, infrastructure, etc.
- *Social-culture context:* Digital illiteracy.

## PORNOGRAPHY AND HORMONES

The young brain lacks a mature prefrontal cortex, and hence there are no brakes to stop the behavior.

The brain is the biggest sexual organ. Internet porn releases dopamine, which stimulates the brain. This leads to changes in the brain that are associated with

## ■ FUTURE DIRECTIONS

*Future directions include:*

- Sexuality education in schools starting from primary schools
- Life skills education including critical thinking, decision-making, and coping with emotions in primary and secondary schools
- Digital literacy, educating about safe and healthy internet use, limiting access to children
- Effective implementation of laws
- Good parent–child communication
- Education of adolescents regarding what healthy love and its safe expression is.

## ■ KEY MESSAGES

- Exposure to pornography is unavoidable as long as adolescents have access to internet be it computers, smart phones, and iPads, but educating them to minimize its side effects is possible.
- Children as low as 8 years have been exposed to online porn. Nearly half of children between the ages of 9 and 16 years experience regular exposure to sexual images.
- There is a relationship between online pornography/ sex material and internet addiction, engagement in online erotica (sex-based Internet chat sites), risky online sexual behaviors (sending online sexually explicit pictures and sexting).

- Pornography and related sexual media can influence sexual violence, attitudes, moral values, and sexual activities.
- The open parent–child communication channels about sexual and media experiences, sex education at home, school and parental participation are all constructive influences
- Warm and open parent–teen relationships can deal with the challenges of sexualized media.
- Pornography and its impacts need to be situated within a broader framework of primary prevention and supporting the sexual safety and well-being of children and young people.

## ■ SUGGESTED READING


1. Collins RL, Strasburger VC, Brown JD, Donnerstein E, Lenhart A, Ward LM. Sexual media and childhood well-being and health. Pediatrics. 2017;140(Suppl 2):S162-6.
2. Cooper A. Sexuality and the Internet: Surfing into the new millennium. CyberPsychology & Behavior. 1998;1(2):187-93. https://doi.org/10.1089/cpb.1998.1.187
3. Srivastava S, Chauhan S, Patel R, Marbaniang SP, Kumar P, Dhillon P, et al. Exposure to pornographic content among Indian adolescents and young adults and its associated risks: Evidence from UDAYA survey in Bihar and Uttar Pradesh. Arch Sex Behav. 2023;52(1);361-72.
4. Wright PJ, Herbenick D, Paul B. Adolescent condom use, parent-adolescent sexual health communication, and pornography: Findings from a U.S. probability sample. Health Commun. 2020;35(13):1576-82.


<br>

# 8.13 POCSO Act 2012 and JJ Act 2015: Impact on Medical Fraternity and Adolescents

*Rashmi Gupta*

## ■ INTRODUCTION

India is a country of vivid population with nearly 40% of people aged below 18 years. They inherit the past and they are the future. Therefore, their overall well-being and security matter for our nation. Statistics show that there is an increasing trend of juveniles falling prey to sexual abuse and also getting trapped in juvenile delinquency because of their poverty, illiteracy, human trafficking, and drug abuse. The children are like wet cement, whatever falls on them they carry lifelong and their immature prefrontal cortex adds to the trouble. Therefore, a stringent law was always needed and the answer to this is the Protection of Children from Sexual Offenses (POCSO) Act and Juvenile Justice (JJ) (Care and Protection of Children) Act.

Doctors, especially pediatricians and adolescent counselors, cannot deny their responsibility ethically because they are the first point of contact with these children, either the victim or the perpetrator. They can play a key role in providing comprehensive and empathetic care to these children and adolescents.

# PROTECTION OF CHILD FROM SEXUAL OFFENSE ACT 2012

It is unfortunate to observe that every 2nd child is exposed to such a heinous crime and at any given point in time, 1 in every 10 children is being abused. This fact was revealed in a study conducted by the Ministry of Women and Child Development in 2007 and accessed in 2014. The United Nations (UN) Convention on the Rights of the Child (11th December 1992) and the Constitution of India mandated all States to undertake measures at all levels to protect the children in their best interest, especially concerning sexual offense, and to ensure their health and security, freedom, and dignity.

- *Purpose of the POCSO Act:* It is an Act to protect anyone under 18 years from sexual abuse and to provide the establishment of special courts for the trial of such offenses and for matters connected. POCSO Act states that any sexual act (consensual or nonconsensual) with a child below 18 years is a sexual offense. The POCSO Act came up on November 14, 2012, and was amended in 2019, 2022, and 2023. It was also published in the Gazette of India (*Bharat ka Raj Patra*) and constitutes 9 chapters, 46 sections, and 13 rules.
- *Magnitude of the problem:* The National Crime Records Bureau (NCRB) report 2021 very well depicts that crime against children is on the rise. In 2016, the data (**Fig. 1.**) says crime against children was around 1 lakh 6 thousand, while in 2021, it reached up to 1 lakh 50 thousand. More than 50% of all crimes against children are related to sexual offenses, which are rising year after year. The incidence of crime is increasing age-wise too. More and more juveniles are in conflict with the law and the conviction rate is very low. In 2021, out of all accused, only 32% of them were convicted.

## Salient Features

- POCSO Act is gender-neutral.
- All efforts are made to ensure physical and mental safety and comfort of the victim.
- Onus lies on the accused to prove himself not guilty.
- Reporting to the special juvenile police unit/local police is mandatory by the institution as well as the guardian.
- Punishment for abetment of the act is similar to that of the perpetrator.
- Police are designated as responsible protectors of the child and also inform the Child Welfare Committee (CWC).
- Police make all arrangements for legal procedures and medical treatment.
- The act empowers CWC to provide a support person to assist throughout the investigation and trial process in the best interest of the child to prevent revictimization.
- There is no time limit for reporting the abuse by the survivor.
- Minimum punishment is prescribed and tailor-made.
- Amendment 2019 stepped up stringent punishment from 10 years to 20 years and may be convicted to the death penalty.

The term aggravated is used for the person sharing the same household, neighbor, close relatives, or any government employee.

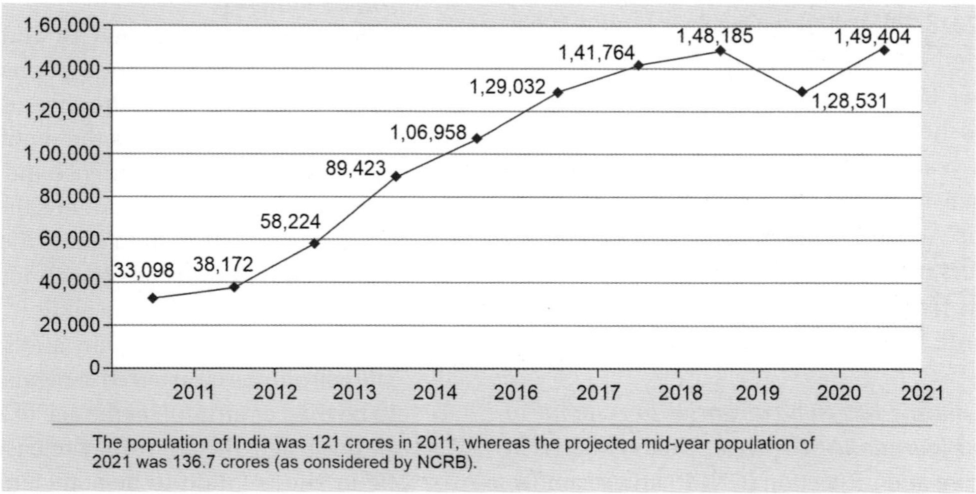



The population of India was 121 crores in 2011, whereas the projected mid-year population of 2021 was 136.7 crores (as considered by NCRB).

**Fig. 1**

- POCSO 2022 further added natural calamity or administered hormones or any other chemical substance to the child to attain puberty to sections 3– to 18 under aggravated offense.
- Through order of a special court, interim compensation is granted within 30 days for which the accused does not need to be convicted.
- Immediate payment for essential needs like food, clothes, and transport is done.
- POCSO 2023 added Fast Track Special courts (FTSCs) for the heaping up cases of POCSO.

## JUVENILE JUSTICE (CARE AND PROTECTION OF CHILDREN) ACT 2015

After the *Nirbhaya* case in 2012, there was a tremendous impact on the public perception regarding JJ Act 2000, because the boy who committed the heinous crime was just a few months younger than the cutoff 18-years-of-age criteria of being a child, and was tried as a juvenile and hardly got any punishment. Finally, the Parliament of India passed the law amidst intense controversy, debate, and protest. It replaced the Juvenile Delinquency Law and JJ Act 2000, which did not incorporate heinous crimes done by the age group 16–18 years who had mental status nearly as an adult.

- *Purpose of JJ Act 2015:* This Act is enacted to adopt a child-friendly approach in the adjudication and disposition of matters in the best interest of children and for their ultimate rehabilitation through various institutions established under the law. It is also an Act to consolidate and amend the JJ law relating to children alleged and found to be in conflict with the law. This Act came up in the year 2015 and implemented on January 15, 2016. Published in Gazette of India, it has 10 chapters and 112 sections.
- *Magnitude of the problem:* The data collected by NCRB established that crimes by children in the age group 16–18 years have increased from 54 to 66% in 2014, especially in certain categories of heinous crime. The previous Acts were ill-equipped to tackle the child offenders in this group in conflict with the law. Therefore, the JJ Act 2015 came up.
- *Salient features:* Juvenile means a child below the age of 18 years.
  - *This Act mainly has two categories to respond to child in the juvenile justice system:* Firstly children in need of care and protection (CNCP) and secondly, the children in conflict with the law (CICL).

- Delinquent behaviors of juveniles need to be understood. According to the psychodynamic theory of Sigmund Freud, a child is born with animal instinct, ego is realization of real life, and superego is developed by the interaction with parents and society. According to social learning theory, the child learns from imitating elders and society. There are theories like genetic and epigenetic theories. Myelination of the brain completes by 24 years. Disorganized rational thinking and risk-taking behavior favor delinquency. Most of the children and youth outgrow delinquent behaviors with age and community support.
- Delinquent behaviors include running away from home, use of vulgar language, wandering on streets, railway stations, marketplaces, begging, stealing, shoplifting, gambling, committing sexual offenses, etc.
- Reporting of these children is mandatory by guardians, police officials, and institutes. Nonreporting entails imprisonment for 6 months or a fine.
- *General principle of care and protection:* The child is presumed to be innocent, and they have the right to live with dignity, worth, health, and security. So, the action should be in the best interest of the child's overall development, health, and security, under the scrutiny of CWC and child foster homes.
- A transfer system was included in 2015, according to which a child who commits an established heinous crime is to be treated as an adult in the court of law.
- *The CICL consists of three categories of offenses:* (1) Petty offenses (a punishment is <3 years of imprisonment), (2) serious offenses (between 3 and 7 years), and (3) heinous crimes (7 years or more of imprisonment).
- A juvenile, aged between 16 and 18 years, who has committed a heinous offense can be tried as an adult only when the Juvenile Justice Board (JJB) justifies that he has the mental and physical capacity to perform the offense and understands its consequences and still commits the crime.
- This assessment is then confirmed by a JJB and CWC before it proceeds to conduct the juvenile's trial as if he or she were an adult.
- If the juvenile is found guilty and sentenced, he or she will only be transferred to regular imprisonment to be tried as an adult at the age of 21 years.
- At this stage, the court may release the juvenile if he or she is found to be sufficiently reformed or rehabilitated and is safe for the society.

## COMPARISON BETWEEN POCSO AND JJ ACTS

| POCSO Act | JJ Act |
|---|---|
| 1. This Act is for age below 18 years but mainly includes punishment where the preparator is considered as accused and onus lies on him to prove himself not guilty. Therefore, the age of minor becomes crucial for the progress of the matter | JJ Act mainly deals with restoration of young criminals below 18 years<br>*There are two classified groups:*<br>1. Children in conflict with the law<br>2. Children in need of care with protection |
| 2. This act does not have any provision to prove the age | This act also provides documents to prove the age |
| 3. This act does not have its own compensation scheme for the victim | Children have provision to demand compensation |
| 4. Though this act is apparently gender-neutral, actually it is a female-centric Act, because when two juveniles are in conflict with the law, then the male is considered accused | Similarly in this Act too, female minor is treated as CNCP and male as CICL |
| 5. Child trafficking is not covered | Child trafficking is not addressed |
| 6. Fast trial special courts were set up in 2023 to deal with a huge burden of pending cases | • Similarly, Juvenile Justice Board (JJB) is constituted which hears only juvenile cases<br>• There are special juvenile prosecutors appointed with an efficient team of medical fraternity with child psychiatrists |

(CICL: children in conflict with the law; CNCP: children in need of care and protection; JJ: juvenile justice; POCSO: protection of children from sexual offenses)

## IMPACT OF ACTS ON MEDICAL FRATERNITY

According to these acts, any hospital, either government or private, cannot refuse to examine or provide medical treatment to the victim of sexual offense or any medical condition under CNCP JJ Act 2015.

- No consultation fee or other expenses must be taken.
- Do not need and cannot demand a requisition from police or magistrate for clinical management.

- Nonreporting or recording by a doctor or whoever knows about the sexual crime or delinquent behavior is a punishable offense for which they can be jailed for 6 months with or without fine and the head of any institution can be jailed for 1 year.
- In case of sexual offense, if examination and medical care are delayed, crucial evidence of a sexual offense may be lost, or the victim may succumb to her or his injuries. Therefore, it is a medicolegal emergency.

### Role of Pediatrician

The pediatricians have dual responsibilities as many times they are the first point of contact and they need to provide comprehensive medical treatment efficiently. The pediatrician is considered as an academically enriched fraternity and is also very popular in nongovernmental organizations (NGOs) active in health awareness programs. Therefore, pediatricians through these programs can generate and impart knowledge to the general public and teaching institutes to create awareness about these acts. Child psychologist and psychiatrist's role is very crucial in care and rehabilitation of these children.

## IMPACT OF ACT ON ADOLESCENTS

Adolescence is a phase of physical, social, and neurobehavioral changes. The limbic system, mainly amygdala, is the site of emotional thinking. It makes them prone to risk-taking behavior. The absence of proper guidance and parenting and poor circumstantial and environmental factors add to the problem. Overruling these facts, both acts criminalize the adolescent sexuality where hormone upsurge plays a major role in the hyperactive limbic system.

## CHALLENGES IN IMPLEMENTATION OF THE LAWS

- NCRB statistics states that 80% of the juvenile delinquents are from families with low economic status. It is observed that juvenile crime has increased from 0.63 to 1.2% after POCSO. It is ironic to state that the conviction rate in juveniles is nearly 87% while the overall conviction rate is 42.5%, which includes consensual sexual behavior among adolescents. Therefore, the juveniles in conflict with the law are in a more worse state than the adult who is on trial for a similar crime because the adult is more mature and manipulative to face the trial.

- The offense and punishment is tailor-made, which needs to take into account socioenvironmental and neurobiological factors. In case of consensual sexual expression, the girl is considered as the victim, which is against the biological frame of the relationship.
- When the act is implemented, corporal punishment in childcare homes and torture in police custody are not uncommon. According to law, the identity of the child is not to be disclosed based on child-friendly provisions, because of which the nature of JJ remains unevaluated. The impact of JJB, CWC, and special juvenile police unit (SJPU) is difficult to assess.
- The juvenile justice system gets only 0.6% of the Union Budget to maintain its vast functions. Due to low resources, the child homes are not equipped well with necessary amenities. Recruiting of staff and regular training of the staff are also difficult in this sanctioned budget. Studies have also revealed that there are not a sufficient number of trained medical staff or women police to understand the complexities of these acts. There is also low investment in community-based programs like family life education programs for adolescents, family, parents, and society, to address the vulnerable risk factors.
- Though India is moving toward being a developed country, the honor of the family still comes first than child safety and the patriarchal society gives less opportunity for the girls to open up.
- Low educational status adds to indifference and low economic status leads to ignorance toward these assaults. Moreover, lack of social awareness about the stringent law and concerned judicial system adds to the problem. The studies have revealed that only about 30% of the medical fraternity know about POCSO and JJ Acts.

## ■ KEY MESSAGES

- Though the POCSO Act 2012 and JJ Act 2015 are amended as requirements of societal factors where they show zero tolerance to accused, they still need a robust support system with a proficient judiciary, a competent police unit with more women force, competent medical staff, and well-functioning child homes with rehabilitation units.
- Psychosocial well-being is also an important aspect for these children and delinquents.
- These Acts need to treat all persons below 18 years under the same framework of CNCP even CICL to avoid atrocities. A relative maturity should not make them devoid of the need for care and protection.
- Adolescents need to be taken into consideration when it comes to consensual sex.

It is a welcome recommendation by the Law Commission of India (September, 2023) for making amendments in POCSO and JJ Act to reduce the age of consent for sexual activity among age group 16–18 years and considering other favorable factors in the best interest of teenagers.

## ■ RECOMMENDED READING

1. Advocating for Adolescent Concerns. (2024). Juvenile Justice. [online] Available from http://pldindia.org [Last accessed April, 2024].
2. Kumar S. (2023). Live law. Supreme Court Monthly Roundup-September 2023 [online] Available from http://www.livelaw.in [Last accessed April 2024].
3. Ministry of Health and Family Welfare. (2014). Guidelines and Protocols: Medico-legal care for survivors/victims of sexual violence.[online] Available from https://main.mohfw.gov.in/sites/default/files/953522324.pdf [last accessed 2024].
4. Ministry of Law and Justice. (2016). The Juvenile Justice (Care and Protection of Children) Act, 2015. [online] Available from https://www.childlineindia.org/pdf/j-j-act. PDF [Last accessed April, 2024].
5. Ministry of Law and Justice. (2019). The Protection of Children from Sexual Offences (Amendment) Act. [online] Available from https://www.mha.gov.in/sites/default/files/2022-12/20-11-2019%5B1%5D.pdf [Last accessed April, 2024].
6. Ministry of Women and Child Development. (2018). Draft National Child Protection Policy. [online] Available from http://www.wcd.nic.in/childabuse.pdf. [Last accessed April, 2024].

# 8.14 Gender Empowerment

*Himabindu Singh*

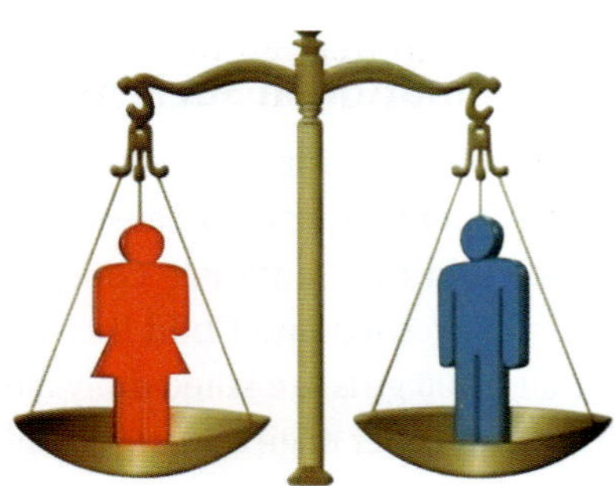

## ◼ DEFINITION

- *Gender:* "It refers to the socially constructed characteristics of women and men such as the norms, roles, and relationships that exist between them." *[World Health Organization (WHO)]*
- *Empowerment:* "Empowerment is a process that fosters power in people for use in their own lives, their communities, and their society by acting on issues they define as important." *(Page and Czuba, 1999)*
- *Gender empowerment:* "An increase in the power of people of any gender, though usually refers to the empowerment of groups that are marginalized on the basis of their gender." *(IGI Global)*

## ◼ THE NEED OF GENDER EMPOWERMENT

### Gender Imbalance

*The world population in 2023 [at midyear, according to the United Nations (UN) estimates]:*
- *Total population:* 8,045,311,447
- *Male population:* 4,042,987,695 or 4,043 million (50.25%)
- *Female population:* 4,002,323,752 or 4,002 million (49.75%)

*According to UN estimates 2023, India population (**Fig.1**):*
- *Total:* 1,440,025,349
- *Male:* 743,523,107 (51.6%)
- *Female:* 696,502,241 (48.4%)

*Birth rate:*
- 17.464/1,000 people (World, 2023), 1.15% decline from 2022

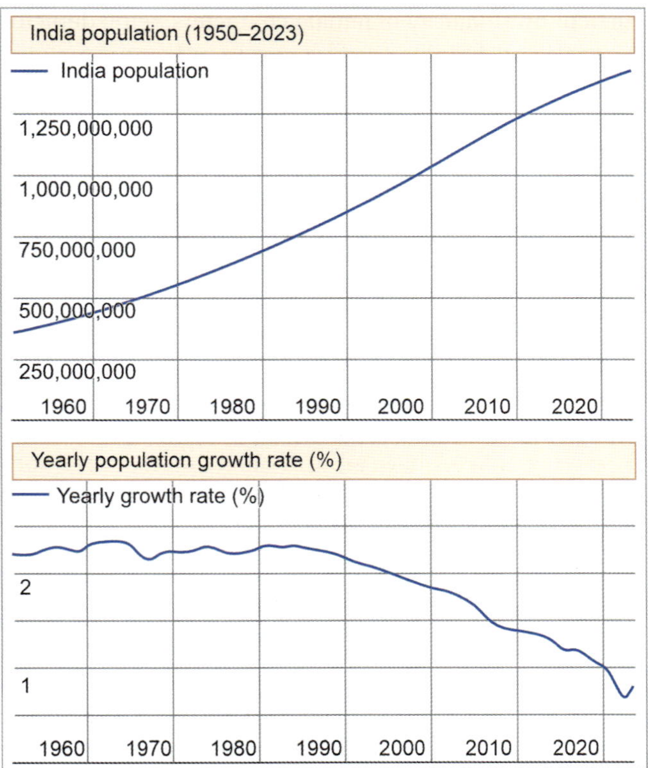


**Fig. 1:** India population (1950–2023).

- 16.949/1,000 people (India, 2023), 1.25% decline from 2022

*Sex ratio:* The National Family Health Survey, 2020–21 (NFHS-5) stated that India's sex ratio is about "1,020 females/1,000 males".

*In India:*
- *Rural Area:* 1,037 females/1,000 males
- *Urban area:* 985 females/1,000 males

*Note:* These statistics show that the female ratio is less compared to the male ratio globally. In India, female ratio is less compared to the male ratio in the urban area.

### Education Inequalities
- Schooling
- Literacy
- Reservations for female students.

### Schooling

In rural India, girls continue to be less educated than boys. According to a 1998 report by the United States (US) Department of Commerce, the chief barriers to female education are inadequate school facilities (such as sanitary facilities), shortage of female teachers, and gender bias in curriculum (majority of female characters being depicted as weak and helpless versus strong, adventurous, and intelligent men with high-prestige jobs.)

### Literacy

In India, education and learning opportunities for girls are comparatively lower than the boys. The misperception of parents is that the girl's education will not support their future. As a result, 129 million girls are out of school, and most drop out at the upper secondary level school [United Nations Children's Fund (UNICEF) 2021].

Literacy rate among men and women in India between 2019 and 2021, by area is illustrated in **Figure 2**.

*Note:* The figure shows that the female literacy rate is less than male literacy rate in urban and rural areas.

### Reservations for Female Students

*Is this a need for gender empowerment?*

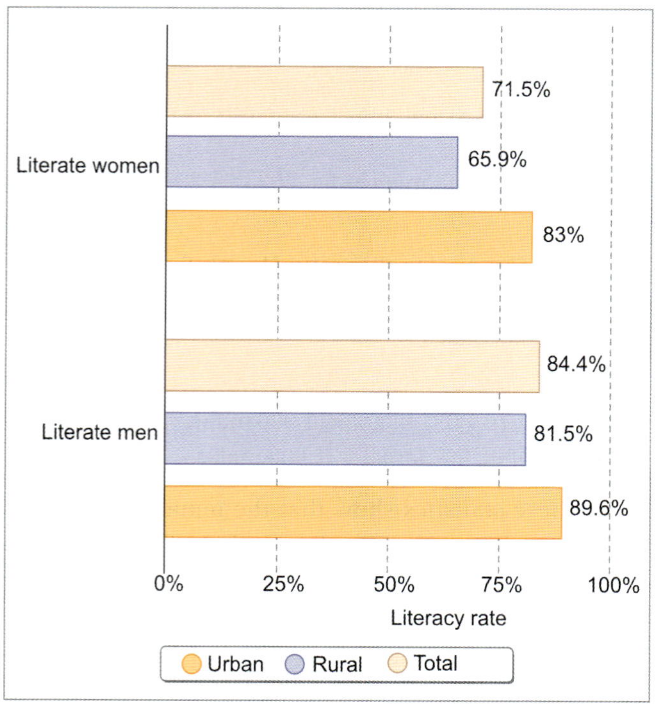


**Fig. 2:** Literacy rate among men and women in India between 2019 and 2021, by area.

- Under a nonformal education program, about 40% of the centers in states and 10% centers in universities are exclusively reserved for females.
- Certain state-level engineering, medical, and other colleges, like in Orissa, have reserved 30% of seats for females.

## Gender Discrimination in Society

- *At birth:* Female foeticide is more common in India compared to other countries because people prefer to raise a male child than a female child due to dowry. The Ministry of Women and Child Development, 2015 reported that 2,000 girls are killed daily and the census shows that the number of girls was 78.8 million in 2001, declining to 75.8 million in 2011.
- *Early marriage/underage marriage:* According to NFHS5, 23.3% girls got married before the age of 18 years.

  According to UNICEF, child marriage is often the result of entrenched gender inequality, making girls disproportionately affected by the practice. Globally, the prevalence of child marriage among boys is just one-sixth among girls. Child marriage robs girls of their childhood and threatens their well-being.
- *Teenage pregnancy:* Lack of adequate sexual education, peer pressure, use of alcohol or drugs, and some of the environmental factors (poverty) are responsible for teenage pregnancy.
- *Health:* Health expenditure is 1.5 times higher in men compared to women. In India, 70% of females cannot take care of their health as they are involved in noneconomic activities like homemaking. Indian women suffer from various health issues, which would affect the development of women in all respects.
- *Gender wage gap:* According to an International Labor Organization (ILO) study, women were paid about 20% less than men globally, due to the stereotypical traditional practice of a male-dominated society where the women are considered less productive than male.
- *Property rights:* According to the Indian Legislation Act, women have equal rights over their parents' property but if a woman tries to entitle her rights, she is termed "greedy". The traditional practice of discriminating with women in sharing property exists throughout the country.
- *Abuse, exploitation, and violence:* According to the NFHS5, nearly one-third of Indian women experience

physical or sexual violence and 30% of women face physical violence since the age of 15.

According to UNdocs (2019), 18% of women face physical violence from their spouses and the above statistics reveal the male dominance in society. At the household level, women are considered as enslaved people and ill-treated.

- *Patriarchy* is a system where men have authority over women in all aspects such as how they should behave, how they should dress up, what kind of jobs they should take, or all the major decisions for their lives.
- *Politics:* Percentage of the women elected to Lok Sabha is 14.94 and the Rajya Sabha is 14.05.
- *Legislation:* The Government of India has passed legislation to secure women's rights like the Protection of Women from Domestic Violence Act, 2005, Protection of Women against Sexual Harassment Bill, 2007, etc., Despite these Acts, women still struggle to ensure their fundamental rights.
- *Gender stereotype:* It is a generalized view or preconception about the attributes or characteristics, or the roles that are performed by women and men.

A gender stereotype is harmful when it limits women's and men's capacity to develop their personal abilities, pursue their professional careers, and/or make choices about their lives.

## Gender Prejudice

Prejudiced actions or thoughts are based on the gender-based perception that women are not equal to men in rights and dignity.

## Low Confidence

Boys are expected to develop self-confidence, whereas if girls show self-confidence, it is considered a breach of traditional gender roles.

*There is a lack of unity among stakeholders to solve the existing problems related to gender inequality.*
- *Problems related to health:*
  - Gender discrimination plays a role in the overall health of an individual.
  - Adolescent girls and women are expected to eat last and left-out food
  - Boys are offered better nutritious food, especially if the family is poor.
  - Anemia is very common in girls due to inadequate dietary intake.

47% of the girls in the age group of 15–19 years had a body mass index (BMI) <18.5 kg/m$^2$.
- *Poverty and ignorance:* The majority of women are poor and ignored due to cultural norms and values, gendered divisions of assets, and power dynamics between men and women.

## THE SPECIAL SIGNIFICANCE OF GENDER DURING ADOLESCENT AGE GROUP

Adolescence is a period of transition between childhood and adulthood.

It is a time of rapid physical, cognitive, social, and emotional maturing as a boy prepares for manhood and a girl prepares for womanhood.

*Salient attributes of adolescence:*
- Physical, psychological, emotional, and social development
- Rapid but uneven physical growth
- Sexual maturity and onset of sexual activity
- Desire for exploration and experimentation
- Development of adult mental process and self-identity
- Transition from dependence to relative independence.

### Period of Transition through Adolescent Years

The period of transition between childhood to adolescence to young adulthood is the period where young minds can be helped.
- Help them with their curiosity about the opposite sex.
- Help them with their struggle for independence and acceptance.
- Help them consolidate their sexual identity.
- Help them develop their thought process and idealism, to identify their feelings, intimacy, commitment, and relationships.

## BARRIERS OF GENDER EMPOWERMENT

Barriers to gender empowerment include the following **(Fig. 3)**.
- *Gender attitudes* such as men do not need to, nor should they access flexible work arrangements or women are not interested in promotions because they have young children
- *Work stereotypes* such as males make better leaders and managers or females cannot do certain jobs
- *Embedded bias* such as overlooking a candidate, in this case, a female in her early 30s because she is put

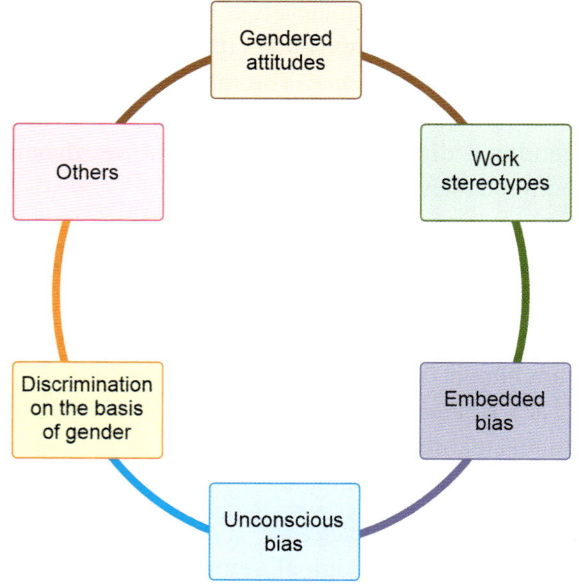



**Fig. 3:** Barriers to gender empowerment.

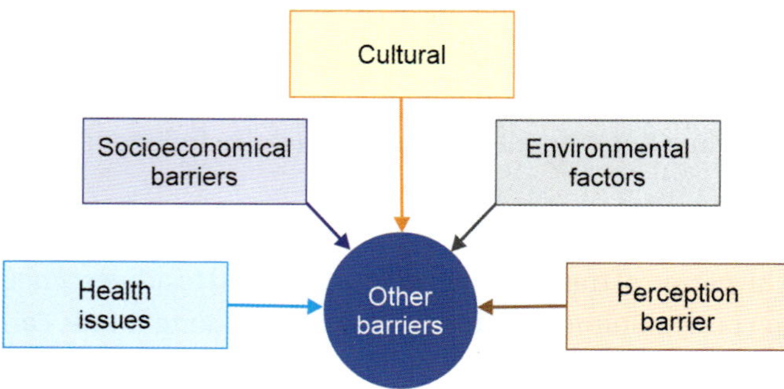



**Fig. 4:** Other barriers to gender empowerment.

in the "will likely have kids and go on maternity leave" category.

- *Unconscious bias:* Where there is bias (conscious or unconscious) in the workplace, we continue to recruit toward someone's opinion more (even if they are not the subject matter expert) whom we have unconscious affinity with.
- *Discrimination on the basis of gender:* Particularly in relation to family and caring responsibilities.

Other barriers are illustrated in **Figure 4**.

## ROLE OF EDUCATING ADOLESCENT BOYS

Gender inequality starts at home, when mothers tell their daughters that they do not need to play with boys or it is their duty to do household jobs and look after the family or when fathers tell their sons that only the man of the house should earn a living and the women need to take care of the children. This preconception of parents' thinking needs to be changed.

*Parents can educate adolescent boys by the following points:*

- *By being a role model:* Teaching boys about the values and behaviors they should honor, by demonstrating those virtues in life.
- *Work as a team with other caregivers:* Whether in a traditional family or nuclear family, it is necessary to connect with the caretakers to reinforce the values that we are trying to build on.
- *Limit potentially harmful influences:* Restrict harmful media and encourage your son to make good friends. Make sure that these families share similar values and are equally committed to raising the young gentlemen. In this way, we can be sure that our son's earliest friends will be good influences in his life.
- *Tell stories about gentlemen:* Positive role models should be provided from books, television, movies, and other media.
- *Balance male and female influences:* Boys should be exposed to both male and female influences in their lives. Female influences can teach boys about treating girls in their own age as any gentleman should.
- *Defending and respecting girls:* Respectful speech, averting eyes when something is inappropriate, being mindful of spatial boundaries, and always asking before assuming are practical ways through which boys learn to know that respect for girls is not "optional".
- *Parents should monitor the aggression of their children from childhood. They should inculcate empathy and encourage emotional expressions in boys.*
- *Setting up a value system is very important:*
  - Promoting good listening skills
  - Being friendly and personable
  - To develop leadership qualities
  - Help him to be a good sport
  - Encouraging boys to use good manners
  - Emphasize the importance of honesty
  - Let him develop a generous spirit
  - Foster a steady work ethic
  - Teach him to turn away from vices and temptations.

## THE ROLE OF PEDIATRICIANS AND OTHER STAKEHOLDERS

*The role of pediatricians:*

- Pediatricians are the largest body; they are strong advocates for children.

- Pediatric care starts at birth and lasts through a child's 21st birthday or longer.
- They start a trustworthy relationship with the child and the family and have a big role to play in their lives.
- They prevent, detect, and manage physical, behavioral, and development issues that affect children.
- They can liaison with the government and its various departments working for children.
- They can collaborate with nongovernmental organizations (NGOs) working in the community.
- They can approach schools, colleges, and address young people.
- They have access to parents and organization.
- They can outreach the community.

## ROLE OF GOVERNMENT

- To create a safe environment for studies, sports, and financial assistance for education.
- Educating society and parents about the importance of education for girl child.
- Formulate different programs to treat and prevent malnutrition in girl child.
- Educate to eliminate the trend of sexual discrimination.

*Top 10 government schemes for ensuring the welfare of the girl child in India.*

Considering the numerous obstacles that come in the way of a girl child, throughout her life, the government has many schemes in place to make sure that she is given the right opportunity and additional aid to help her progress and succeed in life. Some of the top schemes are given below:

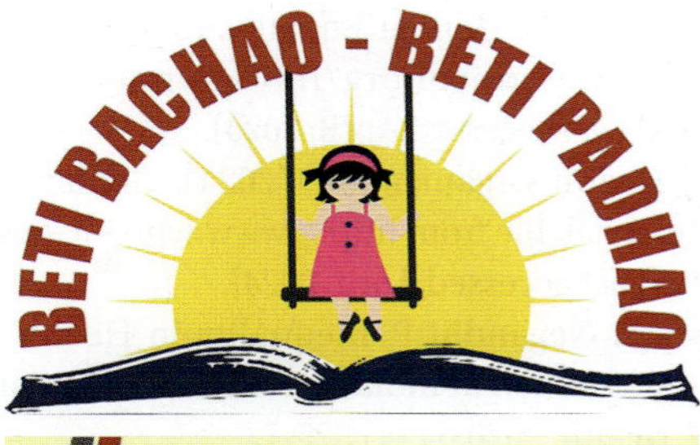


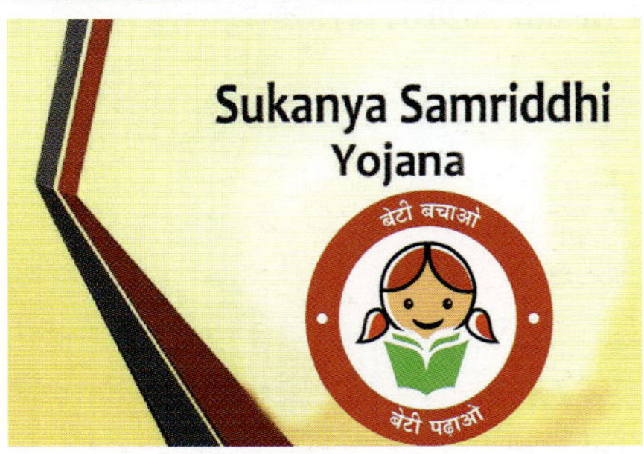


1. Beti Bachao Beti Padhao
2. Sukanya Samriddhi Yojana
3. Balika Samridhi Yojana
4. Mukhyamantri Rajshri Yojana
5. Mukhyamantri Laadli Yojana
6. Central Board of Secondary Education (CBSE) Udaan Scheme
7. National Scheme of Incentives to Girls for Secondary Education
8. Mukhyamantri Kanya Suraksha Yojana
9. Mazi Kanya Bhagyashree Scheme
10. Nanda Devi Kanya Yojana

## THE FUTURE DIRECTION

*UNICEF's Gender Action Plan* specifies how each of our global strategic plan (2022–2025) goal areas will advance gender equality, from before birth through adolescence. This includes plans and targets related to:

- *Maternal health and nutrition*, including human immunodeficiency virus (HIV) testing, prevention, counseling, and care.
- *Gender-responsive education systems*, especially when it comes to equitable access to schooling, STEM (science, technology, engineering, and mathematics) and digital skills for adolescent girls.
- *Harmful practices* (child marriage and female genital mutilation) and violence against girls, boys, and women.
- *Equitable water, sanitation, and hygiene systems*, including services for menstrual health.
- Gender-responsive social protection and care.

### Leadership and Well-being of Adolescent Girls

*This Gender Action Plan reiterates UNICEF's strong commitment to the leadership and well-being of adolescent girls.*

- Quality health and nutrition services, including human papillomavirus (HPV) and HIV prevention
- Skills for the future, especially those related to STEM and digital skills
- Freedom from child marriage and violence
- Social protection and care.

*Gender-transformative workplaces and practices:*

- Gender parity in staffing at all levels
- A minimum of 15% of all funding received to be earmarked for gender-equality priorities

- Zero tolerance for discrimination, sexual exploitation, abuse, or harassment.

## ROLE OF ADOLESCENT HEALTH ACADEMY AND INDIAN ACADEMY OF PEDIATRICS

- Adolescent Health Academy (AHA) and Indian Academy of Pediatrics (IAP) support in advocacy and national programs.
- Capacities building in various national health programs.
- Identification and training of community resource person.
- Advocacy and member in various task forces.
- Evaluation and monitoring of various national programs.
- Organization of community adolescent health care clinics.
- Expert services in private clinics, and school/colleges based or linked clinics.
- Organization of teen clubs.
- School health program.
- Community awareness program.

## KEY MESSAGES

- Discuss gender equality and advancement with family members and children.
- Speak out against gender-based violence.
- Challenge gender stereotypes.
- Address gender discrimination in society.
- The role of educating adolescent boys is very important.
- Raising women's status through education, awareness, literacy, and training should be the way forward.
- There is a big role of government and NGOs in gender empowerment.

## RECOMMENDED READING


1. Chicago Tribune. Los Angeles Times. (2007). Teenage pregnancy just isn't scary enough anymore. [online] Available from http://articles.chicagotribune.com/2007-12-18/news/0712170390_1_teen-pregnancy-abortion-clinic-pregnant-teenagers [Last accessed April, 2024].
2. Countrymeters. (2024). India Population. [online] Available from https://countrymeters.info/en/India [Last accessed April, 2024].
3. Jain S, Bajaj B, Singh A. (2022). Are Indian higher education institutions doing their bit towards empowerment of mid-career women?: A study of public and private universities in India. [online] https://www.researchgate.net/publication/363360519_Are_Indian_Higher_Education_Institutions_Doing_Their_Bit_Towards_Empowerment_of_Mid-Career_Women_A_Study_of_Public_and_Private_Universities_in_India [Last accessed April, 2024].
4. Next IAS. (2022). NFHS-5 Survey. [online] Available from https://www.nextias.com/current-affairs/07-05-2022/nfhs-5-survey/ [Last accessed April, 2024].
5. Page N, Czuba CE. Empowerment: What is it? Journal of Extension. 1999;37(5):1-5.
6. Statista. (2024). Literacy rate among women and men in India between 2019 and 2021, by area. [online] Available from https://www.statista.com/statistics/1303303/india-gender-literacy-rate-by-area/ [Last accessed April, 2024].
7. The Center for Parenting. (2024). Over-indulgence and values:
Values matter: Using your values to raise caring, responsible, resilient children. [online] Available from https://centerforparentingeducation.org/library-of-articles/indulgence-values/values-matter-using-your-values-to-raise-caring-responsible-resilient-children-what-are-values/ [Last accessed April, 2024].
8. UNICEF. (2021) Gender Action Plan, 2022-2025. [online] Available from https://www.unicef.org/executiveboard/documents/UNICEF-Gender-Action-Plan-2022%E2%80%932025-SRS-2021 [Last accessed April, 2024].
9. UNICEF. (2021). Gender Equality. [online] Available from https://www.unicef.org/india/what-we-do/gender-equality [Last accessed April, 2024].
10. World Health Organization. (2024). Gender and health. [online] Available from http://www.who.int/health-topics/gender [Last accessed April, 2024].
11. Zodpey S, Negandhi P. Inequality in Health and Social Status for Women in India–A Long-Standing Bane. Indian J Public Health. 2020;64 (4):325-7.

## 8.15 Sexuality Education and Role of Gatekeepers

*Sumitha Nayak*

### ■ INTRODUCTION

The World Health Organization (WHO) mentions that according to the International Technical Guidance on Sexuality Education, no age is too early to start sex education, as even young children can be taught developmentally appropriate information related to their body parts. This underlines the importance of imparting sexuality education to adolescents. The word sexuality is however different from the words sex and gender, and this needs to be emphasized.

### MEANINGS OF THE WORDS "SEXUALITY" AND "GATEKEEPERS"

According to the Cambridge dictionary, the word "sexuality" refers to a person's ability to experience or show sexual feelings, the fact or action of showing sexual feelings, as well as the attitudes and activities related to sex. Adolescents begin to realize their sexuality or sexual orientation and preferences, as their body evolves.

The word "gatekeeper" refers to a person who is empowered to open and close a gate and hence prevent entry of unauthorized persons. It could also refer to someone who decides who gets particular opportunities or benefits and who does not.

The initial role in sexuality education has to be given by the parents; hence they would be considered as the first gatekeepers.

The other members of the immediate family, including older siblings, grandparents, and uncles and aunts do influence the thoughts and understanding of one's sexuality, and are considered as gatekeepers at the next level.

Once at school, the teachers and the peer group play a major role in influencing the understanding of sexuality and sexual behavior. The teachers are considered an important gatekeeper, as they have the capacity of driving the direction of sexuality related behaviors through the information and teachings that they impart. By providing scientific and correct descriptions and explanations, being there to clear any doubts and to guide the adolescents when they require hand-holding, the teachers play an extremely vital role in imparting healthy sexuality to the future generations.

Policy makers are the final gatekeepers, as they are responsible for proposing the legal aspects related to varied gender identities. This reflects the cultural practices of the region and the nation, and the acceptance or otherwise of deviations in sexuality and gender identity.

### ■ TERMS ASSOCIATED WITH "SEXUALITY"

The term "sex" refers to the physical and psychological assignment as male or female based on the external genital organs and the corresponding internal organs.

"Gender" refers to the social or cultural distinctions that are associated with a particular sex. A category of "intersex" exists, where the individual does not fit into either of the two biological sexes, but is eventually assigned to one of them.

The gender identity refers to the extent to which an individual identifies with the assigned gender and their subjective experience of this identification. While the gender identity is shaped from early life usually around 3–4 years of age, it evolves and may change during adolescence.

When the individual identifies with the assigned gender, they are referred to as "cisgender". When there is a conflict between the assigned physical gender and their identity, they are referred to as "transgender". The term "nonbinary" refers to the uncategorized gender identity. The "gender neutral" individual refers to one who does not consider themselves belonging to any gender.

### ■ SEXUAL ORIENTATION

Sexual orientation of an individual is a part of the spectrum of sexuality and depicts who you are attracted to sexually. This is an interpersonal relationship and need not always be aligned with the assigned sex of the person.

Some expressions of sexuality are included in **Table 1** (*Chapter 8.5*).

## ■ FACTORS AFFECTING SEXUALITY

Adolescent sexuality is explained using the bio-psycho-social model, as many factors are associated with the development of the individual's sexuality.

Biological factors not only influence the physical sex, but also play a role in the psychological sex via genetic and neuroendocrinal factors. Stress and sex hormones are known to influence the brain neurocognition which plays a role in the sexual orientation. These changes are noted in the early infancy period itself. The personality, psychological make up, and temperament also influence the sexuality. Social and environmental factors, including the parental attitudes, parenting styles, peers, and cultural influences affect the sexual attitudes of adolescents. Media reports of crimes, violence and literature reports, movies, and digital media exposure are contributors to affecting an adolescent's perception of their sexuality. Cultural influences have a major impact together with the law of the land, as the natural sexuality tends to be kept hidden and curbed, away from public view. Peer relationships could make the adolescents swing toward a particular identity, at the same time making them wary and fearful of negative outcomes and scorn. Mental health issues such as depression and schizophrenia affect the sexuality of the individual. Depressive disorders tend to have altered sexual orientation related to volition drive deficit, low self-esteem, feelings of worthlessness, and inadequacy.

Childhood sexual abuse leads to the high likelihood of altered sexual self-concept, and the possibility of sexual dysfunction.

## ■ IMPORTANCE OF SEXUALITY EDUCATION

Adolescents have a right to learn about the role of sexuality in their life. Developing a healthy sexuality is a core developmental milestone for adolescents, as the youth need to understand how their sexuality relates to their own body, their family, community, culture, mental health, and relationships.

Studies have shown that adolescents are unprepared for the physical, emotional, and social changes that occur during this phase and several knowledge gaps and misconceptions exist, resulting in fears and anxiety.

A need to access scientifically and medically correct information is essential, that will allow them to understand the physical and hormonal changes that occur in adolescence. These changes, together with the environmental factors, are responsible for the attitude of an individual to sexuality.

Teaching that each one is in charge of making their decisions relating to their body, orientation toward a particular gender, the good touch-bad touch concepts, implications of the outcomes of sexual activity, needs of a healthy future, avoiding sexual abuse, and the need for timely treatment whenever necessary, must all be emphasized.

The education should cover the critical gaps in knowledge of modern contraception, human immunodeficiency virus (HIV) prevention, and complications of sexual intercourse and avoidance of pregnancy. There is a fear of ridicule and nonacceptance in case of nonconformity to the societal norms and rules of gender identity. These fears must be addressed scientifically and nonjudgmentally. Studies have shown that once there is adequate sexuality education, the health outcomes are much better with reduced rates of sexual diseases, unwanted pregnancy, etc.

A need for a robust, correct, unbiased, and nonjudgmental guidance is absolutely essential as the hormonal changes initiate changes in the physical and the mental processes of the individuals.

## ■ MEANS TO IMPART SEXUALITY EDUCATION AND ROLE OF GATEKEEPERS

There is no age that is too early to impart sexuality education. According to the WHO, children and adolescents have a right to receive age and development appropriate education relating to themselves. This is invaluable for their health and wellbeing. The United Nations International Guidance calls for children between 12 and 15 years to be made aware of sexual abuse, sexual assault, intimate partner violence, and bullying being violations of human rights and stresses the need for sexuality education.

The gatekeepers are those who would play a vital role in teaching the adolescents about their sexuality and reproductive health.

- *Parents* should be the first teachers, especially the mother. This education by parents starts right from birth. Parents need to explain the changes that occur as the children grow and especially when puberty hits their offspring. This information must be given ideally well before the onset of menstruation in girls and before the complete development of the secondary sexual organs in both sexes. They must ensure that the correct, scientific information is shared along with details of the gender orientation and sexuality. They should allow the offspring to ask questions, to prevent misconceptions, and the need to address their problems by unsolicited methods and unreliable sources. The parents must be prepared to accept their offsprings' sexuality and gender orientation preferences.

- Family members and elders play a role in teaching to ensure that the adolescents understand the physical, emotional, and psychological changes.
- Teachers and educators play a key role. They are in the best position to offer this education in a group setting. However, they must be trained to address queries related to sexuality and other concerns related to sexual health, in a scientific and nonjudgmental manner.
- Social workers and counselors who work with young people play an important part in ensuring well-being as they are generally considered to have the knowledge required to deal with issues of sexuality, sexual health, and gender.
- Policy makers need to be aware of the challenges faced and the need to create up to date and implementable guidelines, along with adequate training programs, so that the community workers and teachers can learn to handle the problems they would encounter. The laws such as Protection of Children from Sexual Offences (POCSO) that are related to sexuality are useful to prevent and address sexual offences against this vulnerable age group

## ◼ THE WAY FORWARD

There is a definite need for comprehensive sexuality education (CSE) in India. 25% of the population is under the age of 14 years and adolescents and young adults between 10 and 24 years constitute 27% of India's population. The poor knowledge of sexuality and sexual behaviors leads to high-risk behavior and poor health of the youth.

Some of the suggested ways to move ahead include the following:

- The integration of a CSE into the school curriculum is one way of imparting knowledge on the cognitive, social, emotional, and physical aspects of sexuality that can lead to better health, well-being, and dignity of the young people. The program must provide comprehensive education on the different domains of sexuality including gender identity, aiming to bring about a behavioral change in the community.

The CSE program should provide scientifically accurate, age and developmentally appropriate, gender sensitive, and culturally relevant information. It must provide opportunities to explore the attitudes, values, existing norms and rights, and thus promote the acquisition of improved life skills. Sexuality and sexual behavior is one of the key components of the CSE.

- Sexuality education must take place in an environment where the youngsters are comfortable, safe from harassment and their privacy is respected and unbiased and nonjudgmental exchange of information can take place. Studies done in India have shown that following CSE, the risk-taking behavior of the adolescents decreases and there is a more responsible sexual behavior including delayed initiation and reduced frequency of sexual intercourse and increased condom usage.
- Sexuality education can be integrated along with the Rashtriya Kishor Swasthya Karyakram (RKSK) and the Reproductive, Maternal, Newborn, Child and Adolescent (RMNCH+A) Programs of the Government of India. By creating a robust and scientifically sound program, the CSE can be implemented in every nook of the country and will go a long way in remodeling the cultural concepts of sexuality and gender orientation in India.
- Setting up of Adolescent Friendly Health Clinics (AFHS) in all district and major hospitals is another way of dealing with adolescent problems, including sexuality education as a component. Under the RKSK program, the government is attempting to address these issues.

Terminologies of sexuality (Refer to *Chapter 8.5*)

## ◼ KEY MESSAGES

- "Sexuality" refers to a person's ability to experience or show sexual feelings, the fact or action of showing sexual feelings, as well as the attitudes and activities related to sex.
- The bio-psycho-social model plays a major role in the modeling of an individual's gender identity and sexuality.
- There are several nomenclatures for an individual's preferences of gender identity and sexual orientation.

- Parents are the first gatekeepers to provide authentic information and sexuality education from an early age, so also are the family members and elders.
- Teachers and educators have a unique opportunity to impart sexuality education in a group and must be trained with a scientific and nonjudgmental methodology.
- Social workers and counselors who work with young people play an important part in ensuring well-being as they are generally considered to have the knowledge required to deal with issues of sexuality, sexual health, and gender.
- Policy makers need to create up to date and implementable laws and guidelines, along with adequate training programs, so that the community workers and teachers can learn to handle the problems they would encounter.
- The integration of a CSE into the school curriculum is one way of imparting knowledge on the cognitive, social, emotional and physical aspects of sexuality that can lead to better health, well-being, and dignity of the young people.

## ■ RECOMMENDED READING

1. Gilmore D. More questions than answers: factors affecting gender identity and sexual orientation: a mini review. Am J Biomed Res. 2020;10(4):401-4.
2. Joesph JT. Comprehensive sexuality education in the Indian context: challenges and opportunities. Indian J Psychol Med. 2023;45(3):292-6.
3. Kar SK, Choudhury A, Singh AP. Understanding normal development of adolescent sexuality: a bumpy ride. J Hum Reprod Sci. 2015;8(2):70-4.
4. World Health Organization. WHO recommendations on adolescent sexual and reproductive health and rights. Geneva: World Health Organization; 2018.

# 8.16 Comprehensive Sexuality Education

*Shubhada Khirwadkar, Geeta Patil*

## ■ INTRODUCTION

In Indian scenario, early marriages, unplanned pregnancies, gender bias, sexual abuse, patriarchy, and insufficient information regarding sexual behavior and risks are major challenges faced by adolescents. They are exposed to various erotic materials in films, newspapers, magazines, or internet. Adolescents are bubbling with sex hormones, confused with sexual identity, peer pressure, and inadequate information or guidance on sexuality with hardly any family life education. Public discussion of sexuality and sexual behavior is considered taboo in our country and controversial. Adolescents are curious to know many things but neither parents nor school and community clarify their doubts, so they indulge in unsafe ways such as internet, pornography, and peer interaction; which may provide unscientific and age-inappropriate information. This may affect healthy mental and physical growth adversely.

Some other factors such as lack of social buffers, changing values and life style, influence of media, and earlier attainment of puberty adds to problems.

## ■ MYTHS ABOUT SEXUALITY KNOWLEDGE

- Only parents and close relatives can educate the adolescents about sexuality.
- Sexuality education is good for young people, but not for young children.
- Abstinence is the solution.
- Sexuality education should only promote values.
- It leads to promiscuity, experimentation, and irresponsible sexual behavior; and deprives children of their innocence.
- Sexuality education has no place in a country such as India with its rich cultural traditions and ethos.

Comprehensive sexuality education (CSE) is a curriculum-based process of teaching and learning which includes cognitive, emotional, physical, and social aspects of sexuality. It aims to equip adolescents with knowledge, skills, attitudes, and values. This knowledge will empower them to realize their health and well-being with dignity; and develop respectful social and sexual relationships **(Box 1)**.

<table>
<tr><td>

**BOX 1:** Need for comprehensive sexuality education (CSE) in India.

- Promoting healthy relationships
- Preventing teenage and unintended pregnancies
- Reducing sexually transmitted infections (STIs)
- Empowering women and girls
- Foster positive attitudes toward sexuality and relationships
- Addressing taboos and stigmas
- Tackling child sexual abuse
- Promoting inclusive education
- Improving Mental Health
- Meeting the Demands of a Changing Society

</td></tr>
</table>

<table>
<tr><td>

**BOX 2:** Essential components of comprehensive sexuality education (CSE).

- Relationships
- Values, rights, culture, and sexuality
- Understanding gender
- Violence and staying safe
- Skills for health and well-being
- The human body and development
- Sexuality and sexual behavior
- Sexual & Reproductive Health

</td></tr>
</table>

It will also help them to consider how their choices affect their own well-being and that of others; and make teenagers understand and ensure the protection of their rights throughout their lives. Many girls lack access to adequate facilities for menstrual hygiene and with associated social stigma which may lead to school absenteeism and increased dropouts. Because of sociocultural changes, the opportunities for sexual experimentations have increased. Early sexual debut may lead to unintended pregnancy and sexually transmitted infections (STIs). Though child marriages are decreasing in India, early marriages and pregnancy may lead to school drop outs and disruption in social and economic activities. The reason could be lack of knowledge about modern contraceptive methods and services, limited access to timely and relevant information and quality sexual and reproductive health (SRH) services.

Comprehensive sexuality education should be scientifically accurate, incremental, age and developmentally appropriate, curriculum based, comprehensive, and culturally acceptable. It includes sexual and reproductive anatomy, physiology of puberty and menstruation, reproduction, modern contraception, pregnancy and child birth, and sexually transmitted diseases (STDs). The entire approach will be based on human rights approach **(Box 2)**.

There are many challenges during the process, such as:

- *Social opposition* from policy makers, religious beliefs and leaders, teacher's beliefs, and parental (non)cooperation which prevents policy making and implementation.
- *Operational constraints* such as insufficient training of trainers, lack of self-confidence (omit topics which are sensitive), lack of access to authentic curriculum and training resources, funds, overburdened students, and teachers with academics.

## COMPREHENSIVE SEXUALITY EDUCATION: KEY FOR SUSTAINABLE DEVELOPMENT

- *Empowers individuals, especially women and girls:*
  - Reduces the spread of human immunodeficiency virus (HIV)/STIs and unintended pregnancies
  - Promotes gender equality and prevents gender-based violence
  - Enhances education and economic opportunities
  - Improves critical thinking
- *Fosters healthy societies:*
  - Reduces social issues
  - Improves mental health and well-being
  - Improves maternal and child health
  - Promotes inclusive development
  - Empowers to become active and responsible citizenship
- *Promotes environmental protection:* By population control leading to reduction of sustainable consumption.

## METHODOLOGY

- Teachers, doctors, social workers, nurses, parent, and volunteers can take part in teaching of CSE.
- Print and electronic media can be used in appropriate way.
- It can be taught in classroom setup by didactic way or by demonstration, group work, and case study followed by discussion and role plays by guest speakers like doctors.
- It can be effectively delivered by age appropriate and developmentally relevant content by skilled and trained educators, using interactive teaching methods.
- It should be remembered to be taught in culturally sensitive way and by inclusive approach.

- Parental and community involvement is essential in this project.
- Information given should be accurate and up-to-date.
- Creating a safe and confidential learning environment will help to have better learning.
- Always addressing the needs of marginalized groups and those with disabilities have to be kept in mind.
- Sustainable Development Goal 4 (SDG4) (to ensure inclusive and equitable quality education and promote lifelong learning opportunities by 2030) can be achieved by this project.
- Main aim is to impart knowledge, modify attitudes, and help for skill building.

## CONCLUSION

It is essential to strengthen the capacity of adolescents and young people by providing them with age appropriate, scientific, and culturally appropriate information. They should be taught skills to make informed choices and adopt healthy behaviors so that they can overcome gender inequalities, be safe from coercion, exploitation, and all types of violence, and to lead healthy life to realize their potential. This will help to achieve holistic well-being of adolescents.

Adolescent education program is getting revised by the government in the National Council of Educational Research and Training (NCERT) syllabus but pace is very slow.

## KEY MESSAGES

- Our collective aim is to equip children with the correct knowledge, skills, attitudes, and values that will enable them to live life and thrive with good health, well-being, and dignity,
- Involve *education system* to implement comprehensive information about sexuality and reduce *social stigma* around adolescent sexuality.
- Capacity building and training of teachers.
- Create resource, teaching materials, and guiding tools.
- Scale up implementation of CSE program in association with existing programs such as Adolescence Education Program (AEP), Rashtriya Kishor Swasthya Karyakram (RKSK), and School Health and Wellness Program (SHWP).
- *Reach out* to policy makers and relevant stake holders.

## RECOMMENDED READING

1. International Institute for Population Sciences. National Family Health Survey (NFHS-5), 2019–21: India Report. Mumbai: International Institute for Population Sciences; 2022.
2. UNESCO. (2023). Menstrual Health and Hygiene Management, Survey and Gap Analysis Report. [online] Available from https://unesdoc.unesco.org/ark:/48223/pf0000385512. [Last accessed April, 2024].
3. World Health Organization. Global Health Estimates. [online] Available from https://www.who.int/data/global-health-estimates. [Last accessed April, 2024].

# Social Media

**Section Editors:** *Shamik Ghosh, Kripasindhu Chatterjee*

## 9.1 Types of Media

*Shilpi Siddhanta Talukdar*

### ■ INTRODUCTION

Media plays an important role in a teen's life. Teenagers use the media to express themselves and to interact with others by using emails, social networking sites, message boards, dating apps, etc. They find it an easy means to pass their time by gaming, watching videos on YouTube, making reels, blogging, etc. News apps and websites like Wikipedia provide an important source of information.

### ■ WHAT IS MEDIA?

Media can be defined as an important mean of mass communication for the common people. Initially mass communication started as social gatherings and gradually developed into *gurukulams* and organizations. Indigenous media dates back to ages where gatherings, social organizations, direct observation or oral instructions given by the gurus to the students used to be the only means of communication. Other means of communication were records which were verbal, written or carved.

People expanded their reach via the written word, but communication have taken off in unimaginable ways in the twentieth century. While the invention of the telephone changed communication forever, the cell phone was even more transformative.

In the beginning, media was for mass consumption. *Traditional media* which includes the press, television, radio, and films was unidirectional for masses to be consumed. *Digital media* led to bidirectional exchange of digitalized information over internet. Today a single digital reader like Kindle can hold hundreds of books and newspapers. Radio, TV, and movies can be watched on the cell phone or a computer. More importantly, the digital media permits not only consumption but also production and interaction: One can download videos onto YouTube, and converse with others on WhatsApp, Facebook, Instagram, or X. One can play videogames by oneself or as a member of an online group.

Traditional media was available periodically not 24/7 like digital media.

The major source of finance for all this mass communication is advertising. Advertising has become a major industry influencing the habits and shaping the behaviors and fashions of the masses, especially adolescents, as they are less knowledgeable and discriminatory. The media applies direct pressure on adolescents by targeting branded products at them.

There is also indirect media pressure through content on social media like Instagram, Snapchat, TikTok, and YouTube. The presence of violent, sexual, misogynistic, or racial imagery in video games, songs and news media, and of the use of alcohol and drugs of abuse, normalizes these behaviors. While parents and teachers and other leaders of society were expected to influence and guide adolescents on their trek toward adulthood, today this role has been hijacked to some extent by the social media.

## HOW ADOLESCENTS GET ADDICTED TO MEDIA?

Adolescents are at highest risk of falling into addiction because of their impulsive nature, their growing need for social interaction, and the necessity for them to affirm their group identity.

- Some teens spend all their time on social media, due to their fear of missing out (FOMO) on what is happening around them.
- Teens use social media to escape from stress or even depression.
- On this platform it is easier to make friends.
- It is an easy way of passing the time.

## KEY MESSAGES

- The boon of technology is not without its potential risks.

- The crux lies in teaching adolescents to use it wisely and judiciously.
- Rather than asking them to completely cut out social media, it would be a good idea to advise them to limit the time they spend on media and point all the potential risks to them.

## RECOMMENDED READING

1. Bozzola E, Spina G, Agostiniani R, Barni S, Russo R, Scarpato E, et al. The Use of Social Media in Children and Adolescents: Scoping Review on the Potential Risks. Int J Environ Res Public Health. 2022;19(16):9960.
2. Pantic I. Online social networking and mental health. Cyberpsychol Behav Soc Netw. 2014;17(10):652-7.
3. Strasburger VC, Jordan AB, Donnerstein E. Health effects of media on children and adolescents. Pediatrics. 2010;125(4):756-67.

---

# 9.2 Social Media: Benefits and Hazards

*Geeta Patil*

## INTRODUCTION

Electronic media and gadgets have become a part of daily life for everyone, especially for teenagers. The present era may be labeled as the age of "screenagers". Screen use is pervasive even among infants and toddlers, whose caregivers utilize them to keep the children occupied. It should not be a surprise that today the social media is usurping the role of parents, teachers, and religious leaders in shaping the beliefs and practices of society.

Social media is media used for social interaction. It differs from any other media in quality (highly palatable and creates craving), durability (stays in the mind for a long time), reach (phenomenal), usability, and immediacy (immediately available). Unfortunately, this often leads to excessive use and addiction.

Social media provides the social connectedness that adolescents crave. Adolescents with low self-esteem, social anxiety, depression, chronic diseases, and marginalized adolescents are attracted by its ability to help them connect with others, to develop and nurture friendships.

It helps them to create a social identity without parental supervision and knowledge **(Fig. 1)**.

Social media offers easy, fast, and inexpensive connectivity. It provides information about innovations, ideas, entertainment, and job opportunities. Social media campaigns are effective means to promote behavior change, like prevention and control of substance abuse, encouraging physical activities, maintaining healthy diet, and prevention of sexually transmitted infections in adolescents.

Indians are heavy users of many apps. Nearly 10% of WhatsApp users in the world are Indians. WhatsApp addiction may soon become the most common disease of this generation!

There has been growing concern about the increasing amount of time spent by adolescents in viewing and interacting with media in the form of TV, music, video games, social networking sites, and its impact on their health.

When someone experiences something rewarding, neurons in the dopamine-producing areas in the brain

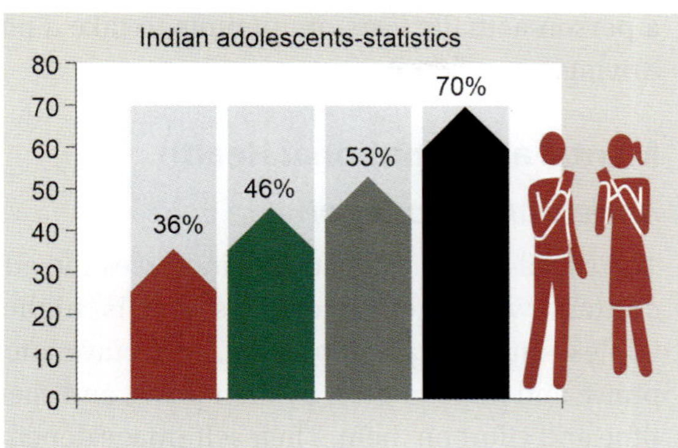


**Fig. 1:** Internet use among adolescents.
*Source:* RKSK guidelines, Participant's handbook, for Training of Medical Officers on Adolescent Friendly Health Services, Chapter 9, Promotion of safe use of Internet, Gadgets and Social Media.

are activated and dopamine levels rise, making them feel good. When a social media user gets a like or a mention, his brain receives a rush of dopamine, causing the individual to feel pleasure. Social media provides an endless stream of immediate rewards in the form of attention from others, for relatively minimal effort. Social media use becomes hazardous when viewing social networking sites becomes an important coping mechanism to relieve stress, loneliness, or depression. As it provides them with the attention that they are not receiving in real life, they engage increasingly in social media use, and gradually they may ignore real life relationships, work or school responsibilities, and even physical health.

This increases their isolation, unhappiness, and stress levels, and initiates a vicious cycle of engaging even more in the social networking behavior. This results in psychological dependency on social media. Social media use should not compromise sleep, study time, physical activity, relationships, and eating.

The effects of social media on adolescents are largely dependent on their personal and psychological characteristics, their preexisting strengths or vulnerabilities, the contexts in which they grow up, their social circumstances, and what they do and **Box 1**. Personal risk factors for excessive social media use include poor self-esteem, low risk perception, ignorance of the consequences of risky behavior, peer pressure, childhood experience of physical and sexual abuse, and emotional, psychological, or social problems. Family factors include low parental control and support, parental risky behavior, parental unemployment, and a family history of substance abuse. Societal factors include excessive media exposure and socioeconomic vulnerability **(Box 2)**.

---

**BOX 1:** Protective factors for social media use.

- Strong offline interests and hobbies
- Help-seeking behavior and access to service providers
- Cyber literacy or social media literacy
- Strong connections with family
- Healthy self-esteem
- Positive offline peer influence/friends

---

**BOX 2:** Risk factors for social media use.

- *Personal factors:* Poor self-esteem, peer pressure, lack of knowledge of preventive behavior and consequences of risky behavior, school drop outs, victims of physical and sexual abuse, developmental changes, and emotional, psychological, or social problems
- *Family factors:* Low parental support and controls, family history of substance abuse, high risk behavior, and unemployment
- *Societal factors:* Affiliation to gangs, access to weapons, media exposure (modeling), sociocultural factors which normalize violence, and unsafe migration due to socioeconomic and environmental reasons

*Source:* RKSK guidelines, Participant's handbook, for Training of Medical Officers on Adolescent Friendly Health Services, Chapter 9 Promotion of safe use of Internet, Gadgets and Social Media.

The risk is greater in adolescents than in adults, as their need for social connectedness and peer recognition is so high, while the capacity for self-control, which requires maturation of the prefrontal cortex, is only fully attained by 25 years of age. Parents should monitor their adolescents and set appropriate limits for social media use.

## ■ SOCIAL MEDIA HAZARDS

There are physical, mental, emotional, and interpersonal relationship issues to consider.

## Physical Health

### Obesity

This results from reduced physical activity and the tendency to consume snacks while using the screen.

### Eye Problems

Prolonged screen time without blinking leads to dryness, irritation, and a burning sensation in the eyes. Sleep deprivation adds to the problem.

### Inadequate Sleep

Blue light emitted by smartphones reduces the secretion of melatonin and delays onset of sleep. The temptation to see the latest messages, photos, and comments leads to sleep deprivation.

### Headaches, Body Aches, Neck Pain, and Pain in the Small Joints

These are more common when one's sitting posture at the computer is less than ideal **(Fig. 2)**. Neck pain often arises from holding the phone between the neck and the shoulder while talking to it. Small joints can hurt from persistent typing on one's mobile with one's thumbs.

### Road Accidents

Using a mobile while driving or even walking increases the chances of traffic accidents. The risk is vastly greater when a person actually texts or attempts to take a photo while driving.

## Mental and Emotional Health

### Anxiety and Depression

The social media dramatically increases the adolescents' contact with their peers. Its use is higher among adolescents who are depressed, who crave attention and praise and hope to get it by their posts, and spend a lot of time and effort on them. Their self-image depends on how many online "friends" they have and how many "likes" their posts receive; hence they accept friend requests from strangers or fleeting acquaintances. They eagerly post messages and photos of themselves, and then wait anxiously in anticipation of the response. They may be inordinately thrilled when a post attracts praise and excitement, but they can be quite upset if it is ignored, and negative comments may leave them in tears **(Fig. 3)**.

Acceptance by peers is an important element of adolescent life. Some adolescents are on multiple social media sites and instantly check notifications due to fear of missing out (FOMO) and feeling of being left out (FOBLO), which are responses caused by a sense of insecurity. They may conclude irrationally that they are being neglected purposefully by their friends, and slip into frank depression.

### Perverted Concepts

Girls may be upset or confused by depictions of the female as a submissive or a sex toy. Excessive exposure to pornography distorts boys' concepts about sexuality and sex, leading to inappropriately sexualized attitudes toward the other sex, and may impact their future relationships toward their spouses.

### Poor School Performance

Excessive social media may reduce the time available for study and sleep. They may spend less time with peers and family in the real world than in the virtual world.

### Cyberbullying

It is discussed in the next *Chapter*.

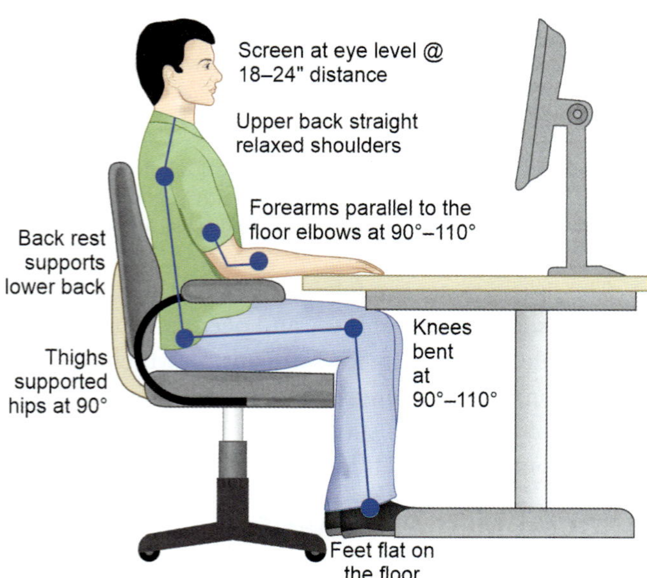


**Fig. 2:** The correct posture while sitting at a computer.

**Fig. 3:** These responses make or break a teenager's life!

## Sexting

The digital world has opened up opportunities in adolescent social life. The use of electronic media for sharing and exchanging content of a sexual nature has become another form of intimate sexual communication. Sexting is the sending, receiving, or forwarding of sexually explicit messages, photographs, or videos. Surveys in the USA reveal that about 20% of girls have posted nude or seminude photographs or videos of themselves. Boys are curious about nudity, and often pressurize their girlfriends into it. Girls indulge in sexting because they want to spark a boy's interest in them as they are in love and trust the boy fully and want to prove their commitment and maintain a relationship, especially if the boy is less committed.

Boys and girls use this as an alternative to sexual activity and indicate their readiness for sexual activity.

Sexting has risks involved. It causes the boy to objectify the girl as a sexual object, and sexual activity often follows. He may be so thrilled and excited that he may boastfully show it to his best friends, or even share it with them, and rarely one of them may post it online.

The vast majority of teen love affairs end within a year, and if it is the girl who ends the affair the boy may feel so upset and angry that he may take revenge by posting the images or videos to all their common friends. This is called revenge porn. The girl may be shamed and ostracized by peers of both sexes, and cyberbullied. She experiences shame and guilt, and may become depressed.

## Effect on Interpersonal Relationships

Conflicts with parents, the family, and friends are an inevitable part of life. Adolescents who have poor interpersonal relationship skills may find it easier and more rewarding to have virtual relationships. The consequence is social media addiction, an unhealthy dependence and uncontrollable urge to use social platforms constantly. This is one form of problematic internet use (PIU), which is sometimes referred to as internet addiction disorder (IAD). It is generally defined as problematic, compulsive use of the internet that results in significant impairment in an individual's function in various aspects of life over a prolonged period of time.

The Bergen Social Media Addiction Scale (BSMAS), a six-item self-report scale, is a brief and effective psychometric instrument for assessing those at risk for social media addiction.

> **BOX 3:** Problematic social media manifests all the features of a typical addiction.
>
> - A tendency to use social media use even when one wants to stop, or realizes it is interfering with necessary tasks such as studies and household chores
> - Spending more time online then intended
> - A need to increase duration of use as time goes by (tolerance)
> - Anxiety and irritability if the internet connection fails or one is offline (withdrawal symptoms)
> - A persistent desire or recurrent unsuccessful attempts to cut down on use
> - Taking extra pains to ensure that they can continuously access social media
> - Reduced social and peer interactions, prefers online friendships
> - Lying or deceptive behavior to retain access to social media use

Among the other variants of PIU, internet gaming disorder is declared as a mental health disorder in Diagnostic and Statistical Manual of Mental Disorders, fifth edition (DSM-5), while internet addiction, online gambling, and social media addiction are under consideration **(Box 3)**.

*Other useful tools include:*
- Internet Addiction Test (refer to Annexure 20)
- Problematic and Risky Internet Use Screening Scale (PRIUSS) (refer to Annexure 21)
- Social Media Use Disorder Scale for Adolescents
- Smartphone Addiction Scale–Short Version (SAS-SV).

## ROLE OF THE PEDIATRICIAN

This includes a Home, Education/Employment, Eating, Activities, Drugs, Sexuality, Suicide/Depression, and Safety (HEEADSSS), counseling adolescents and their parents, and in severe cases referring for management. Anticipatory guidance in office practice should discuss:
- Age-appropriate use of social media based on the adolescent's level of maturity (self-regulation skills, intellectual development, and comprehension of risks).
- Warn about the digital footprint, which may come in the way of admission in the universities and jobs.
- *Cultivate media literacy:* Teenagers should understand that the mass media are often driven by powerful economic or political forces.
- Advise about managing privacy settings online, not to share private information about self and family to strangers, protecting passwords, to refrain from

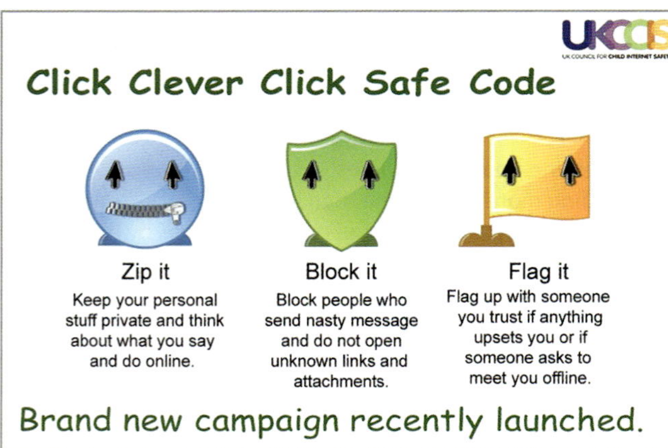


**Fig. 4:** Zip it, block it, and flag it.

opening links from unknown numbers, not to share travel plans, and not to share revealing pictures/selfies/videos.

- Monitor screen time.
- Discuss cyberbullying, and how to handle it.
- Teach them the Click Clever Click Safe Code.
- Advise them on eye hygiene if there is extensive computer use (mentioned elsewhere) and about sleep hygiene.
- *Advise about smartphone use:* Turn off social media notifications, check social media only at specified times when not at school or at work, use apps that limit screen time to specific times of the day, occasionally take a digital detox by staying away from the phone, find creative ways to spend time like learning new things, taking a hobby, spending time with family and friends, and exercising, and practice mindfulness.
- Social media should be used to connect more closely with those whom we know offline, like family and friends, and not to make new friends.
- Online social interaction and education is useful during periods of social isolation, when experiencing stress, when seeking connection with similar developmental, and/or health conditions, especially who experience adversity or isolation in offline environments.
- Bangalore's Service for Healthy Use of Technology (SHUT) clinic in the National Institute of Mental Health and Neurosciences (NIMHANS) has opened doors to adolescents battling tech addiction **(Fig. 4)**.

## ROLE OF PARENTS/CARETAKERS

- Monitoring is required, while giving adolescents appropriate autonomy. They can use tracking software as an aid to supervision and to block offensive websites.
- Parents should realize that the adolescents' online lives are an extension of their offline lives. They should discuss specific issues such as online safety, cyberbullying, and sexting, and check privacy settings and online profiles.
- Parents should be aware of sexting codes which teenager's use to send messages.
- They should help the adolescent balance screen time with other important activities: 1 hour of outdoor physical activity, 8–9 hours of sleep, time for homework, hobbies, peer interaction, and family time.
- Most of the adolescent screen time should be related to education, communication, skill development, and promoting healthy life style.
- Parents should be role models in their online usage.
- They should stay connected to their adolescents and spend adequate time with them.
- They should not use mobiles and TV sets as babysitters or child care takers.
- They should have media-free zones such as the bedroom, dining hall, and toilets.
- Look for subtle signs of distress, and consult an expert urgently when needed.

## ARTIFICIAL INTELLIGENCE BOON OR BANE IN FUTURE

Artificial intelligence refers to the development of computer systems that typically requires human intelligence such as visual perception, speech recognition, decision-making, and language translation. It will play a great role in early diagnosis, monitoring, and management of diseases. Challenges are accuracy of the data, over reliance, reducing creativity, and overdependence/addiction.

## KEY MESSAGES

- The social media can be a blessing or a curse, depending on how we use it.
- The social media is a super power, handle it with utmost responsibility. Judicious use of social media can give excellent returns.
- Social media use should not compromise sleep, relations, physical activity, and study time. Spend less time on social networking service (SNS) and more time in the real world.
- Media literacy and self-discipline are important.
- Parents should implement digital rules and digital hygiene, and nurture responsible digital citizen with good online habits.

- The HEEADSSS screen must include adequate discussion on media use.

## RECOMMENDED READING

1. Boer M, Stevens GWJM, Finkenauer C, van den Eijnden RJJM. The course of problematic social media use in young adolescents: A latent class growth analysis. Child Dev. 2022;93(2):e168-87.
2. Council on Communications and Media. Media use in school-aged children and adolescents. Pediatrics. 2016;138(5):e20162592.
3. Dalwai S, Chawala B. Electronic media and gadgets. In: Dalwai SH, Unni JC, Ahmed S, Multani KS, Deshpande L, Srivastava L (Eds). IAP Handbook of Developmental and Behavioral Pediatrics, 1st edition. New Delhi: Jaypee Brothers Medical Publishers (P) Ltd.; 2022. Pp. 281-6.
4. Galagali PM. Screen time guidelines for parents. In: Ugra D, Gupta P (Eds). 105 IAP Guidelines for Parents and Caregivers. New Delhi: Jaypee Brothers Medical Publishers (P) Ltd.; 2022. p. 35.
5. Kanikar A. Managing the mighty (impact of social media). In: Kanikar A (Ed). From Terrible to Terrific Teens, 1st edition. Chandigarh, India: White Falcon Publishing; 2019. p. 141.
6. Pemde H, Luiz N, Rathi R. Social Media: Do's and Don'ts. Mumbai, India: Indian Academy of Pediatrics; 2022. pp. 925.
7. RKSK guidelines, Participant's handbook, for Training of Medical Officers on Adolescent Friendly Health Services, Promotion of safe use of Internet, Chapter 9, Gadgets and Social Media.

---

<table>
<tr><td>**9.3**</td><td><h1>Cyberbullying: A Digital Menace and Preventive Strategies</h1></td></tr>
</table>

*Prashant Kariya, Geeta Patil*

## INTRODUCTION

Globally, there has been an increase in concern over cyberbullying, and India is not an exception. The prevalence of cyberbullying has increased dramatically among teenagers due to the growing use of digital gadgets and the internet.

## INCIDENCE OF CYBERBULLYING IN INDIA

Cyberbullying is a widespread problem that impacts teenagers in India. According to UNICEF survey, 70% of Indian teenagers between the ages of 15 and 19 years reported having experienced cyberbullying in some capacity. Because of their frequent usage of social media, online gaming, and cell phones, adolescents are especially susceptible to cyberbullying. The concerns have increased in post-COVID (corona virus disease) era.

## DEFINITION

The use of digital communication technologies and platforms to harass, threaten, intimidate, or injure others is known as cyberbullying. This could be posting humiliating or private material online, starting untrue rumors, or sending nasty or threatening comments. Cyberbullying is a serious issue for the mental and emotional health of teenagers because of its extensive reach and anonymity on the internet.

In traditional bullying, we can easily identify the bully and the intention is known. Unless great efforts are taken, it will not spread fast. It is usually done in physical or verbal form. However, the victim of cyberbullying frequently does not know who the bully is and cannot figure out why they are being bullied. It is very quickly and easily disseminated. It remains in the media as a digital footprint for long time. Smartphones are simple tools for this kind of harassment. It is quite upsetting and challenging to manage.

## TYPES OF CYBERBULLYING

Cyberbullying can take various forms, including but not limited to:

- *Harassment:* Repeated, aggressive, and harmful online behavior, such as sending offensive messages or spreading hateful comments on social media
- *Online impersonation:* Creating fake profiles to impersonate the victim and engage in harmful activities, causing damage to their reputation
- *Outing (also called doxing):* Sharing private or sensitive information about the victim without their consent,

leading to emotional distress and potential real-life consequences

- *Cyberstalking:* Consistently monitoring, tracking, or threatening the victim online, causing significant psychological distress
- *Exclusion or ostracism:* Deliberately excluding an individual from online groups, chats, or social circles to isolate and harm them emotionally
- *Trolling:* Posting offensive or derogatory comments with the intention of provoking a negative response from the victim.

## HEALTH HAZARDS OF CYBERBULLYING

The impact of cyberbullying on adolescents' health and well-being is profound and concerning. Some of the health hazards associated with cyberbullying include the following:

- *Psychological and emotional distress:* Adolescents who experience cyberbullying often suffer from anxiety, depression, and lower self-esteem. The constant fear of being targeted can lead to long-term psychological issues.
- *Academic consequences:* Cyberbullying can disrupt a student's ability to focus on their studies, leading to lower academic performance and absenteeism.
- *Suicidal ideation:* In severe cases, the emotional trauma caused by cyberbullying can result in suicidal thoughts or even suicide attempts among adolescents.
- *Social isolation:* Victims of cyberbullying may withdraw from social activities and face difficulty in forming relationships, both online and in real life.
- *Physical health issues:* The stress and anxiety resulting from cyberbullying can manifest as physical health problems, including headaches, insomnia, and digestive issues.

## CHARACTERISTICS OF CYBERBULLY

- Introverts
- Underachievers
- Underdogs
- Low self-esteem
- Feel like victims
- Difficulty expressing anger appropriately
- Tend to use anonymity online
- Use the internet for revenge
- Avoid taking responsibility for their actions

- Cyberbullies:
  - May have parents who are less involved in their lives
  - May have parents less interested in school
  - May have difficulty managing emotions and following rules
  - May be associated with conduct disorders, behavioral problems, substance abuse, attention-deficit/hyperactivity disorder (ADHD), and violence.

## SIGNS OF GETTING CYBERBULLIED

- Becomes angry or distressed when using a cell phone or computer
- Appears anxious when receiving emails or messages
- Avoids discussing their cell phone activities
- Becomes more withdrawn from activities, hobbies, friends, and family
- Experiences a drop in grades without an apparent reason
- Shows reluctance to attend school or specific classes
- Exhibits rapid changes in mood, sleep, appetite, or behavior
- May express suicidal thoughts.

## PREVENTING CYBERBULLYING

Preventing cyberbullying among adolescents in India requires a multifaceted approach involving parents, educators, and the community. Some strategies to tackle this issue effectively are as follows:

- *Education and awareness*: Adolescents should be educated about the risks of cyberbullying and taught online etiquette and responsible internet usage.
- *Open communication*: Create a safe space for adolescents to discuss their online experiences and seek help when needed. Discuss online interactions and enquire about cyberbullying.
- *Parental involvement*: Parents should actively engage in their children's online activities, monitor their internet usage, and set boundaries to ensure responsible online behavior.
- *Reporting mechanisms*: Encourage the use of reporting mechanisms on social media platforms and websites to report cyberbullying incidents. Make sure adolescents know how to use these tools effectively. Report on www.cybercrime.gov.in or call 1930.
- *Counseling and support*: Schools should offer counseling services to victims of cyberbullying,

providing a safe and confidential space to discuss their experiences and seek emotional support.

- *Legal measures:* Strengthen the laws about cyberbullying. Ensure that perpetrators are punished appropriately.
- *Digital literacy:* Promote digital literacy and responsible online behavior through workshops, seminars, and curricular interventions in schools.
- *Empower bystanders:* Encourage bystanders to stand up against cyberbullying and support the victim rather than remain passive observers.

## TEACHING ADOLESCENTS THE SMART WAY TO DEAL WITH CYBERBULLYING

*S:* **Stop the Messengers:** Encourage adolescents to immediately stop communicating with the bully on the platform where the bullying is occurring.

*M:* **Messenger Block:** Teach adolescents how to block the person responsible for the cyberbullying. Blocking the bully can prevent further harassment on that platform.

*A:* **Always Preserve Evidence:** Emphasize the importance of saving evidence of the cyber bullying. Encourage adolescents not to delete any messages, images, or content related to the incident.

*R:* **Retaliate Never:** Stress the importance of not retaliating or responding to the cyberbully with anger or insults. Reacting in a negative way can exacerbate the situation.

*T:* **Take Action and Report:** Teach adolescents to take action by reporting the cyberbullying to the appropriate authorities or platforms. In India, they can report cyberbullying to www.cybercrime.gov.in or call 1930. Reporting is essential to ensure that the incident is properly addressed and the perpetrator held accountable. Every major city has a cybercrime branch.

By following the *SMART* approach, adolescents can better protect themselves from the harmful effects of cyberbullying and contribute to creating a safer online environment.

## KEY MESSAGES

- Cyberbullying among adolescents in India is a serious issue with far-reaching consequences for mental, emotional, and physical health.
- It is imperative that parents, educators, and the community come together to address this problem.
- By raising awareness, fostering open communication, and implementing preventive measures, we can help protect the well-being of adolescents in India and create a safer digital environment for all.

## RECOMMENDED READING


1. Hinduja S, Patchin J. Cyberbullying: Identification, Prevention, & Response [Internet]. 2018. Available from: https://cyberbullying.org/Cyberbullying-Identification-Prevention-Response-2018.pdf
2. Livingstone S, Smith PK. Annual research review: Harms experienced by child users of online and mobile technologies: The nature, prevalence and management of sexual and aggressive risks in the digital age. J Child Psychol Psychiatry, 2014;55(6):635-54.
3. Lessons learned and promising practices in low-and middle-income countries Ending Online Child Sexual Exploitation and Abuse [Internet]. Available from: https://www.unicef.org/media/113731/file/Ending-Online-Sexual-Exploitation-and-Abuse.pdf.
4. Shaw M, Black DW. Internet addiction: definition, assessment, epidemiology and clinical management. CNS Drugs. 2008;22(5):353-65.
5. Zajac K, Ginley MK, Chang R, Petry NM. Treatments for Internet gaming disorder and Internet addiction: a systematic review. Psychol Addict Behav. 2017;31(8): 979-94.

<table>
<tr><td>**9.4**</td><td># Caught in the Web: Exploring Internet Addiction in Adolescents</td></tr>
</table>

*Prashant Kariya, Manmeet Sodhi*

## ■ INTRODUCTION

With the increasing accessibility of digital devices and the internet, adolescents are more exposed to the risks associated with excessive internet use and online harassment.

- In 2023, India had over 1.2 billion internet users, making it the world's second-largest online market after China.
- The number was projected to reach 1.6 billion users by 2050, indicating substantial market potential.
- Internet usage was on the rise in both urban and rural areas, showcasing widespread growth in access.

As a result, internet addiction disorder, characterized by compulsive and uncontrollable internet use, has become a pertinent concern.

Internet addiction disorder is sometimes referred to as problematic internet use or compulsive internet use. Adolescents, in particular, are vulnerable to this issue as they often lack the self-regulation skills needed to manage their online behavior. This addiction can disrupt their daily lives, leading to poor academic performance, social isolation, and mental health problems.

## ▌ INCIDENCE OF INTERNET ADDICTION DISORDER IN ADOLESCENTS

The incidence of internet addiction disorder in adolescents is on the rise. Adolescents are particularly susceptible to developing this disorder due to their increased access to the internet, social media, and online gaming. Studies have shown that the prevalence of internet addiction among adolescents can vary widely depending on the population and diagnostic criteria used. However, it is generally estimated that around 2–10% of adolescents may be affected by internet addiction, and this number is expected to grow as technology continues to advance.

As a behavioral addiction, internet addiction shares similarities with substance-related addictions. It results in symptoms akin to those observed in substance addiction, including mood alteration, heightened importance, increased tolerance, withdrawal symptoms, interpersonal conflict, and the potential for relapse.

## ▌ CRITERIA FOR DIAGNOSING INTERNET ADDICTION DISORDER

Diagnosing internet addiction disorder in adolescents can be challenging, as it is not officially recognized as a mental health disorder in the Diagnostic and Statistical Manual of Mental Disorders (DSM-5). However, numerous assessment tools and diagnostic criteria have been developed to help identify the condition. Commonly used criteria include the following:

- *Preoccupation with the internet:* Adolescents with internet addiction disorder often think about their online activities excessively, and it becomes the dominant focus of their lives.
- *Withdrawal symptoms:* When offline or unable to access the internet, they experience withdrawal symptoms such as irritability, anxiety, and restlessness.
- *Tolerance:* Over time, adolescents may require increasing amounts of time spent online to achieve the same level of satisfaction.
- *Loss of control:* They are unable to control their internet use, often spending more time online than intended, neglecting other responsibilities, and sacrificing sleep and social activities.
- *Neglect of other activities:* Internet addicts often neglect other activities, such as schoolwork, physical exercise, or face-to-face social interactions.
- *Continued use despite negative consequences:* Adolescents continue using the internet excessively, even when it results in negative consequences, such as declining academic performance or strained relationships.
- *Deception and escape:* Some individuals may use the internet to escape from unpleasant emotions or problems in their lives, and they may deceive family members or therapists about the extent of their internet use.
- *Mood swings:* Frequent mood swings, including irritability and depression, can be associated with internet addiction.

- *Relapse:* Even after periods of abstinence, adolescents with internet addiction often relapse, returning to their previous patterns of excessive internet use.

## ASSESSMENT TOOLS

- *Internet Addiction Test (IAT) by Dr Kimberly Young:* IAT is a reliable and valid measure of addictive use of internet, developed by Dr Kimberly Young. It consists of a 20-item (refer to Annexure 20) self-reporting questionnaire. It measures mild, moderate, and severe levels of internet addiction.
- Problematic and Risky Internet Use Screening Scale (PRIUSS) for Adolescents and Young Adults (refer to Annexure 21).

## DISADVANTAGES OF INTERNET ADDICTION IN ADOLESCENTS

Internet addiction disorder can have severe consequences for adolescents in various aspects of their lives, including physical health, mental health, and social well-being. Some of the disadvantages associated with internet addiction in adolescents include the following:

- *Academic performance:* Excessive internet use can lead to poor academic performance as adolescents may neglect their homework and studies.
- *Social isolation:* Internet addicts often withdraw from real-life social interactions, which can lead to loneliness, reduced self-esteem, and difficulties in building relationships.
- *Physical health:* Spending long hours online can lead to sedentary lifestyles, contributing to physical health issues such as obesity, sleep disturbances, and posture-related problems.
- *Mental health issues:* Internet addiction has been linked to mental health problems, including depression, anxiety, and attention deficits.
- *Risky behaviors:* Adolescents with internet addiction may engage in risky online behaviors, including cyberbullying or exposing themselves to inappropriate content.
- *Family conflict:* Excessive internet use can lead to family conflicts, as adolescents may neglect responsibilities, lie about their internet use, or become irritable when their online activities are restricted.
- *Financial consequences:* Online gaming or gambling can lead to financial problems for both adolescents and their families.
- *Decreased productivity:* Internet addiction negatively impacts adolescents' productivity and creativity in other areas of life.

## TREATMENT OF INTERNET ADDICTION DISORDER IN ADOLESCENTS

Treating internet addiction disorder in adolescents is a complex and evolving field. Various therapeutic approaches and interventions have been developed to address the condition. Treatment typically involves a combination of the following strategies:

- *Psychotherapy:* Cognitive-behavioral therapy (CBT) and family therapy are commonly used to help adolescents understand the underlying causes of their addiction and develop coping strategies. These therapies can help individuals manage triggers and cravings.
- *Education and awareness:* Adolescents and their families can benefit from education about the risks associated with excessive internet use. Understanding the consequences of addiction is a crucial first step in recovery.
- *Support groups:* Joining support groups with peers who have experienced similar issues can provide adolescents with a sense of community and encouragement.
- *Parental involvement:* Parental guidance and supervision are essential in helping adolescents overcome internet addiction. Establishing healthy boundaries and monitoring online activities can be effective in preventing relapses.
- *Technology restrictions:* Implementing software and tools that limit internet access can be helpful in controlling online time.
- *Lifestyle changes:* Encouraging physical activity, engaging in hobbies, and building face-to-face social connections can help adolescents replace their excessive internet use with healthier activities.
- *Medication:* In some cases, medication may be prescribed to address co-occurring mental health conditions, such as depression or anxiety.

It is important to tailor treatment approaches to the individual needs of the adolescent, as there is no one-size-fits-all solution. Additionally, ongoing research is needed to develop more effective treatments for internet addiction disorder.

## ■ KEY MESSAGES

- Internet addiction disorder is a growing concern among adolescents due to the widespread availability of the internet and its numerous attractions.
- The incidence of this disorder is on the rise, and its diagnosis remains a subject of debate. Nevertheless, it is clear that internet addiction can have severe disadvantages, affecting academic performance, mental and physical health, and social relationships.
- Addressing this issue requires a multifaceted approach that includes psychotherapy, education, support, and technology restrictions.
- More research is necessary to further refine diagnostic criteria and develop more effective treatments for internet addiction disorder in adolescents.

## ■ RECOMMENDED READING

1. Besser B, Loerbroks L, Bischof G, Bischof A, Rumpf HJ. Performance of the DSM-5-based criteria for Internet addiction: A factor analytical examination of three samples. J Behav Addict. 2019;8(2):288-94.
2. Gabrielli S, Rizzi S, Carbone S, Piras EM. School Interventions for Bullying-Cyberbullying Prevention in Adolescents: Insights from the UPRIGHT and CREEP Projects. Int J Environ Res Public Health. 2021;18(21):11697.
3. Kuss DJ, Griffiths MD, Binder JF. Internet addiction in students: Prevalence and risk factors. Comput Human Behav. 2013;29(3):959-66.
4. Menesini E, Salmivalli C. Bullying in schools: the state of knowledge and effective interventions. Psychol Health Med. 2017;22(suppl 1):240-53.
5. Statista. (2021). Number of internet users in India from 2015 to 2026. [online] Available from https://www.statista.com/statistics/255146/number-of-internet-users-in-india/ [Last accessed April, 2024].
6. Young KS. Internet addiction: The emergence of a new clinical disorder. CyberPsychol Behav. 1998;1(3):237-44.

---

| **9.5** | **Media Education and Literacy: The Need of the Hour in Adolescent Medicine** |

*Prashant Kariya*

---

Media literacy can be remembered by mnemonic DIGITAL.

### D: Determine source credibility

- To ensure a better level of security, verify whether the website address starts with "https://" in order to gauge the credibility of the information source.
- Verify the author's credentials and experience carefully before sending or providing any information.
- Use respectable publications and organizations as your primary sources of information when accessing the information, you are given.

### I: Investigate multiple sources

- To obtain a complete picture, compare data from multiple sources.
- Verify accuracy by cross-referencing facts and data.
- Point out similarities and differences between various sources.
- Use trustworthy fact-checking websites, such as factchecker.in.

### G: Guard your privacy

- Guard your personal information and use caution when sharing it online.
- Become familiar with social media networks' privacy settings.
- Create strong passwords and think about utilizing a password organizer.
- Employ licensed antivirus software and virtual private networks.
- Turn on two-factor verification.
- *Proceed with caution when accepting friend requests:* Grant friendship requests to those you know directly.
- Avoid using the dark web to browse unlawful content.
- When downloading applications
  - Only download apps from official stores, such the Play Store or App Store.
  - Before installing the program, make sure you provide the rights it requests.
  - Make checking the app's release date and reading reviews your first priority.

## *I:* Interpret with critical thinking and check data reliability

- Analyze media content critically, being aware of potential bias. Question the intentions and agenda of the information source. Avoid taking information at face value; think critically about its implications.
- Scrutinize the reliability of statistics and data presented in media. Learn how to discern credible data from unreliable or misleading information. Fact-check claims and figures before accepting them as truth.
- Be vigilant in detecting fake news, hoaxes, and misinformation. Check for reliable sources and corroboration of information. Look for signs of photo or video manipulation, morphs, or misleading visuals.

## *T:* Think before sharing

- Take a moment to think before sharing content online.
- Confirm the information's dependability and correctness.
- Consider the possible repercussions of disclosing information.
- Refrain from acting disrespectfully or cyberbullying others. Prior to making a post online, consider the impact of your words.

Share the information only if it fulfils the below criteria with mnemonic "THINK":

1. Is it *T*rue?
2. Is it *H*elpful?
3. Is it *I*nspirational?
4. Is it *N*ecessary to post?
5. Is it *K*ind?

## *A:* Avoid plagiarism

- *Appropriate citations:* Make sure you properly acknowledge original sources by using the appropriate citation style.
- *Summarize and paraphrase:* Put concepts into your own words and give credit to the original source.
- *Quotation marks:* Properly cite your quotes when using direct text.
- *Thorough records:* Maintain source information for accurate reference.
- *Know guidelines:* Recognize the citation guidelines and plagiarism standards of your university.

## *L:* Limit screen time

- Monitor the amount of time you spend on screens and set sensible limits. Make use of built-in functions such as "Usage Time/Screen Time" on Android smartphones and "Screen Time" on iPhones. To manage screen time, Google provides tools such as the Family Link app that may be connected between parent and kid devices. Think about limiting recreational media consumption to 1 hour throughout the week and up to 2 hours on the weekends.
- Strike a balance between your offline and digital media usage. Make in-person connections and exercise a priority.
- Always have a *Family Media Policy*
  - Who Will Follow—All Family Members. This policy applies to every member of the household, including parents and children.
  - Where to Use Media
    - *Common areas:* Media can be used in shared spaces like the living room or study areas.
    - *Bedrooms:* Limited use is allowed for educational or entertainment purposes.
    - *Designated media spaces:* If available, media should be primarily used in designated areas (e.g., media room).
  - Where not to use media
    - Dining table
    - Bathroom
    - School or work
    - Designated quiet spaces
    - Driving
    - Walking
- Time limit guidelines on media usage
  - *Daily time limits:* Set reasonable daily time limits for media use based on individual needs and responsibilities.
  - *Homework/study first:* Complete homework and study before leisure media use.
  - *Outdoor play:* Encourage outdoor play and physical activity before screen time.
  - *Mealtime restrictions:* No media during meals to promote conversation and healthy eating.
  - *Bedtime curfew:* Establish a media-free 1 hour bedtime in night and 1 hour after getting up in morning.
  - *Weekend/holiday guidelines:* Adapt limits for weekends and holidays but ensure a balance with other activities.
  - *Parental control:* Parents should monitor and enforce these guidelines to ensure compliance.

By incorporating these "DIGITAL " tips into their daily media consumption and online interactions, adolescents can become more informed, responsible, and critical digital citizens and will have better *media literacy.*

The Indian Academy of Pediatrics' guidelines are designed to support children's healthy screentime habits and digital well-being. Key messages of their suggestions are given in the following text.

## ■ KEY MESSAGES

- Turn off devices at least an hour before going to bed to practice mindful screen usage at bedtime. The device's blue light has the ability to inhibit melatonin secretion, which is essential for encouraging sound sleep.
- *Optimal posture and eye care:* When using a computer or smartphone, ensure that your posture is correct. Follow the 20-20-20 rule to reduce eye strain and dryness: After 20 minutes of screen usage, take a 20-second break and concentrate on an object that is 20 feet away.
- *Focused engagement:* Refrain from multitasking, particularly when doing schoolwork. Turn off all screens in order to improve focus.
- Avoid watching or playing violent games or programs if you are content-conscious.
- Install antivirus software, secure search engines, and appropriate privacy settings. If your children are younger, you might want to install safety software to prevent them from seeing inappropriate websites.
- *Make use of "teachable moments":* Take advantage of media exposure to promote family values and healthful living options. Talk about media messages that promote reckless sexual activity as soon as you and your partner see shows that portray such scenarios.
- *Create digital-free zones:* To encourage deeper family connections, set aside particular spaces such as bedrooms, dining tables, kitchens, restrooms, and motorized vehicles as digital-free zones.
- *Scheduled digital fasting:* Assign specific times when no family member uses a gadget to observe a digital fast. Make the most of this time as a family to bond and decide on a timetable that works for everyone.
- *Parental role modeling:* Parents should set an example of responsible media use, make a strategy for the family's media consumption, and teach their kids internet etiquette.

Together, these rules support a thoughtful and balanced approach to kids' and families' digital engagement.

## ■ RECOMMENDED READING


1. Indian Academy of Pediatrics. (2021). Screen time guidelines for parents. [online] Available from https://iapindia.org/pdf/Screentime-Guidelinesfor-Parents-Ch-005.pdf [Last accessed April, 2024].
2. PRAGYATA: guidelines for digital education. Department of School Education and Literacy. Ministry of Human Resource Development Government of India 2021. [online] Available from https://www.education.gov.in/sites/upload_files/mhrd/files/pragyata-guidelines_0.pdf [Last accessed April, 2024].
3. Rideout V, Robb MB. (2019). The Common Sense census: Media use by tweens and teens. Common Sense Media. [online] Available from https://www.commonsensemedia.org/research/the-common-sense-census-media-use-by-tweens-and-teens-2021 [Last accessed April, 2024].
4. Strasburger VC, Jordan AB, Donnerstein E. Health effects of media on children and adolescents. Pediatrics. 2010;125(4):756-67.


**9.6**   **Artificial Intelligence: Boon or Bane**

*Prashant Kariya*

## ■ INTRODUCTION

In November 2022, "Open AI" introduced the revolutionary ChatGPT, a trending AI bot. The ability of machines to demonstrate intelligence—to grasp, synthesize, and draw conclusions from data—is known as artificial intelligence, or AI. For adolescents, artificial intelligence (AI) is a crossroads of promise and hazard, bringing both boons and banes as they navigate a digitally driven world.

Some of the real cases of use of AI by adolescents are as follows:

- Prithvi leveraged the capabilities of AI by seeking assistance from ChatGPT for his school homework, streamlining his academic tasks with the support of advanced technology.
- Faced with peer pressure and struggling to navigate a response, Preeti turned to the Google Gemini AI,

exploring various strategies and approaches to effectively address and communicate her feelings to her friends.

- Sakshi enriched her life skills through an online education platform that utilizes AI, providing personalized and adaptive learning experiences tailored to her individual needs and preferences.
- Aaryan employed AI tools, such as searching on PubMed, to efficiently identify a suitable topic for his dissertation, leveraging the vast resources available through advanced algorithms to streamline his research process.
- Aaryan ingeniously employed AI-generated mnemonics to enhance his memory retention for challenging topics. By tapping into the cognitive support offered by AI, he crafted mnemonic aids that not only facilitated easier recall but also personalized the learning experience, making complex subjects more accessible and memorable.

So on the plus side, AI has shown to be an invaluable educational tool, providing personalized learning experiences tailored to individual needs. Advanced web search engines, such as Google Search, use AI algorithms to give more accurate and relevant results. Recommendation systems, such as those used by YouTube, Amazon, and Netflix, use AI to adapt content choices to individual tastes. The importance of AI extends to interpreting human speech, as demonstrated by virtual assistants such as Siri and Alexa, which use natural language processing to provide smooth interactions.

Furthermore, AI's influence in healthcare is beneficial to teens. AI-powered diagnostics and predictive analytics help to discover health issues earlier, resulting in more effective and timely therapies. Wearable gadgets with AI algorithms can monitor vital signs and warn individuals and healthcare providers to potential health problems. This proactive approach is especially advantageous for teenagers who have chronic diseases, since it allows for better management and a higher quality of life.

But as said, a coin has two sides. The dark side of AI, on the other hand, creates severe issues for youth. The pervasiveness of social media, which is sometimes driven by AI algorithms, can lead to concerns such as addiction, mental health issues, and exposure to unsuitable content. AI-powered platform recommendation systems can generate echo chambers, reinforcing existing opinions and limiting exposure to other perspectives. Such echo chambers can impede the development of critical thinking

abilities in adolescents, who are at a key stage of identity construction.

Another big worry is privacy. The collecting and analysis of massive volumes of personal data by AI systems raises concerns about the security of sensitive information, particularly for a demographic that is still figuring out how to traverse the complexity of the digital realm.

Finally, the impact of AI on adolescents is a two-edged sword. While technology provides a new opportunity for tailored learning and improved healthcare, the potential hazards, ranging from mental health problems to privacy concerns, must not be overlooked. As teenagers continue to grow up in an increasingly AI-driven environment, striking a balance that optimizes the advantages while limiting the hazards is critical.

Positioned as a potential invention of the millennium, its impact on adolescents remains uncertain, and only time will reveal whether it proves to be a boon or a bane for this demographic.

## ◼ KEY MESSAGES

- AI enhances education for adolescents, offering personalized learning experiences.
- AI positively impacts teen healthcare with early diagnostics and predictive analytics.
- Social media, driven by AI, poses risks like addiction and mental health issues for teens.
- AI-generated echo chambers may hinder critical thinking in adolescents.
- Privacy concerns arise from widespread AI data collection, impacting adolescents navigating the digital realm.

## ◼ RECOMMENDED READING


1. Culp WC Jr. Artificial Intelligence and ChatGPT: Bane or Boon for Academic Writing. J Educ Perioper Med. 2023;25(2):E702.
2. Farhat F. ChatGPT as a Complementary Mental Health Resource: A Boon or a Bane. Ann Biomed Eng. 2023. doi: 10.1007/s10439-023-03326-7. Epub ahead of print. PMID: 37477707.
3. Jeyaraman M, K SP, Jeyaraman N, Nallakumarasamy A, Yadav S, Bondili SK. ChatGPT in Medical Education and Research: A Boon or a Bane? Cureus. 2023;15(8): e44316.
4. Kung TH, Cheatham M, Medenilla A, Sillos C, De Leon L, Elepaño C, et al. Performance of ChatGPT on USMLE: Potential for AI-assisted medical education using large language models. PLOS Digit Health. 2023;2:0.

# Adolescent and the School

**Section Editors:** *R N Sharma, Mona M Basker*

## 10.1 Introduction and Adolescent Skill Development

*R N Sharma, Merlin Thanka Jemi*

### ■ INTRODUCTION

A school-going adolescent living in India spends on an average 7–12 hours in school and related scholastic activities. Adolescence is a dynamic and vulnerable phase in development, when they are developing autonomy from a close-knit family environment. During this period, time spent in school can be a positive experience. On the other hand, difficulties in the school milieu need special attention from adults, including parents, teachers, school authorities, and siblings. Adults need to understand what a teen is going through in physical, cognitive, and psychosocial domains.

### BENEFITS OF SCHOOL FOR A GROWING ADOLESCENT

In school and college, an adolescent is presented with opportunities for development, by trying out their skills in the arts, elocution, sports, and interpersonal relationships. They develop critical thinking skills. They interact, work, and play with teachers and school authorities who could be good role models for both academics and personal growth. Peer interaction can pave way for positive lifelong friendships. Teens develop self-esteem, confidence, and identity. Hence, school can have a positive impact on adolescent growth.

### ■ ROLE OF PARENTS AND TEACHERS

School teachers and parents can encourage, motivate, be good role models, and play a crucial role in the development and in shaping their personality. Genuine interest, quality time, support, and involvement in literacy are essential. Maternal support results in a healthy, positive, and good learner. Responsive parents rear humane adolescents who feel secure and loved. Teachers can provide structure, give feedback, provide mentorship, inspire, and create meaningful learning experience.

### Tips for the Role of a Parent or Teacher

- Giving teens full attention, creating a consistent daily routine, and safe and engaging home environment. Switch off TV and mobile, talk about the day's events.
- Create a positive environment, using positive language, empathetic listening, positive instructions, and lots of praise for right work.
- Use positive disciplining, identify change in behavior, discuss consequences, try to understand from their viewpoint, and seek professional help. Avoid physical punishment.
- Fun time with them is essential, with individual time spent with them. Parenting should be socially interactive, joyful, meaningful, and actively engaging with their teen.

- Have realistic expectations and appreciate good work including extracurricular activities.
- Encourage them to talk to you and engage with them.
- Be aware and vigilant about how they spend time in and out of school, especially online.
- Teachers could create an enjoyable milieu, teach concepts, share their own educational experience, partner in learning, nurture individual interests, and assist independence.
- If supportive, teachers often act as mentors, provide strength, support their personal and academic success, and treat them fairly and with appreciation.
- Positive change occurs when parents and teachers work together focusing on the teen. Trust and concern in teacher-parent relationships will pave way for happy learning for the teen. Teachers should recognize and inform parents if a student has special educational needs.

## Key Message

A healthy teacher-parent relationship is essential for a teen to perform better both in academics and extracurricular activities and in overall development.

## SKILL DEVELOPMENT IN THE PHYSICAL DOMAIN

Adolescents are able to move their bodies with better ability and accuracy than younger children. There are two categories of movement skills, gross and fine motor. Gross motor skills refers to movement of large musculoskeletal portions of the body (e.g., running), while fine motor refers to small, precise muscle movements (e.g., texting or typing). The inherent plasticity of brain and the characteristic dynamic changes called "pruning" result in neuroanatomical changes and cognitive benefits. Adolescents given the opportunities and stimulation for developing motor skills, also show structural changes in the gray matter.

## Gross Motor Skills Development

Schools typically offer physical education and sports in a structured, supervised, and safe environment. These help teens develop motor skills, improve physical fitness, and learn the basic rules of the game. Team sports reinforce skills of teamwork, communication, and leadership. Physical education teachers can provide appropriate guidance.

## Fine Motor Skill Development

Fine motor skills evolve while writing, typing, and texting. Extracurricular activities do the same, as in card making, drawing, painting, clay modeling, crafts, origami, knitting, sewing, crocheting, jewelry making, and embroidery. Musical instruments and dance can also enhance fine motor skills.

## SKILL DEVELOPMENT IN COGNITIVE, EMOTIONAL, SOCIAL, MORAL, AND PSYCHOSOCIAL DOMAINS

### Cognitive Development

- Cognitive development during adolescence is rapid.
- Transition from concrete to abstract thinking is salient during teen years (Jean Piaget).
- Adult intelligence progress via application of propositional and hypothetical thinking.

### Emotional Development

- Emotions are triggered by abstract ideas, past events, and anticipating future events.
- Emotions are inconsistent, fluctuating, making them "moody", and difficult to control.
- As teens begin to realize people as "personalities", response to relationships intensify.
- Nail biting, tension, and conflict with adults and peers indicate this heightened emotionality.
- A sense of isolation can lead to feeling alienated, desperate, and overwhelmed.

### Social Development

- Adolescents start considering perspectives of a society/community (Robert Selman).
- Mature social cognition gives them the ability to find acceptance in relationships.
- Belonging to a peer group is important. It indicates adaptation, a developmentally appropriate move to autonomy and loyalty toward friends, in turn building self-esteem.
- Individualized friendships deepen with time, with sharing of secrets with a friend rather than a family member.
- Powerful peer influence can result in positive social interactions, or high-risk behavior.

## Moral Development

As cognition matures, morality stages 3 and 4 (Kohlberg) becomes prevalent, marked by:

- A sense of absolute "right" and "wrong" and a rigid concept of "good" and "bad".
- Purpose of morality is to fulfill duties, respect authority, and maintain social order.

## Psychosocial Development

- Self-concept and new attachments broaden.
- Identity refers to questions of who am I? and what am I going to do with my life?
- Difficulty in answering such questions leads to role confusion.
- A favorable ratio of "role confusion" versus "identity" results in consistency (Erikson).

### ■ RECOMMENDED READING


1. Beukema L, Reijneveld SA, Jager M, Metselaar J, de Winter AF. The role of functional health literacy in long-term treatment outcomes in psychosocial care for adolescents. Eur Child Adolesc Psychiatry. 2020;29(11):1547-54.
2. Fayyaz HN, Hashmi K. Adolescence and Academic Well-being: Parents, Teachers and Students' Perceptions. J Educ Educ Dev. 2022;9(1):27-47.
3. Jin X, Chen W, Sun IY, Liu L. Physical health, school performance and delinquency: a comparative study of left-behind and non-left-behind children in rural China. Child Abuse Neglect. 2020;109:104707.
4. Ministry of Education. Guidelines for Parent Participation in Home-based Learning during School Closure and Beyond. [online] Available from https://www.education.gov.in/sites/upload_files/mhrd/files/MoE_Home_Learning_Guidelines.pdf. [Last accessed April, 2024].
5. Morgan C, King R, Weisz J, Schopler J. Introduction to Psychology, 7th edition. New York: McGraw Hill; 2017.
6. Sadock BJ, Sadock VA, Ruiz P. Kaplan and Sadock's Comprehensive Textbook of Psychiatry, 11th edition. Alphen aan den Rijn, Netherlands: Wolters Kluwer; 2020.
7. Wickrama KA, Lorenz FO, Conger RD. Parental support and adolescent physical health status: a latent growth-curve analysis. J Health Soc Behav. 1997;38:149-63.
8. Wright MS, Wilson DK, Griffin S, Evans A. A qualitative study of parental modeling and social support for physical activity in underserved adolescents. Health Educ Res. 2010;25:224-32.


# 10.2 | Healthy Lifestyle and Physical Illnesses

*Reshmi YS, Ravi Bhatia*

### ■ ADOLESCENT NUTRITION AND PHYSICAL ACTIVITY

Nutritional requirement is highest during adolescence. They develop 45% of bone mass, 25–50% of weight, and 15–25% of final adult height during adolescence. Hence, they require higher energy, protein, vitamins, minerals, calcium for bone health, iron for hemoglobin, and overall growth. A major part of teen diet is eaten during school hours. Hence, school has an important role in promoting healthy eating behavior and ensuring that the requirement is met.

### Balanced Diet

A balanced diet containing essential nutrition to promote growth and development, should include a variety of fruits, vegetables, protein, whole grains, and dairy, providing the right amount of carbohydrates, proteins, fats, vitamins, minerals and fiber. Adolescent boys require 2,400–2,800 kcal a day and girls require 2,100–2,400 kcal, in the form of three major meals and two healthy snacks. Choosemyplate.org has an easy to use pictorial guide for a balanced diet.

### Role of School in Nutrition

- *A healthy breakfast* can improve cognitive performance and concentration. Skipping breakfast can also lead to unhealthy eating throughout the day causing obesity. Starting school in the early hours is a challenge for parents and teens in our country, preventing them from having breakfast. Teachers and school authorities should emphasize the importance of breakfast and ensure adequate recess to help teens have breakfast.

- *Healthy snacking:* Cafeteria should promote only healthy snacking options within school premises, such as whole fruit, salads, milk, yogurt, and traditional whole grain or protein snacks. Sweetened beverages, carbonated, caffeinated drinks, energy drinks, and fast food should be banned. School could implement policies that support healthy eating while the teen is in school.
- *Hydration:* Adolescents need 2–3 liters of water to stay well hydrated, and more during summer and after physical activity. Water is the recommended choice for hydration, and not juices or soft drinks. Potable water should be available in school and teens encouraged to drink.
- *Nutrition education* should be an integral part of curriculum, including the importance of healthy eating, food groups, food labels, portion sizes, and consequences of unhealthy diet. Sessions on application could help, to empower them to make informed healthy choices.
- *School meals:* The "Mid-Day Meal Programme" launched by the government to cater to the primary school in 1995 has been extended to include 8th grade under the National Programme of Mid-Day Meals in October 2007. The 6th to 8th graders receive 700 calories and 20 grams of protein. If it extends to cover high school students, it will benefit school going adolescents of all age groups. School authorities must ensure that meals provided in school are balanced with adequate amount of carbohydrates, proteins, fruits, and vegetables and micronutrients.
- Periodic health screening including growth charts is useful for early identification of underweight, overweight, and micronutrient deficiencies.
- Schools should be empathetic about "adolescents with chronic illness" needing specialized care, have policies for specific nutritional interventions to enable speedy recovery.
- Eating patterns and food content can be monitored daily, unhealthy habits resolved, and diet compliance ensured.
- Food handling and storage for safety should be ensured in cafeterias.

## Physical Education and Physical Activity

Exercise is crucial for the health of adolescents. It helps develop strong bones and muscles, maintain a healthy weight, improve cardiovascular fitness, and mental health. Physical education classes at school and opportunities for extracurricular activities (ECAs) can help adolescents achieve this.

## Recommended Physical Activity

Adolescents need daily 1 hour of moderate to vigorous aerobic exercise, viz., brisk walking, running, swimming, cycling, dancing, and playing sports. They also need bone- and muscle-strengthening exercises 3 days a week, viz., with weights, planks, squats, and resistance workouts with appropriate supervision. Benefits of physical activity include:

- Healthy muscle, bone, body, and mind, and prevention of obesity and metabolic syndrome.
- Good coping skills in facing various challenges and ability to regulate emotions.
- Positive impact on studies through better concentration, memory, and cognitive function.
- Team sports build social skills, viz., teamwork, communication, and sportsmanship.

## Role of Schools in Ensuring Adolescent Physical Activity

- There should be a comprehensive physical education curriculum for all students.
- Daily physical activity of at least 1 hour should be facilitated in school premises. This will help a teen form exercise as a habit, leading to a healthy lifestyle through adulthood.
- Physical education instructors should guide, supervise, and thereby reduce the risk of injuries.
- Exercise should include students with different interests including those with disabilities.
- Team sports bringing students, teachers, and parents together, will foster life skills such as teamwork, communication, and discipline.
- For interested students, the school can facilitate after-school special classes in sports. They should be provided with opportunities to explore sports as their career choice.

## ◼ EXTRACURRICULAR ACTIVITIES

Extracurricular activities are defined as a range of activities organized outside of the school hours and apart from the curriculum. These help a student get involved in school and community and develop particular skills.

Extracurricular activities facilitate positive outcomes via four mechanisms:

1. Transfer paradigm suggests that skills learnt through ECAs are transferred to other areas, viz., classroom.
2. It helps them build positive relationships, self-esteem, and a sense of responsibility.
3. It indicates to teachers/parents, that they possess the intellect needed to participate in community.
4. Absence of ECAs places adolescents at risk for delinquent behavior.

Ideally 1 hour daily should be dedicated to any type of ECA and in balance with curricular activities.

## IMPORTANCE OF SLEEP FOR A SCHOOL GOING TEENAGER

Sleep promotes growth, learning, development, and immunity. Inadequate sleep is associated with obesity, heart disease, and poor academic performance. Sleep plays an important role in adolescent health, both in short and longer term. Improved early recognition of sleep disorders is necessary for a holistic development:

- 8–10 hours of sleep is recommended for an adolescent.
- Insufficient sleep is the most common sleep disorder seen during adolescence.

### Biology of Adolescent Sleep

Sleep occurs in a complex and intricate neurobiological system, regulated by a "two-process model". The homeostatic process (process S) regulates the length and depth of sleep, following an accumulation of adenosine and such sleep promoting cytokines. Endogenous circadian rhythm (process C) influences the internal organization of sleep, timing, and duration of daily sleep wake cycles. From infancy to adolescence, there is a decline in daytime and nighttime sleep duration.

Adolescent sleep is the result of biochemical changes and is not a behavioral quirk, rebellious statement, or a decided attempt to fit in socially. Teens have a delayed release of melatonin, resulting in a delayed sleep onset; they need 8–10 hours of sleep, and so remain sleepy later into the day. Added academic and societal pressures lead to sleep debt on weekdays and increased sleep on weekends.

### Tips for a Healthy Sleep Pattern in Teens

- Wake up and go to bed at the same time.
- Avoid sleeping extra on weekends.
- Naps should be scheduled for mid-afternoon and not be >1 hour.
- Spend time outside.
- Exercise regularly.
- The bed should be used for sleeping only.
- Make 30–60 minutes before bedtime a quiet or wind-down time.
- Do not go to bed hungry.
- Alcohol, sleeping pills, and caffeinated products at dinnertime should be avoided.

### Sleep Problems Seen during Adolescence

- Insufficient sleep
- Delayed sleep–wake phase disorder
- Narcolepsy
- Restless leg syndrome.

Assessing an adolescent for sleep problems could include:

- BEARS scale, a comprehensive and age-specific screening tool for sleep disorders:
    - B—Bedtime problems. Do you have any problems falling asleep at bedtime?
    - E—Excessive daytime sleepiness. Do you feel sleepy a lot during the day? In school?
    - A—Awakening at night. Do you wake up a lot at night? Do you have trouble going back to sleep?
    - R—Regularity and duration of sleep. What time do you go to bed on school nights? Weekends?
    - S—Snoring. Does your teenager snore loudly at night?

## SCREEN TIME

Screen time (ST) defined as the time spent in a day, using computers, laptop, tablets, smart phones, etc., has become an integral part of our lives. Blackboard has been replaced by a smart class room and digital media.

There is a global concern about the ill effects of ST. Exposure to screen starts as early as infancy in most countries. In India, adolescents spend ≥3 hours daily in front of the screen, the hours increase on holidays. Factors affecting ST include:

- Age at which a person is exposed to the screen, younger the age the more the ST.
- Parental ST, if excessive, risk of their child having increased ST is more.
- Digital environment.

Harmful effects of ST include obesity, sleep deprivation, abnormal posture, and cognitive defects. Beneficial effects of ST include, better understanding of concepts and learning, increased abstract thinking and problem-solving skills.

Excessive ST can be prevented by some strategies:
- ST is balanced with academics, 1 hour of physical activity and 8–10 hours of sleep.
- A maximum of 2 hours per day of ST could be allowed.
- Parents should monitor media use by adolescents.
- Of the time spent in ST, a part should be in the real world with friends and family.
- Every home should have a digital free zone, with no laptops or smart phones.

Judicious use of ST is essential for the physical and mental well-being of an adolescent.

## ■ PHYSICAL EFFECTS OF SUBSTANCE USE

Adolescents are vulnerable for high-risk behavior and because of strong peer influences tend to experiment with substances. Currently, schools seem to be a fertile ground for these harmful drugs, distributed by fellow students or drug dealers who prey upon naïve students. Substance abuse usually occurs in the vicinity of a school, due to a lack of adult supervision.

Warning signs of substance abuse can be recognized by parents and teachers as changes in:
- Academic performance, school attendance, truancy, behavioral such as aggression, irritability, mood swings, anhedonia, conduct issues, excessive sadness, and being secretive.
- In their friends' circle.
- In personal hygiene or grooming habits.
- Physical signs, viz., bloodshot eyes, unexplained weight loss, and smell of tobacco/marijuana and other substances on clothing or breath.
- Stealing money or valuables and secretive behavior.

If identified, parents or teachers should talk to the teen and refer to counselor/professionals.

### Role of Schools in Safeguarding Their Students

- Teachers and counselors, as role models can deter teens from starting substance use.
- Schools can implement substance abuse prevention programs and promote awareness.
- Adolescents should be empowered to say "No" to peer pressure and early help seeking.
- Strict policies with dire punishment should be displayed and communicated to students.

- Life skills and counseling for those struggling with substance use.
- Teachers and staff should be able to recognize early signs of substance abuse.

## ■ SEXUAL HEALTH AND SCHOOL

Sexual health education, a vital component of comprehensive health education, can provide students accurate and age-appropriate information. It equips students to make informed decisions.

Role of schools in improving sexual health can be in the form of:
- Comprehensive, culture, and age-appropriate curriculum covering sexual anatomy and physiology, consent, healthy relationships, sexually transmitted infections, teen pregnancy, contraception, and gender identity.
- Abstinence, safe sex practices, and options for pregnancy are important.
- Teaching about consent and the right to say no at any time and empowerment are crucial.
- Easily accessible, confidential, and respectful sexual health services are necessary.
- Protection of Children from Sexual Offences (POCSO) law and the courage to speak up should be taught to students.
- School should be raise awareness about responsible online behavior, risks related to sexting, sexual cyberbullying, and the process of redressal through cyber police.
- Schools should be inclusive of students with gender dysphoria and prevent discrimination, bullying, and mental health problems.
- If they present with a sexual health-related problem, school authorities should confidentially offer appropriate counseling, discuss with close family members they trust and refer to an adolescent friendly healthcare professional.

## ■ ADOLESCENTS LIVING WITH A CHRONIC ILLNESS

This vulnerable and special group of adolescents faces numerous challenges that impact academic performance, emotional well-being, and overall quality of life. They require ongoing support at school which is not only essential for their academic success but also for their overall well-being. School needs to address their unique challenges to enable them to do well academically, physically, and emotionally.

Challenges at school include:

- Missed school days due to hospital visits, hospitalizations, and struggle to catch-up with the course.
- Physical limitations might prevent them from participating in sports and ECAs.
- Illnesses like epilepsy can impact cognition, memory, ability to concentrate, and affect completion of assignments.
- Stigmatization and bullying can negatively affect self-esteem and cause distress, anxiety, and depression.
- Taking medicines in school premises and compliance can be a challenge, especially if the adolescent wants confidentiality. School staff/nurse should ensure compliance while maintaining confidentiality.
- Specific dietary restrictions/needs should be facilitated by the schools authorities.

These challenges can be mitigated by the following considerations:

- Flexible options such as online classes and relaxed timelines for assignments and projects.
- Counseling in the school to help cope with the challenges of living with a chronic illness.
- School nurse could provide medical care, if required.
- Good communication with school staff, parents, and healthcare providers is imperative.
- Educating school staff and students about a particular illness will reduce stigmatization and foster a supportive environment.
- Facilities to accommodate for a student with physical disabilities to move and participate.
- Career counseling should be provided considering their specific challenges.

## KEY MESSAGES

- Adolescent nutrition is crucial for overall health and development. Healthy habits not cultivated during adolescence can lead to adulthood diseases.
- Schools should be responsible to nutrition and safety for their teenaged students.
- Schools play a critical role in promoting physical activity for adolescents.
- The school must establish a well-rounded physical education curriculum, sports programs even after school hours and offer options for teen with varied interests and disabilities.
- Schools play an important role in safeguarding adolescents from substance use and recognizing early warning signs for intervention.
- Prevention programs, counseling services, and an informed and supportive environment will help students make healthier choices and access the support systems if needed.
- Comprehensive sexual education is a much needed part of the school curriculum.
- Empowering teens in this area will enable to make healthy life choices.

## RECOMMENDED READING


1. Council on School Health, American Academy of Pediatrics; Committee on Substance Abuse, American Academy of Pediatrics; Mears CJ, Knight JR. The role of schools in combating illicit substance abuse. Pediatrics. 2007;120(6):1379-84.
2. Gupta P, Shah D, Bedi N, Galagali P, Dalwai S, Agrawal S, et al. Indian Academy of Pediatrics Guidelines on Screen Time and Digital Wellness in Infants, Children and Adolescents. Indian Pediatr. 2022;59(3):235-44.
3. Hagenauer MH, Perryman JI, Lee TM, Carskadon MA. Adolescent changes in the homeostatic and circadian regulation of sleep. Dev Neurosci. 2009;31(4):276-84.
4. Indian Academy of Pediatrics. (2019). Indian Journal of Adolescent Medicine. [online] Available from https://aha.iapindia.org/wp-content/uploads/2020/07/Indian-Journal-of-Adolescent-Medicine-column-July-Dec2019.pdf. [Last accessed April, 2024].
5. Lloyd CB. (2007). The role of schools in promoting sexual and promoting sexual and reproductive health e health among adolescents among adolescents in developing countries. [online] Available from https://knowledgecommons.popcouncil.org/cgi/viewcontent.cgi?article=1076&context=departments_sbsr-pgy. [Last accessed April, 2024].
6. Lum A, Wakefield CE, Donnan B, Burns MA, Fardell JE, Jaffe A, et. al. School students with chronic illness have unmet academic, social, and emotional school needs. Sch Psychol. 2019;34(6):627-36.
7. O'Flaherty M, Baxter J, Campbell A. Do extracurricular activities contribute to better adolescent outcomes? A fixed-effects panel data approach. J Adolesc. 2022;94(6):855-66.
8. Sawyer S, Drew S, Duncan R. Adolescents with chronic illness—the double whammy. Aust Fam Physician. 2005;36(8):622-7.
9. van de Kop JH, van Kernebeek WG, Otten RHJ, Toussaint HM, Verhoeff AP. School-Based Physical Activity Interventions in Prevocational Adolescents: A Systematic Review and Meta-Analyses. J Adolesc Health. 2019;65(2):185-94.

# 10.3 Methods to Improve Learning

*Nirmala Joshi, Sylvia James*

## ■ LEARNING TECHNIQUES

Different learning techniques are used by adolescents, but using the appropriate one will help concentrate, stay motivated, and improve performance. Some may use mnemonics, others may be attentive and register in long-term memory. Learning techniques include understanding concepts, memorizing, and remembering.

### Techniques to Understand Concepts

#### SQ3R

SQ3R helps to learn easily, especially when there are large portions to read.

*SQ3R stands for:*

Survey: Look over the main headings and general content, to get an overview of a chapter and help focus on the subject.

Question: Turn a heading into a question, to help the teen to take an active part in learning, and improving motivation and concentrating.

Read: Read to find the answers to the questions, which you have asked.

Recite: Answer the question, write a summary in your own words, and make brief notes of important ideas and information. Then, read it again and again to answer the question. Reciting helps to remember new material and to check up on how much has been learned.

Review: This helps to see how the material is related, how well the teen has understood and also helps to prepare for tests.

#### Note-taking

Note-taking helps to organize information, summarize key points, and reinforce learning. Key note-taking methods are as follows:

- Cornell's method: This method helps to organize information, note key terms, and summarize content. Here, adolescents should divide their paper into two columns and a row across the bottom. Right column is large and is used to record the notes, the smaller left "cue column" is used to record the questions and the headings, and bottom row is used to write a summary.
- *Charting method of note-taking:* It can be used when the chapter/lecture falls into predictable and well organized pattern.

### Mind Mapping

Visual representation of information is created using mind maps. This helps to see the connections between different concepts and makes the material more accessible.

### Flashcards/Cue Cards

Flashcards are used for training and repeated exposure while learning. These are organizational tools to avoid forgetting key information such as instructions, reminders, prompts, mnemonics, and definitions. Research has shown that using cue cards increases comprehension, aids in remembering, clarifies behavioral expectations, facilitates higher-level cognitive tasks, and self-regulation, particularly goal setting and self-monitoring.

### Retrieval Practice

Retrieval practice is used to remember concepts for a longer duration. Recalling improves learning and memory. Practice tests, using flashcards, and making own questions are some ways of including retrieval in daily study routine.

### Techniques for Improving Memory

The following techniques can be used for improving memory:

- Mnemonics
- Method of loci
- Number and letter peg system
- Stories you tell yourself
- Remembering names and faces
- Chunking

### Studying to Remember

- Plan a time to study

- Rehearsal, mainly maintenance rehearsal and elaborative rehearsal
- Importance of organization during encoding, for example, subjective organization
- Feedback to remember the learned material
- Review before examination
- Overlearning

## TIME MANAGEMENT

Time is one of the most important, indispensable, and irreplaceable resources for accomplishment. It is a precious asset and cannot be recovered once lost. If time is not managed well, a teen can feel frustrated, dissatisfied, and stressed. It is an essential skill that can make the difference between a mediocre and a superior performer.

Managing time is the process of planning and exercising conscious control on time spent on specific activities, to increase efficiency and productivity. Teens face increasing responsibility in academic, social, and personal domains. Good time management contributes to adjustment, academic performance, emotional well-being, social competence, and mental health. A teen should spend their time doing the things that are most valued.

### Benefits of Time Management

The benefits of time management include the following:

- *Stress relief:* Making and following a task schedule reduce stress and anxiety, and make adolescents happy and calm.
- *More time:* This can be spent on hobbies or other personal pursuits.
- *More opportunities:* Prioritizing leads to less time wasted on trivial activities.
- *Ability to realize goals* in a shorter length of time.

*Skills needed for time management include:*

- Prioritization
- Scheduling
- Execution

### Strategies to Improve Time Management Skills

- Know the goals that are most important. These are the maps that give direction to schedule accordingly.
- *Prioritize:* Connect priorities with long-term values and goals. Never allow peer pressure or short-term gratification to help decide.
- *Plan and write it down:* Minutes spent in planning will save the time spent on the task; use a calendar, diary,

and "to-do" lists. A written plan gives the ability to stand back and have a "helicopter vision".

- *Delegate tasks:* It is wise.
- *Work out a system:* Muddle causes unnecessary work. Organize the workspace. Set up a routine. Allot time based on priority. Minimize distractions. Fix deadlines and evaluate yourself periodically is necessary.
- *Don't procrastinate:* It leads simply to storing up more work.
- *Leave slack in your timetable:* Never fill up a timetable completely, always allow some free time.
- *Learn to say "No"* to some demands to offer some control and prevent being controlled by others.
- *Pursue one goal at a time* because all the goals cannot be done at the same time.
- *Identify prime time* for more demanding tasks; when energy levels are lowest, perform the less-demanding tasks.
- *Overcome perfectionism* to prevent getting trapped in small details, and missing out on overall perspective.
- *Keep a balance* between school, home, leisure, physical activity, and mental activity with breaks.

In conclusion, developing good time management skills takes practice and patience. By implementing these strategies, adolescents can effectively manage time and achieve their goals.

*Further reading can be done for the following techniques:*

- The Pomodoro technique
- The Kanban technique
- Getting things done (GTD)
- Eat that frog
- Timeboxing
- Time blocking
- The Eisenhower matrix
- Pareto analysis
- Rapid planning method
- Pickle jar theory
- Specific, measurable, achievable, relevant, and time-bound (SMART) method.

## KEY MESSAGES

- Different learning techniques for understanding the concept, memorizing and remembering can be used by adolescents.
- The important techniques for understanding the concept are: SQ3R, note-taking, mind mapping, flashcards/cue cards, and retrieval practices.

- Adolescents should learn time management also. There are various strategies to improve time management skills.
- Plan and write it down. Learn to say NO. Identify prime time, keep a balance between school, home, leisure, physical activity and mental activity with breaks.
- Further it may be improved by learning various techniques such as Pomodoro Technique etc.

## RECOMMENDED READING

1. Butler G, Grey N, Hope T. Managing Your Mind, 3rd edition. Oxford: United Kingdom: Oxford University Press; 2018.
2. Deshler D, Schumaker JB. Teaching Adolescents With Disabilities: Accessing the General Education Curriculum, 1st edition. Thousand Oaks, CA: Corwin; 2005.
3. Morgan C, King R, Weisz J, Schopler J. Introduction to Psychology. New York, US: McGraw Hill Education; 2017.
4. Powell T. The Mental Health Handbook, revised edition. London, United Kingdom: Routledge; 2000.
5. Skills you need. (2023). Develop The Skills You Need for Life. [online]. Available from www.skillsyouneed.com [Last accessed April, 2024].
6. www.brevedy.com
7. www.myhours.com

# 10.4   Means to Achieve Academic Excellence

*Merlin Thanka Jemi, Ramesh B Dampuri*

## ■ INTRODUCTION

Academic excellence is the ability to perform, achieve, and excel in scholastic activities. Successful students are active, goal-directed, self-regulating, and assume personal responsibility for contributing to their own learning. They participate actively in class, do their task diligently and submit them on time. They do tasks with objectives in mind. They are self-disciplined and responsible in everything they do.

## ■ TIPS FOR A TEENAGED STUDENT

- Know your learning style. There are three types of learners (Barbe VAK model) **(Table 1)**.
- *Developing good study habits:*
  - Attend class regularly.
  - Study with a definite purpose and with an aim of understanding.
  - Discipline your time. Plan and follow a time schedule.
  - Begin to study immediately in the time set aside for this.
  - Avoid distractions and set up a suitable place for studying.
  - Evaluate immediate and remote goals.
  - Begin your study period by reviewing something that you already know.
  - Study only one subject or one part of a subject at a time.
  - Review your subject materials, lecture notes, and reading regularly.
  - Use appropriate learning techniques; learn to take good notes.
  - Take short breaks in-between.

**TABLE 1:** Types of learners.

| Type of learner vs. characteristics | Visual learners | Auditory learners | Kinesthetic learners |
|---|---|---|---|
| Learns by | Seeing | Listening | Doing |
| Has high ability | For visual recall | Auditory recall | Experience/feelings of a physical event |
| Prefers to learn by | Using visual representations such as graphs, posters, maps, and displays | • Repetition and summaries<br>• Benefits from discussions, lectures, stories, and podcasts | Through field trips, physical activity, touch, and manipulating objects |

- Record your assignments, plans for study and appointment in a small notebook.
- Plan one full day free of study each week.
- Ask for help and explanation whenever necessary.
- *Set effective academic goals:*
  - See if the goals are consistent with your highest values.
  - See if the goal is that you really want to accomplish.
  - Is the goal achievable?
  - Is the goal positive?
  - Are the goals in balance?
- *Ways of overcoming procrastination to achieve the academic goal:*
  - Stop worrying.
  - Look for the hidden rewards.
  - Confront the negative beliefs.
  - Take responsibility for each day.
  - Reward yourself for doing activities.

*Role of the teachers in academic achievement of students:*
- Encourage active learning and success; develop learning pedagogy.
- Increase thinking skills and effective learning zones.
- Provide effective feedback.
- Recognize and create learning windows.
- Develop good relationship.
- Enhance motivation and accept individual differences.

*Role of peers:*
- Select friends with similar interests and goals.
- Select friends with higher aspirations to have more positive academic self-concepts.
- Spend time with friends more productively.
- Group learning and discussions.
- Teaching each other to understand the concept better.

## RECOMMENDED READING

1. Azizi Hj. Yahaya. Factors contributing towards excellence in academic performance. [online] Available from chrome-extension://efaidnbmnnnibpcajpcglclefindmkaj/https://core.ac.uk/download/pdf/11782212.pdf [Last accessed April, 2024].
2. Class room psychology: Unit 7—Skill Development.

# 10.5 | Difficulties in Learning

*Swetha Madhuri, Rachna George*

## SCHOLASTIC DETERIORATION

Scholastic deterioration (SD) or school backwardness is defined as repeated failures in grades and academic underachievement securing marks <35%. There are a large number of school drop-outs because of SD. It negatively impacts the development, psychosocial competence, self-esteem, educational outcomes, career opportunities, and interpersonal relationships. SD is complex and influenced by of multiple factors **(Flowchart 1)**. There is a paucity of original research in SD among the Indian population. Nair et al. and Shenoy et al. report the prevalence as 5 and 15%, respectively.

In the hospital setting, teens with SD might present with a primarily physical or behavioral symptoms. Pediatricians and mental health professionals need to work closely with families and teachers for wholistic outcomes.

*Child-specific interventions include:*
- *Assessments standardized for the Indian child and adolescent:* Binet-Kamat scale, Malin's Intelligence Scale for Indian Children, National Institute of Mental Health and Neurosciences (NIMHANS) battery of Specific Learning Disability (SLD), and Wechsler Intelligence Scale for Children-IV
- Screening for neurodevelopmental comorbidities, skill training, and medications when necessary.
- Treatment of psychiatric comorbidity using a biopsychosocial approach.
- Treatment of chronic illness in an adolescent to prevent school absenteeism.
- Study techniques, time management skills, and remedial strategies to be taught.
- Emotional difficulties can be treated using adaptive coping strategies, problem solving techniques,

**Flowchart 1:** Causes for scholastic deterioration.

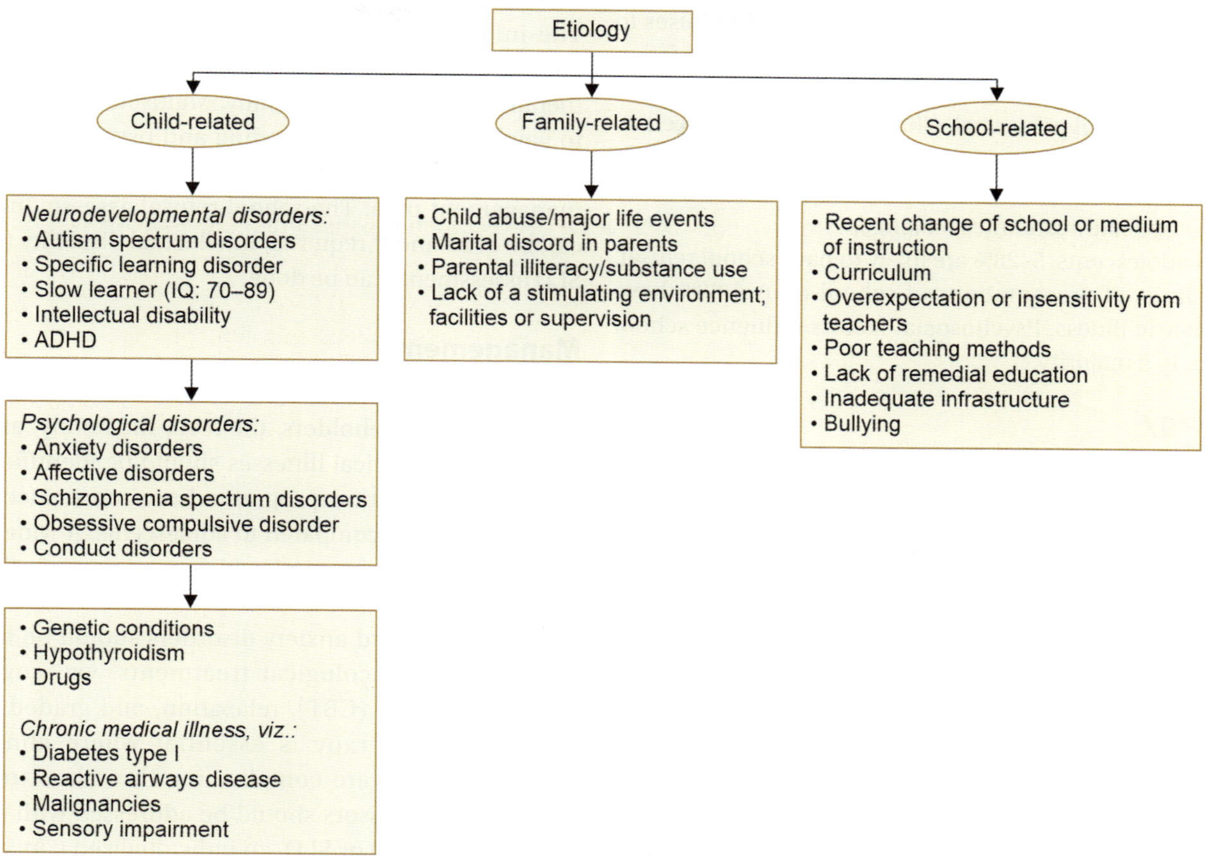

(ADHD: attention-deficit/hyperactivity disorder)

emotion regulation skills, resilience enhancing skills, and social skills.

- Recommendation to the school board for exemptions based on the CBSE or NCERT board guidelines.

*Family interventions include:*

- Explore living conditions, family dynamics, and parental involvement in their education.
- If child abuse or ongoing domestic violence is suspected, district child welfare committee to be involved.
- Assess parental understanding of the teen's difficulties and their expectations.
- Psychoeducation of parents should include exploring subjects other than the mainstream subjects and the need for realistic expectations is crucial.
- Parents should be screened, supported, and treated for their mental health problems.
- Training parents in behavioral interventions to address challenging behaviors.

*School or educational interventions:*

- Collaborate with teachers about the adolescent's work in the school setting.
- Teachers with training in special education can assist in meeting their unique needs.
- School mental health services should be operational, to sensitize and equip staff and students.
- Changes in the structure of class rooms to reduce excessive and distracting sensory input.

Scholastic deterioration is challenging and demands attention from healthcare professionals, teachers, parents, and policy makers. It requires early identification, multimodal assessment, and intervention customized to the teen's unique learning needs for an optimal outcome **(Box 1)**.

# ■ SCHOOL REFUSAL

An ideal school is an environment designed for the wholistic well-being of an adolescent. Acclimatizing to school is a matter of concern for many children. School refusal is a behavioral problem where the child refuses to attend school or finds difficulty in remaining in class for an entire day. It is a challenging problem for children, parents as well as school personnel. Chronic school absenteeism, if unaddressed, is a serious problem that can negatively impact the emotional and social development of the child and complicate academic challenges.

Of adolescents, 5–28% are likely to have school refusal. In a clinic, of presentations of school refusal 88% have psychiatric illness. Psychosocial factors influence school refusal in a majority.

## Etiology

Anxiety disorders and separation anxiety specifically are linked to dysregulation in emotional response system and are one of the most common mechanisms triggering school refusal. If problems, viz. bullying, abuse, or punitive disciplinary, are the reason for school refusal, it is usually the result of post-traumatic stress disorder (PTSD). An underlying neurodevelopmental disorder can also present as school refusal. Avoidance behavior is triggered by a cause and reinforced, this compounds school refusal behavior leading to a cycle of school refusal **(Fig. 1)**.

> **BOX 1:** Simple criteria for screening scholastic backwardness in children.
>
> - A teen fails repeatedly in one or more subjects
> - A teen who is detained in one or more class
> - A teen who is in the lowest 10th percentile
> - A teen identified as difficult to teach by the teachers

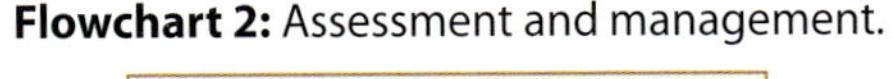


**Fig. 1:** Cycle of school refusal behavior.

## Assessment

The initial consultation should involve the teen and parents to take the teen's perspective and help build a therapeutic alliance with family. Multisource information to gain in-depth understanding and psychoeducational assessment will help formulate an individualized management plan. The school refusal assessment scale can be used and if required, intellectual disability (ID) or SLD assessments can be done.

## Management

A comprehensive management plan should involve the different stakeholders, the teen, the family, and the school team. Medical illnesses should be identified and treated. Intervention programs have more success in younger children compared to adolescents. A wide range of approaches can be employed depending on individual need.

Depression and anxiety disorders should be treated with nonpharmacological treatments, viz. cognitive behavior therapy (CBT), relaxation, and graded exposure. Family therapy is essential where abnormal family dynamics are complicating the school refusal. Psychosocial stressors should be addressed with school authorities. For ID or SLD, an individualized educational plan should be made and communicated to the school team. Pharmacological approaches can be used when appropriate **(Flowchart 2)**. Success of the interventions depends on the teen feeling supported and validated, ensuring a seamless collaboration between the various stakeholders.

## ■ KEY MESSAGES

- Scholastic deterioration requires a compressive multi-dimensional assessment involving the child, family and school.

**Flowchart 2:** Assessment and management.

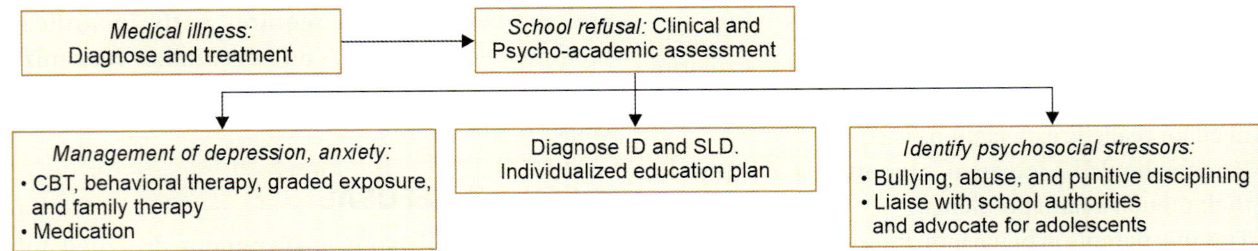


(CBT: cognitive behavior therapy; ID: intellectual disability; SLD: specific learning disability)

- Interventions for scholastic deterioration should be individualized involving the various stakeholders i.e., the child, family, and teachers.
- School refusal needs to be addressed early as it can lead to a cycle of school refusal behavior.

## ■ RECOMMENDED READING


1. Elliott JG, Place M. Practitioner review: School refusal: Developments in conceptualisation and treatment since 2000. J Child Psychol Psychiatr. 2019;60(1):4-15.
2. Hirisave U, Shanti K. Scholastic difficulties with behavioural problems. Indian J Pediatr. 2002;69:963-4.
3. Kearney CA, Bates M. Addressing school refusal behavior: Suggestions for frontline professionals. Child Sch. 2005;27(4):207-16.
4. Kearney CA, Bensaheb A. School absenteeism and school refusal behavior: a review and suggestions for school-based health professionals. J School Health. 2006;76(1):3-7.
5. Kearney CA, Silverman WK. Measuring the function of school refusal behavior: The School Refusal Assessment Scale. J Clin Child Psychol. 1993;22(1):85-96.
6. Nair MKC, Paul MK, Padmamohan J. Scholastic performance of adolescents. Indian J Pediatr. 2003;70:629-31.
7. Prabhuswamy M, Srinath S, Girimaji S, Seshadri S. Outcome of children with school refusal. Indian J Pediatr. 2007;74:375-9.
8. Shashidhar S, Rao C, Hegde R. Factors affecting scholastic performances of adolescents. Indian J Pediatr. 2009;76:495-9.
9. Sukumaran TU. Poor scholastic performance in children and adolescents. Ind Pediatrics. 2011;48(8):597-8.


---

# 10.6 | Examination Stress and Management

*Yatesh Pujar, Mona M Basker*

## ■ INTRODUCTION

Examination stress refers to the physical and emotional pressure experienced by students while preparing for or taking an examination. It is a common response to the demands and expectations associated with examinations.

## ■ COMMON CAUSES OF EXAMINATION STRESS

The causes of examination stress include:

- Fear of failure
- Heavy workload
- Time pressure
- Lack of preparation
- High expectations
- Competitive nature of school
- Perfectionism
- Lack of support
- Cumulative assessments
- Time management challenges
- Limited resources
- Personal factors

## PATHOPHYSIOLOGY OF EXAMINATION STRESS

Examination stress is a complex interplay between psychological, physiological, and behavioral factors. The body activates the "fight-or-flight" response, releasing stress hormones like cortisol, adrenaline, and norepinephrine.

- *Hypothalamic–pituitary–adrenal (HPA) axis activation:* Corticotropin-releasing hormone (CRH) from the hypothalamus stimulates → release of adrenocorticotropic hormone (ACTH) from pituitary → stimulates the adrenals to produce and release cortisol → increased cortisol associated with anxiety and impaired cognition.
- *Sympathetic nervous system activation:* Releases adrenaline and norepinephrine increase in heart rate, blood pressure, and respiratory rate → prepares body for perceived threat, and leads to racing thoughts, restlessness, and difficulty concentrating.
- *Altered neurotransmitter levels:* Serotonin, dopamine, and gamma-aminobutyric acid (GABA) play a crucial role in regulating mood, motivation, focus, and anxiety. Imbalances can lead to anxiety, depression, and loss of concentration and memory.
- *Immune system dysregulation:* Suppression of immunity → increased inflammation, reduced antibody production, and impaired immune response, making individuals more susceptible to illness and infections.

- *Sleep disturbances:* Such as difficulty falling asleep, frequent awakenings, and inadequate sleep duration. Poor quality sleep exacerbates stress and impair cognitive function and memory.

While acute stress can be adaptive and motivating, chronic or excessive stress can have detrimental effects on physical and mental health.

## SYMPTOMS OF EXAMINATION STRESS

Symptoms of examination stress include:
- *Psychological:* Anxiety, excessive worry, feeling overwhelmed, panic, increased irritability, mood swings, difficulty concentrating or remembering, self-doubt, fear of failure or disappointing others, and anhedonia.
- *Physical:* Headaches, migraines, abdominal pain, diarrhea, myalgia, fatigue, difficulty sleeping, tachycardia, shortness of breath, sweating, tremors, and decreased or increased appetite.
- *Behavioral:* Procrastination or avoidance of studying, distraction behaviors (e.g., excessive screen time), difficulty managing time, decreased participation in extracurricular activities or social events, withdrawal from friends or family, and increased sensitivity or emotional outbursts. Some level of stress before examinations is normal and can enhance performance. When these symptoms become overwhelming and significantly interfere with daily functioning, it is important to seek support from family, friends, or professionals.

*Maladaptive coping mechanisms used to deal with pressure include:*
- Procrastination
- Avoidance
- Substance abuse
- Perfectionism
- Overworking
- Test anxiety
- Examination stress, when severe and left unaddressed.

These situations highlight the need for open dialogue, support systems, and appropriate mental health resources. Students with examination stress need immediate help from parents, teachers, counsellors, or mental health professionals.

## COMPLICATIONS OF EXAMINATION STRESS

Complications of examination stress, both in the short- and long-term, include:
- Academic underachievement
- Mental health disorders
- Physically, illnesses, and infections
- Negative impact on relationships
- Substance abuse
- Impaired quality of life
- Future academic and career implications.

## DEALING WITH EXAMINATION STRESS

Assisting students in dealing with examination stress include:
- Encourage open communication.
- Provide information and resources, viz. study strategies, time management techniques, and stress reduction using deep breathing exercises, mindfulness, or meditation. Share resources such as study guides, online resources, or tutoring options.
- Teach stress management.
- Teach effective study skills.
- Offer academic support.
- Provide realistic expectations.
- Encourage self-care, e.g., taking breaks and engaging in hobbies.
- Promote a supportive environment in classroom or school.
- Refer to professional help if needed.

## COPING STRATEGIES TO REDUCE EXAMINATION STRESS

The coping strategies include:
- Time management
- Study techniques
- Relaxation techniques
- Regular exercise
- Adequate sleep
- Healthy lifestyle habits
- Social support
- Relaxation activities
- Positive self-talk
- Seeking help when needed, from teachers, counsellors, or mental health professionals.

Family members play a crucial role in helping students to manage examination stress by:
- Create a supportive home environment.
- Listen actively.
- Offer practical help.
- Provide healthy meals and encourage breaks.
- Encourage regular sleep routine.

- Reinforce positive self-talk.
- Focus on effort and progress, shift the focus from solely outcomes or grades to the effort and progress.
- Celebrate small victories.
- Set realistic expectations.
- Provide a balanced routine between study time and activities they enjoy.
- Emotional support.
- Seek outside support if needed.

*Pediatricians can play a vital a role in the following ways:*
- Physical health assessment and advice
- Sleep guidance
- Medication management
- Referrals
- Parental education and support
- Stress reduction techniques.

Pediatricians typically address the physical aspects but can provide general guidance and referrals to mental health professionals for more specialized support. Collaborating with a mental health professional can ensure a comprehensive approach to addressing examination stress and supporting the overall well-being of the child.

*Spirituality can play a role:*
- *Mind–body connection:* Engaging in activities like meditation or yoga can help reduce stress, promote relaxation, and improve focus, which can all be beneficial during examination periods.
- *Finding meaning and purpose:* With values, beliefs, and a sense of purpose beyond academic performance. This broader perspective can alleviate some of the pressure and provide motivation.
- *Cultivating resilience:* Spirituality can encourage to embrace challenges as opportunities for growth and learning, rather than being overwhelmed by them.
- *Developing a support system:* As spirituality involves community or seeking.
- Creating a sense of peace and calm.

## ■ KEY MESSAGES

- Exam stress is very common among students.
- Hypothalamic–pituitary–adrenal axis becomes overactive to produce distress.
- This distress may make students to underperform in exams and sometimes leads to substance abuse/depression/suicide.
- Healthy coping mechanisms should coached to students.
- Mental health specialists should be involved early, whenever required.

# 10.7 Managing Emotional Problems in School Children

*Rahul Pengoria, Kajal Taneja*

## ■ MANAGING EMOTIONS

Emotional regulation is defined as the use of mechanisms, skills, and strategies to maintain, increase, or suppress an existing emotional state. It implies being aware of own state of emotions and using strategies to manage mood. Strategies used for emotional regulation can be either adaptive or maladaptive. The process model of emotional regulation focuses on two strategies, i.e., cognitive reappraisal and expressive suppression. Cognitive reappraisal is an antecedent-focused strategy and is hypothesized to modify the impact of emotional experience. Expressive suppression is a response-focused strategy that involves inhibiting the ongoing emotion. Greater reliance on cognitive reappraisal is associated with well-being outcomes for most indicators especially life satisfaction, social support perception, and positive affect.

*Emotional regulation processes include:*
- *Situation selection:* Actions to increase or decrease the chances to arrive at a situation to bring forth expected emotions.
- *Situation modification:* Emotional situations are attempted to be modified directly to change their emotional impact.

- *Attentional deployment:* Spread of attention.
- *Cognitive change:* Changing the way we assess the situations we are involved in, changing their emotional significance, by changing how we think about the situation or about our capacity to handle its demands.
- *Response modulation:* Influencing physiological response, experience, or behavior as directly as possible. Sports, relaxation, food, and drugs (alcohol and cigarettes) can be used to modify emotional experiences.

*Practical tips for teens to control emotional problems:*
- Identify and reduce triggers
- Noticing emotions
- Naming your emotions
- Choose your response
- Deep breathing
- Jacobson's progressive muscle relaxation
- Anger management techniques
- Practice mindfulness
- Using problem-solving techniques
- If unmanageable, taking help of a professional.

## CONCLUSION

When adolescents do not learn appropriate self-regulation, they use maladaptive strategies that either numb the experience of emotion, channel it to another form of manageable pain, or avoid the feeling altogether. Some examples of maladaptive behaviors are, "acting out", aggression, substance use, nonsuicidal self-injury, excessive screen time, gaming, etc. Emotional regulation is important for a healthy adolescent lifestyle.

## WAYS TO IMPROVE INTERPERSONAL SKILLS

Interpersonal skills are those that are needed to communicate effectively with another person or a group of people. It is essential for individual well-being. Interpersonal skills promote an atmosphere of confidence and trust, that grows valuable relationships. Skills like respect, helpfulness, integrity, empathy, discretion, openness to other ideas and cultures, effective written and oral communication, and effective body language all contribute to such growth.

### Social Skills

Social skills are the skills needed for communication and interaction with people. They allow teens to succeed in social, academic, personal, and professional areas. They are essential in laying the foundation, establishment, and maintenance of good relationships. These prepare young people to mature and succeed in adult roles within the family, workplace, and community. A few skills to develop include:

- Being patient, kind, and respectful
- Being polite and courteous
- Listening to others
- Praising others and refrain from making negative comments about people
- Waiting for your turn to speak
- Knowing when to use humor
- Knowing what topics of conversation are appropriate for the audience
- Refrain from calling names, swearing, and making obscene gestures
- Respect personal space
- Using good manners
- Develop prosocial behaviors.

### Being Assertive

Assertiveness is the ability to stand up for their rights without violating the rights of others. A skill based on the idea that your needs, wants, and feelings are neither more or less important than those of other people. You should make claims for yourself appropriately, honestly, and clearly. The alternative way to being assertive is either passivity or aggression. Assertiveness involves standing up for one's right, building strength, and steps toward fairness. It improves the sense of identity, confidence, and self-esteem. Being assertive saves energy, reduces tension, and develops healthy relationships.

*Specific skills:*
- *Active listening:* Give undivided attention to the person who is talking to you. Reflect or repeat a few words. Summarize what you have understood. Listen to the end. Do not assume. When you agree say so.
- *Manage criticisms and complaints:* Ask for clarification, refuse to be labeled, agree with the critic (if realistic/constructive criticism), and apologize appropriately. When you want to make a complaint, name the problem, state your feelings or opinions, and specify what you want.
- *Body language:* Your assertiveness is shown in your body posture, eye contact, tone of voice, gestures and movements, facial expression, and the social

distance you maintain. Avoid looking away or looking down. Speak in a firm, relaxed voice, and stand erect, balanced, open body stance.

- *Saying NO:* If someone asks you to do something that you do not want to do, then all you need to do is to say NO. Appreciate their efforts to approach you. Acknowledge the other person's priorities and wishes. Give a clear reason for your refusal. Keep it brief and polite.
- *Negotiating skills:* Choose the right time and place to discuss, present the problem in a constructive way, listen to what the other person has to say, discuss differences, and be prepared to offer a compromise.

## Problem Solving and Decision-making

Problem solving and decision-making are both key life skills, used to address conflicts or to make decisions.

The process involves the following steps:
- Identify and define the problem.
- Brainstorm (think of as many solutions as possible)
- Decide on realistic options.
- Evaluate the pros and cons of the potential solutions.
- Choose the feasible and rewarding solution.
- Plan and prepare strategies to implement.

## Conflict Management

All interpersonal relationships experience conflict at some time and to some degree. Conflict can be good or bad depending on how it is managed. They can be handled in the following ways:
- Use messages that enhance a person's self-image and autonomy.
- Compliment the other person even when in a conflict.
- Make less demands, respect other's time, and give personal person space, especially when in times of conflict.
- Avoid blaming the other person.
- Respect the other's point of view, even when they do not match your own.

- Manage the problems in private (not in front of others/social media).
- Choose the right time for resolving the conflict.
- Avoid being verbally aggressive or attacking the person.

## ■ CONCLUSION

Interpersonal skills leads to all round development of a person and can even give us the opportunity to ask for help when confronted with any adverse situation. Whether it be working more effectively as part of a team or negotiating/reconciling with others or influencing others successfully. Good interpersonal skills can help to be successful in all domains of life.

## ■ KEY MESSAGES

- Emotional problems are the most common mental health problems in childhood and adolescence.
- Cognitive reappraisal and expressive suppression are strategies for emotional regulation.
- Good interpersonal skills help to tide off with the emotional problems effectively.
- Sharpening the interpersonal skills can help to improve both the personal and school life.

## ■ RECOMMENDED READING


1. Aldao A, Nolen-Hoeksema S, Schweizer S. Emotion-regulation strategies across psychopathology: a meta-analytic review. Clin Psychol Rev. 2010;30(2):217-37.
2. Butler G, Grey N, Hope T. Managing Your Mind, 3rd edition. Oxford: United Kingdom: Oxford University Press; 2018.
3. Gross JJ, Ford BQ. Handbook of Emotion Regulation. New York: Guildford Publication; 2014.
4. Koole SL. The psychology of emotion regulation: An Integrative review. Cogn Emot. 2009;23(1):4-41.
5. Powell T. The Mental Health Handbook, revised edition. London, United Kingdom: Routledge; 2000.
6. Skills you need. (2023). Develop The Skills You Need For Life. [online]. Available from www.skillsyouneed.com [Last accessed April, 2024].
7. Verzeletti C, Zammuner VL, Galli C, Agnoli S, Duregger C. Emotion regulation strategies and psychosocial well-being in adolescence. Cogent Psychology. 2016;3(1):1-15.

# Parenting

**Section Editor:** Atul Kanikar

## 11.1 Successful Family Communication Skills

Jugesh Chhatwal

### INTRODUCTION

Family communication involves sharing and exchange of information, thoughts, and feelings, among the family members. Communication within the family is similar to the blood flow in the blood vessels. Whenever there are problems in the blood flow the health of the body is affected. Similarly, whenever the communication within the family is disturbed, the family is affected. Successful and effective communication is essential for healthy and strong relationships and creating harmony within the family. It allows for emotional, psychological as well as physical growth of family members, especially children. Effective communication with teenagers makes happier and connected relationships, and more confidence for having difficult conversations and resolving conflicts. Family communication can involve two aspects, viz. instrumental communication, which concerns information related to day to day family activities such as buying groceries and picking up children, and effective communication, which involves feelings and emotions. For successful family communication, both should be functioning well.

### ROLE OF SUCCESSFUL FAMILY COMMUNICATION

Successful family communication is helpful for the following:
- *Create and maintain connectedness within the family:* This is very important for all but more so for the teenagers as they are more likely to feel alienated and disconnected due to their growing need for independence. Sharing important events of the day and confiding to someone within the family can lead to a stronger sense of connection and intimacy.
- *Building trust and respect:* With successful communication, trust and respect are built, and trust is the foundation of all strong relationships.
- *Resolving conflicts:* Conflicts are bound to happen among all families and need resolution for maintaining harmony. Using appropriate communication skills, conflicts can be resolved effectively.
- *Understand each other:* Frequent and open communication helps for knowing the viewpoints and emotions of the family members. This is useful for creating an understanding between family members, which in turn help in building strong relationships.
- *Tackling difficult situations:* If there are strong relationship with the family, one can rely on them for support during difficult times. Children who trust that their parents will truly listen to them will be more likely to confide in them when they are in trouble.
- *Providing a psychologically safe environment to encourage sharing of thoughts, events, and problems:* When family members feel like they can express themselves without fear of being judged or ridiculed, they are more likely to open up and share their thoughts and feelings. Respecting everyone's opinions, even if one does not agree with them, is important. Adolescent

are more likely to share their view points if they know that their opinions are respected and valued.

## STEPS TO SUCCESSFUL FAMILY COMMUNICATION

Communication involves elements such as verbal 7%, voice 38%, and nonverbal 55%. For successful family communication, appropriate use of all elements of communication is necessary **(Box 1)**. Parents as role models should be aware how their nonverbal communication can be vital in talking with their children, especially the troubled adolescent. The steps for building successful communication including use of nonverbal elements **(Box 2)** are as:

- *Active listening:* It involves being a good listener, giving attention and focusing on what is being said and what the other person might be feeling, and trying to understand their point of view. Sometimes repeating

what the person has said helps in better understanding. Asking clarifying questions and paraphrasing or summarizing what has been said can help. It conveys to another person that they are being heard and responded to. This can help avoid misunderstandings and conflicts.

- *Appropriate language and vocabulary:* Talking within the family requires each one uses clear and appropriate language. No assumptions should be made, instead questions should be asked for clarifying. One of the helpful steps is to use first person, i.e., "I" instead of "You" statements. "You" statements tend to be accusatory and make the other person defensive. Consider "I feel like you are not listening to me." vs. "You do not listen to me."

Thinking and taking the time to decide what one wants to say is also helpful. Avoiding making assumptions about what other family members are thinking or feeling and using direct communication improves communication. Nonjudgmental words help in better interaction.

*Nonverbal communication:* Nonverbal communication of a person is useful in interpreting many aspects.

*Voice modulation:* The tone of voice can communicate a lot about how one is feeling. Speaking loudly at a high volume and pitch or talking very fast indicates anger or aggression. Parents need to avoid sounding angry, judgmental, or sarcastic as this will become a barrier to communication. They can be assertive without being aggressive.

*Visual cues:* Body language can indicate many things about a person. Facial expressions and body posture tell about their thoughts and feelings. Rolled up eyes or crossed arms easily convey the thinking. Similarly, open arms or a smile, eye contact, and leaning toward the person give the confidence to the others that they are welcome to talk and share.

*Proxemic and tactile communication:* Choosing a quiet place without distractions for important conversations is helpful. Also maintaining contact like holding hands or shoulders can give support and confidence to the other person. Touching a family member who is upset or hurt can help them in opening up.

*Family interactions:* In addition to the above conversational issues, building in family interactions allows for better communication. Some of the following can be incorporated in the routine of the family.

---

**BOX 1:** Elements of verbal communication.

- Two-way process
- Active listening
- Appropriate language and vocabulary
- Voice modulation and fluency
- Ask questions
- Paraphrase/summarize

---

**BOX 2:** Elements of nonverbal communication.

*Visual/kinesics' cues:*
- Facial expressions (smile)
- Eye movements (eye contact and glance)
- Gestures (encouraging and inviting)
- Body orientation (listening and attentive posture)
- Breathing (deep exhalation and inhalation to indicate patience)

*Posture:*
- Standing erect and at ease
- Relaxed
- Hands free to emphasize on points spoken

*Vocal/paralinguistic cues:*
- Volume, pitch, and rate
- Inflection (quality, emotion, speaking style, intonation, and stress)
- Vocal nuance

*Gait:* Walking assertively/arrogantly/meekly

*Proxemics cues:*
- Space/place
- Distance between the communicating persons

*Tactile communication:* Touch

*Family meetings:* Regular family meetings to discuss common issues, make decisions, and share information. Involving everyone and hearing their viewpoint without interruptions is important.

*Family games:* Playing games encourages conversation and interaction and can be a fun way to bond and spend time together.

*Family outings:* This can create opportunities for shared experiences and conversations. All must be encouraged to join and also take responsibility in organizing, e.g., like a picnic. It is also important that outings are planned to include everyone's interest.

## BARRIERS TO SUCCESSFUL FAMILY COMMUNICATIONS

- Lack of awareness about communication skills
- Indifferent attitude
- Lack of exposure to good communication
- Introverted personality
- Authoritarian parenting
- Inability to express emotions
- Not listening to others
- Not spending time together as a family
- Biases, prejudices, and assumptions.

## HOW TO OVERCOME THE BARRIERS

- Practice active listening. Lending an ear or listening helps in others expressing themselves and feeling that they are heard.
- Expressing clearly and sharing feelings with family members.
- Asking questions and showing concerns genuinely.
- Honest conversations without antagonizing words. Open and honest conversations build trust.
- Allowing everyone to have their say/viewpoint.
- Not attacking individuals but the situations/problems.
- Communicate frequently—mealtimes, travelling in car, bedtime, etc.
- Communication within the family must consider age and maturity of others.
- Supportive role of family for all, especially teenagers even when they make mistakes. Encourage them to do their own problem solving.

- Maintaining a positive attitude.
- Expressing appreciation and saying thank you.
- Family-based activities.

## KEY MESSAGES

- Family communication involves sharing and exchange of information, thoughts, and feelings, among the family members.
- Successful family communication helps to create and maintain connectedness, build trust and respect, resolve conflicts, understand each other, tackle difficult situations, and provide a psychologically safe environment to encourage sharing of thoughts, events, and problems.
- Successful communication is a two-way process, with active listening, appropriate language, and vocabulary, and one should ask questions and paraphrase.
- Nonverbal communication includes visual cues like a smile, eye contact, encouraging gestures, a listening posture, the right tone of voice, keeping the right distance, relaxed posture, proper gait, and a friendly touch.
- Family meetings, games, and outings can be incorporated in the routine of the family.

## RECOMMENDED READING


1. Epstein NB, Bishop D, Ryan C, Miller, Keitner G. The McMaster model view of healthy family functioning. In: Walsh F (Ed). Normal Family Processes. New York: The Guilford Press; 1993. pp. 138-60.
2. Olsen CS. (2016). Essential Living Skills: Basic Family Communication. Kansas State University. [online] Available from chrome-extension:// efaidnbmnnnibpcajpcglclefindmkaj/https://bookstore. ksre.ksu.edu/pubs/s134e.pdf [Last accessed April, 2024].
3. Peterson R, Green S. Families first: Keys to successful family functioning – Communication. Virginia Cooperative Extension (VCE). [online] Available from http://hdl.handle. net/10919/48300 [Last accessed April, 2024].
4. Rausch A. (2015). "Farm & Family Connections: Balancing Work & Family". Historical Documents of the Purdue Cooperative Extension Service. Paper 1041. [online] Available from https://docs.lib.purdue.edu/agext/1041 [Last accessed April, 2024].

<table><tr><td>**11.2**</td><td># Protective and Risk Factors for the Well-being of Teens and Youth</td></tr></table>

*Sangita Lodha*

## INTRODUCTION

The well-being of teens and youth is influenced by a myriad of factors, and a comprehensive medical perspective takes into account both *protective* and *risk factors*. It is important to consider physical, mental, and social aspects of health. Adolescence is a critical phase, often regarded as a period of transition and transformation, embodying a pivotal juncture where physical, emotional, and cognitive metamorphoses converge.

The well-being of teenagers is a topic of paramount importance in our society. As medical practitioners, it is imperative that we understand and address the influential factors that impact the well-being of teenagers. In doing so, we can contribute to their healthy development and pave the way for brighter futures.

A comprehensive medical perspective recognizes the interconnected nature of these factors and seeks to address them holistically to promote the overall well-being of teens and youth. It involves collaboration between healthcare professionals, educators, families, and communities.

## PROTECTIVE FACTORS (FIG. 1)

- *Social pressures and peer influence:* Adolescents are particularly susceptible to the pressures of conformity and the desire to fit in. Peer influence can lead to risky behavior such as substance abuse, early sexual activity, and engagement in antisocial activities. These actions can have lasting negative impacts on physical and mental health.
- *Technology and screen time:* While technology has opened up new avenues for communication and learning, excessive screen time can lead to isolation, poor sleep quality, and reduced physical activity. Furthermore, the pervasive influence of social media can lead to unhealthy comparisons and contribute to self-esteem issues.
- *Family dynamics:* Turbulent family environments characterized by neglect, abuse, or high levels of conflict can significantly affect a teenager's well-being. Such conditions can contribute to emotional distress, anxiety, and depression.

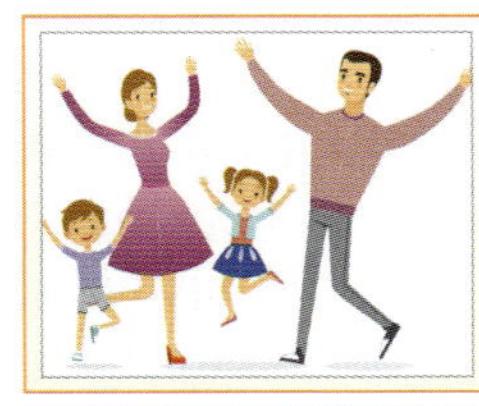


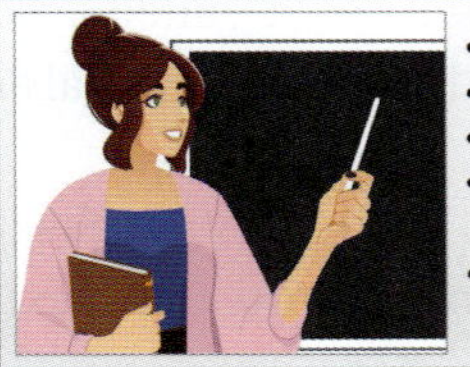


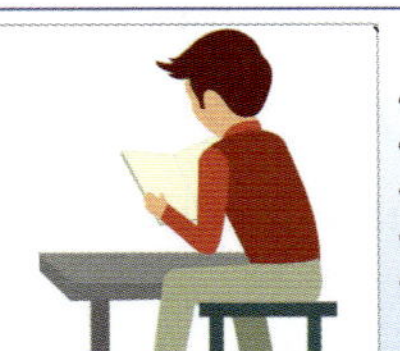


**Fig. 1:** Protective factors for adolescent well-being.

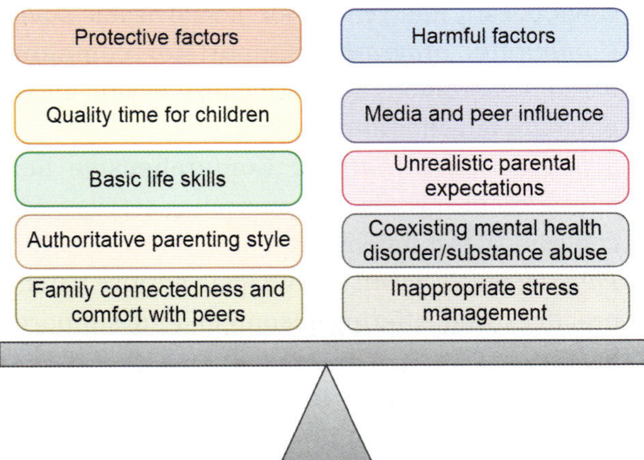


**Fig. 2:** Comparison between protective factors and harmful factors.

- *Academic pressure:* The pursuit of academic excellence is vital, but excessive academic pressure can lead to burnout, anxiety disorders, and feelings of inadequacy. The competitive nature of academic environments can also contribute to a sense of constant stress.

Both sides of the perspective—risk factor and protective factors—are given in **Figure 2**.

## RISK FACTORS

- *Substance abuse:* Use of drugs, alcohol, smoking
- *Unhealthy lifestyle choices:* Poor nutrition and sedentary behavior, lack of physical activity
- *Mental health issues:* Untreated mental health disorders, lack of mental health support
- *Peer pressure:* Negative peer influences and pressure to engage in risky behaviors
- *Family dysfunction:* Family conflict and instability, lack of parental support or involvement
- *Bullying and violence:* Exposure to bullying, both in person and online, involvement in violent situations
- *Poverty and socioeconomic disparities:* Limited access to resources and opportunities, lack of educational and economic support
- *Sexual health:* Ignorance, lack of access to comprehensive sex education, unprotected sexual activity.

## COMPREHENSIVE MEDICAL STRATEGIES

- *Preventive health care:* Regular health checkups, immunizations, and screenings
- *Health education:* Comprehensive sex education and substance abuse prevention programs
- *Mental health services:* Accessible mental health support, early intervention for mental health issues
- *Community programs:* Support for community-based organizations addressing teen health, outreach programs targeting at-risk youth
- *School-based initiatives:* Comprehensive health education in schools and counseling services within educational institutions
- *Parental involvement:* Encouraging positive parenting practices and offering resources and support for parents
- *Legislation and policy:* Implementing and enforcing laws and policies that protect youth, advocating for youth-friendly healthcare services
- *Research and evaluation:* Ongoing research to identify emerging health trends, evaluation of the effectiveness of interventions.

## PROTECTIVE FACTORS

- *Healthy lifestyle choices:*
  - Regular physical activity and exercise promote overall health.
  - A balanced and nutritious diet supports physical and cognitive development.
  - Adequate sleep is crucial for mental and physical well-being.
- *Access to healthcare:* Regular checkups and access to medical care contribute to early detection and prevention of health issues.
- *Mental health support:*
  - Access to mental health services and support systems
  - Resilience and coping skills development
  - Positive peer relationships
  - Supportive friendships and social networks
  - Opportunities for positive social interaction
  - Strong family support
  - Positive family relationships and communication
  - A stable and supportive home environment.
- *Education:*
  - Access to quality education and opportunities for learning
  - Support for educational achievement and aspirations
  - Community engagement
  - Involvement in community activities and organizations
  - Opportunities for civic engagement and volunteering
- *Positive role models:*
  - Exposure to positive adult role models
  - Mentorship and guidance from adults
- *Strong family support:*
  - Healthy family relationships provide a critical buffer against the challenges adolescents face.
  - Supportive families foster emotional resilience, communication skills, and a sense of security that can positively impact mental health (**Figure 3**).

**Warning signs in adolescents**

- Scholastic deterioration
- Avoiding hug and eye contact by parents
- New set of (senior) friends
- Stealing money and valuables
- Wants to be left alone
- Disturbed sleep and appetite
- Disproportionate irritability and mood swings
- Crying constantly or unusually cheerful
- Loss of interest in sports and recreation
- Antisocial behavior

**Mother can be the best clinician at home**

**Fig. 3:** Warning signs in adolescents.

- *Positive peer relationships:* Positive peer connections can serve as sources of emotional support and camaraderie. Encouraging friendships that promote healthy behaviors can contribute to self-esteem and a sense of belonging.
- *Physical activity and nutrition:* Regular physical activity and a balanced diet are essential for physical and mental well-being. Engaging in sports and maintaining proper nutrition not only enhance physical health but also contribute to improved mood and cognitive function.
- *Mental health education*: Comprehensive mental health education in schools and at home can empower teenagers to recognize and manage stress, anxiety, and depression. This knowledge equips them with the tools to seek help when needed and reduces stigma surrounding mental health.
- *Healthy use of technology:* Educating teenagers about responsible technology use can help them navigate the digital world in a balanced and constructive manner. This includes setting limits on screen time and promoting online safety.
- *Community engagement:* Involvement in community activities, volunteering, and extracurricular pursuits fosters a sense of purpose and belonging. It can also enhance social skills, self-esteem, and overall well-being.

In conclusion, as medical professionals, it is our duty to recognize and address the multifaceted factors that influence the well-being of teenagers. By understanding both harmful and protective factors, we can tailor our interventions to create environments that promote positive development and mental health. Collaborative efforts between healthcare providers, educators, families, and communities are essential to ensure that the next generation thrives during the critical phase of adolescence.

In summation, the medical community is entrusted with the task of comprehending and navigating the myriad factors that mold teenage well-being. A holistic understanding of both harmful and protective factors serves as a compass to chart interventions that lay the groundwork for positive development and robust mental health. The harmonious collaboration of healthcare providers, educators, families, and communities serves as a beacon of hope, illuminating the path toward a thriving generation as they traverse the transformative passage of adolescence.

## ■ KEY MESSAGES

- The well-being of teens and youth is influenced by a myriad of protective and risk factors.
- Risk factors include substance abuse, unhealthy lifestyle choices, mental health issues, peer pressure, family dysfunction, bullying and violence, poverty and socioeconomic disparities, and sexual health issues.
- Protective factors include healthy lifestyle choices, access to healthcare, mental health support, education, positive role models, strong family support, positive peer relationships, physical activity and nutrition, mental health education, healthy use of technology, and community engagement.

## ■ RECOMMENDED READING

1. Hurlock EB. Developmental Psychology, 5th edition. New York: McGraw Hill; 2017.
2. Kanikar A, Bhave SY. Parenting of adolescents. In: Bhave's Textbook of Adolescent Medicine. New Delhi: Jaypee Brothers Medical Publishers; 2006.
3. Kanikar A. Risk taking behaviours of teens. Recent Adv Obstet. Gynecol.
4. Nair MKC. Manual of Adolescent Health.
5. World Health Organization. Facilitator's Guide. Program for orientation of Medical Officers.

# 11.3  The Five Basics of Parenting

*Ashim Kumar Ghosh*

## ■ INTRODUCTION

Parenting is both a rewarding and challenging journey that plays a pivotal role in shaping a child's physical, mental, emotional, and cognitive development. With innumerable approaches and strategies available, it is often overwhelming for parents to navigate their way through the complexities of child-rearing. We will explore the five basics of parenting that provide a strong foundation for raising healthy, well-adjusted children.

## ■ FIVE BASICS OF PARENTING

The five basics of parenting are:
1. Love and connect
2. Monitor and observe
3. Guide and limit
4. Model and consult
5. Provide and advocate

### Love and Connect

*Key message for parents: The majority of things in the world are changing for your children but do not let your love for them be one of them.*

Adolescents need their parents to develop and nurture a relationship that offers support and acceptance. On the other hand, parents need to accommodate and affirm the teen's increasing maturity as they assert their own identity and independence.

Studies have found that supportive relationships with parents results in higher levels of self-reliance, better school performance and successful future relationships, and lower risks of substance abuse, depression, and delinquency.

The efforts of teens to establish their own values and identity often results in increased criticism, emotional distancing, and withdrawal from family activities. The challenge for the parents is to provide support at this crucial juncture of life.

*Tips for parents:*
- Express genuine unconditional love, affection, and appreciate your teen.
- Spend time together as a family and find new ways to connect.
- Spend more time in listening than talking to your teen's fears, concerns, interests, ideas, and perspectives.
- Treat your teen as a unique individual distinct from any stereotypes of their or your own generation.
- Appreciate and acknowledge your teen's positive aspects of adolescence such as passions, interests, humor, or intellectual thoughts.
- Provide meaningful roles to your teen for family's well-being.
- Expect increased criticism and debate. Develop skills to discuss ideas and disagreeing on matters without disrespecting both opinions.
- Acknowledge the good times made possible by your teen's personality and growth.

### Monitor and Observe

*Key message for parents: Monitoring your teen's activities still counts.*

A number of studies showed that the monitoring of the teen's whereabouts and activities led to a lower risk of substance abuse, depression, early sexual activity victimization, and delinquency. As our children enter adolescence, our parenting must evolve into new roles.

When they are little, we provide direct supervision. As they enter adolescence we step back and use communication with our teen, observation of their activities, and networking with other adults to guide them. This involves balancing supervision with respect to their privacy.

Monitoring some specific areas has shown to be particularly effective:

*School progress and environment:* Paying attention to teen's grades, progress, and behavior and any disciplinary issues helps in monitoring; to be involved in school events and parent–teacher meetings. Networking with parents of other teens also helps in monitoring.

*Physical and mental health:* To be on the lookout for warning signs of abuse, neglect, depression or mental illness, and poor physical health; talking to teens on ways to properly take care of mind and body; to be a role model for healthy living and seek professional help when necessary.

*Friendships and extracurricular activities:* To get to know teens' friend and romantic partners. To ensure that the activities of the teen match their maturity levels. Network with adults who know the teen like neighbors, friends, teachers, and other parents and ask about teen's behavior.

*Tips for parents:*
- Keep track of teen's whereabouts.
- Keep in touch with other adults.
- Stay informed about teen's progress in school/employment.
- Learn and watch for warning signs of poor physical or mental health.
- To seek proper guidance for the concerns.
- Involve oneself in school events.
- Monitor teen's experiences both inside and outside house.
- Evaluate the challenge levels and the ability of the adolescent to handle them.

## Guide and Limit

*Key message for parents: Loosen up but do not let go control.*

One of the hardest adjustments for parents during adolescence is determining where to set limits and where to let go control. Teens are constantly striving to create their own identity and challenging the status quo. Although it is a natural stage of development, it is hard for the parents to find the balance of keeping their teen safe and maintaining their values, while also encouraging their teen's decision-making skills and respecting their teen's new opinions and beliefs. Teens still need parents to uphold boundaries and family values.

Two key parenting principles in this regard:

1. *To combine rules and expectations with respect and responsiveness:* Parents need to set limits that allow adolescents to develop and maintain their own opinions and beliefs. The reasoning behind the rules needs to be explained.
2. *To combine firmness and flexibility:* All teens need skills to negotiate rules and resolve conflicts with parents in ways that are respectful both to the parent and teen.

Studies have shown that adolescents who feel their parents have consistently violated their individuality through disrespectful, controlling, or manipulative actions have significantly higher rates of problem behaviors.

Physical punishment has been associated with a number of negative effects including rebellion, depression, and aggressive behavior.

*Tips for parents*:
- Maintain family rules and values.
- To communicate expectations which are realistic.
- To use discipline as a tool for teaching not for revenge.
- Restrict punishment that does not cause physical or emotional injury.
- Renegotiate responsibilities and privileges according to teen's changing abilities.

## Model and Consult

*Key messages for parents: Parents still matter, teens still care.*

While teens are influenced by an increasing number of adults and peers during adolescence, parents remain surprisingly influential. Values and beliefs that teens hold on to on major issues tend to be similar to those of parents. Adolescents whose parents model appropriate behavior have better skills and attitudes regarding academic achievement, employment, health habits, individuality, relationships, communication, coping, and conflict resolution. Studies show that parents who have a stronger connection to their teens tend to have more influence on teen's decisions, as do parents who choose ways of imparting ideas that are respectful of the adolescent's developing maturity in thought and action.

Teens need environments and opportunities that enable them to learn from mistakes, as well as try new coping strategies and experience success.

*Tips for parents:*
- Set good example and model behavior.
- Answer teen's queries truthfully while taking into account their level of maturity.
- Maintain or establish traditions—family, cultural, and religious.
- Support teen's educational and vocational training.
- Help teen get information on future options and strategies for education, employment, and lifestyle choices.
- Give teen opportunities to practice reasoning and decision making.
- Model the kind of adult relationships that you would like teens to.

## ■ PROVIDE AND ADVOCATE

*Key messages for parents: You cannot control your teen's world, but you can definitely change it.*

As parents you have responsibility to provide positive resources for your children, such as education, healthcare, guidance, and support. And when they are not receiving them, it is the parent's role to advocate for them. Providing and advocating for resources helps the teen to prepare for the adult world and overcome the societal barriers. For parents, it is a challenge to accomplish these tasks in the face of obstacles like poverty, racism, oppression, unemployment, domestic violence, and a general lack of community resources. It helps parents to address the issues by collaborating with teens and mentoring them by providing with adult support, guidance, and training.

*Tips for parents:*
- Network within the community, schools, family, religious organization, and social services to identify resources for the teens.
- To make informed decisions regarding school and educational programs. Factors to be taken into account would be safety, social climate, community cohesion,

and mentoring opportunities that fit into teen's style of learning.

- To offer constant support for decision making through teaching by example and dialogue.
- Advocate for preventive health care, treatment, and care for mental illness.
- To identify people and organization to support and inform in handling parental responsibilities and the challenges of raising the adolescent.

Finally, by implementing the aforementioned fundamental principles, parents can create a supportive and loving environment that facilitates optimal physical, mental, emotional, and cognitive growth in children.

Parenting teens is an art, not a science. Every family is different and the relationship between the adolescent and parents is determined by their individual personalities. There can never be absolutes or a "one size fits all" parenting method and parenting would thus differ from family to family.

## ■ KEY MESSAGES

- The majority of things in the world are changing for your children, but do not let your love for them be one of them.
- Monitoring your teen's activities still counts.
- Loosen up but do not let go control.
- Parents still matter, teens still care.
- You cannot control your teen's world, but you can definitely change it.

## ■ RECOMMENDED READING

1. Awesome AYA. (2021). Module for parents and teachers. [online] Available from https://aha.iapindia.org/wp-content/uploads/2021/04/Awesome-AYA-Manual-2020.pdf. [Last accessed April, 2024].
2. Raising Teens. (2018). MIT Work life center. [online] Available from https://hr.mit.edu/static/worklife/raising-teens/five-basics.html. [Last accessed April, 2024].

# 11.4 Positive Discipline

*Gayatri Bezboruah*

## ■ INTRODUCTION

The process of discipline involves a series of well-intended efforts by parents and caregivers to inculcate in the child "the art of controlling oneself." If properly learnt and consistently practiced, discipline becomes a very important foundation for the growth of children. It brings self-confidence, feeling of mastery over life, and positive social experience for children even after growing as adults. The positive feelings themselves add up to bring out a well-behaved and confident parent of the future, who would in turn express positive discipline (PD) techniques successfully. The discipline process should act as "vaccination" against untoward effects of peers, media, and other difficult to handle situations in life.

Discipline by definition means "to teach". However, by tradition, we equate this with punishment. Discipline is also encouraging children, guiding them, and helping them feel good about themselves. The root word of discipline is disciple—a person who leads others in the way they should go. Discipline is not what you do to the child, but what you do with and for the child.

Positive discipline is a model in parenting that focuses on the positive points of behavior. It is based on the belief that good behavior in a child can be developed by teaching and reinforcement, while bad behavior can be weaned off without verbal or physical hurt. Negative discipline, in contrast, usually involves angry, destructive, or violent responses to behavior that is considered inappropriate or unacceptable. Dr Jane Nelsen, who authored the book *Positive Discipline*, focuses on an authoritative method of parenting based on encouragement and problem-solving without using yelling, spanking, or severe punishment. According to Dr Nelsen, there are five criteria for effective PD:

1. It is kind and firm at the same time.
2. It helps children feel a sense of belonging and significance.
3. It is effective long term.
4. It teaches valuable social and life skills for good character.
5. It invites children to discover how capable they are and encourages them to use their personal power in constructive ways.

## COMMON MYTHS IN DISCIPLINING CHILDREN

- Discipline means punishment.
- Disciplining children is the school's responsibility.
- The mother has to be blamed, if child misbehaves. The father is anyway very busy.
- Grandparents never understand what is "good" for children.
- Children should never cry or feel unhappy. Costly gifts should be provided to win them back.
- Quiet children are always well behaved.
- Tomorrow onward my children will behave well, because I have disciplined them today.
- Readymade magic recipes are available for bringing up children.
- I am the only one who is in trouble.
- Spare the rod and spoil the child.

## REASONS FOR MISBEHAVIOR

The possible reasons for a child's misbehavior should be considered before taking any action. The reasons could be:

- A physical illness, feeling of rejection or insecurity ("nobody understands me!"), extreme hunger or sleep, and post-TV boredom and lethargy ("what should I do next?").
- Many a times, children simply test the permissible limits of their misbehaviors, and they note what happens if they break the rules.
- On occasion, the misbehavior could be an attempt to attract the attention of parents, especially when they are busy talking to guests, in whose presence they can misbehave safely, because parents cannot do any harm.
- Most commonly, children simply copy the misbehaviors of their parents, e.g., shouting, hitting, and talking back.

Most of us express all forms of parenting styles, sometimes or the other. Depending on our moods and priorities, we would be either a "cane wielding ring-master"—Authoritarian type, "leave them alone"—Liberal type, "leave me alone"—Avoidant type, or "sit across the table"—Negotiator type. What is desired is a good and "time-appropriate" cocktail of these types.

The short-term goal of discipline is to guide everyday behavior and to protect children from hurting themselves and others. However, the long-term goal should be to bring out a confident, self-disciplined individual, responsible for his/her own behavior, who relies upon self, and is comfortable and happy about it.

## CREATING STRUCTURE IN A CHILD'S DAY

All children need and want structure from their parents even when it comes with some sort of protest before it is accepted.

A structure that helps a child behave is a set of routines and rules that are consistent, predictable, and have follow through. This helps when associated with appropriate expectations and limits for the child's behavior.

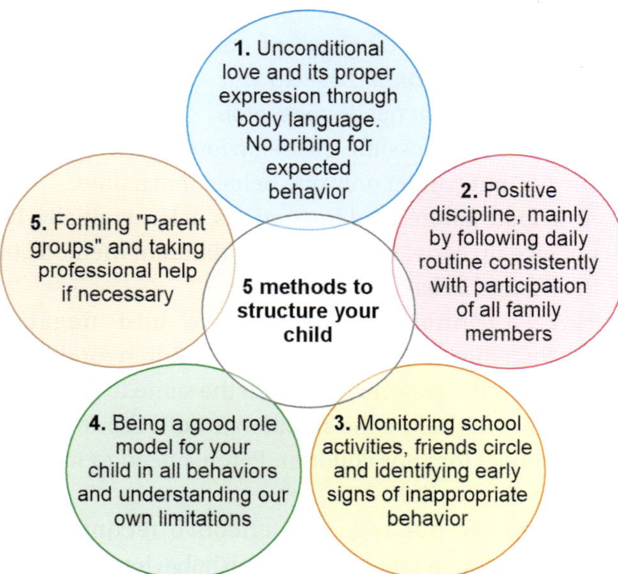


## DO'S AND DON'TS IN DISCIPLINE

- Learn to say "NO" to children, whenever you want to.
- Communicate your expectations very clearly, using only few words. Avoid lectures.
- Ignore minor/harmless behaviors.
- The expectations should be appropriate for the age and developmental stage of the child, culturally acceptable, unanimous, and negotiated well.
- Use positive statements. Avoid saying, "don't". Save "No" or "Don't" for important situations, so the child takes "No" seriously. For example, instead of saying, "don't shout", say, "speak quietly."
- Hold a positive expectation and make children feel responsible and cooperative. The more trust and confidence you place in children, the more they feel worthy of trust and the more trustworthy they become. Never "label" them as bad.

- Acknowledge positive behavior. Praise them *Actively* even for minor good behaviors. Children (even adults) tend to repeat and improve the behavior that is positively noticed by others.
- Lecturing, fighting, impatience, and being punitive only lead to frustration and fatigue for both.
- Be fair, firm, and flexible whenever you make a rule. Make the consequences absolutely clear if the rule is broken, and most importantly follow them.
- Be consistent in whatever strategy is chosen, and involve all the family members.
- Accept your child's feelings, but reinforce your expectations. Active listening is the key.
- Try to separate the behavior from the child. We must give *Unconditional Love* to our children. It is the misbehavior that needs correction.
- Make a list of possible misbehaviors that you want to correct, but correct only one behavior at a time.
- Anticipate failures and frustrations, at least initially. Do not give up early. Keep on trying different methods till the desired behavior is expressed.
- Make rational use of positive and negative reinforcements. Never try to bribe children for desired behavior; the children would do the same to you.
- Take actions before the situation is out of control. Be a role model for your children. Parents need to improve their behavior first.
- Giving time-out is a very effective technique for punishment. In this, following misbehavior, the child is made to remain alone in a nondistracting environment, e.g., a chair facing the wall, for a specified time (usually, 1 minute per year of age is sufficient). During this period, the child is left alone and asked to think about why he is given a time-out.
- Spanking/hitting is best avoided for the reason that we never liked it when we were children. Spanking is blamed for teaching violence to children. Resistance to spanking is fairly common.
  - Spanking is like a nuclear bomb. Always keep, never use. The untoward effects of spanking however are overemphasized nowadays.
- Try to spend quality time with children. Let them know that you also talk to them apart from imparting discipline.
- Be comfortable and consistent with whatever you decide, because whatever you do is right for your child.

There are so many suggestions made by other family members, guests, neighbors, friends, etc., that parents at time get confused, whether they are doing good to themselves and their children? Is the idea of disciplining interfering with the natural child–parent relationship? Our parents never attempted to learn about bringing up children but nothing went wrong, then why should we bother about it now? The answers to these questions could be multidimensional. Family norms are changing. There are only one/two children per family now, and all parents wish to give the best to their children. Nobody wants to accept that every child cannot be at the top. What we are giving to our children is a "filtered" parenting (I keep the troubles with me; my children should never face problems.). In addition, working parents unnecessarily feel guilty for not giving time to their children, but at the same time want their children to win the ever-increasing competitions, may it be studies, sports, or debating.

There are other players in this game, such as grandparents (nowadays rare) and teachers. They have both positive and negative effects and if parents are not unanimous and careful, disciplining soon becomes a topic of conflicts and clashes in the family. Everybody puts the blame on others and eventually avoids the basic aim. In addition, one has to consider the fact that grandparents as well as parents have problems related to their own ages, both physical and psychosocial. The physical capacities are going down; they are at the peak of their careers and have tremendous economic burdens as well. All these factors sometimes lead to a mix-up of strictness and cruelty. Liberal handling and false ideas of "modern" parenting may turn into irresponsibility and risk-taking behaviors.

When the going gets tough, discipline, in combination with understanding, is one of the most precious and lasting gifts parents can give to their children. As they grow up, children will learn the skills necessary to discipline themselves. As parents, we should think back to our childhood. How did we feel when we were ignored? We never felt happy, when somebody shouted at us or spanked us, then why do the same to our children? It is better to stop using words and actions that hurt. Start using words that help.

## ■ AMERICAN ACADEMY OF PEDIATRICS RECOMMENDATIONS

The American Academy of Pediatrics (AAP) recommends PD strategies that effectively teach children to manage their behavior and keep them from harm while promoting healthy development. These include:

- *Show and tell:* Teach children right from wrong with calm words and actions. Model behaviors you would like to see in your children.
- *Set limits:* Have clear and consistent rules your children can follow. Be sure to explain these rules in age-appropriate terms they can understand.
- *Give consequences:* Calmly and firmly explain the consequences if they do not behave. For example, tell her that if she does not pick up her toys, you will put them away for the rest of the day. Be prepared to follow through right away. Do not give in by giving them back after a few minutes. But remember, never take away something your child truly needs, such as a meal.
- *Hear them out:* Listening is important. Let your child finish the story before helping solve the problem. Watch for times when misbehavior has a pattern, like if your child is feeling jealous. Talk with your child about this rather than just giving consequences.
- *Give them your attention:* The most powerful tool for effective discipline is attention, to reinforce good behaviors and discourage others. Remember, all children want their parent's attention.
- *Catch them being good:* Children need to know when they do something bad and when they do something good. Notice good behavior and point it out, praising success and good tries. Be specific (for example, "Wow, you did a good job putting that toy away!").
- *Know when not to respond:* As long as your child is not doing something dangerous and gets plenty of attention for good behavior, ignoring bad behavior can be an effective way of stopping it. Ignoring bad behavior can also teach children natural consequences of their actions. For example, if your child keeps dropping her cookies on purpose, she will soon have no more cookies left to eat. If she throws and breaks her toy, she will not be able to play with it. It will not be long before she learns not to drop her cookies and to play carefully with her toys.
- *Be prepared for trouble:* Plan ahead for situations when your child might have trouble behaving. Prepare them for upcoming activities and how you want them to behave.
- *Redirect bad behavior:* Sometimes children misbehave, because they are bored or do not know any better. Find something else for your child to do.
- *Call a time-out:* A time-out can be especially useful when a specific rule is broken. This discipline tool works best by warning children they will get a time-out if they do not stop, reminding them what they did wrong in as few words—and with as little emotion—as possible, and removing them from the situation for a preset length of time (1 minute per year of age is a good rule of thumb). With children who are at least 3 years old, you can try letting their children lead their own time-out instead of setting a timer. You can just say, go to time-out and come back when you feel ready and in control." This strategy, which can help the child learn and practice self-management skills, also works well for older children and teens.

The concept and meaning of PD can be easily summarized as follows:

- *D:* Daily routine
- *I:* Ignoring minor misbehaviors
- *S:* Setting limits of unacceptable behaviors
- *C:* Consistency
- *I:* Informal talk and methods of disciplining children
- *P:* Patience and persistence
- *L:* Love (unconditional)
- *I:* Involving every family member (including guests)
- *N:* No nagging/labeling or lecturing
- *E:* Empathy and Education by being a good role model.

## ■ KEY MESSAGES

- Discipline involves a series of efforts by parents and caregivers to inculcate in the child "the art of controlling oneself."
- Discipline is teaching the child right behavior rather than punishing him for wrong behavior.
- Misbehavior could be due to a physical illness, feeling of rejection or insecurity ("nobody understands me!"), extreme hunger or sleep, and post-TV boredom and lethargy ("what should I do next?"). It could also be the child's desire to test the limits, an attempt to attract parental attention, or simply imitating parental misbehavior.
- Specific do's and don'ts of discipline have been discussed, and also the AAP guidelines on discipline.

## ■ RECOMMENDED READING

1. AACAP. Parenting: preparing for adolescence. [online] Available from https://www.aacap.org/AACAP/Families_and_Youth/Facts_for_Families/FFF-Guide/Parenting-Preparing-For-Adolescence-056.aspx [Last accessed April, 2024].

2. Adolescent parenting. How and why it is different. Bhave SY, Pratt H, Kanikar A (Eds). In: Parthasarathy S, Bhave SY, Nair MKC, Menon PSN, Greydanus DE (Eds). Bhave's Textbook of Adolescent Medicine. New Delhi: Jaypee Brothers Medical Publishers. pp. 875-85.

3. Kanikar A, Bhave SY. Positive discipline. In: Parthasarathy S, Bhave SY, Nair MKC, Menon PSN, Greydanus DE (Eds). Bhave's Textbook of Adolescent Medicine. New Delhi: Jaypee Brothers Medical Publishers. pp. 854-9.

4. Nair MKC. Parenting adolescents. Indian Pediatr. 2004;41:887-90.

5. Parenting. [online] Available from http://www.focusas.com/parenting.html [Last accessed April, 2024].

6. Parenting. Type of parenting. In: Nair MKC, Pejaver RK (Eds). Adolescent Care 2000 & Beyond. pp. 137-8.

7. Parenting programs. In: Bhave S, Kanikar A (Eds). Course Manual for Adolescent Health. pp. 266-9.

8. Sachs SL, Newby K. Fathering your adolescent: Way to strengthen your relationship. [online] Available from https://ohioline.osu.edu/factsheet/HYG-5298 [Last accessed April, 2024].

9. Shannon L, Sachs HYG. Communicating with your Teen. 5158-96. [online] Available from chrome-extension://efaidnbmnnnibpcajpcglclefindmkaj/https://www.fatherhood.gov/sites/default/files/resource_files/e000002410.pdf [Last accessed April, 2024].

<table>
<tr><td>**11.5**</td><td># Identification and Interventions for a Child/Teenager at Risk</td></tr>
</table>

*Sudhir Mishra*

## ■ INTRODUCTION

Children and adolescents are reared in families and society. Values and culture of the parents' origin as well as the culture in which the family is living at present affect the child-rearing practices. Each family/parent is different in their attitude toward children. In the same family, the manner in which one parent handles the child may be different from the way the other parent inculcates (or does not) discipline. Therefore, it is important for us to understand the parenting styles before we look at the interventions. Protective and risk factors for the teenage and youth are described elsewhere in the chapter.

## ■ PARENTING STYLES

Though parenting styles may be a mix of the described patterns, or vary from one situation to the other, they are generally classified into four types.

1. *Authoritarian parents:* This type of parents create and implement rules strictly. Orders/advice is passed through one-way communication. There is no scope or willingness to understand the child's point of view. Children/adolescents are expected to follow the instructions or comply with the guidance. These children may appear as the most well-behaved children in class. However, they have poor self-esteem and are unable to make decisions for themselves. As these adolescents move out of home, they may become aggressive and tend to indulge in unacceptable behavior, even to the extent of going on the wrong side of the law.

2. *Authoritative parents:* These parents have clearly defined boundaries and goals. Children have a say in deciding the goals and methods or practices adopted to meet the goals. They grow up as self-confident children, capable of making independent decisions, and usually have good academic performance.

3. *Permissive parents:* These parents are warm and caring. They do not set rules, because of which children do not learn self-regulation. As children decide their own snacks, screen time, and bedtime, they run the risk of being indulgent and are likely to suffer from the health effects of unregulated diet and screen time. These children are demanding, impulsive, and lack self-control.

4. *Uninvolved parents:* Sometimes also called negligent parents, they have very little communication regarding expectations from children. There is no disciplining. Children become self-sufficient, out of necessity. They may have good self-esteem. However, coping abilities are not sufficiently developed and they are likely to have a breakdown in a stressful situation. They can move to the wrong side of the law very easily.

## INTERVENTIONS FOR PARENTS

Interventions for parents can be divided into general and targeted interventions. Interventions for parents are based on the knowledge that parents play a crucial and decisive role in adolescent health behavior. Therefore, the interventions are targeted at improving the knowledge and skill sets of parents to modify adolescent health behavior in a positive manner.

Before planning interventions, it is important to know the parental expectations and the area of their interest. There are not many studies on the subject, none from India to the best of my knowledge. A study from the United States of America (USA) explored this aspect, and though limited to certain disadvantaged ethnic groups, provides insight about the expectations of parents. Behavior change (36%) and managing transition years (23%) were described as the most difficult part of parenting. Mental health was considered an issue by 10% parents only and 10% parents had no difficulties. Even then, 87% parents were interested in parenting programs. Areas on which parents wanted guidance were communication with adolescents (65%) and conflict management (50%). The health-related topics where guidance was sought include sex (77%), mental health (75%), and alcohol and drugs (70%). The majority of parents wanted guidance from a pediatrician (61.5%) and clinical psychologist (23%) rather than a social worker or nurse. Written literature and technology like mobile apps or references to websites were considered the preferable method of delivering parental guidance over physical conversation.

## DESIGNING PARENTAL GUIDANCE PROGRAM

The United Nations Children's Fund (UNICEF) provides guidance for developing parenting programs on a large scale like national or state levels. On a smaller scale, Jaccard describes two types of parenting programs. One is a positive adolescent development program where the focus is on maximizing positive development and  adolescent performance in academics and other life skills. The other is to focus on specific problem behavior.

## INTERVENTIONS AT THE INDIVIDUAL LEVEL

At the individual level, the focus of intervention is the issues being faced by the parents/adolescent. This will initially involve assessment of adolescents for various physical, mental, sexual, and academic performance of the child and future goals as envisaged by the child and parents. This last area is important and is often missed in assessment as differences in future goals are more and more frequently seen these days. Even while dealing with individual issues, proactive guidance on communication and identification of mental stress and possible mental disorders should be given, as all parents may not be aware of these issues.

## INTERVENTIONS AT GROUP LEVEL: GENERAL INTERVENTIONS

General interventions at the group level need proper planning with respect to parent groups, place of interaction, method of intervention, time needed, resource person, etc.

For identification of parent groups, schools may be a good starting point. Identification of parents from a school has the advantage of ease of identification. School teachers and administration, however, need to be explained the purpose of intervention and taken on board. Once the school administration and teachers are on board, they can help with the identification of problematic adolescents and apparently healthy adolescents. Although this identification is obviously not foolproof, it can still help in devising parental intervention in a way that is most helpful for the parents. Interaction should take place in a comfortable environment. School premises is usually available, with the help of school administration, and is an excellent place as parents are acquainted with the surroundings. Selection of parents through school also offers the advantage of having parents from more or less similar educational and financial backgrounds, who are likely to have similar issues in dealing with adolescents.

General interventions should focus on communication between parents and adolescents, mental health issues, especially the clues to identify a child in distress or in need of support, sexual health, expectations of parents from the child in academic and other area of child's interest and avoidance of forced education in a stream of the parent's interest.

### Initiation of the Program

In the beginning, there should be a small session on introduction of the resource persons and parents. Appreciation of parents for their presence and that they are doing the best possible for their children is a must.

If relevant, it should be stated that this program is focused on further improvement in adolescent performance rather than correcting issues. If time permits (where the group is small enough), one expectation of parent should be asked for and noted so that the issues can be addressed in the course of interaction. Words of appreciation for school and school administration and teachers must follow. The introduction of the subject involves stressing on the need and importance of the program while still maintaining that most parents already know enough on the subject to allow us to learn from each other.

## Body of the Program

Time management is a real challenge in all such programs. Topics should be prioritized based on the initial interaction with parents. This is required as topics taken up initially invariably get more time, and therefore will have greater satisfaction in the audience. Questions from parents must be answered adequately. In case time constraints does not permit answering all questions, email or phone numbers may be shared for continued interaction.

## Closing

The closing of program should summarize the discussion with a reminder of actionable points.

## PROGRAMS TARGETED AT SPECIFIC PROBLEM BEHAVIOR

The programs targeted at specific problem behavior are more difficult to organize as identification and assembling parents of adolescents with similar problem behaviors are more difficult. However, delivering such program is easier as expectations are limited to one such behavior and all parents are likely to be more interested than the general audience. The basic steps for organizing the program remain the same as stated above and should be followed.

## METHODS OF DELIVERING THE INTERVENTIONS

Parents of adolescents are different from one another in many ways. Most important is the time and availability. Dominant learning styles of different individuals are different. Important ones are auditory, visual, kinesthetic, and reading/writing. Each individual learns by all methods to some extent. However, in adults, the preference becomes more pronounced. Considering this aspect, intervention programs can and should be delivered on multiple platforms. Common and effective methods are classroom-style intervention, educational leaflets and books, technology-driven like videos, audios, blogs, or scientific write up. Given the choice of parent, the platform can and should be used.

## COMMUNICATION BETWEEN PARENTS AND ADOLESCENTS

Many times parents find it difficult to communicate with adolescents, especially on sensitive issues like mental and sexual health. Initiating communication is the key to successful intervention by parents. Various methods may be adopted to initiate communication, for example, reading a small story together or discussing the story after the adolescent has read it. Initiating communication through news items being shown on television, for example, a violence issue or rape story may help parents in initiating conversation on the subject of violence and sex, respectively. Discussion on important holidays like festivals and national holidays, for example, *Rakshabandhan* may be used to inculcate respect for all girls, and 2nd October to discuss violence and its impact. Diwali may be used to discuss environmental issues from where the link with mental health may be taken. World Mental Health Day (10th October) can also be used to discuss mental health issues, and World Human Immunodeficiency Virus (HIV) Day to initiate conversation on HIV leading to other sexual health issues. These are just a few examples to educate parents in identifying appropriate opportunities.

## KEY MESSAGES

- The four classically described parenting styles are authoritarian, authoritative, permissive, and uninvolved parenting. In practice, a mix of styles is common, and it varies with the situation.
- Interventions are targeted at parents to improve their knowledge and skills, so that they can modify their adolescents' health behavior in a positive manner.
- Parents wanted guidance on communication with adolescents (65%) and conflict management (50%). The health-related topics where guidance was sought include sex (77%), mental health (75%), and alcohol and drugs (70%). They preferred guidance from a pediatrician (61.5%) and clinical psychologist (23%) rather than a social worker or a nurse.

- It is comparatively easier to arrange parent groups for such programs in schools through school administrators and teachers.
- As parents find it difficult to communicate with adolescents, especially on sensitive issues like mental and sexual health, they may be advised to initiate the discussion by discussing a story after the adolescent has read it, or news items on television about violence or rape. They can also discuss respect for girls on Rakshabandhan, violence on Gandhi Jayanti, environmental issues at Diwali, Mental health on World Mental Health Day, etc.

## RECOMMENDED READING

1. Atlantic University. (2024). 8 Types of Learning Styles: The Definitive Guide. [online] Available from https://bau.edu/blog/types-of-learning-styles/ [Last accessed April, 2024].
2. Jaccard J, Levitz N. Parent-based interventions to reduce adolescent problem behaviors: New directions for self-regulation approaches. In: Oettingen G, Gollwitzer P (Eds.). Self-Regulation in Adolescence. New York: Cambridge University Press; 2013. pp. 357-88.
3. Jones LD, Grout RW, Gilbert AL, Wilkinson TA, Garbuz T, Downs SM, et al. How can healthcare professionals provide guidance and support to parents of adolescents? Results from a primary care-based study. BMC Health Serv Res. 2021;21(1):253.
4. Masud H, Ahmad MS, Cho KW, Fakhr Z. Parenting styles and aggression among young adolescents: a systematic review of literature. Community Ment Health J. 2019;55(6):1015-30.
5. Sanvictores T, Mendez MD. Types of Parenting Styles and Effects on Children. In: StatPearls [Internet]. Treasure Island (FL): StatPearls Publishing; 2024. [online]. Available from https://www.ncbi.nlm.nih.gov/books/NBK568743/ [Last accessed April, 2024].
6. UNICEF. (2024). Parenting of adolescents programming guidance. [online] Available from https://www.unicef.org/documents/parenting-adolescents-programming-guidance [Last accessed April, 2024].

---

# 11.6    Single Parenting

*Usha Banga*

## WHAT DOES SINGLE PARENTING MEAN?

A single parent is a person who has children but does not have a spouse or live-in partner to support or raise them. 23% of children under the age of 18 years live with a single parents in the United States. Since 1960s, the number of children living with a single parent has increased. This is due to the increase in the number of unmarried women having children and the increasing prevalence of divorce.

## PROBLEMS AND DISADVANTAGES OF A ONE-PARENT FAMILY

Every family's situation is different, yet studies show that children raised in single-parent homes face more struggles and obstacles than those raised in two-parent homes. Some disadvantages of single-parent homes are as follows:

- *Less money:* A single mother/father earns less money than two. This can lead to food insecurity, not being able to provide essential things for children, not having access to a good education, and even slipping into poverty.
- *Lack of meaningful time, support, and attention:* Single parents often have to work multiple jobs to make ends meet and are therefore not always available to their children. This busyness reduces the meaningful time spent together. When the child needs help, the parent is not around. They are not able to pay much attention to the child.
- *Health and behavioral issues:* Single parents often have to do a lot on their own, so problems with their children's health and behavior may arise because there is no extra support to help with parenting. These children may often feel inferior due to the fact that the mother or father is absent from their lives. These emotions can affect the child's behavior and even cause many psychological problems in the child.
- *Concerns about the future:* These children are more likely to have problems that affect their lives as they grow up, such as problems with educational attainment and employment.

## ■ IMPACT ON CHILDREN

Living in a single-parent family can be associated with many problems:

- School failure
- Crime
- Drug problems
- Teenage pregnancy
- Poverty
- Dependence on social assistance and welfare.

Children living with single parents have been found to have worse physical health behavior, mental health, bullying, cultural activities, sports, and family relationships than children from typical families. In contrast, children in a shared parenting arrangement who lived with their divorced mother and father for approximately equal amount of time were found to be better off.

Both British and American researchers show that children without fathers are three times more likely to be unhappy and also more likely to engage in antisocial behavior, substance abuse, and juvenile delinquency.

## ■ ENCOURAGE POSITIVE BEHAVIOR WHEN YOU ARE A SINGLE PARENT

If you are a single parent, a positive relationship with the child will help the child feel secure and loved which makes it easier for them to deal with any family problems. A positive relationship will also improve your mental health. Some ways you can improve your relationship with your child are as follows:

*Make the most of everyday moments:* Spend quality time with your child, anytime, anywhere. Show interest in it. Talk about the child's favorite things, from sports to music to books to how things work. Ask your child to show you his or her favorite app or teach you how to play his or her favorite game. Try going to school performances or sporting events.

*Pay attention to the child:* Respond to the child with warmth and interest no matter how upset you are. This can also happen by smiling, laughing, or hugging the child. You should also show your child through your behavior that you are happy to see them first thing in the morning and greet them with a smile when they come home from school.

*Communicate directly:* If you have more than one child, try to spend some time alone with each child on a regular basis. This could be a book with the younger child before bed or a game with the older child after the younger child falls asleep.

*Set clear rules:* Clear rules and limits will encourage your child to behave appropriately. You should maintain the same standards as you would in a joint family.

*Try to be consistent:* If you guide the child's behavior in a consistent way, he should understand that some rules hold even in changed circumstances.

*Use established routines:* Routines make it clear who should do what, when, in what order, and how often. You should schedule your daily routine according to your work, office, and child's school so that you get enough time to spend with your child.

*Tune into emotions:* Your child may be feeling certain emotions like frustration, anger, shame, or sadness. Behave according to the mental state of the child, ask him questions, and satisfy his curiosity. If you are divorced and the child is grown up, explain your situation to him. If the child is ever agitated with his emotions, you can help him calm down. Sometimes, if the child starts feeling guilty, then talk to him to remove his guilt.

## ■ STAY POSITIVE

Even when it is the only way out, many single parents raise happy, healthy children. Children do well when they are raised to be sensitive, responsive, and warm regardless of whether mother or father is the only one in their life. You can raise your child despite family difficulties:

- Think about ways to meet your child's needs.
- Stay calm and control your emotions and reactions. Do not get nervous.
- Get help from family and friends.

If you are single parenting because of a separation or divorce, reassure the child that both of his or her parents still love him or her and that your separation is not your child's fault.

If you are concerned about your child's behavior, a good first step is to talk to your child's doctor, teacher, or counselor.

## ■ BE KIND TO YOURSELF

As a single parent, people are sometimes hard on themselves. Do not be hard on yourself for doing your best, even when things do not go according to plan.

Being kind to yourself is good for your mental health and well-being. This helps you feel less stressed and less anxious so that you can give your baby the environment he needs to grow well. Remember, raising children is a big job. Other parents find it difficult too—you are not alone in these situations.

In these circumstances, you may forget to take care of yourself, but remember that taking care of yourself physically, mentally, and emotionally will be good for you and your child. As a single parent, your positive attitude, strength, and determination can become an example for your child.

In all families, parents may feel sad, angry, or upset during times of stress. When this happens, it is important to let your child know that you love him or her and that your feelings and reactions are not about him or her. Reassure your child that things will get better and that you have people who will help you.

If your child is old enough to understand, discuss your problems honestly with the child. For example, "I had a bad day at work today" or "I'm not in a good mood right now". By expressing their feelings, children will also easily tell you their feelings and problems. But keep big issues out of discussion with your child. Adult problems—such as money worries, relationship problems, or conflicts with your child's other parent—can cause great distress to the child.

As a single parent, you may need help. Never hesitate in taking or giving help. Choose the right person for help, so that you and your child stay safe. This could be practical help with day-to-day tasks, emotional support for you, or information and advice.

## WHY IS SINGLE PARENTING HARD?

Single parenting is difficult because you have to do everything on your own. You may find yourself feeling frustrated, tired, and stressed at times as you juggle things like cooking dinner and getting the kids' clothes ready for school. There is no one else around to help.

The biggest problem for single parents is finances. Responsibilities become greater when one is alone; everything must be taken care of like education, food, shelter, clothing, and saving for the future. Mothers suffer more from lack of money because not all of them have employment. Single fathers do not often face lack of money because most of them have employment.

There is another difficulty—loneliness. The single parent has no one to talk to about their problems. Loneliness becomes more troubling when children grow up or go away for studies or employment.

## IS IT DIFFICULT TO BE A SINGLE MOTHER IN INDIA?

In India, being a single mother by choice, or having a child out of wedlock, is a very difficult task: Our society still does not accept it.

Many wives of martyred soldiers have raised their children with difficulty. For mothers left alone due to road accidents, illnesses, and other reasons, life is very difficult. Due to lack of money and time, children do not get time to talk with their parents and feel isolated. Due to lack of money, even the things necessary for the life of the child are not available.

## HOW TO BE A CAPABLE SINGLE PARENT?

- Set your goal.
- Stay organized.
- Be flexible.
- Be determined.
- Ask for help.
- Believe in yourself.
- Be optimistic.
- If possible, give something back to the society.

## LEGAL RIGHTS OF A SINGLE MOTHER IN INDIA

The Indian Constitution has tried to equip women with legal rights so that they can take care of the children themselves.

*Right to privacy:* Single mothers are given the right to privacy if they do not wish to disclose the name of the child's father. The right to privacy is inherent in the right to life and liberty guaranteed to the citizens of this country by Article 21. The right to be alone is inherent in it.

Section 13 of the Hindu Maintenance and Guardianship Act, 1956 states that the welfare of the minor shall be paramount. The welfare of the child comes first. There is no obligation for an unmarried mother to reveal the identity of the child's father as she can be the full legal guardian of her child.

*Guardianship rights:* Generally, the mother is the natural guardian of the child till the age of 5 years, but after that the father is the natural guardian. Furthermore, after the death of the father, the mother is granted full guardianship rights. The Guardianship and Wards Act, 1890, and the Hindu Minority and Guardianship Act, 1956 (HMGA), are the two major acts that state the right of guardianship of a parent or any other person. In section 6 of the Hindu Marriage Act, it states that in the case of a married couple, the father is the natural guardian of the child, and the rights of the mother are recognized next to the father. However, when a child is born out of wedlock, the mother becomes the natural guardian, and the father has no legal obligations.

*Right to use the mother's surname:* Every child has the right to use his or her mother's surname as his or her own surname. A single mother providing sole custody of a minor child may give the child her maiden name.

*Child's right to know who his parents are:* The Supreme Court also upheld a child's right to know who his or her parents are, but this information must be kept private, kept in an envelope that is properly sealed, and only then disclosed. This will be done when the court considers it to be in the best interests of the child.

## CONCLUSION: WHO IS MORE IMPORTANT—THE MOTHER OR THE FATHER?

The ideal situation is to have both. Research shows that a father's love and care is as important as a mother's love for children's health and well-being. In fact children are better off when their fathers are sensitive, secure and supportive, as well as close, nurturing and warm.

## ■ KEY MESSAGES

- A single parent is a person who has children but does not have a spouse or live-in partner to support or raise them. The number is increasing due to the increase in the number of unmarried women having children and the increasing prevalence of divorce.
- Some disadvantages of single parenting are having less money, inadequate time to spend with the children, more health and behavioral issues in the children, and concerns about the children's future educational attainment and employment.
- Children living in a single-parent family are more likely to suffer from school failure, crime, drug problems, teenage pregnancy, poverty, and dependence on social welfare.
- To foster a healthy relationship with the children, a single parent should spend quality time with them, behave warmly toward them always, spend a little time alone with each of them, set clear rules and limits, try to be consistent, use established routines, and tune into their emotions.
- *Stay positive:* Many single parents raise happy, healthy children.
- Be kind to yourself, even when things do not go according to plan. It is good for your mental health and well-being and makes you feel less stressed and less anxious so that you can raise your child up in a happy environment.
- Single parenting is difficult because of financial difficulties, having to do everything by oneself, and feeling lonely.
- Being a single parent is more difficult in India because being a single mother by choice, or having a child out of wedlock, is not accepted socially.
- The law protects the legal right of the single mother to privacy if she does not wish to disclose the name of the child's father, guardianship rights if the child is born out of wedlock, and the right to use the mother's surname.

## ■ RECOMMENDED READING

1. Legal Upanishad. Single mother rights in India: Everything you need to know. [online] Available from https://legalupanishad.com/rights-of-a-single-mother-in-india/#:~:text= Section%206%20of%20the%20HMGA, father%20has%20no%20legal%20obligation. [Last accessed April, 2024].

# 11.7 Distant Parenting

*Harinder Singh, Anuradha Bansal*

## ■ INTRODUCTION

Parenting adolescents is often considered a challenging endeavor, but the task becomes even more complex when geographical distance separates parents from their adolescent children. Distant parenting of adolescents can take various forms, such as adolescents staying in hostels for education or those moving abroad for work or studies. According to the Ministry of Statistics and Programme Implementation (MoSPI), nearly 4.1 million adolescents and young adults reside in hostels across the length and breadth of the country (2019–20). Likewise in 2022 alone, 750 thousand adolescents and young adults left India for the purpose of studies or work in foreign nations.

Hence, knowledge about managing distant parenting is the need of the hour for modern-day parents. In this chapter, we will explore the intricacies of distant parenting and delve into strategies to maintain a strong connection and effectively communicate with adolescents in these situations. As pediatricians, we need to equip ourselves with strategies to offer insights and guidance to parents facing this unique parenting challenge.

## UNDERSTANDING ISSUES RELATED TO DISTANT PARENTING

### Early and Mid Adolescence

*Adolescents moving to hostels for education:* Adolescence is a critical developmental stage marked by heightened independence, identity exploration, and the desire for autonomy. When adolescents must stay in hostels for education, they often face a multitude of new experiences, responsibilities, and challenges. Some of them include:

- Feeling of loneliness
- Missing the familiar home atmosphere
- Getting familiar with hostel food
- Getting accustomed to the unfamiliar surroundings and making new friends
- Adaptation to the new teaching–learning system.

All these factors increase the risk of psychological problems in already vulnerable adolescents.

Moreover, the feeling of autonomy, peer pressure, and lack of parental supervision might expose them to the risk of substance abuse and unsafe sexual activity.

For parents too, it is an altogether different experience. Adapting to distant parenting can be emotionally taxing, as they are forced to relinquish some degree of control and face uncertainty about their child's well-being. They are dependent on limited phone conversations and holiday visits to ensure their child's well-being.

### Late Adolescence

*Adolescents moving to hostels or going abroad for higher studies or work:* During late adolescence, many teens move abroad for higher education or better work opportunities. In addition to the challenges of distant parenting mentioned above, these adolescents seek more autonomy. Some of them do not like to stay connected to their family, feeling they are grown up and too busy. It is important to stay connected with them to help them stay on the right path and help them seek support if the need arises.

## ■ MANAGING DISTANT PARENTING

Parents can be advised the following strategies to help their children cope up with the new surroundings in their absence:

### Set Up a Schedule for Phone Calls

It is crucial to stay connected when adolescents are living away from their parents. The quality of parent–child communication positively influences adolescent adjustment. A systematic review recommends positive parent–child communication, characterized by openness, warmth, and freedom of choice, for better well-being of children as well as adolescents.

Technology can be a wonderful tool for bridging the geographical distance in communication. Keeping in mind the time zones and adolescents' school or work as well as extra-curricular schedule, parents should set aside a time for a phone call each day. They should keep this time distraction-free so that they can discuss their child's concerns freely. Keeping a consistent schedule will allow the parent–teen duo to connect regularly.

However, adolescent should be told that in case they run into any trouble (with friends or teachers), face any health issue, or want to share something urgently, they may call their parents anytime. Teens should also be given the option to text their parents, in case neither of the parents is available to pick up phone calls. It is not always necessary to fix the problem for them but listening to their feelings is important.

A family WhatsApp group or chats on Messenger also make a good option to stay connected even if there is little time for phone calls, as in case of late adolescents who are busy with their jobs. This gives a sense of reassurance to the teenager and parents can rest assured to be updated about their children as and when the need arises.

### Setting Up the Calendar

Parents can set their work schedule according to their teen's school calendar. They should try to ensure that they have some free time at hand when their teen comes home during hostel vacation. This gives them a feeling of being wanted and emotional security.

### Show Interest in Their Life

Adolescents need to feel that their parents are genuinely interested in their experiences and challenges. Parents may ask questions about their studies, activities, and social life in a nonjudgemental, friendly manner. Being empathetic and actively listening can help adolescents feel connected and fosters positive outcomes in adolescent development.

### Plan Visits Whenever Possible

Parents can make plans to visit their child at their hostel. This provides an opportunity to experience their environment, meet their friends, and support them in person. These visits can strengthen the parent–teen bond and offer a sense of security.

### Respect Their Privacy

If teens are studying in a hostel, they are definitely going to ask for some more privacy and autonomy. There needs to be a fine balance between freedom and parental support. Parents should respect their boundaries and let the teens make minor decisions themselves. Adolescents who feel

they have control over their lives tend to adapt better to life away from home.

However, for the safety of adolescent, being a silent member of their social media groups and following their social media handles can help keep a watch from a distance.

### Role of Local Guardians

It is preferable to have a local guardian or mentor who is dependable and may be available to the teen in case of an emergency.

### Keeping Note of Special Days

In distance parenting, parents should take special care to wish their children on their birthdays, and note the examination results and any other competitions their teens are participating in. They can text a heartfelt note, send a card, or small meaningful gifts to foster a better connection with their teens.

### Financial Literacy

Teens living away from their parents need to manage their day-to-day finances themselves. It is pertinent to advise them on managing their finances wisely. Keeping a record of daily expenses, differentiating between needs and wants, and saving for the rainy day are some of the strategies that every teen must know.

### Do Not Ignore Their Mistakes

Distance parenting does not mean ignoring the child's mistakes. As parents get to spend very little time with their teen, they might be tempted to be the "fun parents" to cherish the good times with their child. However, discipline and course correction should not take a backseat. Parents need to keep a watch on their teen's behavior and correct them wherever needed in a stern but friendly manner.

### ■ LOOK OUT FOR WARNING SIGNS

The following signs should alert the parents about the well-being of their adolescents. Any of these signs should prompt them to visit their child or discuss the issue with their teachers or mentors:

- Scholastic deterioration
- Avoiding eye contact during video calls
- Wants to be left alone
- Loss of interest in sports and recreation

- Crying constantly or unusually cheerful
- Antisocial behavior
- In case, any abnormal behavior persists longer than 2 weeks, parents must visit the teen and seek help from a pediatrician. If paying a visit is impossible, the local guardian or mentor may be asked to intervene.

## MANAGING PARENTAL ANXIETY AND CONCERNS

It can be overwhelming for parents to send their children away for the sake of education or work. Depression and anxiety are common issues with parent–teen separation. Parents should:

- *Stay informed but avoid overmonitoring:* While it is important to stay informed about their adolescent's well-being, parents should avoid excessive monitoring, which can create feelings of mistrust. Striking a balance between being a concerned parent and respecting their autonomy is crucial.
- *Seek support and counseling:* Parents often experience their own emotional challenges when their adolescents are far away. Seeking support from friends, family, or professional counselors can provide a healthy outlet for concerns and worries **(Fig. 1)**.
- Distance parenting of adolescents staying in hostels or living abroad is a unique and challenging journey. To foster a strong connection and effective communication with adolescents in these situations, parents must adapt their parenting style to accommodate their child's developmental needs. Open communication, empathy, and respect for their emerging autonomy are essential components of successful distant parenting. While geographical distance may create hurdles, with the right strategies and support, parents can maintain meaningful connections with their adolescents and support them as they navigate this crucial stage of development.

## KEY MESSAGES

- Over 4 million adolescents and young adults reside in hostels across the length and breadth of country, and nearly a million leave India annually for the purpose of studies or work in foreign nations.
- Parenting adolescents is a challenging endeavor, but it becomes even more complex when geographical distance separates parents from their adolescent children.
- Some problems the adolescents face are loneliness, missing the home atmosphere, having to get used to hostel food, adjusting to unfamiliar surroundings and making new friends, and adapting to a new teaching–learning system.
- Parents too are stressed, as they are forced to relinquish some degree of control and face uncertainty about their child's well-being. Older adolescents may demand full autonomy and may not want to remain connected to their families.
- Parents can stay connected by having a fixed schedule for a brief daily phone call to the adolescent. Additionally, the adolescent should feel free to phone them anytime there is an urgent need. Parents can form a family WhatsApp group too.
- Parents should show genuine interest in their experiences and challenges, and discuss their studies, activities, and social life in a nonjudgemental, friendly manner. They should keep a note of special days like birthdays, examination days, and competitions. They should be a silent observer of their social media pages. They can arrange a local guardian for emergencies.
- Parents should ensure free time whenever the adolescents come home on vacation, and plan visits whenever possible.
- While giving adolescents more privacy and autonomy, they should continue to be active parents, teach financial literacy, correct their mistakes, and guide them.

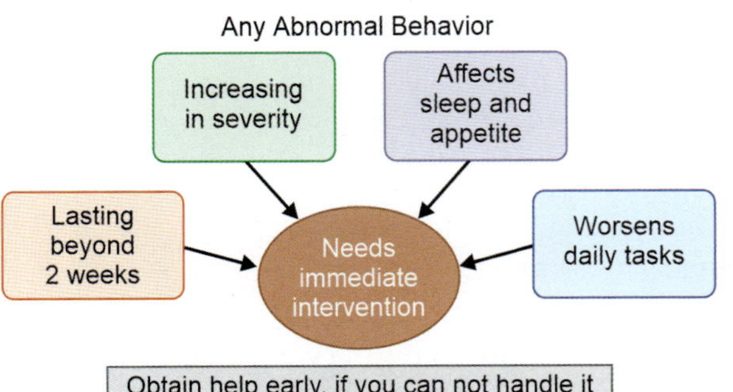


**Fig. 1:** When to seek help for teen issues.

## RECOMMENDED READING

1. Grey EB, Atkinson L, Chater A, Gahagan A, Tran A, Gillison FB. A systematic review of the evidence on the effect of parental communication about health and health

behaviours on children's health and wellbeing. Prev Med. 2022;159:107043.

2. Jovial N. (2023). Why more and more Indian students are going abroad. [online] Available from https://www.theweek.in/theweek/specials/2023/03/18/traps-in-student-migration-causes-challenges [Last accessed April, 2024].

3. National Statistical Office, Ministry of Statistics and Programme Implementation, Government of India. (2022). Statement 45 (c): State-wise number of hostels, intake, and student residing (Based on actual response). Youth in India, 2022. [online] Available from https://mospi.gov.in/sites/default/files/publication_reports/Youth_in_India_2022.pdf [Last accessed April, 2024].

4. Smith LE, Maybach AM, Feldman A, Darling A, Akard TF, Gilmer MJ. Parent and Child Preferences and Styles of Communication About Cancer Diagnoses and Treatment. J Pediatr Oncol Nurs. 2019;36(6):390-401.

# Sports Medicine

***Section Editor:*** *SM Prasad*

## 12.1 Preparticipation Evaluation

*Prashanth MR*

### INTRODUCTION

The Center for Disease Control and Prevention recommends moderate-to-vigorous physical activity on a regular basis for all adolescents. Studies have shown that adolescents who participate in sports have a reduced risk of depression. They are more successful at maintaining healthy relationship with others and maintain heathy lifestyles. Physical activity has favorable effects on hypertension, obesity, and serum lipid levels in youths. Hence, pediatricians should promote physical activity to their patients.

Sports preparticipation examination is to recognize mechanisms of injury and enforcing rules that reduce the likelihood of that mechanism of injury. It is one setting for implementing some of these prevention strategies and for detecting rehabilitated injuries and medical problems that could affect participation in sports is the *Preparticipation Examination* (PPE).

The purposes of the PPE include detecting medical conditions that delay or disqualify athletic participation owing to a risk of injury or death, detecting previously undiagnosed medical conditions, detecting medical conditions that need further evaluation or rehabilitation before participation, providing guidance for sports participation for patients with health conditions, and meeting legal and insurance obligations. If possible, the PPE should be combined with the comprehensive annual health visit with emphasis on preventive health care.

Requirements for how often a youth needs a PPE differ, ranging from annually to entry to a new school level (middle school, high school, and college). At a minimum, a focused, annual interim evaluation should be done on an otherwise healthy young athlete. The PPE is optimally performed 3–6 week before the start of practice.

### HISTORY AND PHYSICAL EXAMINATION

The essential components of the PPE are the history and focused medical and musculoskeletal screening examinations. About 75% of significant findings are identified by the history. History of known medical conditions of the participants is very important to allow proper management of any conditions to minimize risks that physical activity may cause. A standardized questionnaire given to the parent and athlete is important, because the young athlete might not know or might forget important aspects of his or her history. The questionnaire should include questions about previous medical, surgical, cardiac, pulmonary, neurologic, dermatologic, visual, psychologic, musculoskeletal, and menstrual problems, as well as about heat illness, medications, allergies, immunizations, and diet **(Table 1)**.

**TABLE 1:** Sports preparticipatory physical fitness evaluation history.

| | |
|---|---|
| Medical conditions | Diabetes mellitus, asthma, known epilepsy, hypertension, and hepatitis |
| Past history | • Major surgeries (spine, cardiac, abdomen, and genitourinary)<br>• Chronic disease<br>• Heat-related illness |
| Medication utilization (including nutritional supplements) | • Beta-blockers that restrict an increase in heart rate despite physical exertion<br>• Oral hypoglycemic drugs and insulin<br>• Antiepileptic medications<br>• Aspirin may increase trauma-induced bleeding<br>• Anabolic steroids |
| Allergic history | • Any history of allergies and anaphylaxis that may interfere with sports performance like environmental, drug, or food allergy<br>• History of exercise-induced allergies |
| Head and/or neck injuries | • Concussion, a history of neck injuries enquires about persistent numbness, paraesthesias, weakness, or transient quadriplegia<br>• Major surgeries of spine |
| Musculoskeletal conditions | • Musculoskeletal injuries, a history of chronic musculoskeletal pain, and neoplasm or infection |
| Pulmonary | • Asthma<br>• Exercise-related difficulty breathing<br>• Chronic exercise-related cough<br>• Persistent wheezing |
| Cardiovascular disorders | • Family history of sudden cardiac death or known heart disease<br>• Exertional chest discomfort, pain, tightness, and exertional syncope<br>• History of dyspnea or fatigue |
| History of immunizations | Vaccine preventable diseases can be avoided by proper vaccination for diseases like measles, hepatitis A, influenza, and others. Athlete should be vaccinated with tetanus and hepatitis B |
| History of ophthalmologic conditions | Refractive errors, retinal disease, eye injuries, retinal detachment, eye surgery, corneal grafting, etc. |
| Menstrual and gynecologic history | Menarche (age of first menses), last menstrual period, amenorrhea (primary or secondary), dysfunctional uterine bleeding, or dysmenorrhea |

## ■ CLINICAL EXAMINATION

A complete, careful, and thorough physical examination is essential to qualify or disqualify the athletes and also to guide us for further evaluation, if needed. Ideally, the PPE performed preseason that is *at least 4–6 weeks* before the first scheduled practice. It is advised yearly health supervisions for adolescents and also PPE be conducted before the beginning of each new level of competition, e.g., middle school, high school, and college.

- Vital signs' recording is integral part of any examination; it helps us to rule out cardiac disease, hypertension, bradycardia, or tachycardia.
- General physical examination—height, weight, and body mass index (BMI) to rule out obesity and eating disorders; lymph node to rule out infectious diseases, malignancy, etc.; skin examination to identify contagious diseases such as impetigo, herpes, staphylococcal, and streptococcal.
- Sexual maturity rating (SMR) of all adolescent athletes should be done, because an individual with an SMR of 4–5 is stronger than the obese individual with an SMR of 2–3 and also athletes of the same weight but different SMR maturity are not of equal strength, since muscle is stronger than adipose tissue.
- Vision, refractive errors, legal blindness, absent eye, anisocoric eye, and amblyopia.
- Cardiac examination performed both in standing and supine position. Measurement of blood pressure, pulse, cyanosis, heart murmur, heart enlargement, prior surgery, and dysrhythmia.
- Pulmonary examination to rule out recurrent and exercise-induced bronchospasm, chronic lung disease.

**TABLE 2:** Classification of sports by contact.

| Contact or collision | Noncontact |
|---|---|
| • Basketball | • Archery |
| • Boxing | • Badminton |
| • Diving field hockey | • Body building |
| • Martial arts | • Bowling |
| • Rodeo | • Canoeing or |
| • Rugby ski jumping | kayaking (flat water) |
| • Soccer | • Crew or rowing |
| • Team handball water polo | • Curling |
| • Wrestling | • Dancing |
| *Limited contact:* | • Ballet |
| • Baseball bicycling | • Modern |
| • Cheerleading | • Jazz |
| • Canoeing or kayaking (white water) | • Field events |
| • *Fencing field events:* | • Discus, javelin, and |
| – High jump | shotput golf |
| – Pole vault | • Orienteering |
| • Floor hockey football, flag | • Power lifting |
| • Gymnastics handball | • Race walking |
| • Horseback riding | • Riflery |
| *Racquetball skating:* Ice | • Rope jumping |
| • Inline roller | • Running sailing |
| • *Skiing:* | • Scuba diving |
| – Cross-country | • Swimming table |
| – Downhill | tennis |
| – *Water:* | • Tennis |
| - Skateboarding and | • Track |
| snowboarding | • Weight lifting |
| - Softball squash | |
| - Ultimate Frisbee | |
| - Volleyball | |
| - Windsurfing or surfing | |

*Source*: Epidemiology and prevention of injuries. In: Kliegman RM, St. Geme JW III (Eds). Nelson Textbook of Pediatrics, 21st edition, volume 5. Elsevier; 2019. pp. 3678-84.

- Abdomen examination for organomegaly and abdominal mass.
- Genitourinary examination for varicocele, undescended testes, tumor, and hernia.
- Musculoskeletal examination to identify acute and chronic injuries, physical anomalies of spine like scoliosis, limb anomalies, joint hypermobility, deformities, etc.

## LABORATORY STUDIES

There is no routine laboratory or imaging studies recommended. Laboratory studies have not been shown to be cost effective in athletes who are asymptomatic. Routine blood or urine analysis does not identify athletes who require disqualification.

Chest radiographs, electrocardiograms (ECGs), and echocardiograms are not recommended as routine screening tests. If there is a suspicion of heart disease or a history of syncope, presyncope, palpitations, or excessive dyspnea with exercise, or a family history may be subjected for the above evaluation.

## SPORTS CLASSIFICATION

Sports are classified based on the likelihood of contact/collision and according to cardiovascular demands (based on combined static and dynamic components achieved during competition) **(Table 2)**.

## KEY MESSAGES

- History is essential in identifying the potential concerns for fitness evaluation.
- Physical examination and particularly musculoskeletal examination provide highest yield on finding problems.
- The PPE should be done by one provider even if there is a mass screening.
- No routine laboratory tests are recommended in PPE.
- Sports preparticipation examination is to recognize medical problems, mechanisms of injury (including unrehabilitated injuries) and enforcing rules that reduce the likelihood of that mechanism of injury.

## RECOMMENDED READING


1. American Academy of Pediatrics. Preparticipation Physical Evaluation, 5th edition. American Academy of Pediatrics; 2019.
2. Epidemiology and prevention of injuries. In: Kliegman RM, St Geme JW III (Eds). Nelson Textbook of Pediatrics, 21st edition, Elsevier. 2019;5:3678-84.
3. Preparticipation evaluation. In: Fisher M, Elizabeth A, Kreipe RE, Rosenfeld WD (Eds). Textbook of Adolescent Health Care. American Academy of Pediatrics; 2011. pp. 1658-69.
4. Sports participation. In: Bhave S, Menon PSN, Parthasarathy A (Eds). Bhave's Textbook of Adolescent Medicine, 2nd edition. Peepee Publishers; 2016. pp. 263-7.
5. Sports preparticipation evaluation. In: Bhave SY, Patel DR, Greydanus DE (Eds). Handbook of Sports Medicine for Children and Adolescents, 1st edition. New Delhi: Jaypee Brothers Medical Publishers; 2008. pp. 5-10.

# 12.2 Sports Nutrition in Adolescents

*Ramakant Dajiba Patil, Newton Luiz*

## ■ INTRODUCTION

Sports nutrition applies nutrition principles to sport with the intent of maximizing performance. The science of sports nutrition has developed to meet the specific needs of each sport by different eating strategies. Sports nutrition enhances performance by providing enough energy for repair and growth and decreasing fatigue and the risk of disease and injury. Good sports nutrition optimizes training and faster recovery.

The consumption of healthy foods is crucial for all who are involved in exercise and sports. Adolescents involved in sports have increased nutrient demands, but many of them do not meet the adequate requirements their growing bodies need. This can be due to insufficient knowledge of nutrition and its importance in their lives. Furthermore, media, economic, culture, and financial factors can play a critical role on a child and their family in their daily dietary choices. This is why nutrition education is crucial for those involved in sports and to help educate them on the proper nutrient needs for performance before, during, and after practice and competition. However, there is currently a lack of research in this area, particularly for adolescents.

Developing healthy eating and adequate fluid intake habits from the early stages of life maintains long-term health of the adolescent athlete and will enhance performance. A balanced diet will enhance the nutrient value of meals and should have a good proportion of macro- and micronutrients as per the requirement of various sports.

Athletes and adolescents in sports have a higher recommended dietary allowance (RDA) of energy than those who are not into regular exercise or sports. They also need more of certain aspects of macro- and micro-nutrients: Protein, low glycemic index carbohydrates, and micronutrients such as zinc, magnesium, and iron.

## STEPS TOWARD ENHANCING PERFORMANCE IN SPORTS THROUGH NUTRITION

- *Step 1:* Quality of food—make healthy and balanced food choices

- *Step 2:* Quantity of food—how much, when, and how often
- *Step 3:* Recovery and hydration—the right amount of food and fluids to meet the physical requirement during training
- *Step 4:* Supplementation—through proper consultation with the doctor or nutritionist.

## IMPORTANCE OF PROPER NUTRITION IN SPORTS

- To attain the desired weight and body composition for a given sport
- For optimal training
- To assist in recovery after exercise
- To reduce the risk of injury
- For enhanced performance in the sport.

## ■ ENERGY

Between the ages of 13 and 18 years, it is a time of growth spurt, bone and brain development, and pubertal changes. It is therefore essential that young athletes are fueling their bodies with enough energy for these changes to occur properly. To support the extra energy demands for exercise and performance, and to support growth and development, young athletes need to make sure they are eating enough to maximize performance and support recovery. If not, it can lead to tiredness, delayed recovery, poor sleep, hormonal fluctuations, poor athletic performance, and poor concentration in school.

Most athletes are energy deficient up to 30% of their requirement. Growth and protein synthesis happens only in positive energy balance. They have more muscle mass, so resting energy requirement is more in adolescents in physical sports. Repair, growth, and regeneration require enough protein. Quality of calories is equally important. Avoid empty calories from sugary drinks, chocolates, sandwiches with cheese and butter, and burgers. Negative energy balance causes decreased performance, increased injuries, and stress fractures. It causes low insulin growth factor and high cortisol, resulting in low muscle mass, catabolic state, and inflammation.

Energy requirement includes resting energy expenditure + active lifestyle energy requirements + training active energy. A simple formula is (39–44) × weight in kg = 2,660–3,000 calories. Performance is directly related to good energy balance with quality calories.

## FUEL FOR ACTIVITY

The sources of fuel that are used during exercise mainly depend on the duration and intensity of exercise.

- A mixture of fat, glucose, and glycogen are used in low intensity exercises. Carbohydrates and by products like lactates are utilized near-completely in low intensity long exercises without bursts of demand.
- Glycogen depletion is rapid with high intensity, short duration exercise. Once steady state is attained, there is minimal protein utilization with glycogen contribution to the tune of 50–60% and fats 35–40%.
- In a marathon, about 50% of fuel is utilized from fatty acids.

## COMPOSITION OF NUTRIENT INTAKE

### Carbohydrates

Carbohydrates are the preferred source of energy. They should be of high quality, from varied sources, with a good admix of low and high glycemic index. It shall be supplemented with good timing related to training, pre-event, during the event, and post-event.

It is generally recommended that for an average person at least 55% of total calories should come from carbohydrate. Athletes need adequate carbohydrates to store enough fuel for their events, especially for endurance competition. A minimal daily amount of carbohydrates recommended for an athlete is 360 g/day if the total intake is 2,600 kcal (60–90 g/meal).

Requirement of carbohydrates ranges from 30% to 55%, depending on intensity of training and body composition. Female athletes use more fats in training than carbohydrates, so their carbohydrate requirement is comparatively less. Athletes should consume:

- More carbohydrates on game days and less on off days/recovery days of training
- Low glycemic index carbs like vegetables on nontraining or recovery days
- Higher glycemic index carbs around workout time.

### Proteins

Recommended dietary allowance is 0.8 g/kg/day for normal adolescents to maintain positive nitrogen balance, but even 1 g/kg is low for athletes. Consumption of too little or too much protein will have a deleterious effect on the health and performance of an athlete. Hence, utmost care needs to be taken when recommending protein allowances. Townsend documented that increased protein intake by athletes improved bone health in endurance runners, decreased risk of stress fractures, increased muscle protein synthesis, decreased blood triglycerides, stabilized blood sugars, and had higher amounts of micronutrients. For adolescent athletes, the current recommendation is 1.2–1.7 g/kg. Additional recommendations include increasing plant proteins for the added benefits and keeping the percentage to 10–15% of total calories. Weight training athletes need 1.6–2.2 g/kg/day.

If the athlete needs to reduce weight, then the hypocaloric intake should have higher protein intake up to 2.4 g/kg/day with 40% reduction of calories. Still there is 1.2 kg gain in lean muscle mass. So, the current recommendation is not about requirement but about optimization.

It is dangerous to overdose on 2–3 times the recommended amount of protein in nonintense training or weight reduction without training. The hazards are weight gain if too many calories are consumed, dehydration if carbohydrates are not consumed, excess calcium excretion (which can lead to osteoporosis), and possible kidney problems from its excretion. In addition, consumption of high animal protein is associated with a risk of heart disease and colon cancer.

The body uses proteins as a minor source of fuel to meet 2–5% of energy needs during rest and low/moderate exercise, while it provides 10–15% of energy needs during endurance exercise. A carbohydrate-rich diet spares protein from being used as fuel.

Heavy exercise increases protein needs. Intense exercise activates specific enzymes in the muscle that degrade the myofibrillar protein. Protein loss occurs through sweat and urine because of decreased absorption in kidney tubules during heavy exercise.

Protein intake should be divided equally in number of meals and post-workout intake. 100 g protein intake should be taken as 20 g in each of four meals and 20 g within 20 minutes after a workout.

### Fats

Though carbohydrates are the primary source of energy, fat is the primary source of energy in endurance sports like a marathon, as glycogen stores and glucose content are limited. Fats and carbohydrates are oxidized simultaneously. The proportion of which will be used more depends on the prior meal, energy supplementation during exercise, duration, intensity and type of exercise, and fitness level.

## Micronutrients

Iron, calcium, zinc, and magnesium deficiency occur in athletes. Training in hot conditions causes iron and magnesium loss through sweating. Increased physical activity necessitates higher input of vitamins particularly vitamins C, $B_2$, A, and E. Increased input would come from diet if energy expenditure is met from energy input. For most athletes, there is therefore no need for vitamin supplements. Athletes who must restrict body weight and therefore their diet (e.g., gymnasts) may need supplementation for micronutrient inadequacy. Female adolescents have higher iron and calcium needs, and usually need supplementation.

## Hydration

Water intake is very important to regulate temperature, for biochemical reactions, and for transport of waste products. Large amounts are lost in sweating, especially in hot and humid weather. Even mild dehydration drastically reduces physical performance and motivation. Thirst is not adequate to indicate the need to rehydrate a person. A fluid intake of 120–240 mL every 15 minutes is recommended during exercise.

Muscle cramps are believed to be associated with dehydration, electrolyte deficits, and muscle fatigue. Those who sweat profusely, and experience cramps, should take extra care to drink plenty of sodium-containing fluids while exercising. If the diet has a high-salt content, sodium losses after exercise can be replaced with standard postexercise meals. Consuming extra salt in the food if one has high sweat losses can be a smart way to enhance recovery, retain fluid, and stimulate thirst.

*Pre-exercise:* To hydrate well it takes 8 hours and shall have 5–8 mL/kg of fluid before exercise.

*During exercise:* The recommended fluid replacement should have a little sodium to stimulate thirst, a little potassium to help replace sweat losses, and a little carbohydrate (sugar) to provide energy. More precisely, the drink should contain sodium 20–30 mEq/L, potassium 2–5 mEq/L, and 50–100 g/L of carbohydrate. A World Health Organization (WHO) ORS 6 g packet may be diluted in 600 mL rather than 200 mL, and 30 g sugar added in it. Sipping every 10–15 minutes during the workout or event is better than gulping large volumes. Cold water helps dissipate heat.

People who will be exercising for more than 4 hours in the heat should observe the following guidelines to prevent hyponatremia:
- Avoid water loading before the event.
- Eat-salted foods and fluids 90 minutes before you exercise.

*After exercise:* The weight should be checked just before and after exercise. One should consume 1 L of fluid per kg of weight lost, within the next 2–3 hours. Rapid weight loss in exercise is almost 100% water loss. Most athletes can get rehydrated with normal meals and plain water. If significantly dehydrated and need to exercise again within 12 hours, consider a more aggressive rehydration program and sprinkling extra salt on food if one has had high sodium losses through sweat. If dehydrated more during an unusually long and strenuous bout of exercise, one should drink frequently for the next day or two. The body may need 24–48 hours to replace the sweat losses.

## Meals During a Competition

The meal should have high carbohydrate, moderate protein, and low fat content.
- *3-4 hours before the competition*: Have a proper meal, e.g., rice or chapati with boiled dal or chicken. High-carbohydrate, low-fat food that should empty from the stomach rapidly.
- *1-2 hours before the competition*: For example, milk shake, fruit smoothie, a sports bar, and fresh fruit. Rapidly digested and absorbed food.
- *<1 hour before the competition*: A sports drink
- *Within 30 minutes after the competition*: Have a proper meal, e.g., rice or chapati with boiled dal or chicken. Glycogen synthesis is highest within an hour of exercise, so a high-carbohydrate meal is recommended at this time.

## Dietary Supplements

Vitamins and mineral supplements are unnecessary for an adolescent athlete who is having a balanced diet and enough energy intake. Mega doses of vitamins or minerals may be harmful. Creatine is not good for the kidneys and may do harm. Similarly, amino acid preparations like branched chain amino acids or protein supplements are not required and add to expenses. The majority of the supplements available in the market are not researched well, and their safety and efficacy are not substantiated. Herbals may cause anxiety or depression.

The role of supplements is well documented in deficiency states. Athletes who take a low-calorie, high-protein diet may need supplements as their diet may not provide adequate calories. Calcium may be recommended in female athlete albeit limiting it to 1,500 mg/day. Commercial iron preparation may be recommended in females having heavy menstrual flow.

## Energy and Sports Drinks

Energy and sports drinks are most of the time carbonated drinks with caffeine. They may have high sugar and poor electrolytes. They may contain stimulants, which elevate mood temporarily to cause anxiety and depression later. They may contain prohibited substances that are not mentioned.

## ■ KEY MESSAGES

- Different sports have different nutrition strategies.
- Most athletes do not take adequate calories to meet their enhanced requirements.
- Athletes have higher protein needs, and the current recommendation for adolescent athletes is 1.2–1.7 g/kg.
- Overdosing on protein in nonintense training or weight reduction without training is harmful, and may lead to weight gain, dehydration, excess calcium excretion and osteoporosis, kidney problems from the burden of its excretion, and a risk of heart disease and colon cancer.
- It is important to ensure adequate hydration and electrolyte intake before exercise, to take sips of isotonic fluids continually during exercise, and to ensure rehydration and electrolyte balance postexercise.
- Supplements of vitamins, minerals, creatine, amino acids, and proteins are unnecessary unless the patient has a deficiency state.

## ■ RECOMMENDED READING

1. Nutrition and hydration guidelines for excellence in sports performance. [online] Available from http://ilsi-india.org/PDF/Nutrition_&_Hyd_Guidelines_for_Athletes_Final_report.pdf [Last accessed April, 2024].
2. Nutrition and hydration in sports. [online] Available from https://nsnis.org/wp-content/uploads/2020/09/booklet-final_compressed.pdf [Last accessed April, 2024].

---

## 12.3 Sports Injuries

*Prashanth Inna*

## ■ INTRODUCTION

Athletic activities are beneficial both physically and psychologically. Along with the increase in interest and participation in competitive sports, injuries to the components of the musculoskeletal system have become common. The prolonged hours spent and the intensity with which adolescents engage at such a young age contribute to these injuries, in addition to the faulty techniques of playing. Fractures also happen in sports practice. Difference is that they are usually high impact ones. This section elaborates the various aspects of adolescent sports injuries with focus on overuse injuries.

The common aspects of all the injuries will be detailed first. Problems specific to different regions of the body will be dealt with later.

## ■ EPIDEMIOLOGY

While it is difficult to exactly pen down the incidence of injuries among sports players, it is well known that some sports are more damaging. The general incidence of athletes reporting for treatment is in the range of 8–15%. Gymnasts have a higher propensity, up to 45%, to have problems with the wrist.

## ■ ETIOLOGY

Children and adolescents are at particular risk for fractures, given their physes are weaker, muscle imbalance is common during adolescent growth spurt, and coordination is lacking.

For overuse injuries, the cause is multifactorial. More intensive practice and game schedules, participation in multiple same sport leagues, and pressure to perform well along with unprecedented expectations from the parents and coaching staff are blamed for overuse injuries.

Faulty techniques of the sporting actions (e.g., throwing) puts undue and excessive loads on certain parts of the physis producing unwanted consequences.

## ■ PRESENTATION

Fractures present in the usual way with nothing particular in sports injuries.

*What is common to all the overuse injuries are as follows?* Patients complain of gradually increasing local area pain with sporting activities (early stages of overuse) that may progress to pain while at rest (more serious). Acute pain after a particular sporting action is more likely to be an avulsion of the apophysis or a full-blown fracture.

Knowledge of an athlete's training is helpful, as abrupt escalation of the sporting intensity leads to overuse injuries. Growth history should be assessed. 70% of growth of the lower extremity occurs at the distal femoral and proximal tibial epiphyses. During adolescence, this rapid bone growth outpaces the lengthening of the surrounding musculotendinous complexes, resulting in tight hamstrings and quadriceps. This predisposes to traction apophysitis at the muscular attachments.

Often neglected, nutrition and body image are vital components of history. Whether the nutritional input matches the requirements should be assessed.

Clinical examination is region specific. Localized tenderness to palpation can be present. The area of tenderness depends on the area involved; for example, over the anterolateral proximal humerus in little leaguer's shoulder. Certain movements elicit pain; for example, externally rotating the shoulder in Little leaguer's shoulder.

Range of motion of the joints and strength of different muscle groups should be assessed. Movement restrictions are common; for example, internal rotation restriction in shoulder issues, flexion in elbow issues. They may also experience reduction in throwing velocity over time, seen in shoulder and elbow pathologies. Stability of the joint should be checked, eliciting provocative maneuvers, more so in shoulder and knee problems.

Additionally, there may be a flexion contracture and/or a valgus deformity of the elbow with increased laxity of the ulnar collateral ligaments.

The patient may report locking or catching of the elbow, which may indicate loose body formation in the joint. In medial epicondylitis, they may even have features of ulnar nerve damage including weakness, numbness, or tingling of the limb.

## ■ INVESTIGATIONS

Fractures are diagnosed with appropriately taken X-rays or magnetic resonance imaging (MRI).

In overuse injuries, radiographs show widening of the physeal line (sometimes one segment more than the other, depending on the predominant forces while playing), demineralization, sclerosis, cystic changes, and fragmentation of the metaphysis. Separation of the medial epicondylar apophysis can be seen in throwing athletes.

When the X-rays appear normal, imaging the opposite normal side may help pick up subtle changes. Ultrasound shows features of tendinitis and calcium deposits, in lesions of the patellar tendon. MRI is a definite diagnostic tool that should be utilized when in doubt. It may show widening and edema in the involved physis and these are not seen on X-rays.

## ■ COMMON DIFFERENTIAL DIAGNOSES

Since the problems are focal and of long-standing duration, tumor, infection, bone cysts, and possibly stress fractures should be considered as differentials.

## ■ GENERAL TREATMENT

Treatment of fracture and acute physeal injuries follows the general principles of fracture treatment. They are treated surgically, when needed.

For overuse injuries, rest from sports, ice packs, and nonsteroidal anti-inflammatory drugs (NSAIDs) are the initial line of treatment.

Rest is the most essential treatment modality. The duration of cessation of sports depends on the extent and the type of injury. In general, greater the radiographic changes, more is the duration of rest advised. If physeal widening was observed on X-rays, avoidance of sporting activities till the radiographs return to normal is prudent.

Applying plaster casts promotes rest and faster healing, more effective in the upper limbs.

Splints can be used to increase the support while resting or while doing controlled exercises. These are designed keeping in mind the pathology seen, so that particular movements are restricted or particular forces are counteracted (e.g., valgus forces in medial epicondylitis).

While rest is important, strength of the muscles should be preserved by encouraging exercises under the guidance of trained personnel. Complete cessation with no exercises slows down the returning to competitive levels of sports while at the same time, aggressive strengthening exercises do not give adequate rest.

Examining the sporting technique, rectifying the faults, and proper rehabilitation reduce the possibilities of recurrence of the injury.

Surgery is reserved for recalcitrant cases in which there is radiographic evidence of an ununited osseous fragment within the substance of the apophysis, or when there is wide separation of the apophyses as in Little league elbow. Osteochondral fragments need surgery when they have separated completely from their areas of attachment.

## PREVENTION

We need to encourage children participation in sports to counteract the significant problems that the population is facing like obesity, cardiovascular disease, and early-onset diabetes. We must also guide and educate the athletes, their parents, and coaches to ensure safety and prevention of overuse injuries.

The suggestions are:

- Focus on single sports specialization should be reduced. Research supports the recommendation that child athletes avoid early sports specialization until puberty. While success depends on more time spent on training in that particular sport, susceptibility to career threatening injuries also increases with it and should be avoided.
- Short breaks from specific sports are advisable as this will allow for overuse injuries to repair. While the athletes get refreshed both physically and psychologically after these mini breaks, female athletes are additionally noticed to regularize their menstrual routines thereafter. During the breaks, they are encouraged to not lose the physical fitness, by indulging in general strengthening exercises, which are not specific to the sport they specialize in.

It is advisable to train no more than 5 days per week on one specific sport and take off 2–4 consecutive months per year.

- Regulating the duration and severity of training is paramount for future injury prevention and is the single most important intervention. The best example is the pitch count in baseball pitchers.
- The child should be trained to look for the red flag signs that suggest the onset of the injury and report as soon as they are observed.
- Resistance training is safe and even preferred for young athletes if the programs are well designed and supervised by knowledgeable personnel. Strength training can start even during prepubertal period.
- Stretching as part of the daily routine is advised. And warm-up exercises, which are adequate and sports specific, should be regularly done before the sessions.
- Correction of the faulty techniques and improving the biomechanics reduce the overloading or asymmetric loading that can predispose to injuries.
- As a last resort, a drastic decision like changing the sports altogether might be needed. This is undertaken when the symptoms do not resolve and the pathologic changes on the imaging techniques do not revert to normal, despite using all the treatment modalities available.

## SPECIFIC INJURIES

### Growth Plate/Physeal Fractures

Growth plate/physeal fractures account for 20–35% of all fractures in children. The Salter–Harris system, a 5-numbered classification, is commonly used in these injuries. Higher the number, more severe the injury and higher the chances of complications.

The acute bony injuries, namely the physeal injuries and the fractures, are more severe while playing sports, as the impact is more severe. The management is the same as that for any other fractures, with an aim for early rehabilitation and quick return to activities of competitive intensity.

### Little Leaguer's Shoulder

Little league shoulder occurs in adolescent high-performance pitchers between the ages of 11 and 16 years. It is also seen in sports such as volleyball, tennis, and gymnastics. This entity is slightly less common in the Indian context as baseball is not very popular here.

The act of throwing is a very complex activity that exposes the proximal humerus to severe rotational strains, at the high speeds of throwing action. Patients present with lateral shoulder pain with tenderness localized to the lateral aspect of the proximal humerus. Frank tears of the rotator cuff have been surprisingly observed in children.

### Shoulder Internal Impingement and Rotator Cuff Injury

With internal impingement, the rotator cuff, labrum, and joint capsule are repetitively pinched between the greater tuberosity and superior glenoid rim at the extremes of abduction and external rotation, which can occur multiple times in overhead sports.

### Little Leaguer's Elbow

Little league elbow is a broad nomenclature for many conditions associated with throwing activities. Medial epicondylitis is the most common pathology. Others include avulsion fracture of the medial epicondyle, tear of the ulnar collateral ligament, and irregularity in the ossific nucleus of the capitellum. Pain is usually localized to the medial distal humerus. They may even have locking episodes of the elbow or features or ulnar nerve paresis. Regulating the pitch count is important for prevention of this injury.

### Gymnast Wrist

The wrist suffers the maximum in gymnastics as it bears weight on the body, with heavy forces transmitted across it. It is seen between the ages of 8 and 15 years. Extensive compressive forces are transmitted through the radius sometimes ending up with physeal damage and asymmetric deformity of the wrist.

The pain is most often in the dorsal aspect of the wrist and is increased by loading in hyperextension and rotation. Tenderness is also focused on the dorsal distal radioulnar joint (DRUJ) or scaphoid. X-rays might show, in addition to the regular changes, shortening of the radius and positive ulnar variation (distal ulna longer than the radius) due to physeal closure of the distal radius.

### Osgood–Schlatter Disease of the Knee

Osgood–Schlatter disease of the knee is common during periods of rapid growth; commonly between the ages of 10 and 13 years in girls and between the ages of 12 and 14 years in boys. However, it may develop even later.

It may be bilateral in a quarter of the cases. It is a traction apophysitis of the anterior tibial tubercle at the insertion of the distal patellar tendon. Avulsion of bone at attachment sites is however rare.

Patients complain of activity-related pain focused over the tibial tubercle, especially with activities such as jumping, running, climbing stairs, and kneeling activities. Focal tenderness at the patellar tendon attachment on the tibia might be exaggerated by resisted knee extension.

X-rays might show fragmentation or separation of the anterior tibial apophysis (might be normal also!). Complete resolution of the pain might take 12–18 months. Residual bony bulge on the anterior aspect of the knee is common and is never a functional problem.

### Jumper's Knee (Sinding-Larsen-Johansson Syndrome)

Jumper's knee is a tendinopathy of the proximal attachment of the patellar tendon at the inferior pole of the patella, seen in excessive jumping events. Tenderness and swelling are localized to the inferior patellar pole. The patient might have pain with resisted quadriceps extension and with full passive flexion of the knee. X-rays show osteophytes or calcification at the inferior pole of patella.

### Sever's Disease (Calcaneal Apophysitis)

Sever's disease is the inflammation of the calcaneal apophysis at the attachment of the Achilles tendon. It presents as heel pain after high impact loading of the heel, in participants of gymnastics, running, basketball, and football. It is a disease of younger age groups, i.e., 9–12 years. Besides the usual treatment strategies, the addition of padded heel cups to cushion load impact and heel lifts to relax the gastro-soleus complex, thus releasing tension on the calcaneal apophysis can be attempted. Plaster casts in plantar flexion can be used in resistant cases.

### Patellofemoral Pain Syndrome

Patellofemoral pain syndrome is the most common cause of knee pain in adolescents and is commonly attributed to maltracking of the patella in its groove in the distal femur. Giving way or instability is also experienced by few. MRI details the pathologic contributory abnormalities. Surgery to realign the patella is needed in those with frequent dislocations of the patella.

## Osteochondritis Dissecans

It is seen in late teens, at around 13–17 years and is often traumatic in etiology. It can affect any joint. Pathologically, it is an osteochondral lesion that affects the subchondral bone and overlying articular cartilage. This fragment might get detached from its base to form a loose body. Specialized tunnel views of the radiographs of the knee are ordered to show the crescent-shaped radiolucent zone in the medial femoral condyle. MRI is the diagnostic tool of choice.

While milder lesions resolve by periods of nonweight bearing and casting, separated ones need either fixation, removal or either drilling or osteochondral grafting of the bed from where the fragments have detached.

## Spondylolysis

Repetitive hyperextension seen in such activities as gymnastics and weightlifting can place excessive stress on the posterior elements of the spine and create a stress fracture in the pars interarticularis.

## Pelvic Avulsion Injuries

Pelvic avulsion injuries often are the result of an indirect trauma with forceful contraction of the attached muscles avulsing either the anterior superior iliac spine, anterior inferior iliac spine (AIIS), or the ischial tuberosity.

The history is either an acute or acute-on-chronic injury in which a pop or crack is felt about the hip, followed by immediate local pain.

Injuries considered rare in the pediatric population like the anterior cruciate ligament (ACL) tears, meniscus tears of the knee, and rotator cuff tears of the shoulder can be seen in injuries sustained while playing sports. Management principles are no different from the regular injuries.

## ■ SUMMARY

In brief, extensive participation of kids in specialized sports has brought immense health benefits, while exposing them to the risks of overuse injuries. Early diagnosis of the problems and timely preventive strategies ensure an optimal healing of the injuries while allowing early return to competitive levels of sports.

## ■ RECOMMENDED READING


1. Brown T, Moran M. Pediatric Sports-Related Injuries. Clin Pediatr (Phila). 2019;58(2):199-212.
2. French CN, Walker EA, Phillips SF, Loeffert JR. Ultrasound in sports injuries. Clin Sports Med. 2021;40(4):781-99.
3. Strassberg J, Ahmed A. Pediatric Sports Injuries. Clin Podiatr Med Surg. 2022;39(1):89-103.
4. Trentacosta N. Pediatric Sports Injuries. Pediatr Clin North Am. 2020;67(1):205-25.


---

# 12.4 Sports and Mental Health in Adolescence

*Ramakant Dajiba Patil, Shyamkant Chaudhari*

## ■ INTRODUCTION

Sports, athletics, and exercise all lead to physical fitness. They also play a major role in an adolescent's mental health by addressing the physical and psychological aspects of well-being. Sports give adolescents an identity and recognition among peers and significant elders and may even give them entry into academia.

## ■ SPORTS FOR HUMAN DEVELOPMENT

Since ancient times, sports have provided an opportunity for adolescents to:

- Improve self-esteem
- Achieve a range of new skills
- Handle stress in a better way
- Inculcate the value of fair play
- Inculcate cooperation with teammates and coaches, and extrapolate this to society
- Inculcate respect for the opponents and the game.

## ■ SPORTS IMPROVE MENTAL HEALTH

- Vigorous physical activity enhances the production of endorphins from the hippocampus, which elevates mood and leaves the person in a relaxed and positive attitude.
- The release of neurotransmitters like serotonin, dopamine, and norepinephrine helps a person to feel energetic throughout the day.

- Exercise improves the duration and quality of sleep, and results in a sharper memory and better concentration while studying.
- Sports decrease stress and anxiety. They are fun and protect against burnout.
- Yoga is safe and noninjurious, may help in reducing anxiety and depression, and meditation as part of yoga is quite beneficial.
- Physical activity relieves stress and reduces the craving for alcohol and drugs by acting as an enjoyable replacement for them.

## MENTAL HEALTH IMPROVES SPORTS PERFORMANCE

Sports psychologists seek to improve the sports performance of adolescent athletes by making them mentally strong. They teach techniques like:

- *Goal setting:* Goals should be specific, measurable, attainable, relevant, and time-bound (SMART). They should relate to one's performance, which is controllable, not to the outcome.
- *Positive visual imagery:* Often imagine, how it will feel like when you succeed.
- *Awareness of self-talk:* Irrational thoughts like "if I lose, my future is useless," "I will let everyone down," "my opponent is in top form', etc., are self-defeating. Adolescents should realize that winning is not predictable, and it is not everything, and therefore, they should urge themselves to "go all out" and have rational thoughts like "I'll give it my best try".
- *Concentration:* The athlete should learn not to be distracted by fatigue, weather changes, public announcements, the coach, or opponents.
- Systematic relaxation before and after the event.
- Handling stress, and realizing that a little stress is good, but too much is harmful.
- Handling pain.
- Handling defeat and considering, "tomorrow is another day".

## THE DARKER SIDE OF SPORTS

*It can lead to:*
- Injuries
- Violence, when players intentionally try to hurt opponents
- Unequal participation due to high expense and inaccessible venues

- Inequality across groups (socioeconomic, ethnic, geographic, and gender)
- Inadequate safety equipment and precautions
- Increased mental stress due to high levels of competition
- Feeling of rejection when one is not selected for the team
- Cheating and use of performance-enhancing drugs
- Inappropriate expectations of achieving scholarships or a professional career
- Peer pressure from teammates to consume alcohol and drugs after practice
- Some adolescents dislike sports but are pressurized to participate.

### Sports Doping

'Sports doping' is the use of performance-enhancing substances (PESs) in sports. It is commonplace, and some of these substances pose a serious threat to the health and well-being of athletes. Common PESs include anabolic–androgenic steroids, human growth hormone, creatine, erythropoietin and blood doping, amphetamines and stimulants, and β-Hydroxy β-Methyl Butyrate (HMB). Gene doping is a potential future threat.

## ELITE ATHLETES

All the above factors are exacerbated in elite athletes. In addition, they may suffer from the burden of unrealistic expectations, having to travel a lot, having to occasionally train at odd hours, and harsh coaches. This may result in:

- *Anxiety:* Due to high competition and the pressure to achieve
- *Depression:* When they fail and from excessive fatigue.
- *Sleep issues:* Insomnia due to anxiety or depression; disturbed sleep–wake cycle due to touring or training at odd hours.
- *Disordered eating:* Especially in those who need to be slim, like long-distance runners and gymnasts.
- *Alcohol or substance abuse:* When alcohol intake after every competitive event is perceived as the norm among teammates.

## THE FEMALE ATHLETE TRIAD

The female athlete triad consists of the combination of disordered eating, amenorrhea, and osteoporosis. Exercise promotes bone mineralization when associated with adequate energy intake. But, when excessive exercise is combined with inadequate caloric intake, there may be excessive weight loss, which suppresses the hypothalamic–pituitary–adrenal (HPA) axis, resulting in a low estrogen level and amenorrhea. A low estrogen level decreases bone mineralization. In addition, excessive weight loss causes muscle depletion. Exercise is not recommended, if the athlete weighs <85% of the ideal body weight.

The solution is to increase the caloric intake, and decrease physical activity if need be. This will correct the energy status within days or weeks, but it may take months of increased energy intake to establish normal menstruation. Recovery of bone mineral density may take years and may only be partial even with calcium supplementation.

## ■ CODE OF CONDUCT

Coaches and parents must communicate fair play principles through their words and actions, and lead by example. During the natural course of practice and play, fair play values should be inculcated. Praising the player on the field has maximal benefit.

Asking adolescents who are into sports to sign a code of conduct may help in teaching good sports behavior, preventing misbehavior and dealing with it when it occurs. It must be actively promoted by coaches, parents, officials, and organizers. One example is given in **Box 1**.

> **BOX 1:** Code of Conduct.
>
> - I will always play by the rules
> - I would not lose my temper while playing
> - I will cheer good plays made by either team
> - I would not talk trash, tease, or goad opponents
> - Win or lose, I will shake hands with opponents and officials after a game
> - I would not yell at or criticize teammates or coaches for making a mistake
> - I will admit mistakes instead of making excuses or blaming others
> - I will try my hardest on every play, even if the team is losing badly
> - I will point out incorrect calls when they go in our favor
> - I would not argue with calls that go against me
> - I would not show off
> - I will have fun

## ■ KEY MESSAGES

- Participation in sports has the potential to improve both physical and mental fitness.
- It teaches the values of fair play, cooperation with teammates, and respect for opponents.
- Vigorous physical activity improves mental health by releasing endorphins and neurotransmitters like serotonin and dopamine, improving sleep, and relieving stress.
- Sports psychologists help adolescent to improve their mental health in order to improve their sports performance, through goal setting, positive visual imagery, awareness of irrational self-talk, concentration, relaxation, and learning to handle stress, pain, and defeat.
- Some negative aspects of sports are that they can lead to injuries, violence, stress due to high competitiveness, feeling of failure when defeated, cheating and use of performance-enhancing drugs, and peer pressure to consume alcohol or drugs.
- These aspects are exacerbated in elite athletes, who may additionally have to deal with unrealistic expectations, having to travel a lot, and demanding coaches.
- The female athlete triad of disordered eating, amenorrhea, and osteoporosis occurs when female athletes lose weight from excessive exercise and inadequate caloric intake, resulting in amenorrhea, which causes decreased bone mineral deposition.

## ■ RECOMMENDED READING

1. Landry GL. Female athletes: Menstrual problems and the risk of osteopenia. In: Kliegman RM, St Geme III JW, Blum NJ, Tasker RC, Shah SS, Wilson KM (Eds). Nelson Textbook of Pediatrics. 21st edition: Philadelphia: Elsevier Inc; 2020.
2. Sovani A, Bhave SY. Sports psychology. In: Bhave SY, Patel DR, Greydanus DE (Eds). Handbook of Sports Medicine for Children and Adolescents, 1st edition. New Delhi: Jaypee Brothers Medical Publishers; 2008. pp. 57-64.

# 12.5 | Performance-enhancing Drugs

*SM Prasad, Geeta Patil*

## ■ INTRODUCTION

Greeks in the ancient Olympics, and Roman gladiators, used certain wines, herbal teas, and mushrooms to help enhance performance. But it was only after the Second World War that sports doping really took off. It started when European countries discovered a shortcut to winning Olympic medals—the routine state-sponsored use of androgens in elite female athletes. It then spread all over the world. Today, the use of androgens is common even among nonathletic schoolboys who wish to have a masculine physique.

The use of drugs to gain an advantage over others is called doping. The International Olympic Committee (IOC) defined doping as "use of any substance foreign to the body and taken with the sole intention of increasing his or her performance in an unfair manner in competition".

Though these chemicals have not proven to be helpful and are very expensive, but their usage has increased globally.

World Anti-Doping Agency (WADA) was established in 1999. It has a list of >300 drugs and metabolites that are prohibited. In addition, there are prohibited practices in sports, for example, blood product administration.

The objections to the use of these substances are that they may enhance performance illegally (cheating), violate the spirit of sport (unsporting), and are harmful to health (safety). There have been counter-arguments that doping should be permitted officially, to equalize opportunity to all. However, this would result in routine use of such substances among adolescents and convert sports from a healthy to a dangerous activity. Attempts to restrict use by age or dosage, and only on medical prescription, have been considered seriously and rejected as unenforceable.

Advertisements by movie and sports stars influence their mind and sometimes adolescents and young adults yield to the pressure from parents, coaches, and peers.

Manufacturers claim that these products maximize lean body mass and strength, lower fat, improve motor skills, augment aerobic capacity, and enhance antioxidant effects. Many of these claims lack adequate research and evaluation of acute and long-term effects.

In all the sports, this trend is increasing. Teenagers are ignorant of the side effects of these chemicals.

## ■ ANTIDOPING TESTING

- Over 322,000 antidoping tests were done in 2017, of which 1.5% were positive, with 61% detecting the presence of androgens.
- The urine tests done for testing for androgens are effective.
- Blood doping with autologous transfusions and erythropoietin injections, are very common but underdiagnosed. A hemoglobin (Hb) ≥17 g/dL (or hematocrit of ≥0.50) is highly suspicious. An algorithm involving eight parameters [Hb, packed cell volume (PCV), erythrocyte count, reticulocyte count and percentage, mean corpuscular volume (MCV), mean corpuscular hemoglobin (MCH), and mean corpuscular hemoglobin concentration (MCHC)] can detect any form of Hb doping, whether direct or indirect, with good sensitivity.
- As athletes often stop taking the drugs just prior to a competition, it is important to do out-of-competition testing too.
- Due to the wide variety of drugs used in sports doping, it is important to do an increasing number of tests on the samples and to find more sensitive tests.

## ■ ANABOLIC-ANDROGENIC STEROIDS

Androgens act by increasing muscle mass and strength, and are most beneficial in sports that require bulky muscles and massive power like sprinting, throwing, wrestling, and boxing.

There is a wide variety, including androgens (testosterone, methyltestosterone, and danazol), precursors of testosterone [androstenedione and dehydroepiandrosterone (DHEA)], designer androgens that are chemically modified to avoid detection [e.g., tetrahydrogestrinone (THG)], and nonsteroidal specific androgen receptor modulator (SARM) drugs. Recent experiments by athletes include "indirect androgen doping" by using human chorionic gonadotropin (hCG), luteinizing hormone (LH), antiestrogens, and neuro-transmitters involved in the regulation of testosterone and LH secretion.

Testosterone is the hormone responsible for male secondary sexual characteristics and muscle and bone metabolism. It has been proven, by detailed experiments, to increase muscle mass and strength by a massive 20–37% when combined with exercise. Exercise alone causes an increase of 10–20%. Taking testosterone without doing exercise results in a 10% increase. The effect is dose-related, unrelated to age, and applies to both males and females. It probably does not increase endurance. It also decreases body fat, and many nonathletic adolescent boys take it for the lean and muscular body shape that it helps to create.

Adverse effects are many, especially in females. Common side effects include testicular atrophy and low sperm count (by suppressing endogenous testosterone in males), hirsutism and menstrual irregularities in females, acne, and gynecomastia. Dangerous side effects are dilated cardiomyopathy, stroke, blood clots, and liver dysfunction. Anabolic-androgenic steroids (AASs) are banned by the IOC and all major sporting bodies.

Dehydroepiandrosterone (DHEA) and andro-stenedione are injectable testosterone precursors that are used as prescription drugs for certain conditions. They increase testosterone and estrogenic metabolites levels in the blood. While they do have the adverse effects of testosterone, they are not significantly anabolic and are not banned.

## ERYTHROPOIETIN AND BLOOD DOPING

A higher hemoglobin level will increase the oxygen-carrying capacity of the blood, which is especially beneficial in endurance sports. Athletes may deliberately stay and train at high altitudes, which is a natural and legal way to increase their hemoglobin levels. Another technique is to withdraw a pint of blood, wait for the body to automatically compensate for it, and later transfuse it back ("blood doping"). Repeated autologous blood transfusions are safe and effective, and do not have any of the side effects associated with receiving blood transfusions repeatedly from donors. Some athletes prefer erythropoietin injection, which is difficult to detect as it is present in the bloodstream only for a few days, while its benefits last many months as erythrocytes have a lifespan of 120 days.

It is believed that such practices are common in endurance sports. The adverse effects include hypertension, headaches, and an increased risk for a thromboembolic event (myocardial infarction or pulmonary embolism), due to the high hematocrit and viscosity. Blood doping and erythropoietin are banned by the IOC and all major sports bodies. Athletes can escape detection and side effects if they only increase their hemoglobin levels modestly.

## HUMAN GROWTH HORMONE AND GROWTH FACTORS

Human growth hormone (HGH) and growth factors are postulated to be of benefit in contact sports, where rapid recovery from frequent injury during intense physical training is important. hGH increases lipolysis and protein metabolism, and theoretically, this will result in an increase in lean muscle mass and a decrease in body fat. In one study, 0.4% of student-athletes admitted to using hGH in the previous year, with the average age of first use being 14–15 years. But, the beneficial effect is controversial, especially in adolescence, as hGH release is normally pulsatile, and is regulated by a variety of factors like growth hormone (GH)-releasing hormone, exercise, sleep, and arginine. hGH has significant side effects on chronic use; it activates the renin–angiotensin system, causing fluid retention, and leading to arthralgias, carpal tunnel syndrome, pseudotumor cerebri, and also hyperglycemia and hyperlipidemia. It is banned by the IOC and many international federations.

## STIMULANTS

Drugs that improve concentration and reduce fatigue offer an unfair advantage. Commonly used stimulants include amphetamines, caffeine, ephedrine, pseudoephedrine, and phenylephrine. Small studies have suggested that these substances can increase strength, muscular power, speed, acceleration, aerobic power, and anaerobic capacity, and delay the onset of exhaustion. Other studies have shown little benefit. Caffeine has been studied the most, but results have been contradictory.

The side effects of stimulants relate to excessive central nervous system (CNS) stimulation. Dangerous side effects include arrhythmias, heat exhaustion, seizures, myocardial infarction, and sudden death. Minor side effects include agitation, headache, hallucinations, insomnia, and gastrointestinal (GI) upset. Stimulants other than caffeine are banned by the IOC. Antiasthmatics are restricted to therapeutic use. In the United States of America (USA), the National Collegiate Athletic Association (NCAA) has limited caffeine levels in urine to approximately that obtained from six regular cups of coffee.

## ■ CREATINE

Creatine is important for the conversion of adenosine diphosphate (ADP) to adenosine triphosphate (ATP) and serves as an energy substrate for the contraction of skeletal muscle. Not all athletes benefit from it, but those who are "responders" demonstrate an increase in strength, power output, sprint performance, total work to fatigue, peak force, and peak power. This oral supplement is probably safe, though the athlete should watch out for heat stroke and dehydration. Its use is permitted. Creatine is one of the most common sports supplements used today.

## ■ β-HYDROXY β-METHYL BUTYRATE

β-hydroxy β-methyl butyrate (HMB), a metabolite of leucine, is believed to attenuate protein breakdown after workouts. It is suspected to increase muscular mass, strength, and power. The International Society for Sports Nutrition suggests that HMB may enhance recovery by reducing skeletal muscle damage after exercise. Chronic consumption of HMB appears safe. It is available as a nutritional supplement and is permitted.

## ■ GENE DOPING

Gene doping is defined as the "transfer of nucleic acid sequences or the use of normal or genetically modified cells to enhance sports performance". Hypothetically, one day it will be possible to transplant the gene for insulin-like growth factor or erythropoietin into the athlete. Adverse effects might include autoimmune reactions or cancer.

## ■ PROTEIN SUPPLEMENTS

The protein requirement of athletes is higher than that of nonathletes, as they need more protein for building up muscle mass and for tissue repair. Sportspersons should preferably obtain more proteins and amino acids from their diet, but there is no contraindication to their use of protein supplements.

## ■ THERAPEUTIC USE EXEMPTION

Therapeutic use exemption (TUE) may be granted by a national antidoping organization following a stringent, independent, expert review, if an athlete requires treatment using a substance that is banned by the WADA. Care must be taken to ensure there is no unjustified use or overdosage. TUEs may rarely be granted for the treatment of adolescents with testosterone, glucocorticoids, insulin, GH, or erythropoietin. For example, testosterone therapy may rarely be justified for a young male athlete with genuine androgen deficiency who is already on life-long testosterone replacement therapy (e.g., bilateral orchidectomy, severe mumps orchitis, and Klinefelter syndrome). The dosage should be carefully monitored.

## ■ CONCLUSION

One strong motivation for using banned substances is the belief that one's rivals are using them.

Hence, most elite adult athletes welcome the use of routine and rigorous antidoping tests after every event and at random.

## ■ KEY MESSAGES

- The use of performance-enhancing substances is high among adolescent athletes, and poses a threat to their health.
- Anabolic-androgenic steroids are most misused among young athletes, and their use starts as early as 14–15 years.
- Blood doping and erythropoietin use are probably underdiagnosed.
- HGH injection may not be beneficial and has many harmful side effects.
- Stimulants have doubtful efficacy. Most are banned, while the use of caffeine is restricted.
- Creatine is a wildly popular sports supplement that is safe and legal to use. HMB too may be beneficial. Protein supplementation is recommended in adolescent athletes, but they should preferably get a higher protein intake through their diet rather than from protein supplements.

## ■ RECOMMENDED READING

1. Handelsman DJ. Performance-enhancing hormone doping in sport. In: Feingold KR, Anawalt B, Blackman MR, et al (Eds). Endotext [Internet]. South Dartmouth (MA): MDText. com, Inc; 2000. Available from: https://www.ncbi.nlm.nih. gov/books/NBK305894/ [Last accessed April, 2024].
2. Momaya A, Fawal M, Estes R. Performance-enhancing substances in sports: a review of the literature. Sports Med. 2015:45;517-31.

<table>
<tr><td>**12.6**</td><td># Role of the Government</td></tr>
</table>

*SM Prasad*

## INTRODUCTION

The Government firmly believes in the principle of "a sound mind in a sound body", and the National Youth Policy 2021 envisions "a culture of sports and fitness among the youth and achieving national and international eminence".

"Fit India" movement was launched by the Prime Minister in 2019. The goal is to encourage everyone to lead a more physically active lifestyle.

*Fit India plans to:*
- Promote fitness as an easy, fun, and free activity.
- Run awareness campaigns on physical activities that promote fitness.
- Promote fitness in every educational institute and every village and town.
- Encourage traditional tribal and rural sports, for example, *gilli–danda* and *kabaddi.*
- Create a community platform for the common man to share personal fitness stories, and thereby encourage each other to be fit.

"Khelo India" is the national program for development of sports in India. In the last few years, India has begun to do well internationally in the sports arena. The tremendous potential of our large country can be developed by inspiring young talent and giving them high-quality infrastructure and training. The plan is to encourage sports participation at the grassroot level, support traditional and indigenous sports, and provide facilities in every state and district. In addition to physical fitness programs in schools, there should be regular district, state, and national sports competitions, talent search programs, support for sports among women and in rural communities, support for disabled sportspeople, and training of coaches. The Sports Authority of India (SAI) has a major role in this program.

## KEY MESSAGES

- *"Fit India Movement"* launched by the Government encourage everyone to lead a more physically active lifestyle both at educational institutions and community levels.
- It envisages promoting the youth both in urban as well as rural India for better fitness programs at all levels.
- *"Kelo India movement"* encourages the sport activities at individual level exposing the youth talent by providing the infra structure and necessary training. Sports authority of India (SAI) has an important role in this.
- India has begun to do well internationally in the sports arena and with the indigenous programs. More youth from different places have the great opportunities of representing our Nation.

## RECOMMENDED READING


1. Coleman E, Steen SN. The Ultimate Sports Nutrition Handbook. Palo Alto, CA: Bull Publishing Company; 1996.
2. Committee on Sports Medicine and Fitness. American Academy of Pediatrics Policy Statement. Adolescents and anabolic steroids: a subject review. Pediatrics. 1997;99(6):904-8.
3. Greydanus DE, Patel DR. Sports doping in adolescent athlete the hope, hype, and hyperbole. Pediatr Clin North Am. 2002;49(4):829-55.

# 13

# Adolescent Health and the Environment

**Section Editor:** *Somashekar AR*

## 13.1 | Adolescent Health and the Environment

*Swati Y Bhave, Narmada Ashok, Ruth Etzel*

### ■ INTRODUCTION

The environment has changed profoundly in the past 200 years. India has become more industrialized which has resulted in pollution of the air, water, and food. This pollution affects children, who as a group are more vulnerable because their organs are still developing. Children encompass an age group of up to 18 years. The environmental health risks to infants and children at early stages of development have been well analyzed, and significant progress has been made to understand and prevent the same. However, the impact of a polluted environment during adolescence, which is the final stage of maturation, is less known. Adolescence is a unique stage of development with rapid physical, cognitive, and psychosocial growth, and these changes affect the way adolescents interact with the world around them. Though the mortality and morbidity appear to be low in this age group, it is important to focus on adolescents because of their susceptibility to greater exposures due to their risk-taking behaviors. They are particularly vulnerable, for example, to tobacco addiction. Because some of their organs are reaching maturity, adolescents may be less vulnerable than younger children to other environmental risks including outdoor air pollution and water pollution. However, as a result of their risk-taking behavior, they may be inadvertently exposed to hazardous chemicals and waste, radiation, and emerging threats such as e-waste. Exposures of adolescents differ with changes in physical location, types, and amount of foods consumed and stage of development. This chapter will give a brief overview of the impact of environmental changes on adolescent health.

### ■ ENVIRONMENT OF AN ADOLESCENT

Adolescents are influenced by their immediate physical and social environment which interact with each other to influence the adolescent's health. The physical component includes "micro environment" and "macro environment". Macro environment may be the bigger city or geographical area where the adolescent lives and micro environment is unique for each adolescent and depends on the smaller units, such as the particular type of house, the school that the adolescent attends, and the places the adolescent works. Day-to-day circumstances in the social environment under which the adolescent is living and the regulations that exist in this place have a unique influence on the developing adolescent.

### ■ UNIQUE FEATURES OF ADOLESCENTS MAKING THEM VULNERABLE TO ENVIRONMENTAL HAZARDS

#### Environmental Exposures

*Occupational Hazards*

Adolescents are vulnerable to exposure to toxicants because many of them start working and can be employed due to their dexterity in occupations which can be hazardous, e.g., waste segregation. They may also be at an increased risk of skin cancer as they may be employed in tanning units.

## Target Organ Susceptibility

### Lung Function Parameters

The lung functions have a growth spurt similar to their anthropometric measurements, and hence toxic inhalation exposures may be harmful **(Table 1)**.

### Endocrine Disrupters

Growth in the adolescent period is characterized by differentiation and migration of the cells. When cells take on specific tasks in the body, differentiation occurs and hormones can trigger the same. It is possible that chemicals from environmental pollutants can mimic the hormones and alter cell differentiation. These are called endocrine disruptors, and they may have effects on the reproductive system. There are many endocrine disruptors in the diet, skin products, etc., to which adolescents can be exposed during the vulnerable window of their growth **(Table 2)**.

These are associated with early puberty and precocious puberty if the exposure occurs early in childhood **(Table 3)**.

### Hepatic Metabolic Pathway

During adolescence, the hepatic metabolic pathway affecting the cholesterol and steroid hormone pathway is vulnerable to changes due to rapid growth and differentiation. This also can cause protein–calorie malnutrition and micronutrient deficiencies. The toxicant's action in several ways including altered expression of the metal-binding proteins transferrin and metallothionein, which could influence increased deposition of toxic metals, especially in the growing bones, is enhanced by these deficiencies.

## Psychosocial Changes and Risk-taking Behavior

As adolescents gain freedom from parental authority, they venture outside more frequently and may be less protected from exposures. Although their stamina is at a peak, their abstract reasoning skills are still being acquired.

**TABLE 1:** Types of pollution of the air and impact on adolescent health.

| Type of pollution | Sources | Major pollutants | Clinical effects |
|---|---|---|---|
| Air pollution (outdoor) | Large industrial facilities, dry cleaners, gas stations, natural disasters like wildfires, highway vehicles, biomass fuels | • Criteria pollutants—ozone, particulate matter, lead, $SO_2$, CO, and $NO_2$<br>• Toxic chemicals | • Increased respiratory symptoms<br>• Asthma and allergic rhinitis<br>• Decrements in lung function<br>• Asthma exacerbations<br>• Chronic obstructive pulmonary diseases (COPD)<br>• Neuroinflammation<br>• Leukemia |
| Smoking E-cigarettes | • First-hand active smoking<br>• Second-hand exhaled smoke and smoke from smoldering end of cigarettes<br>• Third-hand smoking—residual smoke contamination | • 50 carcinogens including polycyclic aromatic hydrocarbons<br>• Nicotine, volatile organic compounds, metallic nanoparticles (nickel, cadmium, and lead), and tobacco-related carcinogens | • Increased school absenteeism, respiratory disorders, pneumonia, and uncontrolled asthma<br>• Alteration in the development of brain, long-term impairment in executive functioning, memory, and attention span<br>• Tremors and palpitations<br>• Headache and nausea<br>• Acute injuries—facial and limb burns due to vaping devices<br>• Vaping-associated lung injuries (EVALI) |
| Air pollution (indoor) | • Stain repellent carpets and fabrics, polishes, furniture, clothing, food packages<br>• Soap lotions, shampoos, antiperspirants and deodorants, hair straighteners | • Per-polyfluoroalkyl substances (PFAS)<br>• Acrylic polymers, benzocaine, oxybenzone, sodium lauryl sulfate | • Increased liver weight, fatty liver, lipid abnormalities, immunotoxicity, reduced thyroid and testosterone concentrations<br>• Major cause of asthma<br>• Eye irritation |

**TABLE 2:** Various pollutants of water and food and impact on adolescent health.

| Major substances producing the hazard | Sources | Clinical effects |
|---|---|---|
| *Microorganisms and radioactive spills* | | |
| • Harmful microorganisms<br>• Loss of biodiversity and increased oxygen consumption leads to eutrophication—essentially dead zones where life exists—food availability is compromised | • Agricultural practices<br>• Storm water runoff occurring during rainfall carries road salts, oils, grease, chemicals, and debris to waterways<br>• Big oil spills<br>• Radioactive wastes | • Spread of waterborne diseases such as hepatitis, typhoid, and cholera<br>• Nutrient deficiency<br>• Skin diseases—melanosis and keratosis<br>• Neuropsychiatric diseases<br>• Cancer—colorectal, lung, non-Hodgkin's lymphoma |
| *Heavy metals* | | |
| Lead | Lead paints, plumbing, food cans, lead-laden dust, toy jewelry | • Thyroid and steroid hormone disruptor<br>• Nervous system side effects—reduction in cognitive functions, subclinical effects on hearing and attention deficit<br>• Anemia, abdominal pain, constipation, colic, anorexia |
| Cadmium | Industrial application as corrosives, stabilizer, combustion of fossil fuels | • Disruption in bone mineralization, osteoporosis, damage to kidneys, liver, and cardiovascular system with deterioration in sight and hearing<br>• Alteration in steroidogenesis, disorders in menstrual cycle |
| Arsenic | Drinking water and industrial sources | Hyperkeratosis, diabetes, pulmonary disease, precursor to certain cancers of bladder, lungs, and skin |
| Mercury | • Shark, tuna, tile fish from contaminated lakes, rivers, and streams<br>• Skin-lightening creams and soaps, teeth whiteners | • Long-term exposure—insomnia, forgetfulness, tremors, loss of appetite, emotional lability, hypertension<br>• Renal toxicity—proteinuria, nephrotic syndrome, proximal tubular necrosis |
| *Endocrine disruptors* | | |
| Perchlorates | Industrial chemicals found in groundwater | Antagonists—inhibit iodide uptake by thyroid gland—thyrotoxic and interfere with puberty in males |
| Bisphenols | Bisphenol resins may be found in lining of some canned foods and beverages. Used in applications to manufacturing, food packaging, and toys | Agonists xenoestrogens interfere with thyroid pathway, obesogenic, insulin resistance, and antiandrogenic effects |
| Phthalates | Liquid plasticizers and used in industries like food packaging, children's toys, and medical device tubing and cosmetic industry | • Arachidonic acid hormone receptor—agonists/antagonists<br>• Interfere with male reproductive system, induce testicular dysgenesis syndrome, ovarian function interference, premature ovarian failure |
| Phytoestrogens | Naturally occurring excluding soy foods | Estrogen receptor agonists—disruption of hypothalamic–pituitary–gonadal axis |
| Polybrominated diphenyl ethers | Used in furniture foams and carpets | Interfere with thyroid hormone transport, obesity, thyroid disease |

*Contd…*

*Contd...*

| Major substances producing the hazard | Sources | Clinical effects |
|---|---|---|
| Polychlorinated biphenyls | Used in fluids like hydraulic, heat transfer fluids and lubricants. Now banned | • Aryl hydrocarbon receptor agonists<br>• Estrogenic and antiandrogenic effects—decreased sperm motility, and altered sex ratio |
| Triclosan | Previously added in liquid body wash and soaps | Activate the human pregnane X receptor thyroid hormone disruptor |
| *E-Waste*<br>• Heavy metals—lead, mercury, gold, chromium, cadmium, zinc, and nickel<br>• Brominated flame retardants<br>• Polychlorinated biphenyls<br>• Dibenzodioxins and dibenzofurans<br>• Perfluroalkyls<br>• Polyaromatic hydrocarbons | • Computers and monitors<br>• Video cameras<br>• Televisions<br>• Household appliances<br>• Medical devices and electronic devices | May be linked to impaired neurodevelopment and behavior issues, changes to multisystems |

**TABLE 3:** Other types of environmental hazards and effect on adolescent health.

| Type of hazard | Sources | Major substances producing the hazard | Clinical effects |
|---|---|---|---|
| Heat stress due to climatic changes | • Fuel combustion<br>• Vehicle smog | Coal, oil, and gas | • Heat exhaustion, heat stress, and heat cramps<br>• Rhabdomyolysis<br>• Metabolic acidosis and tachypnea |
| Noise pollution | Vehicular traffic, railways, airport, videogames, music devices, and portable listening devices | | Poor academic performance, short attention span, ringing in ears, modification of normal circadian cortisol rhythm |
| Electric and magnetic fields | • Extremely low-frequency waves—electric lines, or transmission towers<br>• Radiofrequency waves—cellular phones and towers, Wi-Fi stations, hair dryers, electric shavers, coffee makers, microwave ovens, mixers, window air conditioners, electric dryers, irons, and digital clocks | | • Stimulation, thermal and nonthermal effects<br>• *Stimulation effects:* Human carcinogenesis<br>• *Thermal effects:* Increase in body temperatures<br>• *Nonthermal effects:* Long-term exposure causes electromagnetic hypersensitivity syndrome and neurodevelopmental disorders |

- They may select physical environments like a pub (often ignoring the risks) or a joint where exposure to loud music and smoking may pose increased risk.
- They are likely to hang out more in the mid or late afternoons when levels of ozone peak and are more likely to be exposed to excessive ultraviolet radiation effects which put them at risk for skin malignancies.

## Vulnerability of the Adolescent Brain

The adolescent brain is still developing. Adolescents may take risks and experiment because their prefrontal cortex is not yet fully developed and the hypothalamic limbic pathway is preponderant. Rapid advance in cognitive skills and intense acquisition of new information occur during adolescence. The maturation of the cerebral cortex is in the final event of development. Two major changes occur during the adolescence period: *Pruning* (a process of decrease in the synaptic density from the peak levels in early childhood to adult maturation) and *connectivity* (occurs due to increased myelination of major intracortical commissures). Dopamine receptor density also changes through late adolescence and is overexpressed in them, which explains their vulnerability to risk-taking behavior. Since adolescents' central nervous systems are vulnerable to the dopamine reward pathway, they become vulnerable to all addictions, be it the gateway drugs tobacco and alcohol or substance abuse.

## Digital Environment

Today's adolescents live in a digital world. They are online for many hours a day. In addition to most of their academic work being online, their active involvement in social media has increased profoundly after the coronavirus disease 19 (COVID-19) pandemic. There is a very wide digital divide between adults and youngsters today. The technology quotient and expertise of children and youngsters in using the internet and various digital devices are very high. Many adults are not tech savvy and are often feel ill-equipped to handle online safety education and its safety measures or protocols. Since both children and adults are inadequately trained in cyber safety, it has led to a very high rate of cybercrimes. Children, due to their adventurous nature, high technology quotient, and easy access to internet are easily becoming vulnerable to the dark web.

Unregulated exposure online leads to a lot of issues such as cyber-bullying, cyber stalking, photo morphing, identity theft, cat fishing, and exposure to adult content sites. This has led to a lot of mental health issues and problems arising from internet addictions that lead to adverse effects like sleep deprivation and being constantly in the virtual world leading to real life social isolation, depression, etc. It also leads to various orthopedic issues due to repeated stress injuries—cervical spondylosis, carpel tunnel syndrome, and trigger thumb, to name a few.

## ▪ WHAT THE PEDIATRICIAN CAN DO

It is imperative that we as pediatricians raise our voices to prevent the adverse impact of environmental exposures on adolescent health. Policymakers and government leaders respect pediatricians and hence we can influence policy makers to take immediate action on environmental degradation and the climate crisis. Apart from the role of advocacy there are several ways in which pediatricians can help:

- Taking a detailed environmental history in cases where exposures to environmental hazards could have contributed to the illness (see: https://www.who.int/publications/m/item/children-s- environmental-record--green-page)

- Influence the local community leaders to undertake measures to mitigate environmental hazards.
- Spread awareness on social media on the relationship of environmental pollution to child and adolescent health, the need for monitoring the air quality index, substituting fossil fuels with renewable energy that is also clean, and measures to control the adverse effects of fossil fuel pollution.
- Spread awareness among other health professionals and child advocacy groups about developing comprehensive strategies to prevent and mitigate the impact of environmental hazards on adolescents.

## ▪ ACTIONS TO PROTECT ADOLESCENT WELL-BEING (FIG. 1)

- *Youth for climate action:* Global movement demanding greater action from government to fight climate changes was started by a 15-year-old girl Greta Thunberg.
- *Fridays for Future:* This was the largest climate protest in history which was organized in 7,500 cities.
- *Adolescents from Rwanda* are playing a major part in nutrition advocacy and receive training for the same.
- *Adolescents in various countries* have sued governments for better life and health using United Nations (UN) Convention on the Rights of the Child.
- *The Lancet Countdown on Health and Climate Change:* The worst impacts of climate change will continue to impact children disproportionately, and the Lancet countdown is a multinational collaboration dedicated to monitoring the evolving health profile of children.

## ▪ PREVENTIVE MEASURES

- *International level:* The adolescent well-being framework designed by the H6 Technical Working Group on Adolescent Health and Wellbeing (which includes the Partnership for Maternal, Newborn and Child Health, United Nations Program on HIV/AIDS, UNESCO, UN Population Fund, UNICEF, UN Major Group for Children and Youth, UN Women, World Bank, World Food Programme and World Health Organization) with major stakeholders identified the measures to be taken at the international level to tackle climate change and environmental effects.
- *Role of healthcare professionals:* Health professionals due to their privileged position can be in the frontline for providing climate and age-sensitive health services

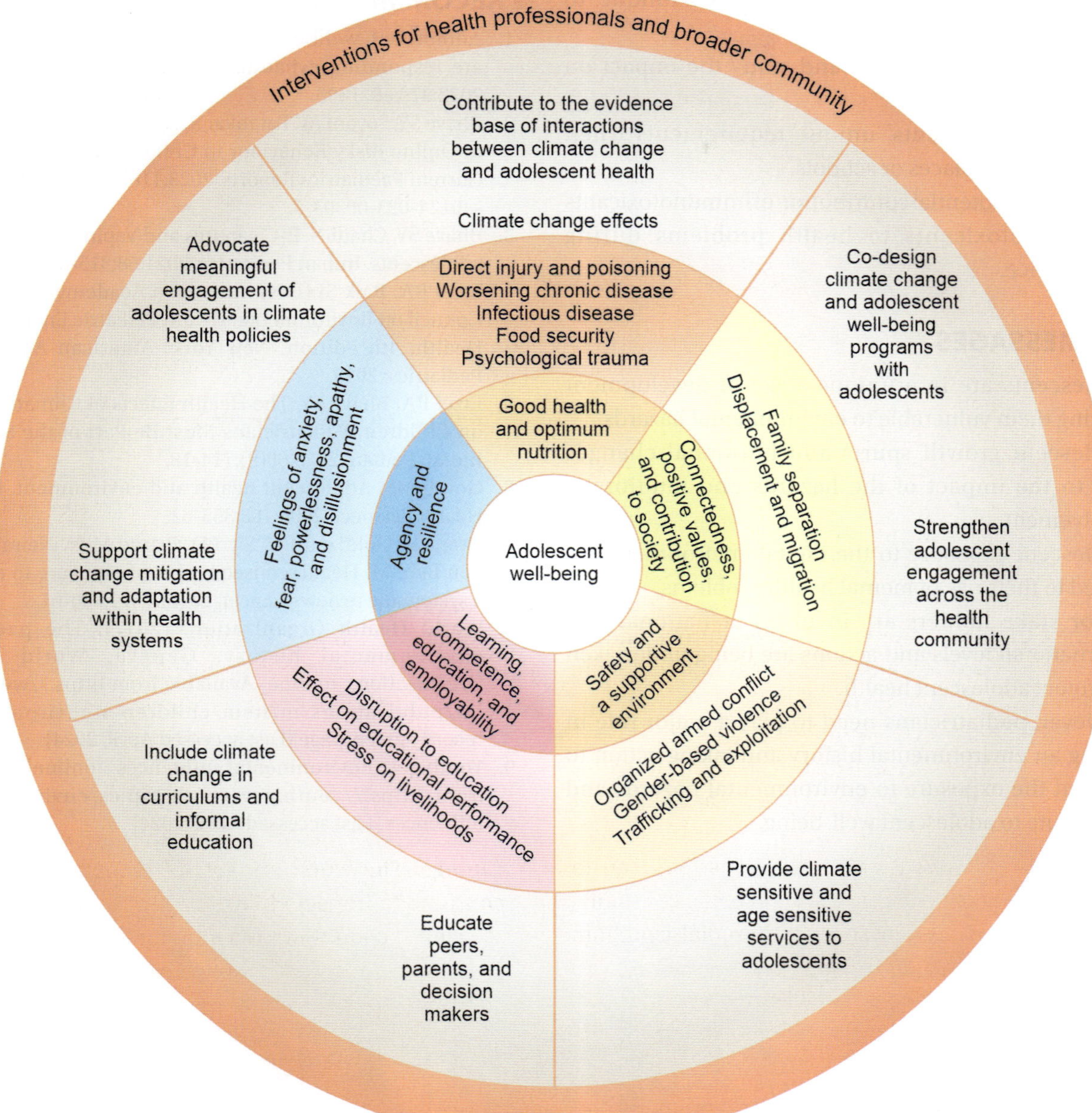



**Fig. 1:** Adolescent well-being framework, described by the H6+ Technical Working Group on Adolescent Health and Wellbeing[*] and adapted to include related climate change effects and interventions at the level of health professionals and the broader community. [*]The H6+ Technical Working Group on Adolescent Health and Wellbeing includes the Partnership for Maternal, Newborn and Child Health, United Nations Programme on HIV/AIDS, UNESCO, UN Population Fund, UNICEF, UN Major Group for Children and Youth, UN Women, World Bank, World Food Programme, and World Health Organization.
*Source:* McGushin A, Gasparri G, Graef V, Ngendahayo C, Timilsina S, Bustreo, F, Costello, A. Adolescent wellbeing and climate crisis: adolescents are responding, what about health professionals? BMJ. 2022;379:e071690.

to adolescents, forefront to support surveillance, analysis, and report of environmental hazards to adolescents. Collaboration with adolescence is needed for advocacy efforts.

## ■ FUTURE DIRECTIONS

- Recognize adolescents and their vulnerability as distinct from other development stages.

- Research to analyze and find hazards unique to adolescents.
- Identify exposure periods and study the impact on adolescents.
- Consider adolescents' unique requirements when designing workplaces or schools.
- Evaluate the potential contribution of immunotoxicants and neurotoxicants to health problems during adolescence.

## KEY MESSAGES

- Adolescents are in a unique stage of development making them vulnerable to environmental hazards.
- Adolescent growth spurts and hormonal changes add to the impact of the hazards and multiorgan involvement.
- Adolescent exposure to the digital environment has added to their risk of mental health problems.
- Major stake holders are involved at national and international levels and actions are being undertaken to protect adolescent health.
- However, pediatricians need to play a major role in asking an environmental history and taking action to prevent the exposure to environmental hazards and contribute to adolescent well-being.

## RECOMMENDED READING


1. Adolescent wellbeing and climate crisis: adolescents are responding, what about health professionals. BMJ. 2022;379:e071690.
2. Bhave SY, Sovani AV, Patankar S. Sexual Exploitation Related to Online Risky Behaviour in Children and AYAs in India. Current Paediatrics Reports. 2023;11(4):1-11. DOI 10.1007/s40124-023-00303-5.
3. Bhave SY, Chadi N. E-Cigarettes and Vaping: a global risk in adolescents. Indian Pediatrics. 2021;58:315-8.
4. Etzel RA, Balk SJ (Eds). American Academy of Pediatrics Council on Environmental Health Pediatric Environmental Health, 4th edition. New York: American Academy of Pediatrics; 2019.
5. Etzel RA, Bhave SY. The Health Effects of Climate Change on Children: Pediatricians Must Be Part of the Solution. Indian Pediatr. 2023;60(9):714-18.
6. Golub MS. Adolescent health and environment. Environ Health Perspect. 2000;108:355-62.
7. Grant K, Goldizen FC, Sly PD, Brune M-N, Neira M, van den Berg M. Health consequences of exposure to e-waste: a systematic review. Lancet. 2013;1(6):E360-61.
8. World Health Organization. (2017). The paediatric environmental history. Geneva: World Health Organization. [online] Available from https://www.who.int/publications/m/item/children-s-environmental-record--green-page [Last accessed April, 2024].
9. Youth.gov. Environmental influences. [online] Available from https://youth.gov/youth-topics/environmental-influences [Last accessed April, 2024].

*Section Editor:* Piyali Bhattacharya

## 14.1 Road Accidents: Causes, Consequences, and Prevention

*NC Prajapati, Bimlesh Kumar*

### INTRODUCTION

Road transport is the dominant mode of transportation in India. The number of vehicles and the length of the road network have increased over the years. However, a negative externality associated with this expansion in the road network, motorization, and urbanization in the country is the increase in road accidents (RAs) and road crash fatalities. Today, road traffic injuries are one of the leading causes of death, disabilities, and hospitalizations in the country, imposing significant socioeconomic costs.

Globally, approximately 1.35 million people lose their lives in RAs each year, with an additional 20–50 million individuals sustaining nonfatal injuries, many of which result in permanent disabilities. According to the World Health Organization (WHO), road injuries are the leading cause of death among individuals aged 5–29 years. Males are three times more likely to die in RAs compared to females, mainly due to their higher involvement in risky driving behaviors and a greater proportion of male drivers and commuters. Low- and middle-income countries (LMICs), despite having 60% of the world's vehicles, account for a staggering 93% of road fatalities, with over half of these fatalities affecting vulnerable road users such as pedestrians, cyclists, and motorcyclists. One reason for this is that an accident involving a motorcycle (the most common vehicle used by adolescents and young adults in developing countries) has a much higher fatality rate than one involving a car.

The problem is increasingly affecting adolescents due to their greater access to motor vehicles, risk-taking behavior, and the lack of effective road safety education. Therefore, it is imperative that road-safety education becomes a mandatory component of school and college curricula.

### PREVALENCE OF ROAD ACCIDENTS IN INDIA

A total of 412,432 RAs were reported from various states and union territories (UTs) of India during the calendar year 2021, resulting in 153,972 fatalities and injuries to 384,448 individuals. These figures equate to an average of 1,130 accidents and 422 deaths daily, or approximately 47 accidents and 18 deaths every hour in the country. The motorized two-wheeler category leads with a share of 30% in accidents and 31% in fatalities, followed by the light vehicle category, which includes cars, jeeps, and taxis, accounting for 16% of total accidents and 16% of total fatalities. Breaking down the age profile, 9% of fatalities occur below 18 years and as many as 24% at age 18–25 years. Individuals in the age group of 18–45 years contribute to 70% of total road accident fatalities.

### CAUSES OF THE ROAD ACCIDENTS

Road accidents can be broadly categorized into those resulting from human error, road and weather conditions, and vehicular conditions.

## Human Errors

### Errors by Drivers

These include overspeeding (40%), which increases the impact during accidents, driving under the influence of alcohol (10%), talking on the mobile while driving (10%), driving on the wrong side (12%), jumping the red light (5%), misunderstanding road signs, and driver fatigue or sleepiness. (See the CRAFFT tool in Annexures, for assessing and guiding adolescents about driving under the influence of alcohol).

While the nonusage of safety devices such as helmets and seat belts do not directly cause accidents, they play a critical role in preventing fatal and grievous injuries in the event of an RA. In Uttar Pradesh (UP), during 2021, a total of 46,593 individuals lost their lives due to not wearing helmets, with 70.6% of them being drivers and 29.4% passengers. Additionally, 16,397 people were killed due to not wearing seat belts, with 48.5% of them being passengers. Nonuse of helmets caused injuries to 93,763 individuals (approximately 28% of all fatalities), and nonuse of seat belts caused injuries to 39,231 (about 16%) individuals during the same year.

### Errors by Pedestrians

These contribute to accidents due to carelessness, illiteracy, crossing at improper locations on the carriageway, and jaywalking.

### Errors by Passengers

These can also influence accidents by projecting their bodies outside vehicles, engaging in distracting behavior with drivers, and boarding or alighting from vehicles on the wrong side or while the vehicle is in motion.

## Road and Weather Conditions

Road conditions are also significant factors contributing to RAs. Potholes, damaged roads, erosion, the merging of rural roads with highways, diversions, unavailability of pedestrian and cyclist facilities, and the presence of illegal speed breakers are some of the leading causes of these accidents. According to a 2021 survey, 34% of RAs occur on national highways, 29% on state highways, and 2% on expressways. Road junctions, where traffic converges, are particularly prone to accidents, with the highest number of accidents occurring at T-Junctions. Effective traffic control measures can help prevent RAs, including the deployment of traffic police and traffic signals. It is worth noting that 74% of RAs happen in areas without proper traffic control. Additionally, road features like sharp curves and steep grades are accident prone, as they demand a high level of skill, extra care, and alertness to navigate safely.

Adverse weather conditions, such as heavy rain, snow, thick fog, strong winds, and hailstorms, can lead to RAs by reducing visibility and making road surfaces slippery.

## Accidents Caused by Vehicle Conditions

Malfunctioning vehicles are also a leading cause of RAs. Issues such as brake or steering failures, tire bursts, inadequate headlights, overloading, and protruding loads can all contribute to accidents. Older vehicles are more prone to malfunctions, leading to an increased risk of RAs. Vehicles that are 15 years or older accounted for 26% of all road accidents. Overloaded vehicles and those carrying protruding or hanging loads pose a significant road traffic hazard, endangering not only themselves but also other road users.

## ■ CONSEQUENCES OF ROAD ACCIDENTS

Road accidents have profound and far-reaching consequences for individuals, families, communities, and healthcare systems. These incidents, although brief, leave enduring marks, including:

- Loss of life
- *Physical injuries:* While minor injuries can be painful, severe injuries can lead to long-term disabilities, often necessitating surgeries and rehabilitation.
- *Psychological trauma:* Significant psychological trauma is a common aftermath of RAs, which can lead to conditions such as post-traumatic stress disorder (PTSD), anxiety, and depression.
- *Economic burden:* Road accidents result in a substantial economic burden, including medical expenses, property damage, lost productivity, legal fees, vehicle repairs/replacements, loss of personal belongings, traffic disruptions, and insurance claims.
- *Disabilities:* Road accidents can cause a range of disabilities, including physical, cognitive, sensory, and psychological impairments.

## ■ PREVENTION OF ROAD ACCIDENTS

Preventing RAs requires a comprehensive approach involving multiple sectors, including transportation, law enforcement, health, education, and political commitment, along with public cooperation.

*Effective interventions include:*

- Incorporating road safety features into urban planning and transportation design
- Ensuring vehicle safety features in all vehicles
- Enforcing laws related to key risks, such as overspeeding, drunk driving, use of unsafe vehicles, and driving on unsafe roads, and effective enforcement of road safety laws including seat belt usage, child restraints, and helmet regulations
- Raising public awareness
- Enhancing postcrash care for accident victims through life-saving measures at the accident scene and rehabilitation services.

The "Decade of Action for Road Safety 2011–2020" adopts a systemic approach, focusing on five pillars: (1) Road safety management, (2) safer roads and mobility, (3) safer vehicles, (4) safer road users, and (5) postcrash care. The State of UP recommends a 4E strategy to address road safety issues, consisting of education, engineering (both road and vehicle), enforcement of safety laws, and emergency care for road accident victims.

## Education Measures

The Ministry of Road Transport and Highways has initiated a scheme called "Grant of Financial Assistance for Road Safety Advocacy and Awards". The program covers themes like road safety audits, pilot projects, and awareness campaigns aimed at enhancing road safety. To raise public awareness about road safety, the Ministry conducts effective publicity and awareness campaigns through various channels, including social media, electronic media, and print media.

## Road Engineering

To reduce RAs, it is crucial to separate vulnerable road users from larger and faster vehicles. Adequate lighting, lane markings, pedestrian crossings, and roadside barriers are essential. Traffic calming measures, such as speed bumps or rumble strips, have proven effective in reducing RAs. The Ministry prioritizes the identification and rectification of accident blackspots on national highways identified based on accident data.

## Vehicle Engineering

Technologies like crash avoidance systems and electronic stability control systems show promise in mitigating road traffic injuries. To ensure the safety of vehicle occupants in the event of a crash, specific crash safety norms have been established, such as automotive industry standard (AIS) 098 for frontal collisions and AIS 099 for lateral collisions. These standards became applicable to new models from October 1, 2017, and to all existing models from October 1, 2019. The Ministry periodically mandates safety technologies to enhance vehicle safety. Some of the mandatory safety technologies include airbags, antilock braking system (ABS), combined braking system (CBS), seat belt reminders for drivers and codrivers, overspeed warning systems, reverse parking sensors, and manual override for central locking doors, effective from July 1, 2019.

## Enforcing Safety Rules

Promoting safe road user behavior involves fostering a culture of responsible road conduct through legislation, which necessitates not just stringent enforcement but also the public's perception of its strength. Research has shown that:

- Enforcing speed limits can lead to a remarkable reduction of up to 34% in road traffic injuries.
- Setting blood alcohol concentration legislative limits at 0.05 g/dL and conducting random breath tests can significantly decrease alcohol-related road traffic injuries.
- Enforcing helmet use can lower the risk of death by 40% and reduce the likelihood of serious head injuries by over 70%.
- Mandating seat belt use is instrumental in reducing the risk of fatal injuries by up to 50% for front-seat occupants and up to 75% for rear-seat occupants.
- The use of child restraints can substantially diminish the likelihood of a fatal crash for children by up to 80%.

## Emergency Management of Road Accident Victims

Providing trauma care within the "golden hour" (the first hour after an accident) greatly enhances the chances of survival. Prehospital care should include prompt communication, treatment, and transportation to healthcare facilities.

- *Immediate care at the scene:* Laypersons can play a crucial role in providing early care after an RA by recognizing emergencies, calling for help, and administering first aid, if possible. Traffic police officers can also serve as first responders and should be sensitized to trauma care and the availability of toll-free services. Promoting information, education, and communication activities can lead to better utilization of these services.

- *Safe and efficient patient transport:* Ambulances designed for patient transport should have sufficient space to keep patients stable and should be accompanied by trained personnel capable of providing care en route.
- *Matching patients to appropriate facilities:* Timely transfer of seriously injured individuals to hospitals with the necessary equipment and personnel is crucial. Designating trauma centers and establishing clear protocols for prehospital providers can ensure that injured persons receive prompt and appropriate treatment, improving overall patient outcomes.
- *Hospital-based emergency care:* Prompt interventions are essential for injury care, and emergency departments should be equipped with specialized staff and the necessary equipment for diagnosis and treatment. Operative care must be readily available at certified trauma centers.
- *Special considerations for injured children:* When children are involved in accidents, legal issues of guardianship and the psychological and developmental needs of children should be considered. Prompt and high-quality injury care is especially beneficial for children.

## EMERGENCY CARE RESEARCH AND DATA COLLECTION

Data on injuries and injury events can inform postcrash services and injury prevention strategies. Trauma registries can help identify risk factors and gaps in quality of care. Trauma registries are underdeveloped in many LMICs, but guidelines and standardized data sets have been developed to facilitate data collection.

## REHABILITATION AND REINTEGRATION

Long-term physical and psychological conditions can affect survivors and their families. Rehabilitation can help alleviate suffering, prevent further harm, and optimize functioning, enabling independence and reintegration into society. Rehabilitation involves a multidisciplinary approach to achieving treatment goals.

## PSYCHOLOGICAL SUPPORT

Road accidents have a profound psychological impact on survivors, often resulting in acute and long-term psychological conditions. Mental health support can mitigate these conditions and prevent them from becoming disabled, facilitating reintegration into work and social life.

## CONCLUSION

India is committed to bring down fatalities from RAs. The RAs are multicausal, which requires multipronged measures to mitigate the problems through concerted efforts of all agencies of both Central Government and State Governments. The Ministry has formulated a multipronged strategy to address the issue of road safety based on education, engineering (both of roads and vehicles), enforcement, and emergency care.

## KEY MESSAGES

- Road transportation is an integral part of our daily lives, but it has led to an increase in the risk of RAs.
- Globally, RAs are a leading cause of death among individuals aged 5–29 years.
- 24% of all fatalities occur in those aged 18–25 years. Men are three times more likely to die in RAs than women, mainly due to their higher involvement in risky driving behaviors and a greater proportion of male drivers and commuters.
- LMICs have 60% of the world's vehicles, but account for 93% of road fatalities, with over half of these fatalities affecting vulnerable road users such as pedestrians, cyclists, and motorcyclists.
- India leads the world in RA deaths, with about 80,000 fatalities annually, contributing to 11% of global RA deaths. Despite a decline in the number of RAs, the death toll has risen due to factors like population density, lax traffic regulation adherence, and inadequate road planning.
- RAs place a substantial burden on public health and the economy, and the problem is increasingly affecting adolescents who lack adequate road safety education.
- Factors such as human error, poor road conditions, and poor vehicular conditions contribute to RAs, with overspeeding being the leading cause.
- Addressing RAs requires a holistic approach, including reducing risk exposure, addressing risk factors, minimizing injury severity, and enhancing postcrash care.

- A systematic approach and comprehensive strategies are essential for preventing road traffic injuries and minimizing their far-reaching impacts, including measures for road users, vehicle safety, road infrastructure, and effective emergency care.

## RECOMMENDED READING


1. Elvik R, Vaa T, Hoye A, Sorensen M (Eds.). The Handbook of Road Safety Measures. UK: Emerald Group Publishing Limited; 2009.
2. GBD 2013 DALYs and HALE Collaborators; Murray CJ, Barber RM, Foreman KJ, Abbasoglu Ozgoren A, Abd-Allah F, Abera SF, et al. Global, regional, and national disability-adjusted life years (DALYs) for 306 diseases and injuries and healthy life expectancy (HALE) for 188 countries, 1990–2013: Quantifying the epidemiological transition. Lancet. 2015;386(10009):2145-91.
3. Kanchan T, Kulkarni V, Bakkannavar SM, Kumar N, Unnikrishnan B. Analysis of fatal Road Accidents in a coastal township of South India. J Forensic Leg Med. 2012;19(8):448-51.
4. Mock CN, Nugent R, Kobusingye O, Smith KR (Eds). Injury Prevention and Environmental Health, 3rd edition. Washington, DC: The International Bank for Reconstruction and Development/The World Bank; 2017.
5. National Crime Records Bureau. Ministry of Home Affairs, Government of India. (2022). Accidental deaths & suicides in India. 2022. [online] Available from https://data.opencity.in/dataset/accidental-deaths-and-suicides-in-india-2022 [Last accessed April, 2024].
6. National Highway Traffic Safety Administration. (2015). The economic and social impact of motor vehicle crashes 2010 (Revised). [online] Available from https://crashstats.nhtsa.dot.gov/Api/Public/ViewPublication/812013 [Last accessed April, 2024].
7. Perel P, Ker K, Ivers R, Blackhall K. Road safety in low- and middle-income countries: A neglected research area. Inj Prev. 2007;13(4):227.
8. World Health Organization. (2011). Global Plan for the Decade of Action for Road Safety 2011–2020. [online] Available from https://www.who.int/publications/m/item/global-plan-for-the-decade-of-action-for-road-safety-2011-2020 [Last accessed April, 2024].
9. World Health Organization. (2017). Global Status Report on Road Safety 2018. [online] Available at https://www.who.int/publications/i/item/9789241565684 [Last accessed April, 2024].


---

## 14.2   Road Etiquette and the Role of Gatekeepers

*Sonia Bhatt, Payal Mittal*

## INTRODUCTION

Road accidents are one of the most important cause of mortality in the pediatric age group throughout the world. Hence, it is the responsibility of society, lawmakers, nongovernment organizations (NGOs), parents, teachers, and other stakeholders to train children and adolescents in road etiquette.

The following are some preventive measures that have been recommended to reduce the incidence of road accidents in children:

- Reducing speed (30 km/h) around schools, parks, and other crowded areas
- Dedicated lanes for child cyclists and exclusive motorcycle lanes
- Vehicle modifications, and child restraint systems (i.e., booster cushions or booster seats)
- Seat belts (children >10 years of age)
- Bicycle and two-wheeler helmets

## ROAD ETIQUETTE

Training should be started as early as possible. Safety skills should be taught according to the mental and neurological understanding of the child.

### Toddlers

Parents should start to teach toddlers about:

- The difference between the footpath and the road
- The importance and significance of zebra crossings and traffic lights
- Holding hands with an adult while on the road
- Stop, look, listen, and think

## Children Aged 5–7 Years

Road safety apps are a fun way of teaching children how to cross the road. Parents and teachers can teach them:

- How pedestrians walk safely on the pavement while vehicles use the road
- How important it is to hold hands with an adult when crossing the road
- Safe versus less safe crossing places
- The stop, look, listen, and think sequence for crossing the road
- Be bright be seen.

  *The stop, look, listen, and think sequence:* Before crossing a road, *Stop* at the edge of the pavement. *Look* and *Listen* for any vehicle on the right, left, and right again. *Think* if there is enough time to cross the road.

## Children Aged 7–11 Years

At this age, parents should consider allowing their children to walk independently on the road, after assessing their mental age and development, and the amount of traffic in a particular area. They should be taught road signs and the Green Cross Code:

- *Find a safe place to cross:*
  - Use a pedestrian crossing if there is one.
  - Choose a place where you can see clearly in all directions.
  - If an obstacle is blocking your view of the road, choose a better place to cross.
- *Stop just before you get to the kerb:*
  - Do not stand on the kerb.
  - If there is no pavement, stand at the edge of the road.
- *Look all around for traffic and listen:*
  - Traffic can come from any direction.
  - Sometimes you can hear traffic before you see it.
  - If you see or hear an emergency vehicle in the distance, let it pass.
- *If traffic is coming, let it pass:*
  - Never run across the road when traffic is coming, even if you think there is time. It can be difficult to judge the speed of traffic.
  - Be aware that traffic may speed up.
- *When it is safe, go straight across the road. Do not run:*
  - Continue to look and listen as you cross.
  - Look out for cyclists and quieter vehicles, you may not hear them approaching.
  - Walk straight across the road.

## ADOLESCENTS AND YOUNG ADULTS AS PEDESTRIANS

Some Indian studies have suggested that adolescents have a reasonably good level of knowledge of the rules of the road. Yet they may still be victims of road accidents while walking on or crossing the road, as they are distractible.

*Despite frequent advice, they may:*

- Walk in a row while talking with friends, blocking most of the road
- Often walk at the center of the road
- Use mobile phones while walking
- Walk with earphones in their ears.

## ADOLESCENTS AND YOUNG ADULTS AS CAR DRIVERS AND MOTORCYCLISTS

There is an urgent need to teach adolescents and young adults about road etiquette while using a vehicle. Risk-taking is common between 15 and 25 years of age, reaching a peak at 18 years and decreasing after 25 years. Accidents are common, but most adolescents treat minor accidents as a normal part of learning to become good drivers. Hence, the recurrence rate is high: One in four teenagers will have a second accident within a year of the first accident.

The most important risk factors for road traffic accidents are driving under the influence of alcohol, cell phone use while driving, and driving while sleepy, especially at night.

### Underage Motorcycle Use

An adolescent in India can get a two-wheeler license at 16 years, and a four-wheeler license at 18 years. Yet underage driving was common in an Indian study. Underage and unlicensed two-wheeler driving was considered acceptable and safe in "low risk" traffic circumstances, such as within colonies or when going at low speeds. It was used for the convenience of shopping, to impress peers, and to learn a new skill.

### Unsafe Practices

Common practices when riding a motorcycle are:

- Reluctance to use a helmet
- Carrying a passenger who does not use a helmet
- Having more than one passenger
- Exchanging seats with your passenger, even though she/he may not have a license
- Overtaking dangerously, swerving in and out of traffic
- Overspeeding
- Using the mobile phone while driving

- Riding a motorcycle after consuming alcohol, because they feel their skills are unimpaired
- Doing stunts on the motorcycle to impress other boys
- Doing stunts on the motorcycle to impress girls, or frighten them, or harass them. This has resulted in death or injury to the rider or the victim.

## THE GATEKEEPERS' ROLE

- The family strongly influences a young person's driving behavior. Adolescents will model their parents if they do not use helmets, or state that it is unnecessary, if they ride motorcycles under the influence of alcohol, if they use a mobile phone while driving, if they drive recklessly, and if they manifest road rage.
- Underage driving is usually done with the permission and often approval of the gatekeepers, i.e., the parents.
- Parents and teachers should educate adolescents on the dangers of road traffic accidents. They should point out that riding a motorcycle is glamorous, but there is nothing glamorous about an accident that damages the motorcycle, makes the adolescent bedridden for months, and leaves horrible scars that last a lifetime.
- "An accident frightens us for a day, then it is back to normal." While it is true that many adolescents forget all about the dangers of overspeeding when seated on a motorcycle, classes in schools have been shown to have a significant impact on adolescent minds, especially when accompanied by scary pictures of road accident victims, and when taken by traffic police.

## PREVENTING ACCIDENTS

- Advertising campaigns about safe driving have better recall among adolescents when humorous, but are more effective when they are somber, and especially if they show scenes of damaged vehicles, accident victims, and the scars that may follow an accident.
- Many countries have adopted a graduated driver licensing program, which has proven successful in reducing accident rates and mortality. Instead of giving the adolescent a blanket license to drive once he is of age and passes a test, he initially gets a license that permits him to drive only under adult supervision, in the daytime, with passenger limits, etc., and the limits are gradually removed over months, if he proves to be a safe driver.
- It has been suggested that advertising and teaching about safe driving would be more effective among adolescents if done through social media like WhatsApp, Facebook, and X (formerly Twitter).

- Underage driving should be punished more severely, not only by a fine, but also by not allowing entry of motorcycles into school, confiscating the vehicle, and making the parents pay the fine to get the motorcycle released. The latter is effective because it discourages wealthy parents who permit their underage adolescents to drive to show off their wealth.

## KEY MESSAGES

- Children and adolescents should be taught about road safety, including the use of helmets while using two-wheelers and seatbelts while in a car.
- Children should be taught the basics of road safety by their parents right from the toddler age group.
- They should learn the stop, look, listen, and think sequence for crossing the road.
- By 7–11 years, they should learn the Green Cross Code for crossing the road independent of adult supervision.
- Adolescents and young adults are prone to distractions and may have an accident when they walk in a row while talking with friends, use mobile phones while walking, and walk with earphones in their ears.
- The most important risk factors for road traffic accidents in adolescents are driving under the influence of alcohol, phone use while driving, and driving while sleepy at night.
- Parents, teachers, and traffic police should firmly discourage underage riding of motorcycles and unsafe practices, which should be firmly punished.

## RECOMMENDED READING


1. Agrawal A, Bhoi S, Galwankar S, Pal R, Deora H, Ghosh A, et al. Safer Roads to School. J Emerg Trauma Shock. 2020;13(1):15-9.
2. Gicquel L, Ordonneau P, Blot E, Toillon C, Ingrand P, Romo L. Description of various factors contributing to traffic accidents in youth and measures proposed to alleviate recurrence. Front Psychiatry. 2017;8:94.
3. Jagnoor J, Sharma P, Parveen S, Cox KL, Kallakuri S. Knowledge is not enough: Barriers and facilitators for reducing road traffic injuries amongst Indian adolescents, a qualitative study. International Journal of Adolescence and Youth. 2020;25(1):787-99.
4. Thakur N, Mahajan P, Misra S, Fayyaz J. Pediatric Trauma Training in India–Need of the Hour. Indian Pediatr. 2023;60(10):800-3.
5. The Royal Society for the Prevention of Accidents. (2024). Teaching road safety: A guide for parents. [online] Available from www.rospa.com/media/documents/road-safety/teaching-road-safety-a-guide-for-parents.pdf. [Last accessed April, 2024].

# Annexures

HEADSS Psychosocial History

## 1 | Key Interventions for School-aged Children

**BOX 1:** Key interventions for school-aged children.

- *Infectious diseases:*
  - Immunization with routine, boosters, and catch-up vaccines
  - Education about water, sanitation, and hygiene conditions
  - Oral rehydration solution for diarrhea management
  - Screening and treatment of common illnesses
  - Deworming
- *Nutrition and healthy lifestyle:*
  - Healthy lifestyle promotion by healthy eating, physical activity, and decreasing sedentary behavior
  - School meal programs and micronutrient supplementation
  - Oral health and hygiene education
- *Noncommunicable disease:*
  - Early identification and management of chronic noncommunicable disease
  - Screening of blood pressure and body mass index for early detection of hypertension and obesity
- *Mental health and positive development:*
  - Mental health promotion by meditation and yoga, and targeted interventions for prevention mental illness and substance use
  - Prevention of school bullying, violence, and gender-based violence
- *Unintentional injuries:*
  - Traffic safety rules for prevention of road traffic accidents
  - Swimming lessons for prevention of drowning
  - General first-aid and resuscitation education
  - Prevention strategy from fire, poisons, and injuries
- *Sexual and reproductive health and rights:*
  - Age-appropriate sexual and reproductive health education
  - Prevention of sexually transmitted diseases
  - Prevention of abuse, early marriage, and adolescent pregnancy

<table>
<tr><td>**2**</td><td colspan="2"><h1>HEEADSSS Psychosocial History</h1></td></tr>
</table>

| *Psychosocial domain* | *Sample questions* |
| --- | --- |
| Home | • Who lives at home with you?<br>• How is your relationship with each family member?<br>• Do you have a separate room?<br>• Do you sleep alone?<br>• Has there been a recent change in living arrangement?<br>• If I was invisible and you were having a disagreement with your parent, what would I hear?<br>• How would I see your parent disciplining you? |
| Education/employment | • Are you studying/working?<br>• How is the situation at school/work place?<br>• How has your performance been in school this year compared to last? Are you satisfied with your performance?<br>• How is your relationship with teachers and peers at school?<br>• Has anybody ever spoken to you in a way that you have not liked?<br>• Who helps you with school work?<br>• Please share details regarding your study habits.<br>• Where do you see yourself 5 years from now? |
| Eating | • Recall your dietary intake on a typical day.<br>• How often do you eat out/drink sugar sweetened beverages?<br>• How do you stay healthy? What do you think about your diet?<br>• How do you feel about your body?<br>• Do you ever feel that food controls you rather than vice versa? Has there been any change in your appetite lately? |
| Activities | • What do you do for fun?<br>• How much time do you spend in structured or unstructured outdoor/physical activity?<br>• What are your hobbies? Do you attend special hobby classes?<br>• Are you happy with your performance? Do you have friends you socialize with?<br>• Where do you and your peers hang around for fun? How is your relationship with friends?<br>• Which digital devices do you use and own?<br>• For what purpose do you use your digital devices? Are you a member of social media sites? Which ones?<br>• Do you feel the media device controls your life? Do you get into trouble with family and friends for using media excessively?<br>• For how many hours do you sleep?<br>• Do you have any sleep-related problems?<br>• Are you a part of a religious community? How often do you participate in religious activities?<br>• What role does religion have in your life? Do you have personal spiritual beliefs? What aspects of spirituality or spiritual practices do you find most useful?<br>• Have you lately lost interest in activities that you enjoyed previously? If yes, since how many days or months? |
| Drugs | • What is your attitude toward drug usage? How do you feel about this issue?<br>• Do your friends smoke, drink, or use drugs?<br>• Have you ever tried? If yes, which drug and how often? |
| Sexuality | • When did you attain menarche? When was your last menstrual period? What is the length of your menstrual cycle and for how long does the bleeding last? How many pads do you use in a cycle? Do you have any problems during menstruation?<br>• I ask all teenagers a few questions pertaining to sexual health, which is an important component of general health. Are you ok with that? You could let me know anytime if you are uncomfortable or embarrassed. |

*Contd...*

*Contd...*

| Psychosocial domain | Sample questions |
| --- | --- |
|  | • Are you in a romantic relationship?<br>• Have you been physically intimate with somebody? If yes, with whom? What do you do in intimate moments?<br>• Are you married? Do you use any contraceptive method? Have you ever been pregnant?<br>• Do you have any vaginal/penile discharge or itching? Do you have burning micturition or pain in the abdomen?<br>• Has anybody touched you in a way that you did not like? |
| Suicide/depression | • Have you ever felt hopeless, sad, and a failure in life?<br>• Has there been a recent change in your mood, behavior, sleep, appetite, or academic performance?<br>• For how long have you been feeling low?<br>• What would make you feel better?<br>• What do you do when you feel sad?<br>• Do you confide your problems in someone?<br>• Sometimes when young people are in unbearable pain or trouble they wish that they could end it all.<br>• Have you ever wished the same?<br>• Have you ever tried to end your life? |
| Safety | • Do you feel safe at home, school, and while playing in the neighborhood?<br>• Do you drive a vehicle? If yes, which one?<br>• Do you wear a helmet/seat belt while riding/driving a vehicle?<br>• Have you ever got into a physical fight with anybody?<br>• Have you ever been hurt during fights?<br>• Have you ever got into trouble with law? |

# 3 | Perceived Stress Scale (PSS)

A more precise measure of personal stress can be determined by using a variety of instruments that have been designed to help measure individual stress levels. The first of these is called the *Perceived Stress Scale (PSS)*.

The PSS is a classic stress assessment instrument. The tool, while originally developed in 1983, remains a popular choice for helping us understand how different situations affect our feelings and our perceived stress. The questions in this scale ask about your feelings and thoughts during the last month. In each case, you will be asked to indicate how often you felt or thought a certain way. Although some of the questions are similar, there are differences between them and you should treat each one as a separate question. The best approach is to answer fairly quickly. That is, do not try to count up the number of times you felt a particular way; rather indicate the alternative that seems like a reasonable estimate.

For each question, choose from the following alternatives:

0—never; 1—almost never; 2—sometimes; 3—fairly often; 4—very often

1. In the last month, how often have you been upset because of something that happened unexpectedly?
2. In the last month, how often have you felt that you were unable to control the important things in your life?
3. In the last month, how often have you felt nervous and stressed?
4. In the last month, how often have you felt confident about your ability to handle your personal problems?
5. In the last month, how often have you felt that things were going your way?
6. In the last month, how often have you found that you could not cope with all the things that you had to do?
7. In the last month, how often have you been able to control irritations in your life?
8. In the last month, how often have you felt that you were on top of things?
9. In the last month, how often have you been angered because of things that happened that were outside of your control?
10. In the last month, how often have you felt difficulties were piling up so high that you could not overcome them?

## ■ FIGURING YOUR PSS SCORE

You can determine your PSS score by following these directions:

- First, reverse your scores for questions 4, 5, 7, and 8. On these four questions, change the scores like this:
  0 = 4, 1 = 3, 2 = 2, 3 = 1, 4 = 0.
- Now add up your scores for each item to get a total. *My total score is_______________________.*
- Individual scores on the PSS can range from 0 to 40 with higher scores indicating higher perceived stress.
  - Scores ranging from 0 to 13 would be considered low stress.
  - Scores ranging from 14 to 26 would be considered moderate stress.
  - Scores ranging from 27 to 40 would be considered high perceived stress.

The PSS is interesting and important, because your perception of what is happening in your life is most important. Consider the idea that two individuals could have the exact same events and experiences in their lives for the past month. Depending on their perception, total score could put one of those individuals in the low stress category and the total score could put the second person in the high stress category.

***Disclaimer***: *The scores on the following self-assessment do not reflect any particular diagnosis or course of treatment. They are meant as a tool to help assess your level of stress.*

# 4   Generalized Anxiety Disorder 7 (GAD-7)

| Over the last 2 weeks, how often have you been bothered by the following problems? | Not at all | Several days | More than half the days | Nearly every day |
|---|---|---|---|---|
| 1. Feeling nervous, anxious, or on edge | 0 | 1 | 2 | 3 |
| 2. Not being able to stop or control worrying | 0 | 1 | 2 | 3 |
| 3. Worrying too much about different things | 0 | 1 | 2 | 3 |
| 4. Trouble relaxing | 0 | 1 | 2 | 3 |
| 5. Being so restless that it is hard to sit still | 0 | 1 | 2 | 3 |
| 6. Becoming easily annoyed or irritable | 0 | 1 | 2 | 3 |
| 7. Feeling afraid, as if something awful might happen | 0 | 1 | 2 | 3 |

Column totals __________ + __________ + __________ + __________ = 

Total score__________

If you checked any problems, how difficult have they made it for you to do your work, take care of things at home, or get along with other people?

| Not difficult at all | Somewhat difficult | Very difficult | Extremely difficult |
|---|---|---|---|
| 0 | 1 | 2 | 3 |

## ■ SCORING GAD-7 ANXIETY SEVERITY

This is calculated by assigning scores of 0, 1, 2, and 3 to the response categories, respectively, of "not at all," "several days," "more than half the days," and "nearly every day."

GAD-7 total score for the seven items ranges from 0 to 21.

*0–4:* Minimal anxiety
*5–9:* Mild anxiety
*10–14:* Moderate anxiety
*15–21:* Severe anxiety

---

<table>
<tr><td rowspan="2">**5**</td><td colspan="2"># Screen for Child Anxiety Related<br>Disorders (SCARED)</td></tr>
<tr><td colspan="2">### CHILD Version—Page 1 of 2 (to be filled out by the CHILD)</td></tr>
</table>

**Name:** ___________________________________________________________ **Date:** ______________

**Directions:**

Below is a list of sentences that describe how people feel. Read each phrase and decide if it is "Not True or Hardly Ever True" or "Somewhat True or Sometimes True" or "Very True or Often True" for you. Then, for each sentence, fill in one circle that corresponds to the response that seems to describe you *for the last 3 months*.

| | 0<br>*Not True or*<br>*Hardly Ever True* | 1<br>*Somewhat True*<br>*or Sometimes True* | 2<br>*Very True or*<br>*Often True* | |
|---|---|---|---|---|
| 1. When I feel frightened, it is hard to breathe. | O | O | O | **PN** |
| 2. I get headaches when I am at school. | O | O | O | **SH** |
| 3. I don't like to be with people I don't know well. | O | O | O | **SC** |
| 4. I get scared if I sleep away from home. | O | O | O | **SP** |
| 5. I worry about other people liking me. | O | O | O | **GD** |
| 6. When I get frightened, I feel like passing out. | O | O | O | **PN** |
| 7. I am nervous. | O | O | O | **GD** |
| 8. I follow my mother or father wherever they go. | O | O | O | **SP** |
| 9. People tell me that I look nervous. | O | O | O | **PN** |
| 10. I feel nervous with people I don't know well. | O | O | O | **SC** |
| 11. I get stomachaches at school. | O | O | O | **SH** |
| 12. When I get frightened, I feel like I am going crazy. | O | O | O | **PN** |
| 13. I worry about sleeping alone. | O | O | O | **SP** |
| 14. I worry about being as good as other kids. | O | O | O | **GD** |
| 15. When I get frightened, I feel like things are not real. | O | O | O | **PN** |
| 16. I have nightmares about something bad happening to my parents. | O | O | O | **SP** |
| 17. I worry about going to school. | O | O | O | **SH** |
| 18. When I get frightened, my heart beats fast. | O | O | O | **PN** |
| 19. I get shaky. | O | O | O | **PN** |
| 20. I have nightmares about something bad happening to me. | O | O | O | **SP** |

# Screen for Child Anxiety Related Disorders (SCARED)
## CHILD Version—Page 2 of 2 (to be filled out by the CHILD)

| | 0<br>Not True or<br>Hardly Ever True | 1<br>Somewhat True<br>or Sometimes True | 2<br>Very True or<br>Often True | |
|---|---|---|---|---|
| 21. I worry about things working out for me. | O | O | O | GD |
| 22. When I get frightened, I sweat a lot. | O | O | O | PN |
| 23. I am a worrier. | O | O | O | GD |
| 24. I get really frightened for no reason at all. | O | O | O | PN |
| 25. I am afraid to be alone in the house. | O | O | O | SP |
| 26. It is hard for me to talk with people I don't know well. | O | O | O | SC |
| 28. People tell me that I worry too much. | O | O | O | GD |
| 29. I don't like to be away from my family. | O | O | O | SP |
| 30. I am afraid of having anxiety (or panic) attacks. | O | O | O | PN |
| 31. I worry that something bad might happen to my parents. | O | O | O | SP |
| 32. I feel shy with people I don't know well. | O | O | O | SC |
| 33. I worry about what is going to happen in the future. | O | O | O | GD |
| 34. When I get frightened, I feel like throwing up. | O | O | O | PN |
| 35. I worry about how well I do things. | O | O | O | GD |
| 36. I am scared to go to school. | O | O | O | SH |
| 37. I worry about things that have already happened. | O | O | O | GD |
| 38. When I get frightened, I feel dizzy. | O | O | O | PN |
| 39. I feel nervous when I am with other children or adults and I have to do something while they watch me (for example: read aloud, speak, play a game, play a sport). | O | O | O | SC |
| 40. I feel nervous when I am going to parties, dances, or any place where there will be people that I don't know well. | O | O | O | SC |
| 41. I am shy. | O | O | O | SC |

**SCORING:**

A total score of ≥**25** may indicate the presence of an **Anxiety Disorder**. Scores higher than 30 are more specific. TOTAL =

A score of **7** for items 1, 6, 9, 12, 15, 18, 19, 22, 24, 27, 30, 34, 38 may indicate **Panic Disorder** or **Significant Somatic Symptoms.** PN =

A score of **9** for items 5, 7, 14, 21, 23, 28, 33, 35, 37 may indicate **Generalized Anxiety Disorder.** GD =

A score of **5** for items 4, 8, 13, 16, 20, 25, 29, 31 may indicate **Separation Anxiety SOC.** SP =

A score of **8** for items 3, 10, 26, 32, 39, 40, 41 may indicate **Social Anxiety Disorder.** SC =

A score of **3** for items 2, 11, 17, 36 may indicate **Significant School Avoidance.** SH =

*For children ages 8 to 11, it is recommended that the clinician explain all questions, or have the child answer the questionnaire sitting with an adult in case they have any questions.*

*The SCARED is available at no cost at www.wpic.pitt.edu/research under tools and assessments, or at www.pediatric bipolar.pitt.edu under instruments.*

March 27, 2012

## ■ SCORING SHEET FOR SCARED ANXIETY QUESTIONNAIRE

In the table below, enter the score for each question to the right of the question number. Add the scores in each column and enter the total at the bottom of the column. Add the scores across the "TOTAL" row to calculate the overall score.

| Panic Disorder or Significant Somatic Symptoms | | Generalized Anxiety Disorder | | Separation Anxiety Disorder | | Social Anxiety Disorder | | Significant School Avoidance | | |
|---|---|---|---|---|---|---|---|---|---|---|
| Question number | Score | Question number | Score | Question number | Score | Question number | Score | Question number | Score | |
| #1 | | #5 | | #4 | | #3 | | #2 | | |
| #6 | | #7 | | #8 | | #10 | | #11 | | |
| #9 | | #14 | | #13 | | #26 | | #17 | | |
| #12 | | #21 | | #16 | | #32 | | #36 | | |
| #15 | | #23 | | #20 | | #39 | | | | |
| #18 | | #28 | | #25 | | #40 | | | | |
| #19 | | #33 | | #29 | | #41 | | | | |
| #22 | | #35 | | #31 | | | | | | |
| #24 | | #37 | | | | | | | | |
| #27 | | | | | | | | | | |
| #30 | | | | | | | | | | |
| #34 | | | | | | | | | | |
| #38 | | | | | | | | | | Overall Score |
| TOTAL | = | + | = | + | = | + | = | + | = | |

A total score of ≥**25** may indicate the presence of an **Anxiety Disorder**. Scores higher than 40 are more specific. ⬚ TOTAL = 

A score of **7** for items 1, 6, 9, 12, 15, 18, 19, 22, 24, 27, 30, 34, 38 may indicate **Panic Disorder** or **Significant Somatic Symptoms**. ⬚ PN = 

A score of **9** for items 5, 7, 14, 21, 23, 28, 33, 35, 37 may indicate **Generalized Anxiety Disorder**. ⬚ GD = 

A score of **5** for items 4, 8, 13, 16, 20, 25, 29, 31 may indicate **Separation Anxiety Disorder**. ⬚ SP = 

A score of **8** for items 3, 10, 26, 32, 39, 40, 41 may indicate **Social Anxiety Disorder**. ⬚ SC = 

A score of **3** for items 2, 11, 17, 36 may indicate **Significant School Avoidance**. ⬚ SH = 

Developed by Boris Birmaher MD, Suneeta Khetarpal MD, Marlane Cully MEd, David Brent MD, and Sandra McKenzie PhD. Western Psychiatric Institute and Clinic, University of Pittsburgh (October, 1995). E-mail: birmaherb@upmc.edu

# 6

# Screen for Child Anxiety Related Disorders (SCARED)
## Parent Version—Page 1 of 2 (To be filled out by the PARENT)

**Name:** _______________________________________________ **Date:**______________

**Directions:**

Below is a list of statements that describe how people feel. Read each statement carefully and decide if it is "Not True or Hardly Ever True" or "Somewhat True or Sometimes True" or "Very True or Often True" for your child. Then for each statement, fill in one circle that corresponds to the response that seems to describe your child *for the last 3 months*. Please respond to all statements as well as you can, even if some do not seem to concern your child.

| | 0 Not True or Hardly Ever True | 1 Somewhat True or Sometimes True | 2 Very True or Often True |
|---|---|---|---|
| 1. When my child feels frightened, it is hard for him/her to breathe. | O | O | O |
| 2. My child gets headaches when he/she is at school. | O | O | O |
| 3. My child doesn't like to be with people he/she doesn't know well. | O | O | O |
| 4. My child gets scared if he/she sleeps away from home. | O | O | O |
| 5. My child worries about other people liking him/her. | O | O | O |
| 6. When my child gets frightened, he/she feels like passing out. | O | O | O |
| 7. My child is nervous. | O | O | O |
| 8. My child follows me wherever I go. | O | O | O |
| 9. People tell me that my child looks nervous. | O | O | O |
| 10. My child feels nervous with people he/she doesn't know well. | O | O | O |
| 11. My child gets stomachaches at school. | O | O | O |
| 12. When my child gets frightened, he/she feels like he/she is going crazy. | O | O | O |
| 13. My child worries about sleeping alone. | O | O | O |
| 14. My child worries about being as good as other kids. | O | O | O |
| 15. When he/she gets frightened, he/she feels like things are not real. | O | O | O |
| 16. My child has nightmares about something bad happening to his/her parents. | O | O | O |
| 17. My child worries about going to school. | O | O | O |
| 18. When my child gets frightened, his/her heart beats fast. | O | O | O |
| 19. He/she gets shaky. | O | O | O |
| 20. My child has nightmares about something bad happening to him/her. | O | O | O |

# Screen for Child Anxiety Related Disorders (SCARED)
## Parent Version—Page 2 of 2 (To be filled out by the PARENT)

|  | 0<br>Not True or Hardly Ever True | 1<br>Somewhat True or Sometimes True | 2<br>Very True or Often True |
|---|---|---|---|
| 21. My child worries about things working out for him/her. | O | O | O |
| 22. When my child gets frightened, he/she sweats a lot. | O | O | O |
| 23. My child is a worrier. | O | O | O |
| 24. My child gets really frightened for no reason at all. | O | O | O |
| 25. My child is afraid to be alone in the house. | O | O | O |
| 26. It is hard for my child to talk with people he/she doesn't know well. | O | O | O |
| 27. When my child gets frightened, he/she feels like he/she is choking. | O | O | O |
| 28. People tell me that my child worries too much. | O | O | O |
| 29. My child doesn't like to be away from his/her family. | O | O | O |
| 30. My child is afraid of having anxiety (or panic) attacks. | O | O | O |
| 31. My child worries that something bad might happen to his/her parents. | O | O | O |
| 32. My child feels shy with people he/she doesn't know well. | O | O | O |
| 33. My child worries about what is going to happen in the future. | O | O | O |
| 34. When my child gets frightened, he/she feels like throwing up. | O | O | O |
| 35. My child worries about how well he/she does things. | O | O | O |
| 36. My child is scared to go to school. | O | O | O |
| 37. My child worries about things that have already happened. | O | O | O |
| 38. When my child gets frightened, he/she feels dizzy. | O | O | O |
| 39. My child feels nervous when he/she is with other children or adults and he/she has to do something while they watch him/her (for example: read aloud, speak, play a game, play a sport). | O | O | O |
| 40. My child feels nervous when he/she is going to parties, dances, or any place where there will be people that he/she doesn't know well. | O | O | O |
| 41. My child is shy. | O | O | O |

**SCORING:**

A total score of ≥**25** may indicate the presence of an **Anxiety Disorder.** Scores higher than 30 are more specific.

A score of **7** for items 1, 6, 9, 12, 15, 18, 19, 22, 24, 27, 30, 34, 38 may indicate **Panic Disorder** or **Significant Somatic Symptoms.**

A score of **9** for items 5, 7, 14, 21, 23, 28, 33, 35, 37 may indicate **Generalized Anxiety Disorder.**

A score of **5** for items 4, 8, 13, 16, 20, 25, 29, 31 may indicate **Separation Anxiety Disorder.**

A score of **8** for items 3, 10, 26, 32, 39, 40, 41 may indicate **Social Anxiety Disorder.**

Developed by Boris Birmaher MD, Suneeta Khetarpal MD, Marlane Cully MEd, David Brent MD, and Sandra McKenzie PhD. Western Psychiatric Institute and Clinic, University of Pittsburgh (October, 1995). E-mail: HYPERLINK „mailto:birmaherb@msx.upmc.edu"birmaherb@msx.upmc.edu

# 7   Patient Health Questionnaire PHQ-2

| PATIENT HEALTH QUESTIONNAIRE 2 | | | | |
| --- | --- | --- | --- | --- |
| *A score of 3 or greater has good sensitivity and specificity for detecting major depression in adolescents.* | | | | |
| **Over the past 2 weeks, how often have you been bothered by any of the following?** | *Not at all* | *Several days* | *More than half the days* | *Nearly every day* |
| Little interest or pleasure in doing things | 0 | 1 | 2 | 3 |
| Feeling down, depressed, or hopeless | 0 | 1 | 2 | 3 |

*Source:* Richardson LR et al.

# Patient Health Questionnaire PHQ-9: Modified for Teens

**8**

**Name:**________________________ **Clinician:**________________________________________ **Date:**________________

*Instructions:* How often have you been bothered by each of the following symptoms during the past 2 weeks? For each symptom, put an "X" in the box beneath the answer that best describes how you have been feeling.

| | 0<br>Not at all | 1<br>Several days | 2<br>More than half the days | 3<br>Nearly every day |
|---|---|---|---|---|
| 1. Feeling down, depressed, irritable, or hopeless? | ☐ | ☐ | ☐ | ☐ |
| 2. Little interest or pleasure in doing things? | ☐ | ☐ | ☐ | ☐ |
| 3. Trouble falling asleep, staying asleep, or sleeping too much? | ☐ | ☐ | ☐ | ☐ |
| 4. Poor appetite, weight loss, or overeating? | ☐ | ☐ | ☐ | ☐ |
| 5. Feeling tired, or having little energy? | ☐ | ☐ | ☐ | ☐ |
| 6. Feeling bad about yourself, or feeling that you are a failure, or that you have let yourself or your family down? | ☐ | ☐ | ☐ | ☐ |
| 7. Trouble concentrating on things like school work, reading, or watching TV? | ☐ | ☐ | ☐ | ☐ |
| 8. Moving or speaking so slowly that other people could have noticed?<br>Or the opposite—being so fidgety or restless that you were moving around a lot more than usual? | ☐ | ☐ | ☐ | ☐ |
| 9. Thoughts that you would be better off dead, or of hurting yourself in some way? | ☐ | ☐ | ☐ | ☐ |

In the *past year*, have you felt depressed or sad most days, even if you felt okay sometimes?

[ ] Yes          [ ] No

If you are experiencing any of the problems on this form, how difficult have these problems made it for you to do your work, take care of things at home, or get along with other people?

[ ] Not difficult at all          [ ] Somewhat difficult          [ ] Very difficult          [ ] Extremely difficult

Has there been a time in the past month when you have had serious thoughts about ending your life?

[ ] Yes          [ ] No

Have you ever, in your whole life, tried to kill yourself or made a suicide attempt?

[ ] Yes          [ ] No

**If you have had thoughts that you would be better off dead or of hurting yourself in some way, please discuss this with your *Health Care Clinician, go to a hospital emergency room or call 911.*

**Office use only:**________________________________________ **Severity score:**________________________________

## ■ SCORING THE PHQ-9 MODIFIED FOR TEENS

Scoring the PHQ-9 modified for teens is easy but involves thinking about several different aspects of depression.

To use the PHQ-9 as a diagnostic aid for major depressive disorder (MDD):
- Questions 1 and/or 2 need to be endorsed as a "2" or "3".
- Need five or more positive symptoms (positive is defined by a "2" or "3" in questions 1–8 and by a "1", "2", or "3" in question 9).
- The functional impairment question (How difficult....) needs to be rated at least as "somewhat difficult."

To use the PHQ-9 to screen for all types of depression or other mental illness:
- All positive answers (positive is defined by a "2" or "3" in questions 1–8 and by a "1", "2", or "3" in question 9) should be followed up by interview.
- A total PHQ-9 score ≥10 (see below for instructions on how to obtain a total score) has a good sensitivity and specificity for MDD.

To use the PHQ-9 to aid in the diagnosis of dysthymia:
- The dysthymia question (In the past year...) should be endorsed as "yes."

To use the PHQ-9 to screen for suicide risk:
- All positive answers to question 9 as well as the two additional suicide items *must be* followed up by a clinical interview.

To use the PHQ-9 to obtain a total score and assess depressive severity:
- Add up the numbers endorsed for questions 1–9 and obtain a total score.
- See Table below:

| *Total score* | *Depression severity* |
| --- | --- |
| 0–4 | No or minimal depression |
| 5–9 | Mild depression |
| 10–14 | Moderate depression |
| 15–19 | Moderately severe depression |
| 20–27 | Severe depression |

---

*Source*: Modified with permission by the GLAD-PC team from the PHQ-9 (Spitzer, Williams, & Kroenke, 1999), Revised PHQ-A (Johnson, 2002), and the CDS (DISC Development Group, 2000).

# 9 — Beck's Depression Inventory (BDI)

*This depression inventory can be self-scored. The scoring scale is at the end of the questionnaire.*

**1.**
0 I do not feel sad.
1 I feel sad.
2 I am sad all the time and I cannot snap out of it.
3 I am so sad and unhappy that I cannot stand it.

**2.**
0 I am not particularly discouraged about the future.
1 I feel discouraged about the future.
2 I feel I have nothing to look forward to.
3 I feel the future is hopeless and that things cannot improve.

**3.**
0 I do not feel like a failure.
1 I feel I have failed more than the average person.
2 As I look back on my life, all I can see is a lot of failures.
3 I feel I am a complete failure as a person.

**4.**
0 I get as much satisfaction out of things as I used to.
1 I do not enjoy things the way I used to.
2 I do not get real satisfaction out of anything anymore.
3 I am dissatisfied or bored with everything.

**5.**
0 I do not feel particularly guilty.
1 I feel guilty a good part of the time.
2 I feel quite guilty most of the time.
3 I feel guilty all of the time.

**6.**
0 I do not feel I am being punished.
1 I feel I may be punished.
2 I expect to be punished.
3 I feel I am being punished.

**7.**
0 I do not feel disappointed in myself.
1 I am disappointed in myself.
2 I am disgusted with myself.
3 I hate myself.

**8.**
0 I do not feel I am any worse than anybody else.
1 I am critical of myself for my weaknesses or mistakes.
2 I blame myself all the time for my faults.
3 I blame myself for everything bad that happens.

**9.**
0 I do not have any thoughts of killing myself.
1 I have thoughts of killing myself, but I would not carry them out.
2 I would like to kill myself.
3 I would kill myself if I had the chance.

**10.**
0 I do not cry any more than usual.
1 I cry more now than I used to.
2 I cry all the time now.
3 I used to be able to cry, but now I cannot cry even though I want to.

**11.**
0 I am no more irritated by things than I ever was.
1 I am slightly more irritated now than usual.
2 I am quite annoyed or irritated a good deal of the time.
3 I feel irritated all the time.

**12.**
0 I have not lost interest in other people.
1 I am less interested in other people than I used to be.
2 I have lost most of my interest in other people.
3 I have lost all of my interest in other people.

**13.**
0 I make decisions about as well as I ever could.
1 I put off making decisions more than I used to.
2 I have greater difficulty in making decisions more than I used to.
3 I cannot make decisions at all anymore.

**14.**
0 I do not feel that I look any worse than I used to.
1 I am worried that I am looking old or unattractive.
2 I feel there are permanent changes in my appearance that make me look unattractive.
3 I believe that I look ugly.

**15.**

   0 I can work about as well as before.

   1 It takes an extra effort to get started at doing something.

   2 I have to push myself very hard to do anything.

   3 I cannot do any work at all.

**16.**

   0 I can sleep as well as usual.

   1 I do not sleep as well as I used to.

   2 I wake up 1–2 hours earlier than usual and find it hard to get back to sleep.

   3 I wake up several hours earlier than I used to and cannot get back to sleep.

**17.**

   0 I do not get more tired than usual.

   1 I get tired more easily than I used to.

   2 I get tired from doing almost anything.

   3 I am too tired to do anything.

**18.**

   0 My appetite is no worse than usual.

   1 My appetite is not as good as it used to be.

   2 My appetite is much worse now.

   3 I have no appetite at all anymore.

**19.**

   0 I have not lost much weight, if any, lately.

   1 I have lost more than five pounds.

   2 I have lost more than ten pounds.

   3 I have lost more than fifteen pounds.

**20.**

   0 I am no more worried about my health than usual.

   1 I am worried about physical problems like aches, pains, upset stomach, or constipation.

   2 I am very worried about physical problems and it is hard to think of much else.

   3 I am so worried about my physical problems that I cannot think of anything else.

**21.**

   0 I have not noticed any recent change in my interest in sex.

   1 I am less interested in sex than I used to be.

   2 I have almost no interest in sex.

   3 I have lost interest in sex completely.

## INTERPRETING THE BECK DEPRESSION INVENTORY

Now that you have completed the questionnaire, add up the score for each of the 21 questions by counting the number to the right of each question you marked. The highest possible total for the whole test would be 63. This would mean you circled number three on all 21 questions. Since the lowest possible score for each question is zero, the lowest possible score for the test would be zero. This would mean you circles zero on each question.

You can evaluate your depression according to the Table below.

| Total score | Levels of depression |
| --- | --- |
| 1–10 | These ups and downs are considered normal |
| 11–16 | Mild mood disturbance |
| 17–20 | Borderline clinical depression |
| 21–30 | Moderate depression |
| 31–40 | Severe depression |
| Over 40 | Extreme depression |

*Source:* http://www.med.navy.mil/sites/NMCP2/PatientServices/SleepClinicLab/Documents/Beck_Depression_Inventory.pdf

# 10 — ASQ Suicide Risk Screening Tool

## ■ ASK SUICIDE-SCREENING QUESTIONS

### Ask the Patient

1. In the past few weeks, have you wished you were dead?      O Yes      O No
2. In the past few weeks, have you felt that you or your family would be better off if you were dead?      O Yes      O No
3. In the past week, have you been having thoughts about killing yourself?      O Yes      O No
4. Have you ever tried to kill yourself?      O Yes      O No

   If yes, how?_______________________________________________
   When?_____________________________________________________
   *If the patient answers Yes to any of the above, ask the following acuity question:*
5. Are you having thoughts of killing yourself right now?      O Yes      O No
   If yes please describe: ______________________________________

## Next Steps

- If patient answers "No" to all questions 1 through 4, screening is complete (not necessary to ask question #5). No intervention is necessary (*Note: Clinical judgment can always override a negative screen*).
- *If patient answers "Yes" to any of questions 1 through 4, or refuses to answer, they are considered a* positive screen. Ask question #5 to assess acuity:
  - "Yes" to question #5 = *acute positive screen* (imminent risk identified)
    - *Patient requires a STAT safety/full mental health evaluation. Patient cannot leave until evaluated for safety.*
    - Keep patient in sight. Remove all dangerous objects from room. Alert physician or clinician responsible for patient's care.
  - "No" to question #5 = *nonacute positive screen* (potential risk identified)
    - *Patient requires a brief suicide safety assessment to determine if a full mental health evaluation is needed. Patient cannot leave until evaluated for safety.*
    - Alert physician or clinician responsible for patient's care.

## Provide Resources to All Patients

- 24/7 National Suicide Prevention Lifeline 1-800-273-TALK (8255) En Español: 1-888-628-9454
- 24/7 Crisis Text Line: Text "HOME" to 741-741

ASQ Suicide Risk Screening Toolkit      **NATIONAL INSTITUTE OF MENTAL HEALTH (NIMH)**

<table><tr><td>**11**</td><td># Counseling Questionnaire</td></tr></table>

**Name:**_______________________________ **Age:**___________ **Phone Number:** ___________________

**Address:** _____________________________________________________________________

*(You can tick more than one option for the following multiple choice questions)*

1. **Who has suggested you to see me?**
   a. No one. I came on my own.
   b. Friend (mention name and contact number)
   c. Parent/relative (mention name and contact number)
   d. School/college/teacher

2. **What was your first feeling when you entered my clinic?**
   a. Anxious           b. Confused
   c. Irritated          d. Indifferent
   e. Hopeful          f. None of the above

3. **Do you feel that you should have come earlier?**
   a. Yes
   b. Not at all
   c. May be
   d. Delayed due to lack of family support
   e. Cannot say

4. **Which feelings/thoughts daunt you often?**
   a. Worry about future, career, and health problem
   b. Fear about specific thing/object/person/place/animal (mention which ones)
   c. Serious concern about home/parents/family member/friend
   d. Feeling of being useless, helpless, neglected, or inadequate
   e. Stress that has become unbearable
   f. Sadness due to loss of close relative, break up, conflicts with friends/sibling/parent/teacher

5. **Do you have any of the following?**
   a. Disturbed sleep and appetite
   b. Terrible boredom
   c. Excess worry, poor concentration, irritability, and unexplained aches and pains
   d. Dislike for family/friends, self-hatred
   e. Panic attacks (sweating, pounding heart, tremors, restlessness, etc.)
   f. A feeling that somebody is against you and making plans to harm you

6. **How much time do you spend on mobile/laptop/TV?**
   a. <2 hours        b. 2–4 hours
   c. >4 hours
   d. Life will be boring and unbearable without media

7. **What could be the main hindrances for your desired goal or progress?**
   a. Time constraints
   b. Lack of certain skills and poor concentration
   c. Disturbed home environment
   d. Laziness due to excess media use and inadequate sleep
   e. Bad intentions of friends/teacher
   f. Mention if any other

8. **How do you see yourself after few days/months/years/decades?**
   a. I do not know
   b. Better than what I am now.
   c. Worse and without any hope
   d. Disastrous and I do not wish to think about it.

9. **Have you ever been troubled or harassed on social media or by any other person?**
   a. Not at all
   b. Not much
   c. I have experienced it in the past.
   d. I am currently being harassed and threatened.
   e. I do not use mobile and internet.

10. **I would like to have information regarding:**
    a. Specific life skills
    b. Growth, nutrition, or sexuality related issues
    c. Study skills and career guidance
    d. Social media safety and hazards
    e. Drug abuse in teenagers and young adults

11. **As far as my current stress level goes:**
    a. I do not have any particular stress/tension.
    b. I can manage on my own, but it is getting difficult day by day.
    c. I have given up, because there is no hope for me and my future.
    d. I want to get out of this state instantly.
    e. None of the above

12. **Share any other information which you think is essential and needs to be discussed.**

*Your name and signature:*      *Parent's name and mobile number:*      *Date and time:*

# 12 | Questionnaire for Parents/Guardian

**Name:**___________________________ **Age:**__________ **Phone Number:** ___________________________
**Address:** ________________________________________________________________________________

*(You can tick more than one option for the following multiple choice questions)*

**Whom you have come for: My son/daughter/relative/self**

1. **Who has suggested you to see me?**
   a. Friend (mention name, address, and contact number)
   b. Relative (mention name, address, and contact number)
   c. Doctor (mention name, address, and contact number)
   d. School/college/teacher (mention name and contact details)
   e. No one. I came on my own.

2. **Do you feel that you should have come earlier?**
   a. Yes
   b. Not at all
   c. May be
   d. Cannot say

3. **Which things about your child bother you often?**
   a. Future and career
   b. Disobedience, anger, and rebelliousness
   c. Poor academic performance
   d. Media addiction, drug habit, and sexual experimentations
   e. Mention any other specific concern

4. **Do you have any of the following?**
   a. Lack of active support from spouse, in-laws, or other family members
   b. Blame game at home
   c. Time constraints and physical restrictions
   d. Feeling of being inadequate or a failure as a parent/guardian
   e. Your own unfulfilled ambitions which you wish your child should accomplish
   f. Stress which you are not able to handle

5. **What according to you is most vital for your child?**
   a. Academic excellence and bright career
   b. Extracurricular activities and creativity
   c. Good physical, mental, and social health
   d. None of the above
   e. All of the above

6. **How do you intend to contribute for betterment of your child?**
   a. Rescheduling time, changing priorities, and learning certain skills
   b. Discussions with trustworthy friends or professionals
   c. Patience, persistent efforts, and practice
   d. None of the above
   e. All of the above

7. **How do you see your child after few days/months/years/decades?**
   a. I am confused.
   b. Better than the present state.
   c. Worse and without any hope.
   d. Disastrous and I do not wish to think about it.

8. **Will you follow the recommendations/suggestions offered here today?**
   a. May be, I will try
   b. Depends (mention on what)
   c. Surely
   d. Not at all

9. **I would like to have information regarding:**
   a. Specific parenting skills
   b. Growth, incomplete vaccination, nutrition, or sexuality related issues of my child
   c. Study skills and career guidance
   d. Social media safety and hazards
   e. Drug abuse in teenagers and young people

10. **Share any other information which you think is essential.**

*Your name and signature:*          *Your child's name and age:*          *Date and time:*

# 13   IAP Growth Charts

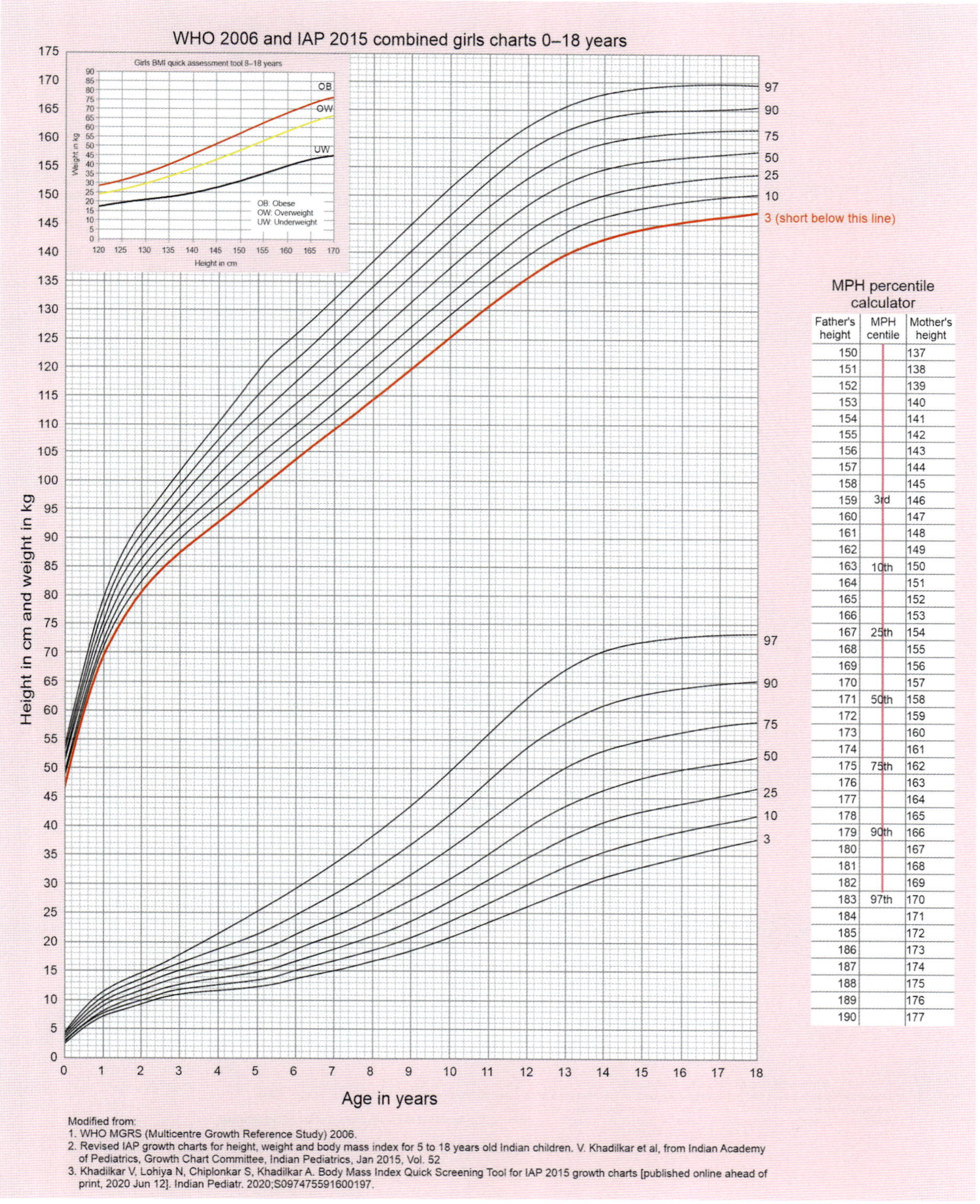



Modified from:

1. WHO MGRS (Multicentre Growth Reference Study) 2006.
2. Revised IAP growth charts for height, weight and body mass index for 5 to 18 years old Indian children. V. Khadilkar et al, from Indian Academy of Pediatrics, Growth Chart Committee, Indian Pediatrics, Jan 2015, Vol. 52
3. Khadilkar V, Lohiya N, Chiplonkar S, Khadilkar A. Body Mass Index Quick Screening Tool for IAP 2015 growth charts [published online ahead of print, 2020 Jun 12]. Indian Pediatr. 2020;S097475591600197.

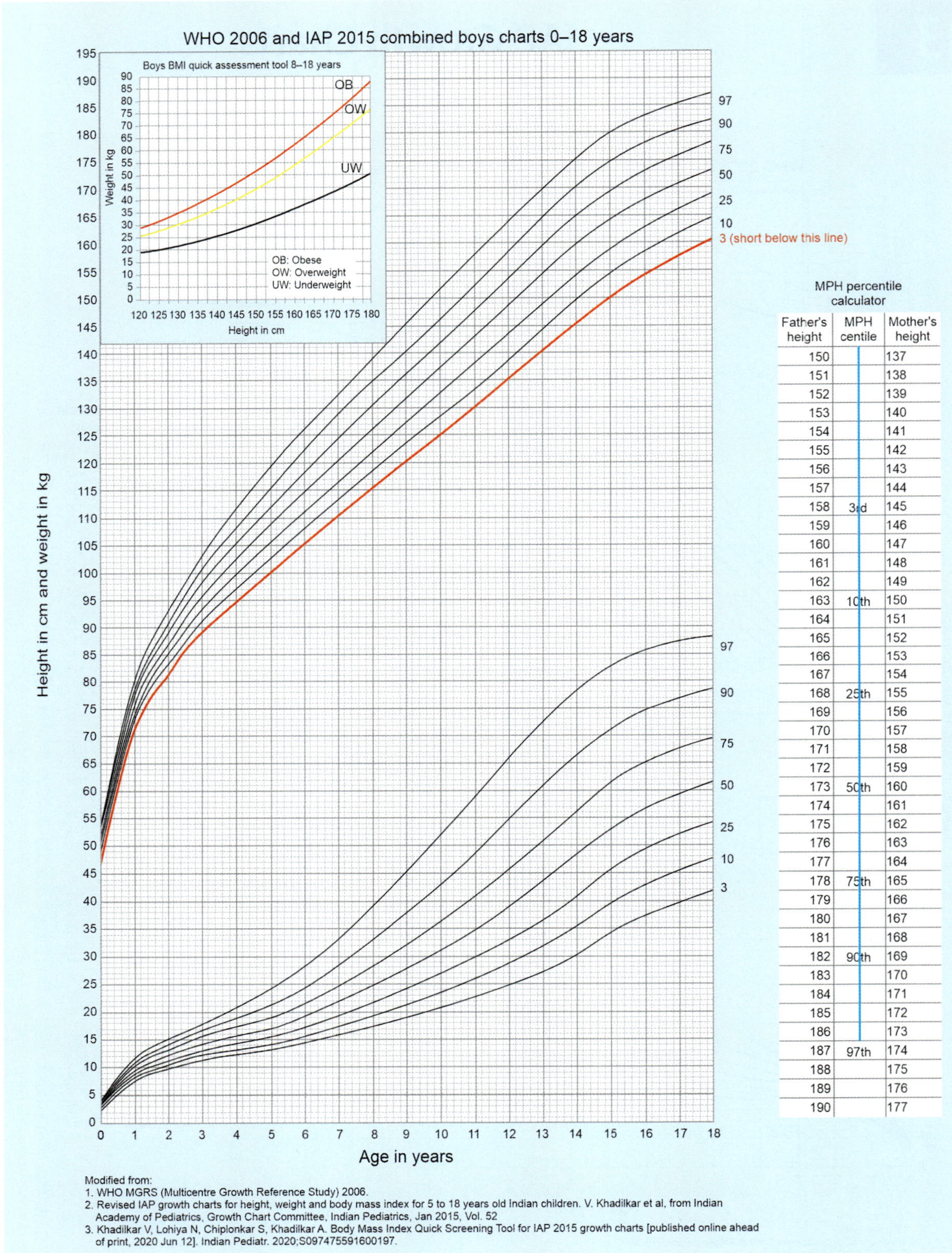



## MPH percentile calculator

| Father's height | MPH centile | Mother's height |
|---|---|---|
| 150 | | 137 |
| 151 | | 138 |
| 152 | | 139 |
| 153 | | 140 |
| 154 | | 141 |
| 155 | | 142 |
| 156 | | 143 |
| 157 | | 144 |
| 158 | 3rd | 145 |
| 159 | | 146 |
| 160 | | 147 |
| 161 | | 148 |
| 162 | | 149 |
| 163 | 10th | 150 |
| 164 | | 151 |
| 165 | | 152 |
| 166 | | 153 |
| 167 | | 154 |
| 168 | 25th | 155 |
| 169 | | 156 |
| 170 | | 157 |
| 171 | | 158 |
| 172 | | 159 |
| 173 | 50th | 160 |
| 174 | | 161 |
| 175 | | 162 |
| 176 | | 163 |
| 177 | | 164 |
| 178 | 75th | 165 |
| 179 | | 166 |
| 180 | | 167 |
| 181 | | 168 |
| 182 | 90th | 169 |
| 183 | | 170 |
| 184 | | 171 |
| 185 | | 172 |
| 186 | | 173 |
| 187 | 97th | 174 |
| 188 | | 175 |
| 189 | | 176 |
| 190 | | 177 |

Modified from:
1. WHO MGRS (Multicentre Growth Reference Study) 2006.
2. Revised IAP growth charts for height, weight and body mass index for 5 to 18 years old Indian children. V. Khadilkar et al, from Indian Academy of Pediatrics, Growth Chart Committee, Indian Pediatrics, Jan 2015, Vol. 52
3. Khadilkar V, Lohiya N, Chiplonkar S, Khadilkar A. Body Mass Index Quick Screening Tool for IAP 2015 growth charts [published online ahead of print, 2020 Jun 12]. Indian Pediatr. 2020;S097475591600197.

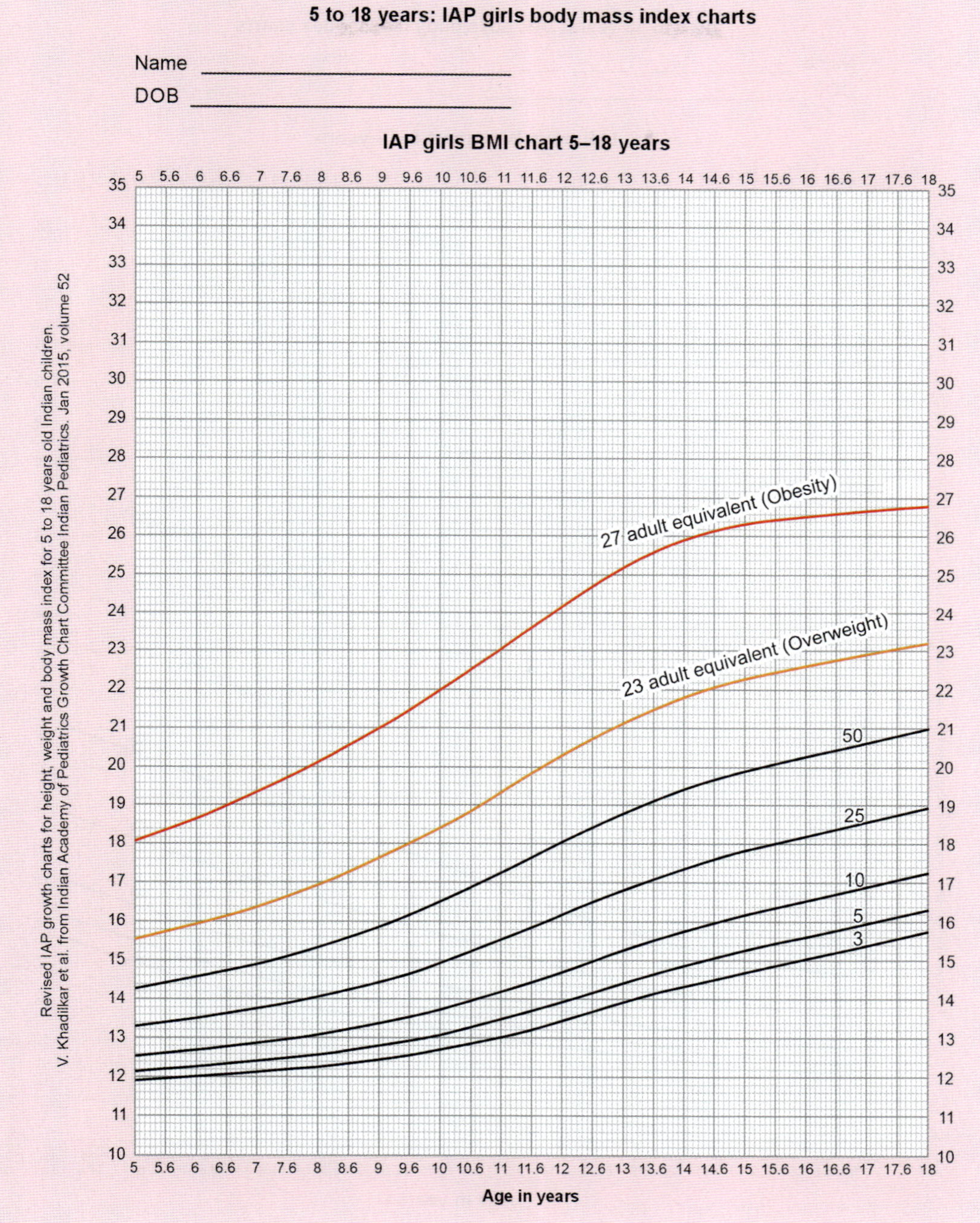

5 to 18 years: IAP girls body mass index charts
Name
DOB
IAP girls BMI chart 5–18 years
27 adult equivalent (Obesity)
23 adult equivalent (Overweight)
50
25
10
5
3
Age in years
Revised IAP growth charts for height, weight and body mass index for 5 to 18 years old Indian children.
V. Khadilkar et al. from Indian Academy of Pediatrics Growth Chart Committee Indian Pediatrics. Jan 2015, volume 52

## 5 to 18 years: IAP boys body mass index charts

Name ___________________________

DOB ___________________________

### IAP boys BMI chart 5–18 years

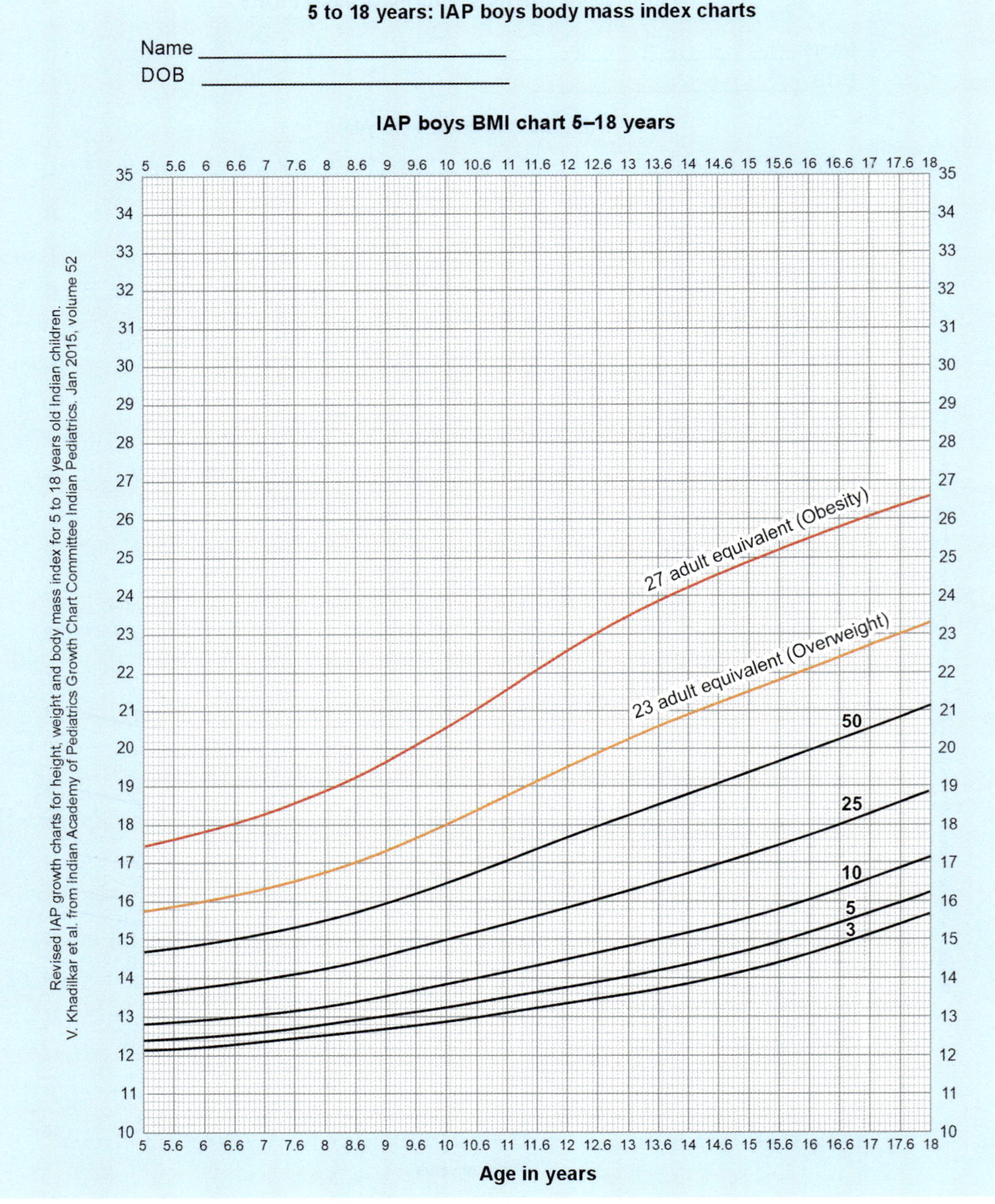

# 14   Useful Puberty Charts and Referral Criteria

## ■ TANNER STAGING [ALSO CALLED SEXUAL MATURITY RATINGS (SMR)]

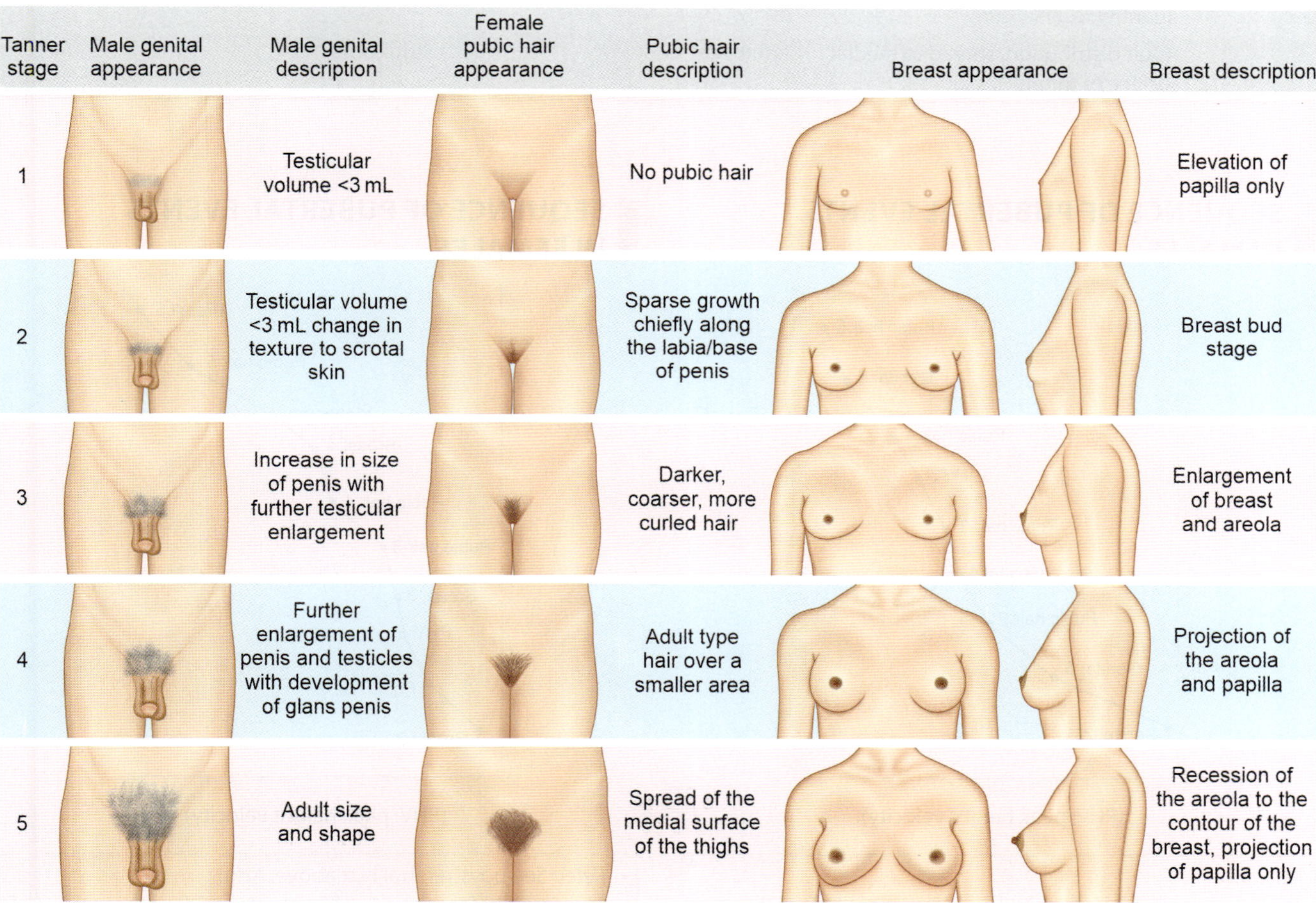



**Fig. 1:** Tanner stages of development.

## ■ CLASSIFICATION OF SEXUAL MATURITY STATES IN GIRLS

| SMR stage | Pubic hair | Breasts |
|---|---|---|
| 1 | Preadolescent | Preadolescent |
| 2 | Sparse, lightly pigmented, straight, medial border of labia | Breast and papilla elevated as small mound; diameter of areola increased |
| 3 | Darker, beginning to curl, increased amount | Breast and areola enlarged, no contour separation |
| 4 | Coarse, curly, abundant, but less than in adult | Areola and papilla form secondary mound |
| 5 | Adult feminine triangle, spread to medial surface of thighs | Mature, nipple projects, areola part of general breast contour |

## ◼ CLASSIFICATION OF SEX MATURITY STATES IN BOYS

| SMR stage | Pubic hair | Penis | Testes |
|---|---|---|---|
| 1 | None | Preadolescent | Preadolescent |
| 2 | Scanty, long, slightly pigmented | Minimal change/enlargement | Enlarged scrotum, pink, and texture altered |
| 3 | Darker, starting to curl, small amount | Lengthens | Larger |
| 4 | Resembles adult type, but less quantity; coarse, curly | Larger; glans and breadth increase in size | Larger, scrotum dark |
| 5 | Adult distribution, spread to medial surface of thighs | Adult size | Adult size |

## ◼ SEQUENCE OF PUBERTAL EVENTS IN MALES

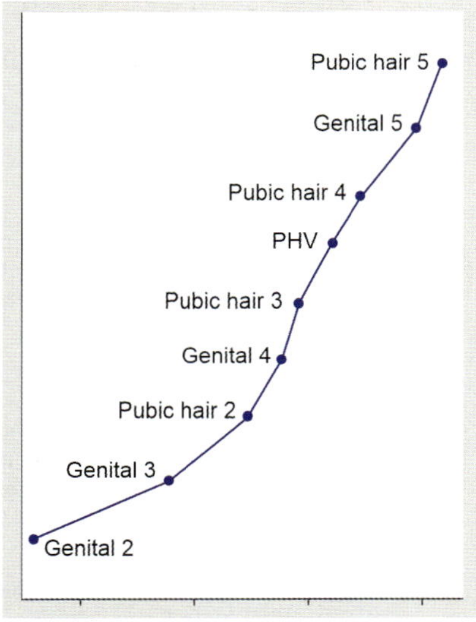


(PHV: peak height velocity)

*Refer:*
- Penile growth and/or testicular enlargement before the age of 9 years
- Steep upward growth trend (increasing across one or more centile spaces—e.g., below 50th to above 75th centile), in 3–6 months
- New onset polydipsia/polyuria, headaches, or visual disturbances
- History of central nervous system (CNS) disorders or injury, e.g., meningitis, irradiation, hypoxic ischemic injury, and neurofibromatosis

## ◼ SEQUENCE OF PUBERTAL EVENTS IN FEMALES

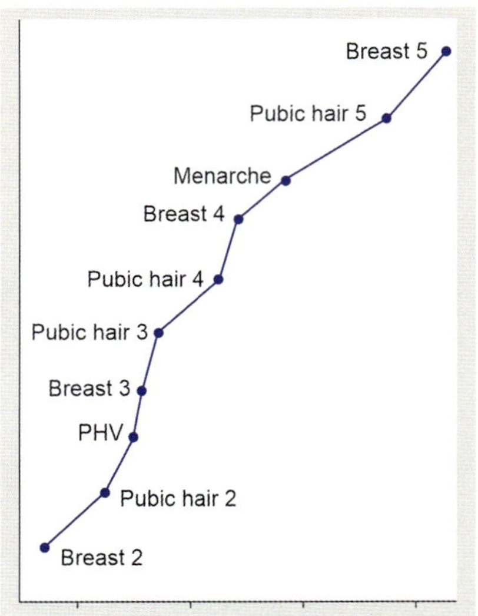


(PHV: peak height velocity)

- *Refer:* See boys' referral box above. Also:
- Menarche before the age of 8 years (consider other causes of vaginal bleeding)
- Progressive breast enlargement before the age of 8 years, over a period of 4–6 months, along with upward crossing of height centile(s)
- Clitoromegaly
- Café au lait macules (McCune Albright?)
- Presence of pubic hair in infancy, with or without breast development

## ■ MEASURING TESTICULAR VOLUME

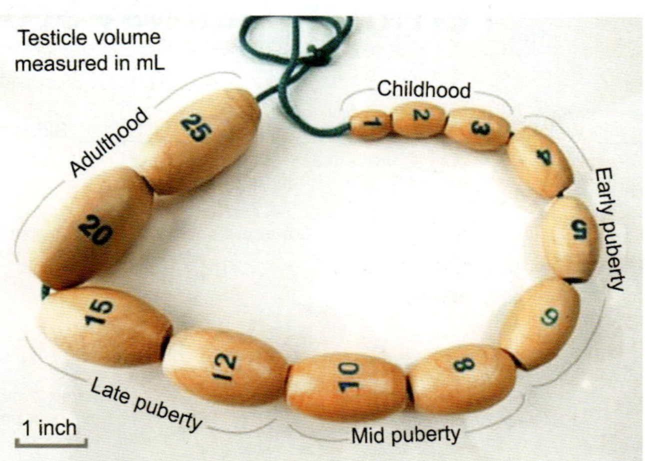


*Length 2.5 cm = 4 mL = early puberty*

Testicular volume calculator available at http://tvcalculator.nchri.org/. Measure the width of the testis (cm) and assess the Tanner/SMR stage of genital development. Plug both these into the online calculator to get the volume (mL).

---

*Source:* From Tanner JM (Ed). Growth At Adolescence, 2nd edition. England, Oxford: Blackwell Scientific; 1962.

# 15 Ferriman-Gallway Score

Age ____________ Height ____________ Weight ____________ Body mass index ____________ Blood pressure ____________

Caucasion ☐    African American ☐    Asian ☐    N. American Indian ☐    Mediterranean ☐

| Upper lip | Sideburn area | Chin | Lower jaw and neck | Upper back | Lower back | ←Subtotal |
|---|---|---|---|---|---|---|
| **1** Small number of terminal hairs over upper lip and outer lip border | **1** Sparse terminal hairs | **1** Sparse terminal hairs on chin | **1** Sparse terminal hairs over lower jaw and upper neck | **1** Sparse terminal hairs over upper back | **1** Sacral area with hair coverage less than 4 cm wide | |
| **2** Thin moustache covering less than 50% of upper lip or at the outer border | **2** Sparse terminal hairs with small thickened areas | **2** Sparse terminal hairs with small thickened areas | **2** Sparse terminal hairs with small thickened areas | **2** Increased number of spread terminal hairs | **2** Increased sides coverage | |
| **3** Moustache covering 50% from outer margin of the lip or 50% the lip height | **3** Light hair growth over sideburn area | **3** Entire chin covered with light growth | **3** Entire area covered with light growth | **3** Entire area covered with light growth | **3** 75% of lower back covered with terminal hairs | |
| **4** Moustache covering most of upper lip and crossing the midline lip | **4** Thick growth over sideburn area | **4** Entire chin covered with heavy growth | **4** Entire area covered with heavy growth | **4** Entire area covered with heavy growth | **4** Entire area covered with heavy growth | |

| Upper arm | Thigh | Chest | Upper abdomen | Lower abdomen | Perineum | ←Subtotal |
|---|---|---|---|---|---|---|
| **1** Scattered terminal hairs over less than 25% of upper arm | **1** Scattered terminal hairs over less than 25% of the thigh | **1** Circumareolar or midline terminal hairs | **1** Scattered midline terminal hairs | **1** Small number of scattered midline terminal hairs the length of linea alba | **1** Scattered perianal terminal hairs | |
| **2** Increased but incomplete coverage | **2** Increased but incomplete coverage | **2** Circumareolar and midline terminal hairs | **2** More terminal hairs, still midline | **2** Midline concentration of terminal hair the length of the linea alba | **2** Spread of terminal hair to the gluteal cleft | |
| **3** Entire area covered with light growth | **3** Entire area covered with light growth | **3** 75% of chest covered with terminal hairs | **3** 50% of upper abdomen covered | **3** A midline thickened band of terminal hair less than ½ width of pubic hair at base | **3** 75% of perineum covered with terminal hairs | |
| **4** Entire area covered with heavy growth | **4** Entire area covered with heavy growth | **4** Entire area covered with terminal hair growth | **4** Entire area covered with terminal hair growth | **4** An inverted V-shaped coverage ½ width of pubic hair at base | **4** Entire area covered with terminal hair growth | |

**Total score =**

# 16   Immunization Card

## ■ IMMUNIZATION CARD FOR ADOLESCENTS OF 9–18 YEARS OLD

(Recommended by Adolescent Health Academy) 2023

**Name:**_______________________________________________________________

**Age:**_________________________________________ **Gender:** _______________________________

**Mother:** _____________________________________________________________

**Father:** ______________________________________________________________

**Address:** _____________________________________________________________

_______________________________________________________________________

**Dr.** __________________________________________________________________

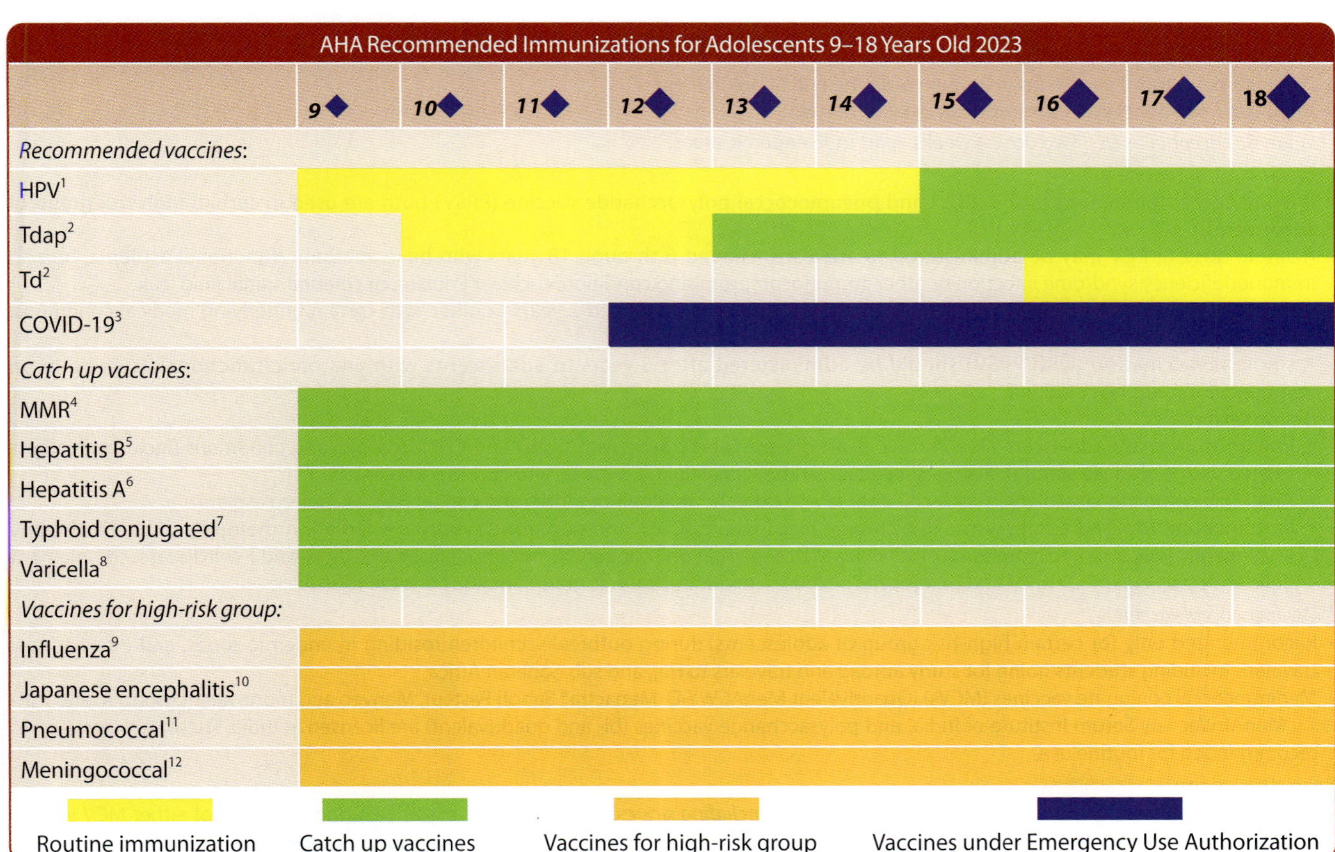



[1]*HPV vaccines*
*Routine vaccination:*
*Minimum age:* 9 years
- HPV4-SII and HPV9 are recommended in a two-dose series (0 and 6 months) for females and males aged 9–14 years of age.
- HPV4 is recommended in a three-dose series (0, 2, and 6 months) for females aged 15–45 years.
- HPV9 is recommended in a three-dose series (0, 2, and 6 months) for females aged 15–26 years.
- HPV4 SII is recommended in a three-dose series (0, 2, and 6 months) for both males and females aged 15–26 years.
- The vaccine series can be started beginning at age 9 years.

*Catch-up vaccination:*
- Administer the vaccine series to females (HPV-4) at the age of 13 years onward if not previously vaccinated.
- Administer the second dose 2 months after the first dose and the third dose 6 months after the first dose (at least 24 weeks after the first dose).

[2]*Tdap/Td:* Tdap at 10–12 years. Catch up up to 18 years. One dose of Td at 16–18 years.

[3]*COVID-19 vaccine:* Vaccines approved in India under Emergency Use Authorization are Covaxin, Corbevax, Covovax, and ZyCov-D. Covaxin and Corbevax are given in two dose schedule 4 weeks apart. Covovax also is given in two-dose schedule but 3 weeks apart, whereas ZyCov-D is licensed as three-dose schedule 28 days apart. All the vaccines are rolled out in adolescents more than 12 years.

[4]*MMR:* Two doses at 4–8 weeks interval. One dose if previously vaccinated with one dose.

[5]*HBV:* Three doses 0, 1, and 6 months.

[6]*Hepatitis A:* Two doses at 0 and 6 months up to 18 years of age [prior check for anti-hepatitis A virus (HAV) immunoglobulin G (IgG) may be cost-effective in children of age more than 10 years] for inactivated vaccine. Those who have previously received one dose at age 12 months or older should receive dose 2 at least 6 months after first dose. Live vaccine is recommended as single dose.

[7]*TCV:* Single dose up to 45 years.

[8]*Varicella:* Two doses 12 weeks apart. Adolescents more than 13 years of age two dose may be given at 4–8 weeks interval.

[9]*Influenza:* Annual dose as vaccine for high-risk cases only. Risk factors include:
- Adults 65 years and older.
- Diseases like asthma, chronic lung disease [chronic obstructive pulmonary disease (COPD) and cystic fibrosis], endocrine disorders (diabetes mellitus), heart disease [congestive heart failure (CHF) and coronary artery disease (CAD)], kidney diseases, and liver disorders.
- Obese with a body mass index (BMI) of 40 kg/m$^2$ or higher, long-term aspirin- or salicylate-containing medications.
- Blood disorders (sickle cell disease).
- Immunodeficiency like human immunodeficiency virus (HIV) or acquired immunodeficiency syndrome (AIDS), leukemia or on chemotherapy or radiation treatment for cancer, corticosteroids.
- Pregnant people and people up to 2 weeks after the end of pregnancy.
- Healthcare personnel and those working in laboratories.

[10]*Japanese encephalitis (JE):* Two dose 4 weeks apart in JE endemic areas.

[11]*Pneumococcal vaccines:*
- Pneumococcal conjugate vaccine (PCV) and pneumococcal polysaccharide vaccine (PPSV) both are used in certain high-risk group of adolescents.
- A single dose of PCV may be administered to adolescents aged 6 through 18 years who have anatomic/functional asplenia, human immunodeficiency syndrome infection or other immunocompromising condition, cochlear implant, or cerebral spinal fluid leak.
- Administer PPSV at least 8 weeks after the last dose of PCV to children aged 2 years or older with certain underlying medical conditions, including a cochlear implant.
- A single revaccination (with PPSV) should be administered after 5 years to adolescents with anatomic/functional asplenia or an immunocompromising condition.
- *Risk group includes:*
  - Immunocompetent adolescents like chronic heart disease (particularly with CCHD and CHF), chronic lung conditions (including asthma treated with high-dose steroid), diabetes mellitus, cerebrospinal fluid (CSF) leak, and cochlear implant.
  - Anatomic or functional asplenia: Sickle cell disease and other hemoglobinopathies, and congenital or acquired asplenia.
  - Immunocompromised adolescents: HIV, chronic renal failure (CRF), and nephrotic syndrome, radiation therapy and chemotherapy (malignancy, leukemia and lymphoma or solid organ transplantation), congenital immunodeficiencies: B-cell and T-cell disease, complement deficiency particularly C1 to C4 and phagocytic disorders [excluding chronic granulomatous disease (CGD)].

[12]*Meningococcal vaccine:*
- Recommended only for certain high-risk group of adolescents, during outbreaks, children residing in endemic zones, and international travelers, including students going for study abroad and travelers to Hajj and sub-Saharan Africa.
- Meningococcal conjugate vaccines (MCVs) (Quadrivalent MenACWY-D, Menactra® Sanofi Pasteur, Menveo and monovalent group A, and PsA-TT, MenAfriVac® by Serum Institute of India) and polysaccharide vaccines (bi- and quadrivalent) are licensed in India. These vaccines are not recommended for routine use.

*Special situations:*
- *Adolescents with functional/anatomic asplenia/hyposplenia (including sickle cell disease):* Administer two primary doses of either MCV with at least 8 weeks between doses for age 2–55 years. Vaccination should ideally be started 2 weeks prior to splenectomy. Boosters every 5 years thereafter throughout life as long as the person remains at increased risk for meningococcal disease.
- *Persons with human immunodeficiency virus:* Administer two doses at least 8 weeks interval and booster every 5 years as long as the person remains at increased risk for meningococcal disease.
- *Laboratory personnel and healthcare workers:* (Those working regularly with *Neisseria meningitidis* in solutions) Single dose of MCV is recommended. A booster dose should be administered every 5 years if exposure is ongoing.
- *Adjunct to chemoprophylaxis:* In close contacts of patients with meningococcal disease (healthcare workers in contact with secretions, household contacts, day care contacts) single dose of appropriate group MCV is recommended.
- *Healthy adolescent who received a single dose for travel:* Boosters are not recommended (e.g., a healthy child who received a single dose for travel to a country where meningococcal disease is endemic).

# 17   Nutrition

**TABLE 1:** Recommended dietary allowances (RDAs)* for energy, protein, and micronutrients: Indian Council of Medical Research (ICMR) 2024.

| Age group | Gender | Energy kcal/day | Protein g/day | Fiber g/day | Calcium mg/day | Magnesium mg/day | Iron mg/day | Zinc mg/day | Iodine µg/day |
|---|---|---|---|---|---|---|---|---|---|
| 10–12 years | Boys | 2,220 | 32 | 33 | 850 | 240 | 16 | 8.5 | 100 |
| | Girls | 2,060 | 33 | 30 | 850 | 250 | 28 | 8.5 | 100 |
| 13–15 years | Boys | 2,860 | 45 | 43 | 1,000 | 345 | 22 | 14.3 | 140 |
| | Girls | 2,400 | 43 | 36 | 1,000 | 340 | 30 | 12.8 | 140 |
| 16–18 years | Boys | 3,320 | 55 | 50 | 1,050 | 440 | 26 | 17.6 | 140 |
| | Girls | 2,500 | 46 | 38 | 1,050 | 380 | 32 | 14.2 | 140 |

*There is no RDA for energy. Instead, estimated average requirement (EAR) is given. EAR for energy is equivalent to estimated energy requirement (EER). Adequate intake (AI) is given for dietary fiber.

**TABLE 2:** Recommended dietary allowances for vitamins—ICMR 2024.

| Age group | Gender | Thiamine mg/day | Riboflavin mg/day | Niacin mg/day | Vitamin $B_6$ mg/day | Folate µg/day | $B_{12}$ µg/day | Vitamin C mg/day | Vitamin A µg/day | Vitamin D IU/day |
|---|---|---|---|---|---|---|---|---|---|---|
| 10–12 years | Boys | 1.5 | 2.1 | 15 | 2.0 | 220 | 2.2 | 55 | 770 | 600 |
| | Girls | 1.4 | 1.9 | 14 | 1.9 | 225 | 2.2 | 50 | 790 | 600 |
| 13–15 years | Boys | 1.9 | 2.7 | 19 | 2.6 | 285 | 2.2 | 70 | 930 | 600 |
| | Girls | 1.6 | 2.2 | 16 | 2.2 | 245 | 2.2 | 65 | 890 | 600 |
| 16–18 years | Boys | 2.2 | 3.1 | 22 | 3.0 | 340 | 2.2 | 85 | 1,000 | 600 |
| | Girls | 1.7 | 2.3 | 17 | 2.3 | 270 | 2.2 | 70 | 860 | 600 |

**TABLE 3:** Quantity of suggested food groups for a balanced diet to meet EAR for adolescents.

| Age | Gender | Cereals (g) | Pulses (g) | GLV (g) | Vegetables (g) | Roots and Tubers (g) | Fruits (g) | Nuts (g) | Milk (mL) | Fats and oils (g) |
|---|---|---|---|---|---|---|---|---|---|---|
| 10–12 years | Boys | 280 | 90 | 100 | 200 | 100 | 100 | 30 | 400 | 35 |
| 10–12 years | Girls | 250 | 85 | 100 | 200 | 100 | 100 | 30 | 400 | 30 |
| 13–15 years | Boys | 390 | 130 | 100 | 200 | 100 | 100 | 40 | 400 | 45 |
| 13–15 years | Girls | 300 | 100 | 100 | 200 | 100 | 100 | 35 | 400 | 40 |
| 16–18 years | Boys | 450 | 150 | 100 | 200 | 100 | 150 | 50 | 400 | 55 |
| 16–18 years | Girls | 315 | 105 | 100 | 200 | 100 | 150 | 40 | 400 | 40 |

(EAR: estimated average requirement; GLV: green leafy vegetables)

**TABLE 4:** Tolerable upper limit of nutrients for the adolescents.

| Age | Gender | Protein (PE ratio) | Calcium mg/day | Magnesium mg/day | Iron mg/day | Zinc mg/d | Iodine µg/day | Folate µg/day | Vitamin C mg/d | Vitamin A µg/day | Vitamin D IU/day |
|---|---|---|---|---|---|---|---|---|---|---|---|
| 10–12 years | Boys | <15% | 3,000 | 350 | 40 | 23 | 600 | 600–800 | 1,050 | 1,700 | 4,000 |
| 10–12 years | Girls | <15% | 3,000 | 350 | 40 | 23 | 600 | 600–800 | 1,300 | 1,700 | 4,000 |
| 13–15 years | Boys | <15% | 3,000 | 350 | 45 | 34 | 900 | 600–800 | 1,550 | 2,800 | 4,000 |
| 13–15 years | Girls | <15% | 3,000 | 350 | 45 | 34 | 900 | 600–800 | 1,800 | 2,800 | 4,000 |
| 16–18 years | Boys | <15% | 3,000 | 350 | 45 | 34 | 1,100 | 600–800 | 1,950 | 2,800 | 4,000 |
| 16–18 years | Girls | <15% | 3,000 | 350 | 45 | 34 | 1,100 | 600–800 | 2,000 | 2,800 | 4,000 |

*Source:* Adapted from Revised Short Summary Report 2024, ICMR—NIN Expert Group on Nutrient Requirements of Indians, RDA and EAR 2020.

# 18 | Noncommunicable Diseases in Adolescents: A Closer Look

**TABLE 1:** Prevalence of metabolic risk factors for NCDs in Indian adolescents (Refer to Annexure 17, Tables 1–4).

| Condition | Value | Prevalence |
|---|---|---|
| Prediabetes | Fasting plasma glucose >100 mg/dL or HbA1c 5.7–6.4% | 10% |
| Diabetes mellitus | Fasting plasma glucose >126 mg/dL | 1% |
| High total cholesterol | >200 mg/dL | 4% |
| High LDL cholesterol | >130 mg/dL | 4% |
| Low HDL cholesterol | <40 mg/dL | 28% |
| High serum triglycerides | >130 mg/dL | 16% |
| Hypertension | Systolic BP >140 mm Hg or diastolic BP >90 mm Hg | 5% |
| Risk for CKD | Serum creatinine >1.0 mg/dL | 7% |

**Flowchart 1:** Health promotion approach.

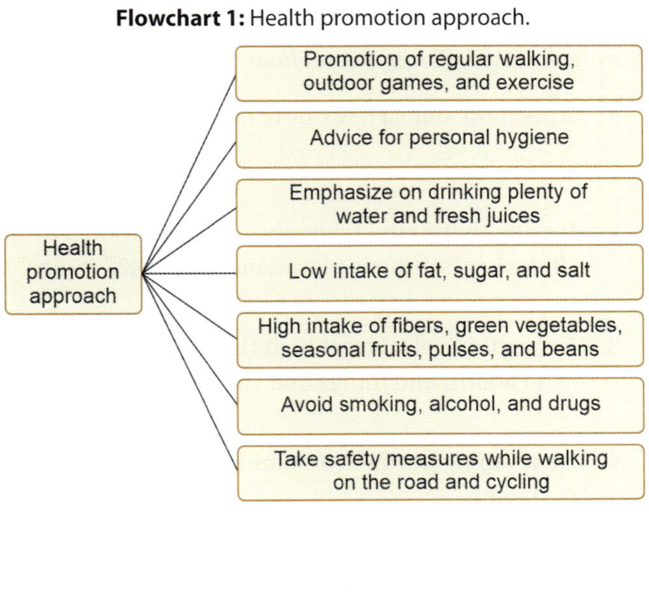


Comprehensive National Nutritional Survey, 2016–2018. Ministry of Health, Government of India. Chapter 8: Markers of noncommunicable diseases. Pp. 213–46; Annex1—pp. 259.

# 19 | The CRAFFT+N Questionnaire

**To be completed by patient**

Please answer all questions *honestly*; your answers will be kept *confidential*.

*During the PAST 12 months, on how many days did you*:

1. Drink more than a few sips of beer, wine, or any drink containing alcohol? Put "0" if none.

    # of days

2. Use any marijuana (cannabis, weed, oil, wax, or hash by smoking, vaping, dabbing, or in edibles) or "synthetic marijuana" (like "K2," "Spice")? Put "0" if none.

    # of days

3. Use anything else to get high (like other illegal drugs, pills, prescription or over-the-counter medications, and things that you sniff, huff, vape, or inject)? Put "0" if none.

    # of days

4. Use a vaping device* containing nicotine and/or flavors, or use any tobacco products[†]? Put "0" if none.

    # of days

*Such as e-cigarettes, mods, pod devices like JUUL, disposable vapes like puff bar, vape pens, or e-hookahs.*
[†]*Cigarettes, cigars, cigarillos, hookahs, chewing tobacco, snuff, snus, dissolvables, or nicotine pouches.*

Read these instructions before continuing:

- If you put "0" in ALL of the boxes above, answer question 5 below, then stop.
- If you put "1" or more for questions 1, 2, or 3 above, answer questions 5–10 below.
- If you put "1" or more for question 4 above, answer all questions on back page.

*Circle one*

5. Have you ever ridden in a *car* driven by someone (including yourself) who was "high" or had been using alcohol or drugs? — No   Yes

6. Do you ever use alcohol or drugs to *relax*, feel better about yourself, or fit in? — No   Yes

7. Do you ever use alcohol or drugs while you are by yourself, or *alone*? — No   Yes

8. Do you ever *forget* things you did while using alcohol or drugs? — No   Yes

9. Do your *family* or *friends* ever tell you that you should cut down on your drinking or drug use? — No   Yes

10. Have you ever gotten into *trouble* while you were using alcohol or drugs? — No   Yes

**NOTICE TO CLINIC STAFF AND MEDICAL RECORDS:**
The information on this page is protected by special federal confidentiality rules (42 CFR Part 2), which prohibit disclosure of this information unless authorized by specific written consent.

**© John R. Knight, MD, Boston Children's Hospital, 2020.**
Reproduced with permission from the Center for Adolescent Behavioral Health Research (CABHRe), Boston Children's Hospital.
For more information and versions in other languages, see **www.crafft.org**

*The following questions ask about your use of any vaping devices containing nicotine and/or flavors, or use of any tobacco products.* Circle your answer for each question.

*Circle one*

1. Have you ever tried to quit using, but could not? — Yes No
2. Do you vape or use tobacco now, because it is really hard to quit? — Yes No
3. Have you ever felt like you were addicted to vaping or tobacco? — Yes No
4. Do you ever have strong cravings to vape or use tobacco? — Yes No
5. Have you ever felt like you really needed to vape or use tobacco? — Yes No
6. Is it hard to keep from vaping or using tobacco in places where you are not supposed to, like school? — Yes No
7. When you have not vaped or used tobacco in a while (or when you tried to stop using)...
   a. Did you find it hard to concentrate because you could not vape or use tobacco? — Yes No
   b. Did you feel more irritable because you could not vape or use tobacco? — Yes No
   c. Did you feel a strong need or urge to vape or use tobacco? — Yes No
   d. Did you feel nervous, restless, or anxious because you could not vape or use tobacco? — Yes No

# 20 Internet Addiction Test (IAT)

Name:_______________________________________________  Male ☐  Female ☐  Age:________

Years Online:___________________ Do you use the Internet for work?  Yes ☐  No ☐

This questionnaire consists of 20 statements. After reading each statement carefully, based upon the 5-point Likert scale, please select the response (0, 1, 2, 3, 4 or 5), which best describes you. If two choices seem to apply equally well, circle the choice that best represents how you are most of the time during the past month. Be sure to read all the statements carefully before making your choice. The statements refer to offline situations or actions unless otherwise specified.

*0* = Not applicable
*1* = Rarely
*2* = Occasionally
*3* = Frequently
*4* = Often
*5* = Always

1. How often do you find that you stay online longer than you intended?
2. How often do you neglect household chores to spend more time online?
3. How often do you prefer the excitement of the Internet to intimacy with your partner?
4. How often do you form new relationships with fellow online users?
5. How often do others in your life complain to you about the amount of time you spend online?
6. How often do your grades or school work suffer because of the amount of time you spend online?
7. How often do you check your email before something else that you need to do?
8. How often does your job performance or productivity suffer because of the Internet?
9. How often do you become defensive or secretive when anyone asks you what you do online?
10. How often do you block out disturbing thoughts about your life with soothing thoughts of the Internet?
11. How often do you find yourself anticipating when you will go online again?
12. How often do you fear that life without the Internet would be boring, empty, and joyless?
13. How often do you snap, yell, or act annoyed if someone bothers you while you are online?
14. How often do you lose sleep due to being online?
15. How often do you feel preoccupied with the Internet when off-line, or fantasize about being online?
16. How often do you find yourself saying "just a few more minutes" when online?
17. How often do you try to cut down the amount of time you spend online and fail?
18. How often do you try to hide how long you have been online?
19. How often do you choose to spend more time online over going out with others?
20. How often do you feel depressed, moody, or nervous when you are off-line, which goes away once you are back online?

## ■ SCORING

The IAT total score is the sum of the ratings given by the examinee for the 20 item responses. Each item is rated on a 5-point scale ranging from 0 to 5. The maximum score is 100 points. The higher the score is, the higher is the severity of your problem. Total scores that range from *0 to 30* points are considered to reflect a normal level of Internet usage; scores of *31 to 49* indicate the presence of a mild level of Internet addiction; *50 to 79* reflect the presence of a moderate level; and scores of *80 to 100* indicate a severe dependence upon the Internet.

# 21 | Problematic and Risky Internet Use Screening Scale (PRIUSS)

Please answer the questions below based on how you have felt and conducted yourself regarding your Internet use over the *past 6 months*. Please do your best to interpret these questions as they apply to your own experiences and feelings.

When considering your Internet use time, think about *any time you spend online*, whether you are using a computer or a mobile device. Do not include time you spend texting unless you are *using text messages to interact with an online application,* such as Facebook or Twitter.

| Place a ✓ in the box which best describes your answer | Never | Rarely | Sometimes | Often | Very Often |
|---|---|---|---|---|---|
| *How often …* | | | | | |
| 1. Do you choose to socialize online instead of in-person? | 0 | 1 | 2 | 3 | 4 |
| 2. Do you have problems with face to face communication due to your internet use? | 0 | 1 | 2 | 3 | 4 |
| 3. Do you experience increased social anxiety due to your internet use? | 0 | 1 | 2 | 3 | 4 |
| 4. Do you fail to create real-life relationships because of the internet? | 0 | 1 | 2 | 3 | 4 |
| 5. Do you skip out on social events to spend time online? | 0 | 1 | 2 | 3 | 4 |
| 6. Do your offline relationships suffer due to your internet use? | 0 | 1 | 2 | 3 | 4 |
| 7. Do you feel irritated when you are not able to use the internet? | 0 | 1 | 2 | 3 | 4 |
| 8. Do you feel angry because you are away from the internet? | 0 | 1 | 2 | 3 | 4 |
| 9. Do you feel anxious because you are away from the internet? | 0 | 1 | 2 | 3 | 4 |
| 10. Do you feel vulnerable when the internet is not available? | 0 | 1 | 2 | 3 | 4 |
| 11. Do you experience feelings of withdrawal from not using the internet? | 0 | 1 | 2 | 3 | 4 |
| 12. Do you put internet use in front of important, everyday activities? | 0 | 1 | 2 | 3 | 4 |
| 13. Do you avoid other activities in order to stay online? | 0 | 1 | 2 | 3 | 4 |
| 14. Do you neglect your responsibilities because of the internet? | 0 | 1 | 2 | 3 | 4 |
| 15. Do you lose motivation to do other things that need to get done because of the internet? | 0 | 1 | 2 | 3 | 4 |
| 16. Do you lose sleep due to nighttime internet use? | 0 | 1 | 2 | 3 | 4 |
| 17. Does time on the internet negatively affect your school performance? | 0 | 1 | 2 | 3 | 4 |
| 18. Do you feel you use the internet excessively? | 0 | 1 | 2 | 3 | 4 |
| Add columns | + | + | + | + | = Total score |

## ■ SCALE DESCRIPTION

The PRIUSS has 18 items and three subscales: (1) *Social Impairment* (items 1–6), which assesses the impact of internet use on both offline and online social interactions; (2) *Emotional Impairment* (items 7–11), which assesses degree of emotional attachment to Internet use, and (3) *Risky/Impulsive Internet Use* (items 12–18), which assess salient problematic behaviors regarding Internet use.

## ■ SCORING GUIDELINE

A cut-off of 25 for the overall scale score is proposed for identifying those at risk for PIU. Screening studies have suggested that 11% of adolescents may be at risk for PIU, as measured by the PRIUSS and using this scoring guideline.

# Index